# SOCIAL PSYCHOLOGICAL FOUNDATIONS OF CLINICAL PSYCHOLOGY

# SOCIAL PSYCHOLOGICAL FOUNDATIONS OF CLINICAL PSYCHOLOGY

Edited by
JAMES E. MADDUX
JUNE PRICE TANGNEY

THE GUILFORD PRESS
New York London

A Division of Guilford Publications, Inc.
72 Spring Street, New York, NY 10012
www.guilford.com



Printed in the United States of America

This book is printed on acid-free paper.

Last digit is print number: 9 8 7 6 5 4 3 2 1

**Library of Congress Cataloging-in-Publication Data**

Social psychological foundations of clinical psychology / edited by James E. Maddux, June Price Tangney.
p. cm.
Includes bibliographical references and index.
ISBN 978-1-60623-679-6 (hardcover : alk. paper)
1. Clinical psychology. 2. Social psychology. I. Maddux, James E. II. Tangney, June Price.
RC467.S63 2010
616.89—dc22

2010015992

# About the Editors

**James E. Maddux, PhD,** is University Professor of Psychology at George Mason University in Fairfax, Virginia, and former director of its clinical doctoral program. A Fellow of the American Psychological Association's Divisions of General, Clinical, and Health Psychology, Dr. Maddux is coauthor (with David F. Barone and C. R. Snyder) of *Social Cognitive Psychology: History and Current Domains* and coeditor (with Barbara A. Winstead) of *Psychopathology: Foundations for a Contemporary Understanding*. He is former Editor of the *Journal of Social and Clinical Psychology* and has served on the editorial boards of the *Journal of Applied Social Psychology, Self and Identity,* and the *International Journal of Cognitive Psychotherapy.* Dr. Maddux's major interest is the integration of theory and research from clinical, social, and health psychology. His research is concerned primarily with understanding the influence of beliefs about personal effectiveness and control on psychological adjustment and health-related behavior.

**June Price Tangney, PhD,** is University Professor of Psychology at George Mason University. A Fellow of the American Psychological Association's Division of Personality and Social Psychology and of the American Psychological Society, Dr. Tangney is coauthor (with Ronda L. Dearing) of *Shame and Guilt,* coeditor (with Jessica L. Tracy and Richard W. Robins) of *The Self-Conscious Emotions: Theory and Research,* and coeditor (with Mark R. Leary) of the *Handbook of Self and Identity.* She is Associate Editor of *American Psychologist* and has served as Associate Editor of *Self and Identity* and Consulting Editor of the *Journal of Personality and Social Psychology, Personality and Social Psychology Bulletin, Psychological Assessment,* the *Journal of Social and Clinical Psychology,* and the *Journal of Personality.* Her research on the development and implications of moral emotions has been funded by the National Institute on Drug Abuse, the National Institute of Child Health and Human Development, the National Science Foundation, and the John Templeton Foundation. Dr. Tangney's current work focuses on moral emotions among incarcerated offenders. A recipient of George Mason University's Teaching Excellence Award, she strives to integrate service, teaching, and clinically relevant research in both the classroom and her lab.

# Contributors

**Jonathan M. Adler, PhD,** Department of Psychology, Franklin W. Olin College of Engineering, Needham, Massachusetts

**Lauren B. Alloy, PhD,** Department of Psychology, Temple University, Philadelphia, Pennsylvania

**Susan M. Andersen, PhD,** Department of Psychology, New York University, New York, New York

**Roy F. Baumeister, PhD,** Department of Psychology, Florida State University, Tallahassee, Florida

**Lorna Smith Benjamin, PhD,** Department of Psychology, University of Utah, Salt Lake City, Utah

**Abraham P. Buunk, PhD,** Department of Psychology, University of Groningen, Groningen, The Netherlands

**Patrick W. Corrigan, PsyD,** Institute of Psychology, Illinois Institute of Technology, Chicago, Illinois

**Ronda L. Dearing, PhD,** Research Institute on Addictions, University at Buffalo, The State University of New York, Buffalo, New York

**Rene Dickerhoof, PhD,** ICON Clinical Research, Lifecycle Sciences Group, San Francisco, California

**Pieternel Dijkstra, PhD,** Department of Psychology, University of Groningen, Groningen, The Netherlands

**Celeste E. Doerr, MS,** Department of Psychology, Florida State University, Tallahassee, Florida

**Carol S. Dweck, PhD,** Department of Psychology, Stanford University, Stanford, California

**Sopagna Eap, PhD,** Department of Psychology, Pacific University, Forest Grove, Oregon

**Elaine S. Elliott-Moskwa, PhD,** private practice, Princeton, New Jersey

**Donelson R. Forsyth, PhD,** Jepson School of Leadership Studies, University of Richmond, Richmond, Virginia

**Howard N. Garb, PhD,** Psychology Research Service, Medical Center, Lackland Air Force Base, San Antonio, Texas

**Frederick X. Gibbons, PhD,** Department of Psychology, Iowa State University, Ames, Iowa

**Robyn L. Gobin, MS,** Department of Psychology, University of Oregon, Eugene, Oregon

**Peter M. Gollwitzer, PhD,** Department of Psychology, New York University, New York, New York, and University of Konstanz, Konstanz, Germany

**Gregory Haggerty, PhD,** Department of Psychology, Nassau University Medical Center, Syosset, New York

**Gordon C. Nagayama Hall, PhD,** Department of Psychology, University of Oregon, Eugene, Oregon

**Martin Heesacker, PhD,** Department of Psychology, University of Florida, Gainesville, Florida

**Brian M. Iacoviello, PhD,** Mental Illness Research, Education and Clinical Center, James J. Peters VA Medical Center, and Mount Sinai School of Medicine, Bronx, New York

**Neil P. Jones, PhD,** University of Pittsburgh Medical Center, Pittsburgh, Pennsylvania

**Ethan Kross, PhD,** Department of Psychology, University of Michigan, Ann Arbor, Michigan

**Sachiko A. Kuwabara, MA,** Bloomberg School of Public Health, Johns Hopkins University, Baltimore, Maryland

**Brian Lakey, PhD,** Department of Psychology, Grand Valley State University, Allendale, Michigan

**Jonathon E. Larson, EdD,** Institute of Psychology, Illinois Institute of Technology, Chicago, Illinois

**Mark R. Leary, PhD,** Department of Psychology and Neuroscience, Duke University, Durham, North Carolina

**Sonja Lyubomirsky, PhD,** Department of Psychology, University of California, Riverside, Riverside, California

**James E. Maddux, PhD,** Department of Psychology, George Mason University, Fairfax, Virginia

**Dan P. McAdams, PhD,** Department of Psychology, Weinberg College of Arts and Sciences, Northwestern University, Evanston, Illinois

**Megan C. McCrudden, MA,** Department of Psychology and Neuroscience, Duke University, Durham, North Carolina

**Regina Miranda, PhD,** Department of Psychology, Hunter College, New York, New York

**Walter Mischel, PhD,** Department of Psychology, Columbia University, New York, New York

**Janet Ng, MS,** Department of Psychology, University of Oregon, Eugene, Oregon

**Gabriele Oettingen, PhD,** Department of Psychology, New York University, New York, New York, and University of Hamburg, Hamburg, Germany

**Chandylen Pendley, BS,** Department of Social and Behavioral Sciences, University of Florida, Gainesville, Florida

**Paul B. Perrin, MS,** Department of Psychology, University of Florida, Gainesville, Florida

**James O. Prochaska, PhD,** Cancer Prevention Research Center, University of Rhode Island, Kingston, Rhode Island

**Janice M. Prochaska, PhD,** Pro-Change Behavior Systems, Inc., West Kingston, Rhode Island

**John H. Riskind, PhD,** Department of Psychology, George Mason University, Fairfax, Virginia

**Peter Salovey, PhD,** Department of Psychology, Yale University, New Haven, Connecticut

**William G. Shadel, PhD,** RAND Corporation, Pittsburgh, Pennsylvania

**Yuichi Shoda, PhD,** Department of Psychology, University of Washington, Seattle, Washington

**Hal S. Shorey, PhD,** Institute for Graduate Clinical Psychology, Widener University, Chester, Pennsylvania

**Caleb Siefert, PhD,** Massachusetts General Hospital/Harvard Medical School, Boston, Massachusetts

**Denise M. Sloan, PhD,** National Center for PTSD, Boston VA Healthcare Systems, Boston, Massachusetts

**Mary B. Smith, PhD,** Department of Psychology, University of Florida, Gainesville, Florida

**Timothy J. Strauman, PhD,** Department of Psychology and Neuroscience, Duke University, Durham, North Carolina

**June Price Tangney, PhD,** Department of Psychology, George Mason University, Fairfax, Virginia

**Eleanor B. Tate, MA,** Department of Psychology, University of Southern California, Los Angeles, California

**Cheryl Twaragowski, MS,** Research Institute on Addictions, University at Buffalo, The State University of New York, Buffalo, New York

**Joel Weinberger, PhD,** Derner Institute, Hy Weinberg Center, Adelphi University, Garden City, New York

# Preface

In the 30 years since the publication of the first issue of the *Journal of Social and Clinical Psychology,* research on the application of social psychological theories and concepts to understanding the development and treatment of psychological problems has grown tremendously. Numerous written and edited books have been published dealing with some aspect or other of this interface, but there has yet to appear a book designed specifically as a textbook for graduate students in psychology and related fields who are interested in this topic. This book is an attempt to meet this need.

This book had its beginning 7 years ago when our clinical doctoral program made some major changes in its focus and curriculum in an attempt to design a clinical psychology training program emphasizing social psychology and community psychology—both nontraditional and nonmedical model approaches to clinical psychology. One of the new courses that we developed as a result of this change in focus was one dealing specifically with the social psychological foundations of clinical psychology, a course that each of us has now taught several times. We realized that there was no suitable textbook for such a course and that the only previous book that might have been suitable at one time, Snyder and Forsyth's (1991) *Handbook of Social and Clinical Psychology,* was out of date. In addition, we had our own ideas of the topics that we wanted to address in the course, and nothing out there seemed to fill the bill. We first constructed the course around journal articles, and then after getting a clearer sense of what we believed such a course should cover, we decided to design our own book to meet the needs of this course. Because coverage of social bases of behavior is required of all clinical programs that wish to be accredited by the American Psychological Association, we hoped and believed that such a book would be useful to programs other than ours.

We designed the book specifically to be a textbook for graduate students in clinical and counseling psychology, although we believe that it will also find a home in other types of programs, especially programs in social psychology that have an applied focus. Although not explicitly designed for advanced researchers or experienced practitioners, we believe that these audiences will find its up-to-date summaries of the empirical literature useful as sources for research ideas and clinical interventions. We also did not design this volume to be an update of Snyder and Forsyth's groundbreaking and comprehensive book, which includes every possible topic at the interface of social and clinical, abnormal, and counseling psychology. Instead, based on our combined 50 years of experience working with clinical doctoral students, we selected for coverage those topics that we believe are most relevant to clinical and counseling psychology training. Our goal was not to cover everything but to cover the basics—hence the word *foundations* in the title. Our ideas about what these foundations are were shaped not only by our experience in working with clinical students over the years but also our experience in teaching this course and getting input from the students concerning what they found relevant and useful.

Our experience has been that clinical students often have difficulty initially seeing the connections between the various broad subfields of psychology and applied clinical work. This book was an attempt to make more explicit the connections between social psychology and clinical practice. We hope that the book will be especially welcome in clinical and counseling psychology programs that adhere to the emerging clinical science model of training.

The book is organized around the three basic questions that confront clinical and counseling psychologists:

1. How do psychological problems develop? (Part II: Psychological Health and Psychological Problems)
2. How can we understand and evaluate them? (Part III: Social Psychology of Psychological Assessment and Diagnosis)
3. How can we design effective interventions for ameliorating them? (Part IV: Social Psychology of Behavior Change and Clinical Interactions)

Each section offers a selection of chapters that take an important social psychological theory or concept that offers an answer to one of these questions. We asked our chapter authors not only to be scholarly in approaching their topics but also to keep in mind the need to make their chapters accessible to and of value to students and practitioners. We believe that they have succeeded admirably, and we hope that the readers will agree.

James E. Maddux
June Price Tangney

## REFERENCE

Snyder, C. R., & Forsyth, D. R. (Eds.). (1991). *Handbook of social and clinical psychology: The health perspective.* New York: Pergamon.

# Contents

# SOCIAL PSYCHOLOGICAL FOUNDATIONS OF CLINICAL PSYCHOLOGY

# PART I

# INTRODUCTION

# 1 Social Psychological Foundations of Clinical Psychology

## *History and Orienting Principles*

James E. Maddux

This chapter attempts to build a foundation for the application of theory and research from social psychology to clinical psychology. According to Baron, Byrne, and Branscombe (2006), social psychology is "the scientific field that seeks to understand the nature and causes of individual behavior and thought in social situations" (p. 6). According to the Society of Clinical Psychology (Division 12 of the American Psychological Association, [APA] *www.apa.org/divisions/div12/aboutcp.html*), the field of clinical psychology "integrates science, theory, and practice to understand, predict, and alleviate maladjustment, disability, and discomfort as well as to promote human adaptation, adjustment, and personal development [and] focuses on the intellectual, emotional, biological, psychological, social, and behavioral aspects of human functioning across the life span, in varying cultures, and at all socioeconomic levels."

Both of these definitions are wide-ranging and cover a lot of territory. In fact, it is difficult to imagine a situation involving any human being that does not involve the "actual, imagined, or implied presence" of another human being. Likewise it is difficult to imagine a situation involving any human being that does not involve some aspect or another of "the intellectual, emotional, biological, psychological, social, and behavioral aspects of human functioning." Can we, therefore, draw any meaningful distinctions between social and clinical psychology? Perhaps not. Although social psychology traditionally has been concerned with more or less "normal" social and interpersonal behavior, and clinical psychology traditionally has been concerned with "abnormal" or "pathological" social and interpersonal behavior, the differences between the fields depend largely on our ability to draw distinctions between normal and abnormal behavior. As discussed below, research strongly suggests that this distinction is difficult, if not impossible, to draw. The field of social psychology has become more difficult to define as social psychologists have become more concerned with topics traditionally viewed as "clinical" (e.g., the cognitive and interpersonal aspects of depression and anxiety). In addition, the field of clinical psychology has become increasingly difficult to define over the past several decades as we have learned more about the generality of psychological change processes, the relationship between normal and maladaptive development, and the continuity between "normal" and "abnormal" and between healthy and unhealthy psychological functioning.

## A HISTORY OF THE INTERFACE BETWEEN SOCIAL AND CLINICAL PSYCHOLOGY

For most of the 20th century, social and clinical psychology remained separate enterprises. Not only were they concerned with what seemed to be different human phenomena (normal social behavior vs. psychological disorders), but they also employed different methods of investigation (controlled experiments vs. case studies). Philosophical and conceptual differences hindered attempts to bridge the two disciplines. Although these differences remain today, to some degree, since the late 1970s theorists and researchers from both sides have focused more on the commonalities between social and clinical psychology than on the differences. The result has been a wealth of conceptual and empirical articles, chapters, and books that have attempted to describe and empirically explore an interpersonal and cognitive approach to understanding psychological adjustment and to developing psychological interventions.

The term *clinical psychology* was first used by Lightner Witmer (1907/1996), who founded the first psychological clinic in 1896 at the University of Pennsylvania. Witmer and the other early clinical psychologists worked primarily with children who had learning or school problems. These early practitioners were influenced more by developments in the new field of psychometrics, such as tests of intelligence and abilities, than by psychoanalytic theory, which did not begin to take hold in American psychology until after Freud's visit to Clark University in 1909 (Korchin, 1976). Soon after Freud's visit, however, psychoanalysis and its derivatives came to dominate not only psychiatry but also the fledgling profession of clinical psychology. During most of the first half of the 20th century, psychoanalytic and derivative psychodynamic models of personality, psychopathology, and psychotherapy were the predominant perspectives. By midcentury, however, behavioral voices (e.g., Skinner; Dollard & Miller) and humanistic voices (e.g., Carl Rogers) were beginning to speak.

The two World Wars greatly hastened the development of the practice of clinical psychology. During World War I, psychologists developed group intelligence tests, which were needed by military services to determine individual differences in abilities. Woodworth developed his Psychoneurotic Inventory to identify soldiers with emotional problems (Korchin, 1976). Clinical psychology was given an even bigger boost by World War II because of the unprecedented demand for mental health services for military personnel during and after the conflict (Korchin, 1976). Of particular concern was the treatment of "shell shock," which had become recognized by the early 1920s as a psychological response to stress (Reisman, 1991). In the mid-1940s, the Veterans Administration recognized clinical psychology as a health care profession, and this recognition spurred the development of doctoral training programs in the field. By 1947, 22 universities had such programs, and by 1950, about half of all doctoral degrees in psychology were being awarded to students in clinical programs (Korchin, 1976). In 1946 Virginia became the first state to regulate the practice of psychology through certification.

In 1949 a conference on the training of clinical psychologists was held at Boulder, Colorado (Maher, 1991). An outgrowth of earlier reports by APA committees in 1945 and 1947, it included representatives from the APA, the Veterans Administration, the National Institute of Mental Health, university psychology departments, and clinical training centers (Raimy, 1950). At this conference, the concept of the clinical psychologist as a *scientist-professional* or *scientist-practitioner*—first developed in 1924 by the APA's Division of Clinical Psychology—was officially endorsed. According to the new standards, a clinical psychologist was to be a psychologist and a scientist first and a practicing clinician second. Clinical programs were to provide training in both science and practice. Clinical practitioners were to devote at least some of their efforts to the development and empirical evaluation of effective techniques of assessment and intervention. However, the integration of research and clinical work often has been more an ideal than a reality. For example, a 1995 survey (Phelps, Eisman, & Kohout, 1998) found that less than one-third of practicing psychologists bother to measure treatment outcome. A more recent survey (Boisvert & Faust, 2006) found that, despite the increasing emphasis over the past decade on empirically supported treatments and evidence-based practice (APA, 2006), practicing psychologists in general have only a "modest familiarity with research findings" (p. 708).

When the scientist-practitioner model was adopted, social psychology was a required part of the training of clinical psychologists and remains so today. Several social cognitive and interactional approaches to personality and adjustment were available during clinical psychology's early years, including the theories of Julian Rotter (1954), George Kelly (1955), Harry Stack Sullivan (1953), and Timothy Leary (1957). Despite these alternatives, clinical psychology remained, for the most part, wedded to psychoanalytic notions. Social psychology had a limited influence on clinical practice because the academic training of clinical students took place in universities, whereas their clinical skills training (in particular, their internships) occurred mostly in psychiatric hospitals and clinics. In these setting, clinical psychologists worked primarily as psychodiagnosticians under the direction of psychiatrists, whose training was primarily biological and psychoanalytic. Therefore, despite required exposure to social, cognitive, and interpersonal frameworks, clinical psychology adopted the individualist, intrapsychic, and medical–biological orientations of psychiatry rather than an interpersonal and contextual orientation grounded in social psychology (Sarason, 1981).

By midcentury the practice of clinical psychology had become characterized by at least four assumptions about the scope of the discipline and the nature of psychological adjustment and maladjustment. First, clinical psychology is the study of psychopathology. That is, clinical psychology is concerned with describing, understanding, and treating psychopathology—deviant, abnormal, and obviously maladaptive behavioral and emotional conditions. Psychopathology is a phenomenon distinct from normal psychological functioning and everyday problems in living. Clinical problems differ in kind from nonclinical problems, and clinical populations differ in kind from nonclinical populations.

Second, psychological dysfunction is analogous to physical disease. This medical analogy does not hold that psychological dysfunctions are caused by biological dysfunctions, although it does not reject this possibility. Instead, it holds that painful and dysfunctional emotional states and patterns of maladaptive behavior, including maladaptive interpersonal behavior, should be construed as symptoms of underlying psychological disorders, just as a fever is a symptom of the flu. Therefore, the task of the psychological clinician is to identify (diagnose) the disorder (disease) exhibited by a person (patient) and prescribe an intervention (treatment) that will eliminate (cure) the disorder.

Third, psychological disorders exist in the individual. Consistent with both intrapsychic and medical orientations, the locus of psychological disorders is *within* the individual rather than in his or her ongoing interactions with the social world.

Fourth, the primary determinants of behavior are intrapersonal. People have fixed and stable properties (e.g., needs or traits) that are more important than situational features in determining their behavior and adjustment. Therefore, clinical psychologists should be concerned more with measuring these fixed properties (e.g., by intellectual and personality assessment) than with understanding the situations in which the person functions.

An early union between social and clinical psychology was attempted in 1921 when the *Journal of Abnormal Psychology*, founded by Morton Prince in 1906, was transformed into the *Journal of Abnormal and Social Psychology*. Clinical psychologist Prince (the journal's editor) and social psychologist Floyd Allport (its managing editor) envisioned an integrative journal that would publish research bridging the study of normal interpersonal processes and abnormal behavior. The vision, however, did not become a reality. In the revamped journal's first two decades, few of its articles dealt with connections between social and abnormal psychology (Forsyth & Leary, 1991). The social psychological research published by the journal became increasingly theory-driven, whereas the clinical research was primarily professional in nature and usually had little relevance to theory (Hill & Weary, 1983).

The failure of this early attempt at integration is not surprising in light of the different paths taken by social and clinical psychologists during this time. Clinical psychology was developing as a discipline with scientific ambitions, but it continued to be dominated by psychodynamic perspectives that did not lend themselves to empirical testing and that emphasized the individual's inner life over interpersonal, situational, and sociocultural influences. For example, despite the best efforts of Kurt Lewin and the Yale Institute of Human Relations (IHR) group, psychoanalysis resisted efforts to be integrated with research-based general psychology. Maher (1991) wrote that, in the 1950s, "as a contributing discipline to psychopathology, psychoanalysis was scientifically bankrupt" (p. 10). At the same time, social psychology, however, was becoming more rigorously empirical and experimental, and thus increasingly irrelevant to the practice of clinical psychology.

Thus, by the 1950s, social psychologists and clinical psychologists were pursuing different paths that rarely crossed, even in the journal devoted to their integration. The questions raised by social psychologists focused largely on the situational determinants of normal social behavior and the cognitive constructions of presumably normal people. The questions raised by clinical psychologists dealt with the intrapsychic determinants of abnormal behavior (psychopathology) and the treatment of clinical disorders. Social psychologists conducted research from a nomothetic perspective that attempted to develop and test elementary principles of social behavior. Practicing clinical psychologists typically employed an idiographic approach with their clients and were concerned with what works with what client and what problem and were less concerned with trying to determine the independent influences of these various factors that seemed to explain a client's problems and of the various strategies that seemed to work. Social psychologists were concerned with the discovery of general principles of social behavior through the use of objective and empirical methods and the analysis of group data. Clinical practitioners were concerned with the subjective experiences of individual clients and with using their own subjective experiences as a tool for understanding clients. Social psychologists were concerned with quantitative descriptions of people; clinical psychologists' descriptions of people were largely qualitative. Finally, social psychologists emphasized internal validity through controlled experiments. Clinical psychologists preferred naturalistic research with high external and ecological validity (Leary & Maddux, 1987).

As a result of these differences, Prince's experiment in social–clinical integration was aborted in 1965 when the *Journal of Abnormal and Social Psychology* was split into *Journal of Abnormal Psychology* and the *Journal of Personality and Social Psychology*. Thirty years later it was remarked that "no act better symbolizes the increasing specialization and fragmentation of psychological science" than this dissolution (Watson & Clark, 1994, p. 3). Like its predecessor, even the new *Journal of Personality and Social Psychology* gave first billing to the traditional study of fixed properties of the individual and second billing to the study of the individual's social world.

Despite this split, some social, clinical, and counseling psychologists continued to pursue integration. As noted previously, clinical psychology began to be influenced by learning theory and research (Dollard & Miller, 1950; Rotter, 1954). Many clinical psychologists, however, were skeptical of the animal-conditioning models on which learning theories were based, and so the influence of these models was limited. In the 1960s several attempts were made to construct connections between social psychology (as opposed to learning theory) and clinical psychology. Frank (1961) argued that all psychological change—including faith healing, religious conversion, and psychotherapy—could be explained by a few basic interpersonal and cognitive processes, such as a trusting relationship with a helping person and positive expectations of help. Goldstein (1966) described the relevance to psychotherapy of research on expectancy, attraction, authoritarianism, cognitive dissonance, norm setting, and role theory. Goldstein, Heller, and Sechrest (1966) offered a social and cognitive analysis of the therapist–client relationship and group psychotherapy and interpreted resistance in psychotherapy as being similar to reactions against attempts at attitude change. Strong (1968, 1982; Strong & Claiborn, 1982) presented an analysis of psychotherapy and counseling as a social influence process and later conducted a program of research on interpersonal processes in psychotherapy. Carson (1969) described the role of disordered social interactions in the origin of psychological problems and argued that psychological difficulties are best explained by *inter*personal rather than *intra*personal processes. This theme was also central to Ullman and Krasner's (1969) influential abnormal psychology text.

Three publications in the 1970s contributed much to the definition of the emerging interface of social and clinical psychology. Two were chapters on social psychological approaches to psychotherapy (Goldstein & Simonson, 1971; Strong, 1978) in the first and second editions of the *Handbook of Psychotherapy and Behavior Change* (Garfield & Bergin, 1971, 1978). The third was a 1976 book by Sharon Brehm that focused on the clinical implications of the theories of reactance, dissonance, and attribution. Since 1976, social and clinical research on the first two theories has declined, but research on attributions has flourished, such as research on the role of attributions in depression (see Riskind, Alloy, & Iacoviello, Chapter 15, this volume). The wave of interest sparked by these publications continued into the 1980s with work on the interpersonal origins of psychological problems, interpersonal approaches to psychological assessment, and interpersonal influence in psychotherapy (Leary & Miller, 1986; Maddux, Stoltenberg, & Rosenwein, 1987; Weary & Mirels, 1982). At the same time, social psychological researchers increasingly studied topics of clinical relevance, such as self-concept, self-regulation, persuasion, and cognitive processes in a variety of psychological problems, as is evident throughout this volume.

A milestone in the development of a more "social" clinical psychology was the publication of the of the first issue of the *Journal of Social and Clinical Psychology* in 1983. Founded by social psychologist John H. Harvey, this new journal provided an outlet specifically for research at the interface of social and clinical psychology. A few years later, Brehm and Smith's (1986) chapter in the third edition of the *Handbook of Psychotherapy and Behavior Change* (Garfield & Bergin, 1986) broadened the perspective offered in Strong's 1978 chapter. (Unfortunately, the most recent edition of this handbook does not include a chapter on social psychological approaches.) An *American Psychologist* article by M. Leary and Maddux (1987) provided a set of basic assumptions for the social–clinical interface and summarized the major developments and issues in the field. The *Handbook of Social and Clinical Psychology: The Health Perspective* (Snyder & Forsyth, 1991) provided the most comprehensive compendium at that time of the application of social psychological theory and research to clinical issues and problems. More recent but less comprehensive volumes include *Social Cognitive Psychology: History and Current Domains* (Barone, Maddux, & Snyder, 1997) and Kowalski and Leary's *The Social Psychology of Emotional and Behavioral Problems* (2000) and *Key Readings in Social-Clinical Psychology* (2003).

In tandem with the publications noted above, professional developments during the past several decades have led to a greater awareness and appreciation by social and clinical psychologists of each others' work and greater opportunities for collaboration.

First, counseling psychology established itself as a field specializing in normal adjustment problems rather than severe psychopathology, and it shifted gradually from intrapsychic to interpersonal models (Tyler, 1972). As a result, counseling psychologists found many concepts and models in social psychology compatible with their approaches to understanding adjustment and psychological interventions. Many important studies on crucial psychotherapy issues, such as therapist–client matching, therapist credibility, the client–therapist relationship, and interpersonal influence, have been published in the past several decades in counseling psychology journals. Clinical psychologists interested in these issues were thus exposed to many psychotherapy-related studies based on social psychological models and concepts.

Second, behavior therapy, the part of clinical psychology most closely linked with general experimental psychology, became more cognitive. A glance at any recent clinical journal or book with *behavior* or *behavioral* in the title provides evidence of the cognitive evolution of behavioral clinical psychology. In fact, behavior therapy became so "cognitive" that several years ago the Association for the Advancement of Behavior Therapy changed its name to the Association for Cognitive and Behavioral Therapy. Cognitive and cognitive-behavioral psychotherapies, developed in the 1950s by psychoanalytically trained psychotherapists Albert Ellis and Aaron Beck, are concerned with many of the same basic issues of concern to social psychological theorists and researchers, such as the relationships among cognition, affect, and behavior and the impact of the situation on behavior. Cognitive-behavioral case formulations draw largely on social psychological principles and constructs. In fact, clinical and counseling psychologists trained in cognitive-behavioral models may feel greater commonality with theorists and researchers in social psychology than with psychodynamic and humanistic clinical and counseling psychologists.

Third, the emergence and tremendous growth of health psychology expanded the traditional boundaries of both social and clinical psychology and provided a forum for the collaboration of researchers and practitioners from both areas. Basic theoretical questions about the relationship between emotional health and physical health and the practical problem of getting people to change their behavior in health-enhancing ways are ideal material for social–clinical collaboration. In fact, most health psychologists are social, clinical, or counseling psychologists who are interested in problems encountered in health and medical settings. The emphasis on health psychology extends beyond the traditional topics of psychopathology, and now much mainstream social psychology is concerned, once again, with understanding and solving important human problems.

Fourth, social psychology has changed in ways that have moved it toward integration with clinical psychology. The "crisis of confidence" in social psychology about the ecological validity of its laboratory findings (Sarason, 1981) resulted in a renewal of interest in applied research and real-world problems. This crisis and renewal set the stage for the entry of social psychologists into the study of clinical problems and issues. Social psychological research increasingly has merged the study of cognitive processes with the study of emotional interpersonal processes and the self. Social psychologists have become more concerned with understanding *social cognition*—how people construe social situations and the effects of these construals on social behavior, as evidenced throughout this volume. The study of social cognition has become central to current approaches to understanding personality, individual differences, interpersonal behavior, and emotions (Fiske & Taylor, 2007; Moskowitz, 2004; Kross, Mischel, & Shoda, Chapter 20, this volume; Shadel, Chapter 18, this volume), as revealed in any recent issue of the *Journal of Personality and Social Psychology*, *Personality and Social Psychology Bulletin*, or the *Journal of Social and Clinical Psychology*. This cognitive evolution includes cognitive approaches to understanding relationships. The study of relationships has shifted from concern with bargaining between strangers in the laboratory to concern with real-life intimacy, love, and marriage. Much of this recent work involves the study of psychological adjustment and dysfunctional behavior. As a result, the relevance of social psychological theory and research to clinical theory, research, and practice has increased immensely, along with the collaborations of social and clinical psychologists.

Fifth, disorders of personality, as formal diagnostic categories, were introduced into the official nosology of psychiatric and psychology disorders with the publication of the third edition of the American Psychiatric Association's (1980) *Diagnostic and Statistical Manual of Mental Disorders, Third Edition* (DSM-III). The inclusion of these categories reflects the notion that personality can be disordered or dysfunctional and is worthy of attention independent of the broad traditional clinical notions of neuroses (e.g., depressive disorders, anxiety disorders) and psychoses (e.g., the schizophrenic disorders; Millon, 1981). Of course, the very notion that we can separate personality into normal and abnormal types (disorders) and the notion that we can neatly categorize types of abnormal personalities are largely inconsistent with a social psychological perspective. However, the definition of this new general category and the diagnostic criteria for the various specific disorders rely heavily on the *interpersonal* (rather than the intrapersonal) manifestations of the individual's dysfunction.

Personality disorders are noted more for the disruption they cause in the individual's relationships and social world than for the inner turmoil of the individual. Thus, this new set of diagnostic entities gave a greater *official* recognition to the importance of the *social* aspects of psychological dysfunction than ever before.

Since the publication of the DSM-III, hundreds of studies have been published examining various aspects of personality disorders. Because of the emphasis on interpersonal functioning in these disorders, research in social psychology and personality has assumed a new and greater relevance to the understanding of psychological adjustment and dysfunction. For example, research on the relationship between "normal" personality and these personality "disorders" strongly suggests that so-called personality disorders are extreme variants of normally distributed dimensions of individual difference rather than disorders discontinuous with normal personality (e.g., Widiger, 2007). This research supports the notion that the study of normal interpersonal behavior and dysfunctional interpersonal behavior involves the study of essentially the same problems and processes.

## ORIENTING PRINCIPLES

It has been over 40 years since the partitioning of the *Journal of Abnormal and Social Psychology* and the symbolic partitioning of social and clinical psychology. It also has been 25 years since the publication of the first issue of the *Journal of Social and Clinical Psychology.* During this time, clinical psychology has become more rigorously empirical while maintaining its focus on understanding psychological adjustment and problems in living; social psychology has become more concerned with psychological adjustment and problems in living while maintaining its empirical rigor. Thus have the fields come to complement one another both in content (what they study) and method (how they study it). Social psychological journals such as the *Journal of Personality and Social Psychology* and the *Journal of Social and Clinical Psychology* regularly publish studies that are relevant to clinical issues, and some clinical and counseling journals (e.g., *Cognitive Therapy and Research*, *Journal of Counseling Psychology*) publish studies that deal with basic social psychological processes.

The following set of implicit assumptions regarding the nature of psychological problems and their treatment, which can be gleaned from the work of numerous theoreticians and researchers over the past several decades, provides a foundation for the application of social psychology to clinical psychology.

### Psychological Problems Are Interpersonal Problems

Behavioral and emotional problems are essentially interpersonal problems. The majority of people who seek psychological services do so because they are concerned about their relationships with other people. Common adjustment problems such as depression, anxiety, marital discord, loneliness, and hostility consist primarily of interpersonal beliefs and behaviors that are expressed in interpersonal settings and make little sense when examined outside an interpersonal context. This assumption does not deny that some psychological problems may have strong biological roots, but it affirms that even biologically based problems are influenced by interpersonal forces.

### "Normal" Behavior Is Sometimes Dysfunctional

Because much of social psychological research and theory deals with how people misperceive, misattribute, and subsequently "misbehave" in their relations with others, much of social psychology involves the study of what Freud (1901/1965) called "the psychopathology of everyday life." Cognitive dissonance theory, reactance theory, and attribution theories, for example, each describes cognitive and motivational processes of normal people, processes that are often illogical, unreasonable, or biased and that lead to poorly reasoned decisions. Therefore, even "normal" social cognitions and their affective and behavioral consequences are sometimes dysfunctional. The clinical or counseling psychologist with an in-depth knowledge of the social cognition literature, especially the errors made by normal people in social perception and judgment, is likely to have a greater awareness of the normality of seemingly pathological thought and behavior. Because the terminology in social psychology is less pathological and less dispositional in connotation, such awareness should lead to a decreased tendency to overpathologize.

### Social Norms Determine the Distinction between Normality and Abnormality

The distinction between normality and abnormality is essentially arbitrary and is the product of social norms that are derived from, and enforced in, social settings. Thus, understanding how attitudes and beliefs become norms, how they change and how they are acquired and enforced, is essential to understanding how and why certain behaviors (including those with biological etiologies) are viewed as abnormal and others are not.

### Abnormal Social Behaviors Are Distortions of Normal Behaviors

The vast majority of so-called abnormal social behaviors are essentially distortions or exaggerations of normal patterns that are displayed at times and in places considered by others to be inappropriate. Thus, many behaviors given pathological labels are governed by the same interpersonal processes that determine behaviors that escape the stigma of being labeled as deviant.

### Clinical Judgment Involves the Same Processes as Everyday Social Judgment

Clinical judgment is a process of social cognition and person perception that involves the same processes as everyday social and person perception. Most important, clinicians make errors in clinical judgment that are similar to errors made by nonclinicians in nonclinical contexts (Leary & Miller, 1986). Thus, the study of social inference, problem solving, and decision making is crucial to understanding clinical assessment and diagnosis (e.g., Garb, Chapter 16, this volume.)

### Clinical Interventions Focus on Social Cognitions

Most, and possibly all, clinical interventions, regardless of theoretical foundation, focus on changing what people think about, how they feel, and how they behave toward others. Marital therapy, family therapy, parenting skills training, assertiveness training, social skills training, interpersonal and cognitive therapies, and other interventions are concerned primarily with helping people get along with other people and feel better about their interpersonal relationships. Indeed, most clinical and counseling psychologists trained in the last 20 years or so (i.e., those trained in social learning or cognitive-behavioral models) are essentially "applied social psychologists" in the sense that they are concerned with the reciprocal interactions of social cognitions (attitudes, self-beliefs, attributions, expectancies), emotion, and behavior.

### Psychotherapy Is a Social Encounter

Psychotherapy, counseling, and other behavior change strategies, either dyadic or group, are interpersonal encounters, first and foremost, albeit social encounters with a specific goal—one person trying to help another. This assumption dictates that the foundation for psychological intervention is an understanding of interpersonal behavior, particularly relationship development and interpersonal influence processes (e.g., Brehm & Smith, 1986; Strong & Claiborn, 1982).

### Social Psychological Theories Provide a Basis for Models of Behavior Change

Successful psychotherapy and behavior change strategies, regardless of theoretical foundation, have in common a relatively small number of features that explain their effectiveness (Frank, 1961). Because they propose general explanations for a broad range of human behavior, social psychological theories can provide the foundation on which to build an inclusive and comprehensive model of therapeutic behavior change.

## OVERVIEW OF BOOK

This book deals with the three basic challenges that confront clinical and counseling psychologists: (1) understanding the causes of psychological problems, (2) evaluating and assessing psychological problems, and (3) designing effective interventions for ameliorating them. The chapters are organized not around psychiatric diagnoses (e.g., depression, anxiety, personality disorders) but around social psychological theories and concepts. Each chapter focuses on an important social psychological theory or concept that can offer a fresh framework for addressing clinically relevant questions.

## REFERENCES

American Psychiatric Association. (1980). *Diagnostic and statistical manual of mental disorders* (3rd ed.). Washington, DC: Author.

American Psychological Association Presidential Task Force on Evidence-Based Practice. (2006). Evidence-based practice in psychology. *American Psychologist*, *61*, 271–285.

Baron, R. A., Byrne, D., & Branscombe, N. R. (2006). *Social psychology* (11th ed.). Boston: Pearson.

Barone, D., Maddux, J. E., & Snyder, C. R. (1997). *Social cognitive psychology: History and current domains.* New York: Plenum Press.

Boisvert, C. M., & Faust, D. (2006). Practicing psychologists' knowledge of general psychotherapy research findings: Implications for science–practice relations. *Professional Psychology: Research and Practice*, *37*, 708–716.

Brehm, S. S. (1976). *The application of social psychology to clinical practice.* Washington, DC: Hemisphere.

Brehm, S. S., & Smith, T. W. (1986). Social psychological approaches to psychotherapy and behavior change. In S. L. Garfield & A. E. Bergin (Eds.), *Handbook of psychotherapy and behavior change* (3rd ed., pp. 69–115). New York: Wiley.

Carson, R. C. (1969). *Interaction concepts of personality*. Chicago: Aldine.

Dollard, J., & Miller, N. (1950). *Personality and psychotherapy: An analysis in terms of learning, thinking and culture*. New York: McGraw-Hill.

Fiske, S. T., & Taylor, S. E. (2007). *Social cognition: From brains to culture.* New York: McGraw-Hill.

Forsyth, D. R., & Leary, M. R. (1991). Metatheoretical and epistemological issues. In C. R. Snyder & D. R. Forsyth (Eds.), *Handbook of social and clinical psychology: The health perspective* (pp. 757–773). Elmsford, NY: Pergamon Press.

Frank, J. D. (1961). *Persuasion and healing: A comparative study of psychotherapy.* Baltimore: Johns Hopkins University Press.

Freud, S. (1965). *The psychopathology of everyday life.* New York: Norton. (Original work published 1901)

Garfield, S. L., & Bergin, A. E. (Eds.). (1971). *Handbook of psychotherapy and behavior change: An empirical analysis.* New York: Wiley.

Garfield, S. L., & Bergin, A. E. (Eds.). (1978). *Handbook of psychotherapy and behavior change: An empirical analysis* (2nd ed.). New York: Wiley.

Garfield, S. L., & Bergin, A. E. (Eds.). (1986). *Handbook of psychotherapy and behavior change: An empirical analysis* (3rd ed.). New York: Wiley.

Goldstein, A. P. (1966). Psychotherapy research by extrapolation from social psychology. *Journal of Counseling Psychology*, *13*, 38–45.

Goldstein, A. P., Heller, K., & Sechrest, L. B. (1966). *Psychotherapy and the psychology of behavior change*. New York: Wiley.

Goldstein, A. P., & Simonson, N. R. (1971). Social psychological approaches to psychotherapy research. In S. Garfield & A. Bergin (Eds.), *Handbook of psychotherapy and behavior change* (pp. 154–195). New York: Wiley.

Hill, M. G., & Weary, G. (1983). Perspectives on the *Journal of Abnormal and Social Psychology*: How it began and how it was transformed over the years. *Journal of Social and Clinical Psychology*, *1*, 4–14.

Kelly, G. A. (1955). *The psychology of personal constructs: A theory of personality* (2 vols.). New York: Norton.

Korchin, S. J. (1976). *Modern clinical psychology*. New York: Basic Books.

Kowalski, R. M., & Leary, M. R. (Eds.). (2000). *The social psychology of emotional and behavioral problems: Interfaces of social and clinical psychology.* Washington, DC: American Psychological Association.

Kowalski, R. M., & Leary, M. R. (Eds.). (2003). *Key readings in social-clinical psychology*. New York: Psychology Press.

Leary, M. R., & Maddux, J. E. (1987). Progress toward a viable interface between social and clinical-counseling psychology. *American Psychologist*, *42*, 904–911.

Leary, M. R., & Miller, R. S. (1986). *Social psychology and dysfunctional behavior.* New York: Springer-Verlag.

Leary, T. (1957). *Interpersonal diagnosis of personality*. New York: Ronald Press.

Maddux, J. E., Stoltenberg, C. D., & Rosenwein, R. (Eds.). (1987). *Social processes in clinical and counseling psychology*. New York: Springer-Verlag.

Maher, B. A. (1991). A personal history of clinical psychology. In M. Hersen, A. E. Kazdin, A. S. Bellack (Eds.), *The clinical psychology handbook* (2nd ed.). New York: Pergamon.

Millon, T. (1981). *Disorders of personality: DSM-III, Axis II.* New York: Wiley.

Moskowitz, G. B. (2004). *Social cognition: Understanding self and others.* New York: Guilford Press.

Phelps, R., Eisman, E. J., & Kohout, J. (1998). Psychological practice and managed care: Results of the CAPP practitioner survey. *Professional Psychology: Research and Practice, 29,* 31–36.

Raimy, V. C. (Ed.). (1950). *Training in clinical psychology.* New York: Prentice-Hall.

Reisman, J. R. (1991). *A history of clinical psychology* (2nd ed.). New York: Brunner-Routledge.

Rotter, J. B. (1954). *Social learning and clinical psychology.* Englewood Cliffs, NJ: Prentice-Hall.

Sarason, S. (1981). *Psychology misdirected.* New York: Free Press.

Snyder, C. R., & Forsyth, D. R. (1991). *Handbook of social and clinical psychology* (pp. 438–468). New York: Pergamon Press.

Strong, S. R. (1968). Counseling: An interpersonal process. *Journal of Counseling Psychology, 15,* 215–224.

Strong, S. R. (1978). Social psychological approach to psychotherapy research. In S. L. Garfield & A. E. Bergin (Eds.), *Handbook of psychotherapy and behavior change: An empirical analysis* (2nd ed., pp. 101–135). New York: Wiley.

Strong, S. R., & Claiborn, C. D. (1982). *Change through interaction: Social psychological processes of counseling and psychotherapy.* New York: Wiley.

Sullivan, H. S. (1953). *Conceptions of modern psychiatry.* New York: Norton.

Tyler, L. (1972). Reflecting on counseling psychology. *Counseling Psychologist, 3,* 6–11.

Ullman, L. P., & Krasner, L. (1969). *A psychological approach to abnormal behavior.* Englewood Cliffs, NJ: Prentice-Hall.

Watson, D., & Clark, L. A. (1994). Emotions, moods, traits, and temperaments: Conceptual distinctions and empirical findings. In P. Ekman & R. J. Davidson (Eds.), *The nature of emotion: Fundamental questions* (pp. 89–93). New York: Oxford University Press.

Weary, G., & Mirels, H. L. (Eds.). (1982). *Integrations of clinical and social psychology.* New York: Oxford University Press.

Widiger, T. A. (2007). Classification and diagnosis: Historical development and contemporary issues. In J. E. Maddux & B. A. Winstead (Eds.), *Psychopathology: Contemporary issues, theory, and research* (2nd ed.). New York: Taylor & Francis.

Witmer, L. (1996). Clinical psychology. *The Psychological Clinic, 1,* 1–9. (Original work published 1907)

# PART II

# PSYCHOLOGICAL HEALTH AND PSYCHOLOGICAL PROBLEMS

# Self and Identity

# 2 The Role of Self-Awareness and Self-Evaluation in Dysfunctional Patterns of Thought, Emotion, and Behavior

Mark R. Leary
Eleanor B. Tate

The emergence of self-awareness was an exceptionally important milestone in the history of human evolution. Although scholars do not agree about precisely when human beings acquired their current ability to self-reflect, most concur that the appearance of self-awareness was among the seminal events that set human beings on such a different trajectory from all other animals (Leary & Buttermore, 2003). A handful of other species (chimpanzees, bonobos, gorillas, orangutans, and possibly dolphins) show evidence of being able to recognize and consciously think about themselves (Mitchell, 2003), but none appears to think about and evaluate itself in the complex and abstract ways that characterize human beings.

The importance of this ability becomes clear when we consider the range of human activities that require self-awareness, such as conscious planning, introspection, self-evaluation, insight, perspective taking, and deliberate self-regulation. Self-awareness undoubtedly contributes to human productivity and well-being in many ways, and most uniquely human features of our lives—such as government, philosophy, science, religion, and education—would not be possible without the capacity for conscious self-relevant thought. Yet, the ability to self-reflect also sets the stage for a variety of emotional and behavioral problems that arise from the ways in which people think about themselves (Leary, 2004a). The goal of this chapter is to examine theory and research in social psychology that deal with the processes involved in self-awareness, self-representation, and self-evaluation, with an emphasis on self-processes that may contribute to psychological difficulties.

## SELF-AWARENESS AND EMOTION

For animals that lack self-awareness, emotional experiences are elicited by features of their physical or social environment. Emotions occur when threats, opportunities, harms, or benefits are perceived, and they abate when the threat or opportunity is no longer present, often because the animal has taken some kind of action (e.g., by fleeing, hiding, or attacking). Of course, human beings also respond emotionally to stimuli in their immediate environments, but, unlike animals without self-awareness, people also generate emotions in their own minds through self-relevant thought. By consciously thinking about past experiences, their current situation, the future, or their own qualities, people can evoke almost any emotion in their own minds (Leary, 2007). Sometimes these self-generated emotions are pleasant and beneficial, as when people are motivated to pursue success by anticipating its positive emotional consequences or make judicious decisions by imagining how a current action will make them feel at some future time. However, many of these self-created emotions are not only functionally useless, in that they do not prepare people to respond to actual threats and opportunities, but many imagined events that cause strong emotions never actually come to pass. As a result, a great deal of unhappiness is fueled by self-relevant thoughts that do not contribute to people's physical, psychological, or social well-being (Leary, 2004a).

### Self-Discrepancies

Duval and Wicklund (1972) are usually credited with initiating contemporary research on self-awareness. Their original version of self-awareness theory proposed that people who are in a state of self-attention automatically and invariably evaluate themselves according to salient standards. Furthermore, because people often find that their current actions and outcomes fall short of their standards, their self-evaluations are typically unfavorable, resulting in negative affect. Subsequent research has shown that self-awareness does not necessarily reveal discrepancies between one's behaviors and standards, nor does it always result in negative emotion. Even so, it is certainly true that perceiving discrepancies between one's standards, goals, or values, on one hand, and one's behavior or outcomes, on the other, can elicit a variety of emotions.

Although ideas regarding self-discrepancy have had a long history in psychology (e.g., Rogers, 1954), the role of self-discrepancies in emotion has been developed most fully by Higgins (1987). According to his self-discrepancy theory, people sometimes experience discrepancies between their actual self (their representation of the attributes that they actually possess) and either their ideal self (their representation of the attributes they would like to possess) or their "ought self" (their representation of the attributes that they should or ought to possess due to their duties, obligations, or responsibilities). According to the theory, discrepancies between one's actual and ideal selves are associated with dysphoric emotions (e.g., sadness, hopelessness), whereas discrepancies between the actual and ought selves result in agitation-related emotions (e.g., anxiety).

Several studies have supported the general prediction that actual–ideal self-discrepancies tend to lead to dejection-related emotions (e.g., depression) and that actual–ought self-discrepancies lead to agitation-related emotions (e.g., anxiety) (Higgins, 1987, 1999; Higgins, Klein, & Strauman, 1985; Moretti & Higgins, 1990; Scott & O'Hara, 1993; Strauman, 1989). However, other predictions of the theory have not been supported. For example, a study by Tangney, Neidenthal, Covert, and Barlow (1998) did not confirm the predictions of self-discrepancy theory regarding the nature of the self-discrepancies that underlie shame versus guilt, and they also failed to replicate earlier studies showing that particular types of self-discrepancies were uniquely related to particular emotions (Higgins et al., 1985). In response, Higgins (1999) acknowledged that unique relationships between particular self-discrepancies and emotions are not always found.

A second approach to self-discrepancies was offered by Ogilvie (1987), who proposed that people also use the undesired self—the self at its worst—as a standard for self-evaluation (see also, Carver, Lawrence, & Scheier, 1999). For example, Ogilvie and Clark (1992) found that discrepancies between people's actual and undesired selves operated separately from discrepancies between their actual and ideal selves. More importantly, actual–undesired self-discrepancies correlated more strongly with people's life satisfaction than actual–ideal discrepancies (Ogilvie, 1987; Rahakrishnan & Chan, 1997). Put simply, people's evaluations of how they are faring, compared to feared outcomes and identities, exert a stronger impact on their emotions than their evaluations of how they are faring compared to their ideal outcomes and identities.

Overall, research supports the general idea that people's self-relevant beliefs are tied to their emotional well-being and that discrepancies between their self-beliefs and what they desire, ought, and fear to become predict particular patterns of emotion. The details of these processes are open to debate, but the importance of self-beliefs and self-discrepancies is not.

## Self-Rumination

Typically, self-reflective emotions wax and wane as people's self-related thoughts change. However, when people cannot stop themselves from thinking emotionally laden thoughts, they may become locked in a particular emotion. Rumination involves unintentional, repetitive, perseverative thoughts on a particular theme that occur despite the fact that the immediate environment does not cue the thoughts (Martin & Tesser, 1996). Although not all rumination is self-focused, a great deal of it involves recurrent thoughts about one's own behaviors, characteristics, life circumstances, or future. At present, it is not clear whether self-focused ruminative thought involves only a high and intractable level of inner self-talk or a motive to think about potential threats in hopes of avoiding them (Silvia, Eichstaedt, & Phillips, 2005; Trapnell & Campbell, 1999). In either case, becoming locked in ruminative thought can extend negative emotions long past the point at which they serve any function.

### *Self-Rumination about the Present*

Most investigations of rumination have focused on patterns of negative thoughts that lead to depression and then sustain depression through passive and persistent thoughts about one's depressive symptoms (Fresco, Frankel, Mennin, Turk, & Heimberg, 2002; Nolen-Hoeksema & Morrow, 1991). These studies suggest that rumination not only causes depression but also intensifies and prolongs depressive symptoms, because rumination about one's depression may amplify pessimistic thinking, interfere with attention and concentration, and inhibit behaviors that might work the person out of his or her depressive episode (see Nolen-Hoeksema, 1987, 1991).

The role of rumination in depression is further supported by research showing that problem solving among depressed people improves when they change from a state-focused ruminative style to a process-oriented style. Watkins and Baracaia (2002) instructed participants to consider hypothetical social problems, such as having an argument with their partner, either by asking themselves state-focused, ruminative questions about the problem (e.g., "What am I doing wrong?", "Why can't I do better?") or questions that focus on the *process* of dealing with the problem (e.g., "How am I deciding on a way to solve this problem?", "How do I know that this is a good thing to do?"). Results showed that depressed participants who were induced to use the latter, process-oriented approach solved the social problems as effectively as people who were not depressed. However, both depressed participants and those who had recovered from depression showed deficits in their ability to solve these social problems in the state-focused ruminative thought condition, whereas nondepressed participants did not. Breaking depressed people's ruminative style by focusing them on the process of solving problems appeared to benefit them.

### *Self-Rumination about the Past*

Although most research on rumination has focused on its relationship to depression, self-focused perseveration can lead to other emotions as well. For example, rumination about past events may prolong or magnify regret for previous actions and stymie progress toward overcoming circumstances that one currently regrets. In a longitudinal study of regret (Stewart & Vandewater, 1999), middle-age women who took steps to change life circumstances that they regretted (e.g., choosing a different profession) reported greater well-being a decade later. In contrast, women who experienced regret in their 30s but did not change their circumstances subsequently reported lower well-being, greater depression, and poorer physical health in middle age than those who had taken steps to combat the source of regret. Importantly, rumination mediated the relationship between regret and well-being for women who made no behavioral changes. The authors concluded that, although regret can motivate goal setting, rumination may hinder the behavioral changes needed to pursue one's goals (Stewart & Vandewater, 1999).

When people look back on their lives (yet another activity that requires self-awareness), they tend to regret failures to take action more than to regret actions that were taken. Although regrettable actions and inactions are equally painful immediately after the instigating event, the potency of regrettable actions wanes over time, whereas the potency of regrettable inactions does not, and may even increase (Gilovich & Husted Medvec, 1995; Landman & Manis, 1992). Clearly, how people think about themselves in the past has important implications for the quality of their lives in the present.

### *Self-Rumination about the Future*

Although some researchers have linked rumination specifically to depression (Fresco et al., 2002), others suggest that ruminating about future events is a leading source of the form of anxiety that is often called *worry*. Not only may rumination about real and imagined future events generate negative affect, but self-preoccupation uses up valuable cognitive resources and thereby undermines cognitive and behavioral performance at the present time. For example, anxiously thinking about how one will introduce oneself to a group of people interferes with one's memory for other people's introductions of themselves (Bond & Omar,

1990), and students who experience test anxiety perform poorly because they ruminate about their own future failure and its implications rather than devote full attention to the test (Wine, 1971).

Some researchers have conceptualized worry and rumination as distinct yet related processes. Studies employing the widely used Response Styles Questionnaire to measure rumination suggest that rumination is more closely associated with depression than with worry (Borkovec, Ray, & Stöber, 1998; Fresco et al., 2002; Nolen-Hoeksema & Morrow, 1991; Watkins, 2004). However, this issue may be more semantic than real, depending on how one defines rumination. If rumination is conceptualized as recurrent, unintentional thoughts on a particular theme (Martin & Tesser, 1996), then certain patterns of rumination lead to depression, whereas other patterns lead to anxiety; in essence, *worry* is merely rumination about a feared future event. Indeed, structural equation modeling suggests that worry and rumination may be subsumed under a latent *repetitive thought* variable that is associated with negative moods (Brosschot, Gerin, & Thayer, 2006; Segerstrom, Tsao, Alden, & Craske, 2000).

## SELF-EVALUATION

Most research that deals with self-evaluation has focused on self-esteem—people's evaluatively based feelings about themselves. Although people's feelings about themselves vary across situations and time (state self-esteem), most research has focused on individual differences in people's general feelings about themselves across situations (trait self-esteem). Unfortunately, researchers do not agree on many fundamental issues about self-esteem. For example, disagreements exist regarding the function of self-esteem, whether high self-esteem is generally beneficial, whether people are inherently motivated to protect and enhance their self-esteem, and whether people benefit from self-enhancing biases that help them to maintain their self-esteem (see Kernis, 2006, for a comprehensive look at many of these issues).

### Self-Enhancing Biases

A great deal of research shows that people tend to think about themselves in ways that seem intended to help them maintain their self-esteem. For example, studies have shown that people are apt to rate themselves more positively than they objectively deserve (Colvin, Block, & Funder, 1995; Robins & Beer, 2001); take more responsibility for their successes than for their failures (Blaine & Crocker, 1993); perceive themselves as better than average on most dimensions (Alicke, Klotz, Breitenbecher, Yurak, & Vredenburg, 1995); selectively seek information that maintains their self-esteem (Ditto & Lopez, 1993); idiosyncratically define their traits in ways that cast them in a positive light (Dunning & Cohen, 1992); overvalue people, places, and things with which they are associated (Pelham, Mirenberg, & Jones, 2002); interpret other people's behaviors and traits in ways that reflect well on them personally (Dunning & Beauregard, 2000); compare themselves with others who are worse than they are (Wood, Giordano-Beech, & Ducharme, 1999); derogate other people to feel good about themselves (Fein & Spencer, 1997); distance themselves from those who outperform them (Tesser, 1988); and deny that they possess these sorts of self-enhancing tendencies (Pronin, Lin, & Ross, 2002).

One pervasive debate has involved whether these kinds of self-serving biases are beneficial or detrimental to people's well-being. Some theorists have argued that self-enhancing biases promote well-being, effective behavior, and success (Taylor & Brown, 1988). In support of this claim, high-trait self-esteem is associated with a variety of positive outcomes, including lower depression, higher confidence, lower stress, and greater success, whereas low-trait self-esteem tends to be associated with problems such as anxiety, drug abuse, delinquency, and depression (Taylor & Brown, 1988, 1994; Taylor, Lerner, Sherman, Sage, & McDowell, 2003a, 2003b).

Others counter that self-enhancing biases and the effort to pursue self-esteem have notable drawbacks (Block & Colvin, 1994; Colvin et al., 1995; Crocker & Park, 2004; Robins & Beer, 2001). In an extensive review of the self-esteem literature, Baumeister, Campbell, Krueger, and Vohs (2003) concluded that the relationships between high self-esteem and positive outcomes are far weaker than many have claimed, and that, moreover, research has revealed several drawbacks of having high self-esteem. For example, under some circumstances, people with high self-esteem make risky decisions, treat others badly, and react aggressively (Baumeister, Heatherton, & Tice, 1993; Baumeister, Smart, & Boden, 1996; Heatherton & Vohs, 2000; Johnson, Vincent, & Ross, 1997). Self-serving biases may also lead people to overestimate the accuracy of their views of themselves and of other people and to conclude that other people are less accurate, objective, and fair than they are (Pronin et al., 2002; Pronin, Gilovich, & Ross, 2004). In addition, other people tend to view self-enhancing individuals negatively, suggesting that self-enhancement can undermine interpersonal relationships (Bonanno, Field, & Kovacevic, 2002; Bonanno, Rennicke, & Dekel, 2005; Colvin et al., 1995; Leary, Bednarski, Hammon, & Duncan, 1999; Robins & John, 1997).

Part of the difficulty in resolving this debate stems from the fact that many studies claiming to demonstrate beneficial effects of self-enhancement do not actually assess whether people's positive self-views are actually self-enhancing or justifiably positive (Kwan, John, Kenny, Bond, & Robins, 2004; Taylor & Armor, 1996). Research that has distinguished self-esteem from self-enhancement suggests that, although self-enhancing biases often make people feel good about themselves and have other short-term benefits, they can undermine people's interpersonal relationships and well-being in the long run (Colvin et al., 1995; Crocker & Park, 2004; Kwan et al., 2004; Paulhus, 1998; Paulhus, Harms, Bruce, & Lysy, 2003; Robins & Beer, 2001). Furthermore, as Baumeister et al. (2003) suggested, many of the assumed benefits of self-esteem—such as academic achievement and social success—actually reflect causes of self-esteem rather than its effects.

Swann, Chang-Schneider, and McClarty (2007) have recently disputed the notion that self-esteem is only weakly related to important life outcomes, arguing that people's self-views are more strongly related to behavior, emotion, and well-being than critics suggest. However, Swann et al. focused primarily on people's beliefs about themselves rather than self-esteem per se. Failing to distinguish people's thoughts about themselves (i.e., self-views, self-beliefs, or self-concept) from their feelings and evaluations about themselves (i.e., self-esteem) obscures the relationships among self-relevant thoughts, feelings, motives, and behavior.

## The Function of Self-Esteem

Whether self-enhancement is viewed as a benefit or liability, people undoubtedly appear to be motivated to maintain, if not enhance, their self-esteem. However, researchers do not agree about the source of this motivation. Among social psychologists, two explanations of self-esteem have received the greatest attention in the past decade: terror management theory and sociometer theory.

### *Terror Management Theory*

Terror management theory (TMT; Solomon, Greenberg, & Pyszczynski, 1991) is based on the notion that people seek self-esteem because it helps to buffer them against existential anxiety. According to the theory, awareness of one's own mortality creates paralyzing terror unless people construct beliefs about themselves and their worlds indicating that they are important and valuable. When people's faith in their cultural worldview and in their own goodness are undermined (e.g., by threats to important beliefs or their own worth), they experience intense anxiety. TMT suggests that people who have high self-esteem are protected against this terror because they believe that they are living up to important cultural values and, thus, feel assured that they will achieve either literal or symbolic immortality. In brief, people engage in behaviors that promote self-esteem to minimize death-related terror.

In support of TMT, studies show that people defend their worldviews when reminded of their own mortality (Florian & Mikulincer, 1997; Greenberg et al., 1990; Rosenblatt et al., 1989). Furthermore, people with high self-esteem react less strongly to reminders of mortality and other threatening stimuli than those with low self-esteem (Greenberg, Solomon, et al., 1992; Harmon-Jones et al., 1997), and making death salient seems to increase people's desire to have high self-esteem (Greenberg, Simon, Pyszczynski, Solomon, & Chatel, 1992). However, evidence that the function of self-esteem is specifically to protect people against terror is weaker than evidence for other parts of the theory (for contrasting views, see Leary, 2002, 2004b; Pyszczynski, Greenberg, & Solomon, 2004).

### *Sociometer Theory*

A second perspective on the function of self-esteem is offered by sociometer theory (Leary, 2006; Leary & Baumeister, 2000: Leary & Downs, 1995). According to this theory, self-esteem is part of a psychological system that monitors people's relational value. Because people's well-being requires that they be valued and accepted by others, people monitor their social worlds for indications that other people may not value them as social interactants, group members, and relationship partners. When the sociometer detects cues that reflect potential social devaluation or rejection, people experience an aversive loss of state self-esteem, which alerts them to the potential relational problem, motivates them to take steps to correct it, and guides their future interpersonal choices. According to the theory, events that lower people's self-esteem—such as failure, rejection, humiliating events, and immoral actions—do so because these events may result in their devaluation or rejection (Leary, Tambor, Terdal, & Downs, 1995). Furthermore, according to sociometer theory, people are not motivated to maintain or enhance their self-esteem for its own sake, as has often been assumed. Rather, people are motivated to behave in ways that help them to avoid rejection. Thus, when people appear to be protecting their self-esteem, they are actually trying to increase their value and acceptance in the eyes of other people.

The central aspects of sociometer theory have received considerable research support. In laboratory studies, experimental manipulations that convey rejection, disapproval, or disinterest consistently lower participants' state self-esteem (Leary, Cottrell, & Phillips, 2001;

Leary, Haupt, Strausser, & Chokel, 1998; Leary et al., 1995; Nezlek, Kowalski, Leary, Blevins, & Holgate, 1997). Similarly, rejecting events in everyday life are associated with lowered self-esteem (Baumeister, Wotman, & Stillwell, 1993; Leary et al., 1995), and longitudinal research shows that perceived relational value prospectively predicts changes in self-esteem (Srivastava & Beer, 2005). Even people who claim to be unconcerned with other people's approval and acceptance show declines in self-esteem when they are rejected (Leary et al., 2003).

### Culture and Self-Evaluation

The majority of studies on self-esteem have been conducted in the United States, Europe, and Australia, leaving open the question of whether people in other cultures also self-enhance. Some theorists propose that people in certain cultures, such as Japan, do not show the same self-enhancing tendencies as people in the United States (Heine, Lehman, Markus, & Kityama, 1999). For example, Japanese participants more readily accept negative feedback about themselves (whereas Westerners tend to reject it) and tend to be modest rather than self-enhancing (Heine, Kitayama, & Lehman, 2001; Heine, Kitayama, Lehman, Takata, et al., 2001; Heine & Lehman, 1995). Other theorists have argued that people in all cultures prefer to feel good rather than bad about themselves and, thus, behave in ways that promote self-esteem (Sedikides, Gaertner, & Toguchi, 2003). However, because different cultures value different characteristics, people may promote their self-esteem in culturally defined ways. According to this view, either self-criticism or self-enhancement can make a person feel good about him- or herself, depending on what the person's culture values.

Along these lines, Sedikides et al. (2003) found evidence that both American and Japanese participants self-enhance but that they use different tactics to do so. American participants in this study self-enhanced primarily with respect to individualistic attributes (e.g., *unique*, *independent*, and *self-reliant*), whereas Japanese participants self-enhanced primarily on collectivist attributes (e.g., *agreeable*, *compromising*, and *cooperative*). This pattern suggests that self-enhancement is expressed differently in different cultures (see Kurman, 2001). The Japanese individual who downplays his or her positive traits may be just as self-serving and feel as good about him- or herself as the American who exaggerates them. In both cultures the person's perceptions and actions are biased in ways that promote social acceptance and foster positive self-feelings.

### Self-Criticism and Impostorism

The research literature on self-esteem, self-enhancement, and self-serving biases might lead one to conclude that human beings are universally and pervasively egotistical, but other research portrays people quite differently. In addition to demonstrating biases that reflect well upon them, people can often be quite self-critical, sometimes evaluating themselves far more negatively than the objective evidence seems to warrant.

Research on self-deprecating biases has focused primarily on their role in clinical disorders such as depression and social anxiety disorder (e.g., Blatt, D'Afflitti, & Quinlan, 1976; Cox, Fleet, & Stein, 2004), so we know relatively little about the garden-variety of self-criticism that we see in otherwise well-adjusted people. However, in a daily diary study conducted on a nonclinical sample, Dunkley, Zuroff, and Blankstein (2003) found that self-criticism was associated with higher negative affect, lower positive affect, and avoidant coping on a daily basis.

One puzzling phenomenon that runs counter to the tendency for people to self-enhance involves the impostor syndrome. So-called impostors acknowledge that other people view them as capable and successful—and indeed they often admit that their own record of success is exemplary—yet they maintain that others' perceptions of them are overly positive. Believing that they are not as competent as they appear to others leads these otherwise successful people to feel like an impostor or fraud and to fear that their inadequacies will eventually come to light (Clance & Imes, 1978; Cozzarelli & Major, 1990; Kolligian & Sternberg, 1991).

The irony is that, according to most conceptualizations, impostors live in fear that their personal deficiencies will eventually be discovered, yet they are quite vocal in asserting that they are not as good as others believe. A series of studies by Leary, Patton, Orlando, and Funk (2000) addressed this apparent paradox, and their results raise questions about previous conceptualizations of impostorism. Their findings suggested that impostors' self-critical claims of feeling like an impostor are partly interpersonal, self-presentational strategies that are intended to minimize the implications of poor performance. People who doubt their ability to sustain their previous successes may try to lower others' expectations by preemptively denying that their success is a reflection of high ability. To openly accept one's success as evidence of one's ability would put the insecure impostor in jeopardy if his or her performance declined in the future. In addition, underplaying one's ability may win points for modesty and elicit affirming support from other people. This conclusion does not deny that people sometimes truly believe that they are not as competent as other people think but rather points to the role of interpersonal motives in the manifestation of self-criticism and impostorism.

## REDUCING EXCESSIVE SELF-AWARENESS AND RECRIMINATING SELF-EVALUATIONS

As we have seen, self-awareness and self-evaluation underlie certain patterns of negative emotion and maladaptive behavior. In light of this relation, people who are plagued by self-preoccupation, self-recrimination, or self-doubt may seek ways to reduce problems that can arise from self-awareness. People can escape these self-created difficulties by either reducing how much they are thinking about themselves (i.e., by lowering self-awareness) or changing their self-evaluations to make them less negative. Some ways of counteracting the "curse of the self" (Leary, 2004a) involve positive or benign methods of reducing self-thought (e.g., exercising, meditating, sleeping, watching TV), but people may also turn to dysfunctional means of lowering self-talk and self-evaluation. Behaviors as varied as alcohol and drug use, procrastination, violent behavior, binge eating, risk-taking activities, masochism, and even suicide have been linked to people's efforts to escape the dual curses of excessive self-awareness and negative self-evaluation (Baumeister, 1991; Hull, Young, & Jouriles, 1986; Leary, 2004a).

Of course, clinical and counseling psychologists have also recognized that many emotional and behavioral problems for which clients seek professional help may benefit from approaches that reduce self-awareness or negative self-evaluations. Space does not permit a full discussion of these perspectives, so we will mention only two broad approaches briefly—one focusing on self-awareness and the other on self-evaluation.

## Reducing Self-Awareness

First, therapists and researchers have devoted attention to approaches that focus on lowering self-awareness and quieting self-related thought. Trying to reduce self-awareness creates a therapeutic quandary, however, because people must employ conscious self-awareness in ways that eventually lead to a reduction in self-awareness (see Leary, Adams, & Tate, 2006).

Treatments that promote mindfulness have become particularly popular as a way to teach clients to lower self-awareness, quiet their minds, and develop a more objective relationship with their own thoughts and emotions. Whether measured as a trait, induced as a temporary state, or developed over time through extensive training, mindfulness is associated with a variety of positive psychological outcomes (see Brown, Ryan, & Creswell, 2007), many of which are probably due to the effects of mindfulness on self-awareness and self-evaluation.

An increasing number of therapists are using mindfulness training to help clients reduce stress, excessive self-awareness, and problematic self-chatter that underlie a number of psychological and physical complaints (e.g., Davidson et al., 2003). For example, *detached mindfulness* is a therapeutic treatment aimed at teaching clients to become aware of the times they engage in rumination or worry and to observe their worries in a detached fashion rather than engaging with them (Wells & Matthews, 1994). Similarly, *dialectical behavior therapy* (DBT) uses mindfulness and present-moment awareness to encourage people to accept the reality in which they find themselves while, at the same time, maintaining the motivation to change or improve (Robins, Ivanoff, & Linehan, 2001). The DBT therapist helps the client acknowledge and accept his or her current situation and emotions and to reframe the problem in a nonjudgmental, behaviorally specific way (Foertsch, Manning, & Dimeff, 2003). Because clients' emotions are accepted as valid, they do not need to suppress any self-relevant thoughts, thereby leading to less rumination and more adaptive behavior. Along the same lines, *acceptance and commitment therapy* (ACT; Hayes, Strosahl, & Wilson, 1999) integrates acceptance and mindfulness-based strategies with commitment and behavior change techniques to help people develop the psychological flexibility to behave in ways that meet the demands of the current situation while remaining consistent with their core values.

Interventions that employ mindfulness are quite diverse, involving one or more of five distinct components (as well as features that are unrelated to mindfulness). As a result, we do not yet know which components are responsible for treatment effectiveness or the psychological processes that mediate those effects (Leary & Tate, 2007). For example, although all mindfulness interventions involve training people to focus their attention "mindfully," treatments differ regarding where and how mindful attention should be directed. Some treatments stress attending to stimuli in one's external environment, others emphasize directing attention to one's inner states (e.g., sensations, feelings, thoughts), and others train people to have an open receptivity to all external and internal stimuli. Furthermore, some mindfulness training instructs people to be mindful with no inner commentary (and thus minimal self-awareness), whereas other interventions teach people to investigate their subjective experiences in order to understand themselves (so self-awareness is high). Advances in understanding mindfulness, as well as the role of self-awareness in causing and ameliorating psychological problems, will require researchers to distinguish among the various components of mindfulness (Leary & Tate, 2007).

### Restructuring Self-Evaluations

For many years cognitive-behavioral therapists have offered treatments that modify self-evaluations for clients experiencing depression, social anxiety disorder, and other problems in which low self-esteem is implicated (Mruk, 1995). These approaches typically make no effort to reduce self-talk in general (as mindfulness-based approaches often do) but rather focus on reducing the frequency of clients' negative self-evaluations. Modifying clients' self-talk is undoubtedly important and, in many cases, quite effective, yet practitioners have often found it difficult to change people's habitual self-perceptions and self-evaluations (Swann, 1997).

As a result, theorists have recently suggested focusing on clients' self-compassion rather than promoting positive self-evaluations and self-esteem (Gilbert & Irons, 2005). Self-compassion involves treating oneself kindly in the face of the failures, rejections, losses, and humiliations that we all face (see Neff, 2003a). Research shows that self-compassion moderates people's reactions to negative events and that even weak experimental inductions of state self-compassion create changes in self-evaluations, attributions, emotion, and dysfunctional behavior (Adams & Leary, 2007; Leary, Tate, Adams, Allen, & Hancock, 2007; Neff, 2003a, 2003b). Because it may be easier to help clients bolster self-compassion than to directly enhance their self-esteem, self-compassion training holds promise as a means of reducing certain patterns of negative self-thought and accompanying problematic emotions and behaviors.

## CONCLUSION

Social psychologists draw a fundamental distinction between states in which people consciously think about themselves and those in which they respond in an automatic or habitual fashion with little or no self-thought. When people think consciously about themselves—that is, when they are self-aware—their self-relevant thoughts exert a strong influence on their emotions and behaviors. Indeed, from a psychological standpoint, people's reactions would be virtually incomprehensible if we did not take into account their perceptions and evaluations of themselves, the feelings that their self-beliefs engender, their aspirations and expectations for themselves, their egocentric perspective, and their nearly incessant tendency to talk to themselves in their own minds. Social psychological theory and research involving self-awareness, self-representation, and self-evaluation provide important insights into the role of the self in both adaptive and maladaptive behavior.

## REFERENCES

Adams, C. E., & Leary, M. R. (2007). Promoting self-compassionate attitudes toward eating among restrictive and guilty eaters. *Journal of Social and Clinical Psychology*, *26*, 1120–1144.

Alicke, M. D., Klotz, M. L., Breitenbecher, D. L., Yurak, T. J., & Vredenburg, D. S. (1995). Personal contact, individuation, and the better-than-average effect. *Journal of Personality and Social Psychology*, *68*, 804–825.

Baumeister, R. F. (1991). *Escaping the self*. New York: Basic Books.

Baumeister, R. F., Campbell, J. D., Krueger, J. I., & Vohs, K. D. (2003). Does high self-esteem cause better performance, interpersonal success, happiness, or healthier lifestyles? *Psychological Science in the Public Interest*, *4*, 1–44.

Baumeister, R. F., Heatherton, T. F., & Tice, D. M. (1993). When ego threats lead to self-regulation failure: Negative consequences of high self-esteem. *Journal of Personality and Social Psychology*, *64*, 141–156.

Baumeister, R. F., Smart, L., & Boden, J. M. (1996). Relation of threatened egotism to violence and aggression: The dark side of high self-esteem. *Psychological Review*, *103*, 5–33.

Baumeister, R. F., Wotman, S. R., & Stillwell, A. M. (1993). Unrequited love: On heartbreak, anger, guilt, scriptlessness, and humiliation. *Journal of Personality and Social Psychology*, *64*, 377–394.

Blaine, B., & Crocker, J. (1993). Self-esteem and self-serving biases in reaction to positive and negative events: An integrative review. In R. F. Baumeister (Ed.), *Self-esteem: The puzzle of low self-regard* (pp. 55–85). New York: Plenum Press.

Blatt, S. J., D'Afflitti, J., & Quinlan, D. (1976). Experiences of depression in young adults. *Journal of Abnormal Psychology*, *65*, 383–389.

Block, J., & Colvin, C. R. (1994). Positive illusion and well-being revisited: Separating fiction from fact. *Psychological Bulletin*, *116*, 28.

Bonanno, G. A., Field, N. P., & Kovacevic, A. (2002.) Self-enhancement as a buffer against extreme adversity: Civil war in Bosnia and traumatic loss in the United States. *Personality and Social Psychology Bulletin*, *28*, 184–196.

Bonanno, G. A., Rennicke, C., & Dekel, S. (2005). Self-enhancement among high-exposure survivors of the September 11th terrorist attack: Resilience or social maladjustment? *Journal of Personality and Social Psychology*, *88*, 984–998.

Bond, C. F., & Omar, A. S. (1990). Social anxiety, state dependence, and the next-in-line effect. *Journal of Experimental Social Psychology*, *26*, 185–198.

Borkovec, T. D., Ray, W. J., & Stöber, J. (1998). Worry: A cognitive phenomenon intimately linked to affective, physiological, and interpersonal behavioral processes. *Cognitive Therapy and Research*, *22*, 561–576.

Brosschot, J. F., Gerin, W., & Thayer, J. F. (2006). The perseverative cognition hypothesis: A review of worry, prolonged stress-related physiological activation, and health. *Journal of Psychometric Research*, *60*, 113–124.

Brown, K. W., Ryan, R. M., & Creswell, J. D. (2007). Mindfulness: Theoretical foundations and evidence for its salutary effects. *Psychological Inquiry*, *18*, 211–237.

Carver, C. S., Lawrence, J. W., & Scheier, M. F. (1999). Self-discrepancies and affect: Incorporating the role of feared selves. *Personality and Social Psychology Bulletin*, *25*, 783–792.

Clance, P. R., & Imes, S. A. (1978). The impostor phenomenon in high-achieving women: Dynamics and therapeutic intervention. *Psychotherapy: Theory, Research, and Practice*, *15*, 241–247.

Colvin, C. R., Block, J., & Funder, D. C. (1995). Overly positive self evaluations and personality: Negative implications for mental health. *Journal of Personality and Social Psychology*, *68*, 1152–1162.

Cox, B. J., Fleet, C., & Stein, M. B. (2004). Self-criticism and social phobia in the U.S. National Comorbidity Survey. *Journal of Affective Disorders*, *82*, 227–234.

Cozzarelli, C., & Major, B. (1990). Exploring the validity of the impostor phenomenon. *Journal of Social and Clinical Psychology*, *9*, 401–417.

Crocker, J., & Park, L. E. (2004). The costly pursuit of self-esteem. *Psychological Bulletin*, *130*, 392–414.

Davidson, R. J., Kabat-Zinn, J., Schumacher, J., Rosenkranz, M., Muller, D., Santorelli, S. F., et al. (2003). Alterations in brain and immune function produced by mindfulness meditation. *Psychosomatic Medicine*, *65*, 564–570.

Ditto, P. H., & Lopez, D. A. (1993). Motivated skepticism: Use of differential decision criteria for preferred and nonpreferred conclusions. *Journal of Personality and Social Psychology, 63*, 568–584.

Dunkley, D. M., Zuroff, D. C., & Blankstein, K. R. (2003). Self-critical perfectionism and daily affect: Dispositional and situational influences on stress and coping. *Journal of Personality and Social Psychology, 84*, 234–252.

Dunning, D., & Beauregard, K. S. (2000). Regulating others to affirm images of the self. *Social Cognition, 18*, 198–222.

Dunning, D., & Cohen, G. L. (1992). Egocentric definitions of traits and abilities in social judgment. *Journal of Personality and Social Psychology, 63*, 341–355.

Duval, S., & Wicklund, R. A. (1972). *A theory of objective self-awareness.* New York: Academic Press.

Fein, S., & Spencer, S. J. (1997). Prejudice as self-image maintenance: Affirming the self through derogating others. *Journal of Personality and Social Psychology, 73*, 31–44.

Florian, V., & Mikulincer, M. (1997). Fear of death and the judgment of social transgressions: A multidimensional test of terror management theory. *Journal of Personality and Social Psychology, 73*, 369–380.

Foertsch, C., Manning, S. Y., & Dimeff, L. (2003). Difficult-to-treat patients: The approach from dialectical behavior therapy. In R. L. Leahy (Ed.), *Roadblocks in cognitive-behavioral therapy: Transforming challenges into opportunities for change* (pp. 255–273). New York: Guilford Press.

Fresco, D. M., Frankel, A. N., Mennin, D. S., Turk, C. L., & Heimberg, R. G. (2002). Distinct and overlapping features of rumination and worry: The relationship of cognitive production to negative affective states. *Cognitive Therapy and Research, 26*, 179–188.

Gilbert, P., & Irons, C. (2005). Therapies for shame and self-attacking, using cognitive, behavioural, emotional imagery, and compassionate mind training. In P. Gilbert (Ed.), *Compassion: Conceptualisations, research, and use in psychotherapy* (pp. 263–325). London: Routledge.

Gilovich, T., & Husted Medvec, V. (1995). The experience of regret: What, when and why. *Psychological Review, 102*, 379–395.

Greenberg, J., Pyszczynski, T., Solomon, S., Rosenblatt, A., Veeder, M., & Kirkland, S. (1990). Evidence for terror management theory II: The effects of mortality salience on reactions to those who threaten or bolster the cultural worldview. *Journal of Personality and Social Psychology, 58*, 308–318.

Greenberg, J., Simon, L., Pyszczynski, T., Solomon, S., & Chatel, D. (1992). Terror management and tolerance: Does mortality salience always intensify negative reactions to others who threaten one's worldview? *Journal of Personality and Social Psychology, 63*, 212–220.

Greenberg, J., Solomon, S., Pyszczynski, T., Rosenblatt, A., Burling, J., Lyon, D., et al. (1992). Assessing the terror management analysis of self-esteem: Converging evidence of an anxiety-buffering function. *Journal of Personality and Social Psychology, 63*, 913–922.

Harmon-Jones, E., Simon, L., Greenberg, J., Pyszczynski, T., Solomon, S., & McGregor, H. (1997). Terror management and self-esteem: Evidence that self-esteem reduces mortality salience effects. *Journal of Personality and Social Psychology, 72*, 24–26.

Hayes, S. C., Strosahl, K., & Wilson, K. G. (1999). *Acceptance and commitment therapy: An experimental approach to behavior change.* New York: Guilford Press.

Heatherton, T. F., & Vohs, K. D. (2000). Interpersonal evaluations following threats to self: Role of self-esteem. *Journal of Personality and Social Psychology, 78*, 725–736.

Heine, S. J., Kitayama, S., & Lehman, D. R. (2001). Cultural differences in self-evaluation: Japanese readily accept negative self-relevant information. *Journal of Cross-Cultural Psychology, 32*, 434–443.

Heine, S. J., Kitayama, S., Lehman, D. R., Takata, T., Ide, E., Leung, C., et al. (2001). Divergent consequences of success and failure in Japan and North America: An investigation of self-improving motivations and malleable selves. *Journal of Personality and Social Psychology, 81*, 599–615.

Heine, S. J., & Lehman, D. R. (1995). Cultural variation in unrealistic optimism: Does the West feel more invulnerable than the East? *Journal of Personality and Social Psychology, 68,* 595–607.

Heine, S. J., Lehman, D. R., Markus, H. R., & Kitayama, S. (1999). Is there a universal need for positive self-regard? *Psychological Review, 106,* 766–794.

Higgins, E. T. (1987). Self-discrepancy: A theory relating self and affect. *Psychological Review, 94,* 319–340.

Higgins, E. T. (1999). When do self-discrepancies have specific relations to emotions? The second-generation question of Tangney, Niedenthal, Covert, and Barlow (1998). *Journal of Personality and Social Psychology, 77,* 1313–1317.

Higgins, E. T., Klein, R., & Strauman, T. (1985). Self-concept discrepancy theory: A psychological model for distinguishing among different aspects of depression and anxiety. *Social Cognition, 3,* 51–76.

Hull, J. G., Young, R. D., & Jouriles, E. (1986). Applications of the self-awareness model of alcohol consumption: Predicting patterns of use and abuse. *Journal of Personality and Social Psychology, 51,* 790–796.

Johnson, E. A., Vincent, N., & Ross, L. (1997). Self-deception versus self-esteem in buffering the negative effects of failure. *Journal of Research in Personality, 31,* 385–405.

Kernis, M. H. (Ed.). (2006). *Self-esteem: Issues and answers.* New York: Psychology Press.

Kolligian, J., & Sternberg, R. J. (1991). Perceived fraudulence in young adults: Is there an impostor syndrome? *Journal of Personality Assessment, 56,* 308–326.

Kurman, J. (2001). Self-enhancement: Is it restricted to individualistic cultures? *Personality and Social Psychology Bulletin, 12,* 1705–1716.

Kwan, V. S. Y., John, O. P., Kenny, D. A., Bond, M. H., & Robins, R. W. (2004). Reconceptualizing individual differences in self-enhancement bias: An interpersonal approach. *Psychological Review, 111,* 94–111.

Landman, J., & Manis, J. D. (1992). What might have been: Counterfactual thought concerning personal decisions. *British Journal of Psychology, 83,* 473–477.

Leary, M. R. (2002). The interpersonal basis of self-esteem: Death, devaluation, or deference? In J. Forgas & K. D. Williams (Eds.), *The social self: Cognitive, interpersonal, and intergroup perspectives* (pp. 143–160). New York: Psychology Press.

Leary, M. R. (2004a). *The curse of the self: Self-awareness, egotism, and the quality of human life.* New York: Oxford University Press.

Leary, M. R. (2004b). The function of self-esteem in terror management theory and sociometer theory: Comment on Pyszczynski et al. (2004). *Psychological Bulletin, 130,* 478–482.

Leary, M. R. (2006). Sociometer theory and the pursuit of relational value: Getting to the root of self-esteem. *European Review of Social Psychology, 16,* 75–111.

Leary, M. R. (2007). How the self became involved in affective experience: Three sources of self-reflective emotions. In J. L. Tracy, R. W. Robins, & J. P. Tangney (Eds.), *The self-conscious emotions: Theory and practice* (pp. 38–52). New York: Guilford Press.

Leary, M. R., Adams, C. E., & Tate, E. B. (2006). Hypo-egoic self-regulation: Exercising self-control by diminishing the influence of the self. *Journal of Personality, 74,* 1803–1831.

Leary, M. R., & Baumeister, R. F. (2000). The nature and function of self-esteem: Sociometer theory. In M. P. Zanna (Ed.), *Advances in experimental social psychology* (Vol. 32, pp. 1–62). San Diego: Academic Press.

Leary, M. R., Bednarski, R., Hammon, D., & Duncan, T. (1997). Blowhards, snobs, and narcissists: Interpersonal reactions to excessive egotism. In R. M. Kowalski (Ed.), *Aversive interpersonal behaviors* (pp. 111–131). New York: Plenum Press.

Leary, M. R., & Buttermore, N. (2003). The evolution of the human self: Tracing the natural history of self-awareness. *Journal for the Theory of Social Behaviour, 33,* 365–404.

Leary, M. R., Cottrell, C. A., & Phillips, M. (2001). Deconfounding the effects of dominance and social acceptance on self-esteem. *Journal of Personality and Social Psychology, 81,* 898–909.

Leary, M. R., & Downs, D. L. (1995). Interpersonal functions of the self-esteem motive: The self-esteem system as a sociometer. In M. Kernis (Ed.), *Efficacy, agency, and self-esteem* (pp. 123–144). New York: Plenum Press.

Leary, M. R., Gallagher, B., Fors, E. H., Buttermore, N., Baldwin, E., Lane, K. K., et al. (2003). The invalidity of disclaimers about the effects of social feedback on self-esteem. *Personality and Social Psychology Bulletin, 29*, 623–636.

Leary, M. R., Haupt, A., Strausser, K., & Chokel, J. (1998). Calibrating the sociometer: The relationship between interpersonal appraisals and state self-esteem. *Journal of Personality and Social Psychology, 74*, 1290–1299.

Leary, M. R., Patton, K., Orlando, A., & Funk, W. W. (2000). The impostor phenomenon: Self-perceptions, reflected appraisals, and interpersonal strategies. *Journal of Personality, 68*, 725–756.

Leary, M. R., Tambor, E. S., Terdal, S. K., & Downs, D. L. (1995). Self-esteem as an interpersonal monitor: The sociometer hypothesis. *Journal of Personality and Social Psychology, 68*, 518–530.

Leary, M. R., & Tate, E. B. (2007). The multifaceted nature of mindfulness. *Psychological Inquiry, 18*, 251–255.

Leary, M. R., Tate, E. B., Adams, C. E., Allen, A. B., & Hancock, J. (2007). Self-compassion and reactions to unpleasant self-relevant events: The implications of treating oneself kindly. *Journal of Personality and Social Psychology, 92*, 887–904.

Martin, L., & Tesser, A. (1996). Some ruminative thoughts. In R. Wyer, Jr. (Ed.), *Ruminative thoughts: Vol. 11. Advances in social cognition* (pp. 1–47). Hillsdale, NJ: Erlbaum.

Mitchell, R. W. (2003). Subjectivity and self-recognition in animals. In M. R. Leary & J. P. Tangney (Eds.), *Handbook of self and identity* (pp. 567–593). New York: Guilford Press.

Moretti, M., & Higgins, E. T. (1990). Relating self-discrepancy to self-esteem: The contribution of discrepancy beyond actual-self ratings. *Journal of Experimental and Social Psychology, 26*, 108–123.

Mruk, C. (1995). *Self-esteem: Research, theory, and practice*. New York: Springer.

Neff, K. (2003a). Self-compassion: An alternative conceptualization of a healthy attitude toward one-self. *Self and Identity, 2*, 85–102.

Neff, K. (2003b). The development and validation of a scale to measure self-compassion. *Self and Identity, 2*, 223–250.

Nezlek, J. B., Kowalski, R. M., Leary, M. R., Blevins, T., & Holgate, S. (1997). Personality moderators of reactions to interpersonal rejection: Depression and trait self-esteem. *Personality and Social Psychology Bulletin, 23*, 1235–1244.

Nolen-Hoeksema, S. (1987). Sex differences in unipolar depression: Evidence and theory. *Psychological Bulletin, 101*, 259–282.

Nolen-Hoeksema, S. (1991). Responses to depression and their effects on the duration of depressive episodes. *Journal of Abnormal Psychology, 100*, 569–582.

Nolen-Hoeksema, S., & Morrow, J. (1991). A prospective study of depression and posttraumatic stress symptoms after a natural disaster: The 1989 Loma Prieta earthquake. *Journal of Personality and Social Psychology, 61*, 115–121.

Ogilvie, D. M. (1987). The undesired self: A neglected variable in personality research. *Journal of Personality and Social Psychology, 52*, 379–385.

Ogilvie, D. M., & Clark, M. D. (1992). The best and worst of it: Age and sex differences in self-discrepancy research. In R. P. Lipka & T. M. Brinthaupt (Eds.), *Self-perspectives across the lifespan*. Albany, NY: State University of New York Press.

Paulhus, D. L. (1998). Interpersonal and intrapsychic adaptiveness of trait self-enhancement: A mixed blessing? *Journal of Personality and Social Psychology, 74*, 1197–1208.

Paulhus, D. L., Harms, P. D., Bruce, M. N., & Lysy, D. C. (2003). The over-claiming technique: Measuring self-enhancement independent of ability. *Journal of Personality and Social Psychology, 84*, 890–904.

Pelham, B. W., Mirenberg, M. C., & Jones, J. T. (2002). Why Susie sells seashells by the seashore:

Implicit egoism and major life decisions. *Journal of Personality and Social Psychology*, *82*, 469–487.

Pronin, E., Gilovich, T., & Ross, L. (2004). Objectivity in the eye of the beholder: Divergent perceptions of bias in self versus others. *Psychological Review*, *3*, 781–799.

Pronin, E., Lin, D. Y., & Ross, L. (2002). The bias blind spot: Perceptions of bias in self versus others. *Personality and Social Psychology Bulletin*, *28*, 369–381.

Pyszczynski, T., Greenberg, J., & Solomon, S. (2004). Why do people need self-esteem? A theoretical and empirical review. *Psychological Bulletin*, *130*, 435–468.

Rahakrishnan, P., & Chan, D. (1997). Cultural differences in the relationship between self-discrepancy and life-satisfaction. *International Journal of Psychology*, *32*, 347–359.

Robins, C. J., Ivanoff, A. M., & Linehan, M. M. (2001). Dialectical behavior therapy. In W. J. Livesley (Ed.), *Handbook of personality disorders: Theory, research, and treatment* (pp. 437–459). New York: Guilford Press.

Robins, R. W., & Beer, J. S. (2001). Positive illusions about the self: Short-term benefits and long-term costs. *Journal of Personality and Social Psychology*, *80*, 340–352.

Robins, R. W., & John, O. P. (1997). The quest for self-insight: Theory and research on the accuracy of self-perception. In H. Hogan, J. Johnson, & S. Briggs (Eds.), *Handbook of personality psychology* (pp. 649–679). New York: Academic Press.

Rogers, C. R. (1954). The case of Mrs. Oak: A research analysis. In C. R. Rogers & R. F. Dymond (Eds.), *Psychotherapy and personality change* (pp. 259–348). Chicago: University of Chicago Press.

Rosenblatt, A., Greenberg, J., Solomon, S., Pyszczynski, T., & Lyon, D. (1989). Evidence for terror management theory: I. The effects of mortality salience on reactions to those who violate or uphold cultural values. *Journal of Personality and Social Psychology*, *57*, 681–690.

Scott, L., & O'Hara, M. W. (1993). Self-discrepancies in clinically anxious and depressed university students. *Journal of Abnormal Psychology*, *102*, 282–287.

Sedikides, C., Gaertner, L., & Toguchi, Y. (2003). Pancultural self-enhancement. *Journal of Personality and Social Psychology*, *84*, 60–79.

Segerstrom, S. C., Tsao, J. C. I., Alden, L. E., & Craske, M. G. (2000). Worry and rumination: Repetitive thought as a concomitant predictor of negative mood. *Cognitive Therapy and Research*, *24*, 671–688.

Silvia, P., Eichstaedt, J., & Phillips, A. G. (2005). Are rumination and reflection types of self-focused attention? *Personality and Individual Differences*, *38*, 871–881.

Solomon, S., Greenberg, J., & Pyszczynski, T. (1991). A terror management theory of social behavior: The psychological functions of self-esteem and cultural worldviews. In M. Zanna (Ed.), *Advances in experimental social psychology* (Vol. 24, pp. 91–159). Orlando, FL: Academic Press.

Srivastava, S., & Beer, J. S. (2005). How self-evaluations relate to being liked by others: Integrating sociometer and attachment perspectives. *Journal of Personality and Social Psychology*, *89*, 966–977.

Stewart, A. J., & Vandewater, E. A. (1999). "If I had it to do over again ... ": Midlife review, midcourse corrections, and women's well-being in midlife. *Journal of Personality and Social Psychology*, *76*, 270–283.

Strauman, T. J. (1989). Self-discrepancies in clinical depression and social phobia: Cognitive structures that underlie emotional disorders? *Journal of Abnormal Psychology*, *98*, 14–22.

Swann, W. B., Jr. (1997). The trouble with change: Self-verification and allegiance to the self. *Psychological Science*, *8*, 177–180.

Swann, W. B., Jr., Chang-Schneider, C., & McClarty, K. (2007). Do our self-views matter: Self-concept and self-esteem in everyday life. *American Psychologist*, *62*, 84–94.

Tangney, J. P., Neidenthal, P. M., Covert, M. V., & Barlow, D. H. (1998). Are shame and guilt related to distinct self-discrepancies? A test of Higgins' (1987) hypotheses. *Journal of Personality and Social Psychology*, *75*, 256–268.

Taylor, S. E., & Armor, D. A. (1996). Positive illusions and coping with adversity. *Journal of Personality*, *64*, 873–898.

Taylor, S. E., & Brown, J. D. (1988). Illusion and well-being: A social psychological perspective on mental health. *Psychological Bulletin, 103*, 193–210.

Taylor, S. E., & Brown, J. D. (1994). Positive illusions and well-being revisited: Separating fact from fiction. *Psychological Bulletin, 116*, 21–27.

Taylor, S. E., Lerner, J. S., Sherman, D. K., Sage, R. M., & McDowell, N. K. (2003a). Are self-enhancing cognitions associated with healthy or unhealthy biological profiles? *Journal of Personality and Social Psychology, 85*, 605–615.

Taylor, S. E., Lerner, J. S., Sherman, D. K., Sage, R. M., & McDowell, N. K. (2003b). Portrait of the self-enhancer: Well adjusted and well liked or maladjusted and friendless? *Journal of Personality and Social Psychology, 84*, 165–176.

Tesser, A. (1988). Toward a self-evaluation model of social behavior. *Advances in Experimental Social Psychology, 21*, 181–227.

Trapnell, P. D., & Campbell, J. D. (1999). Private self-consciousness and the five-factor model of personality: Distinguishing rumination from reflection. *Journal of Personality and Social Psychology, 76*, 284–304.

Watkins, E. (2004). Appraisals and strategies associated with rumination and worry. *Personality and Individual Differences, 37*, 679–694.

Watkins, E., & Baracaia, S. (2002). Rumination and social problem solving in depression. *Behavior Research and Therapy, 40*, 1179–1189.

Wells, A., & Matthews, G. (1994). *Attention and emotion: A clinical perspective*. Hove, UK: Erlbaum.

Wine, J. D. (1971). Test anxiety and direction of attention. *Psychological Bulletin, 76*, 92–104.

Wood, J. V., Giordano-Beech, M., & Ducharme, M. J. (1999). Compensating for failure through social comparison. *Personality and Social Psychology Bulletin, 25*, 1370–1386.

# 3 Autobiographical Memory and the Construction of a Narrative Identity

## *Theory, Research, and Clinical Implications*

Dan P. McAdams
Jonathan M. Adler

Going back to Freud, clinicians have listened to, tried to understand, and tried to change the stories their patients tell them. Different therapeutic approaches have tended to privilege different kinds of stories and to suggest different strategies for interpretation and intervention. Classic psychoanalysis, for example, has traditionally sought to unmask the disguised meanings of manifest dream narratives. Carl Rogers taught an empathic stance toward life narrative: Therapists were to encourage and affirm their clients' autobiographical recollections, holding back critical judgment and expressing the necessary unconditional positive regard through which a client might eventually actualize the good inner self. Cognitive-behavioral therapists pay careful attention to personal narratives, too, as they work to reframe negativistic and depressogenic life stories in more positive, productive, and life-affirming terms. Cutting across a wide range of theoretical orientations, many therapists implicitly know that human beings are natural storytellers, that autobiographical stories reflect personal issues, that therapy involves working with the stories people bring to the session, and that to change a person's life story is, in effect, to change the person. Indeed, this perspective has led some to contend that narrative ought to serve as "a non-trivial point of convergence for the therapy field" (Angus & McLeod, 2004, p. 373).

Although it has developed largely within the fields of personality and lifespan developmental psychology, the broad theory described in this chapter, as well as the growing body of research it has generated, is simpatico with what many psychotherapists know, feel, and experience in their daily work: *Human beings create stories and then live according to them.*

Over the past 20 years, one of us (McAdams) has articulated a life-story model of adult identity, which proposes that people living in modern societies begin, in their late-adolescent and young-adult years, to construe their lives as ongoing autobiographical stories, reconstructing the past, interpreting the present, and imagining the future in such a way as to provide life with some semblance of unity, purpose, and meaning (McAdams, 1985, 1993, 2001, 2006). A person's *narrative identity* is the internalized and evolving story of the self that he or she is implicitly working on, a story that continues to develop as the person moves through the adult life course. The life-story model of identity anticipated a broad turn toward narrative in the social and behavioral sciences over the past two decades (e.g., Bruner, 1990; Josselson & Lieblich, 1993) while reflecting parallel theoretical developments in cognitive, social, developmental, industrial-organizational, and cultural psychology. The model sets forth a conceptual agenda for understanding the development of narrative identity over time, the place of narrative in personality and culture, the different kinds of stories people tell and live by, the role of narrative in making sense of human suffering and loss, and the role of life narrative in mental health. Picking up on the last point, the life-story model of adult identity resonates with the emergence, in recent years, of *narrative therapy* within clinical circles (e.g., Angus & McLeod, 2004; White & Epston, 1990) and suggests implications for understanding many forms of psychotherapy and counseling as narrative interventions (Lieblich, McAdams, & Josselson, 2004).

## STARTING POINT: THE PROBLEM OF IDENTITY

In his famous eight-stage model of psychosocial development, Erik Erikson (1963) argued that adolescents and young adults face the challenge of constructing a unifying and purposeful ego identity. Erikson argued that *identity versus role confusion* defines the central psychosocial problem for this period in the human life course. The problem stems from many sources. The first is sex. The eruption of puberty, the emergence of primary and secondary sexual characteristics, the resurgence of the adolescent libido, the thrall and the anxiety that accompany the full realization of one's own sexual potential—all of this and more usher in new concerns about the self: "Who am I now? I no longer feel like a child, but am I really an adult?"

Second, taking his lead from Piaget, Erikson asserted that the adolescent mind is a newly abstract and ideological mind. Blessed now with what Piaget (1970) called formal operational thinking, the adolescent is able to reason about his or her life in highly abstract and hypothetical terms. The self becomes an object of abstract speculation—and fascination. "What might I be? How might my life be different if I were black instead of white? Male instead of female? An atheist instead of a Catholic?" As a result of their new cognitive powers, many adolescents and young adults become interested in philosophical and ideological issues. "What do I really believe? What is true for me? What does my life mean?" These kinds of questions make no sense to an 8-year-old. Children may know who they are, Erikson argued, but they do not know that such knowing is potentially problematic. Before adolescence, we do not really have an identity because we are not endowed with the cognitive software required to understand that having an identity is a really big, contested, and complex psychological deal.

Third, and arguably most important, identity emerges as an issue in adolescence and young adulthood because society mandates that this is indeed the right time for its emergence, especially in modern Western societies (Giddens, 1991). Compulsory schooling ends in the teenage years. It is now time to leave home, get a job, go off to college or the military, or take some other demonstrable step toward the autonomy and the responsibilities that come with adulthood. Parents, teachers, counselors, friends, and others encourage the adolescent to begin to think about his or her life from a broader, more abstract, and more long-term perspective. Identity becomes an on-time developmental task. "What are you going to do now? What kind of life are you going to make?" These kinds of questions may motivate the adolescent to rethink the truisms of childhood, even to rebel against norms, standards, conventions, and assumptions that were taken for granted in the past. Erikson suggested that many adolescents and young adults enter a period of *psychosocial moratorium*, wherein they experiment with new values, beliefs, aspirations, and goals for the future. Whether through outright rebellion or concerted introspection, the adolescent or young adult endeavors to find and/or create a psychosocial niche in the adult world. Among the most important components of the niche are ideology, occupation, and intimacy. As we move into adulthood, Erikson argued, we come to define ourselves, in part, through what we believe, what we do for a living, and with whom we come to share our lives.

The optimal development of ego identity helps to *integrate* the self and meaningfully situate the person in the adult world. The psychosocial integration of which Erikson wrote seems to have two forms (McAdams, 1985). First, identity integrates a life *synchronically*. It helps to organize the many contemporaneous roles, talents, proclivities, interests, goals, and situational demands that characterize a person's inner and outer lives into a more or less coherent pattern. With the achievement of identity, the person comes to feel that he or she is authentic in some sense, that he or she is living in such a way that seems both intrinsically right (true to the self) and more or less consistent with what society, or some valued group within society, expects. Second, identity integrates a life *diachronically*, that is, in time. Erikson contended that identity challenges the individual to discern threads of continuity between the past, present, and imagined future. Within a coherent, integrative identity, who I am now should make sense in terms of who I believe I was in the past and who I anticipate being in the future.

## IDENTITY AS AN AUTOBIOGRAPHICAL STORY

Identity, then, is a self-constructed configuration or patterning of the self that integrates disparate psychological elements—talents, needs, beliefs and values, goals, important memories, important roles—in such a way as to provide a person with a sense that his or her life is more or less unified over time and across life contexts and meaningfully situated within the ideological, economic, social, and cultural ecology of the adult world. What form might such a configuration take? If identity were a tangible thing, what might it look like? How might it be structured? Psychologists have looked long and hard for a guiding metaphor to capture the rich meaning of Erikson's concept of identity. For example, one line of thinking holds that identity itself is structured like a *theory* (Epstein, 1973). People construct theories of themselves, complete with axioms, models, and testable hypotheses. The identity-as-theory view recalls George Kelly's (1955) conception of human beings as lay scientists, seeking to predict and explain the world and themselves, testing hypotheses as they move through life. In a similar vein, a large number of cognitively oriented perspectives in psychology underscore the ways in which people process self-relevant information, imagining the self as something like a schema or frame or network of associations within which mental representations of self-relevant phenomena are organized.

There are at least two fundamental problems, however, with efforts to translate Erikson's concept of identity into purely cognitive, information-processing terms. First, the resultant metaphors seem rather bloodless and effete when set up against the experientially rich and emotionally complex configuration that Erikson describes. Adolescents and young adults may indeed be formulating new theories about themselves, but, psychosocially speaking, they seem to be doing so much more. Second, most cognitive conceptions of identity fail to capture the sense in which identity integrates a life *in time*. Erikson argued that identity arranges the self in such a way as to show how the past has given birth to the present and how the present will give birth to the future. The configuration or patterning that Erikson viewed as identity itself seems to be organized, in large part, along temporal lines. As such, identity explains who I once was, how I came to be who I am today, and where my life may be headed in the future. It is fundamentally about beginnings, middles, and endings. Thinking about Erikson's conception in this way leads naturally to a metaphor that seems rather more organic and dynamic than what is typically offered by cognitive psychology: the metaphor of *identity as a story*.

McAdams (1985) first proposed that identity can be viewed as an internalized and evolving story of the self—a personal myth—that persons living in modern societies begin to construct in late adolescence and young adulthood. The story is situated within an *ideological setting*, or backdrop of fundamental belief and value upon which the plot unfolds. The plot contains key autobiographical scenes, what Singer and Salovey (1993) called *self-defining memories*. These are vivid and often emotionally charged episodes from the past, such as high points, low points, and turning points in life. The story also features central characters or personal *imagoes* (McAdams, 1985). An *imago* is an idealized personification of the self that captures a select group of important traits, goals, roles, relationships, or identifications in a person's life and serves to function as one of the main characters in the story—the self-as-loving-father, for example, or the self-as-tough-guy-who-grew-up-on-the-wrong-side-of-town. As Erikson knew, modern adults play many different roles in life and express many different, and often contradictory, psychological qualities. Therefore, a life story may contain many different imagoes, many different personifications of the self, each serving as a character in the same story. As Bruner (1990) argued, characters strive to accomplish goals and overcome obstacles over narrative time. Among the most compelling goals are those linked to power and love, or what Bakan (1966) called *agency* and *communion*, respectively. McAdams (1985) proposed that agency (with its attendant strivings for power, achievement, autonomy, self-improvement, self-expansion, self-insight) and communion (encompassing erotic love, friendship, intimacy, caregiving, belongingness, community) are the two most general and most common *thematic lines* in adults' life stories.

Although life stories begin to emerge in consciousness in late adolescence and young adulthood, people implicitly gather material for the stories they will eventually create from the first day of life onward (McAdams, 1993; Tomkins, 1979). For example, the quality of early attachment bonds may ultimately come to shape how the person makes narrative sense of life in the adult years. Insecure attachments may predispose a person to construct a life story with a relatively negative or tragic narrative tone, a story in which characters do not enjoy the confidence that their world is secure and that their best intentions will lead to happy endings. By contrast, secure attachments in infancy may pave the way for the construction of more positive—comic and romantic—personal stories in adulthood. Early experiences of many sorts may eventually become the grist for the narrative mill of identity. (See also, Shorey, Chapter 9, this volume.)

But identity is not simply determined by past experience. Instead, the past is open to constant reinterpretation—to the selective, creative, and adaptive powers of the storytelling self. Anticipating contemporary research on autobiographical memory, Erikson (1963) argued that people work hard to transform the past into something that makes sense in terms of who they are today and who they may be in the future. Like revisionist historians, self-storytellers recast the past into a meaningful and convincing narrative, a myth that explains the self's origins and its destiny. Erikson described it best in this passage:

> To be adult means among other things to see one's own life in continuous perspective, both in retrospect and prospect. By accepting some definition as to who he is, usually on the basis of a function in an economy, a place in the sequence of generations, and a status in the structure of society, the adult is able to *selectively reconstruct* his past in such a way that, step for step, it seems to have planned him, or better, he seems to have planned *it*. In this sense, psychologically we *do* choose our parents, our family history, and the history of our kings, heroes, and gods. By making them our own, we maneuver ourselves into the inner position of proprietors, of creators. (1958, pp. 111–112, some emphasis added)

In hundreds of studies cognitive psychologists have documented the selective and interpretive nature of autobiographical memory (e.g., Conway & Pleydell-Pearce, 2000; Rubin, 2006). As far as memory goes, the personal past is nothing like a long videotape that can be readily played back at the push of a button. Most of the events in a person's life are forgotten soon after they occur, and those that are remembered may be subject to a wide range of biases, mistakes, and distortions. Whereas people usually remember well the thematic and emotional gist of important events from the distant past, memory for specific details is typically less reliable. Furthermore, what is summoned forth from the autobiographical storehouse is often shaped and contoured according to current concerns and future goals (Conway & Pleydell-Pearce, 2000). In an important psychological sense, the past is always up for grabs in autobiographical memory. People do not consciously misremember or create fantasies out of thin air, but they do implicitly and naturally give their recollections of the past narrative form, smoothing out inconsistencies, sharpening transitions, embellishing characters, and introducing drama, tension, conflict, climax, resolution, and the many other features expected of good stories.

Narrative identity summons forth and organizes those relatively few autobiographical memories that seem (to the person who remembers them) most important for the formation of the self and links those memories to both the person's understanding of his or her current station in life and his or her aspirations, dreams, hopes, and plans for the future. Therefore, a life story is not synonymous with the whole of one's autobiographical memory but instead is a highly selective and reorganized subset of recollections from the personal past that is linked in narrative to how the person sees the present and imagines the broad outlines of the future. Narrative identity is comprised of the stories that stick around. As a collection, these stories demonstrate how a person came to be, who a person is now, and where a person's life is going.

Research has shown that it is not until late adolescence and young adulthood that people are able and motivated to use autobiographical memory in the service of constructing full life stories (Habermas & Bluck, 2000). Therefore, it is during that same period in the life course, when identity steps to the fore, that the human mind focuses its powers on the construction of a coherent narrative of the self, an autobiographical story that provides a single life, situated in time and culture, with some degree of unity, purpose, and meaning. With further development and life experience, people continue to work on their life stories, reconstructing the autobiographical past and reimagining the future, as they move into and through their middle-adult years and beyond. At least through late midlife, adults' life stories develop in the direction of greater narrative richness, thematic coherence, and integration of the self (McAdams, 1993; Pasupathi & Mansour, 2006).

## DIFFERENT KINDS OF STORIES AND THEIR PLACE IN PERSONALITY AND CULTURE

People tell many different kinds of stories about their lives. Researchers have examined variations in structure and content of life stories, and they have linked these variations to a wide range of psychological and social variables. Empirical findings strongly suggest that individual differences in narrative identity relate to other important aspects of personality, to psychological well-being, and to socially consequential life outcomes.

Some narrative accounts are relatively simple in structure whereas others exhibit high levels of complexity, differentiation, and integration. More complex life stories have been linked to higher levels of ego development and the personality trait of openness to experience. For example, McAdams (1985) found that people who score relatively high on Loevinger's (1976) measure of ego development—indicating a more nuanced and mature perspective on the self and the world—tended to construct life narratives with a greater number of plots, characters, and interrelated themes. Ego development predicts greater complexity in narrative accounts of one's life in full and in more circumscribed narrations of particular domains in life. For example, McAdams, Booth, and Selvik (1981) found that religious college students scoring high in ego development tended to construe their own religious development as a story of struggle, ambivalence, and exploration. Those scoring at relatively low levels of ego development, suggesting a less nuanced and more conformist perspective on self and world, tended to tell stories of continuity in religious development, showing how their beliefs and values had remained the same over time, even in the face of challenge and doubt. In addition, McAdams et al. (2004) found that students high on the self-reported trait of openness to experience constructed self-defining autobiographical memories that expressed more motivational conflict, emotional complexity, and multiple points of view, than did students lower in openness to experience.

A number of studies have linked thematic lines of agency and communion in life stories to power and intimacy motivation, respectively (e.g., McAdams, 1982; Woike, Gersekovich, Piorkowski, & Polo, 1999). People who score high on measures of the need for power tend to construct life stories that showcase strong and assertive protagonists who seek to effect big changes in their instrumental and interpersonal worlds—classic imagoes of the warrior, the sage, and the adventurer. People with strong needs for intimacy display more communal imagoes, like the caregiver, the friend, and the lover, and they tailor their life stories to accentuate attachment bonds and their connections to human communities. Some life stories feature strong tendencies toward both agency and communion, sometimes narrating dramatic conflicts between these two thematic lines. Life stories that show high levels of both agentic and communal content are often associated with personality and social characteristics indicative of a strong commitment to both parental and occupational roles as well as high levels of community involvement and what Erikson (1963) called *generativity*, or an adult's concern for and commitment to promoting the well-being of future generations (Ackerman, Zuroff, & Moscowitz, 2000; McAdams, 2006).

A growing body of research links individual differences in life narratives to psychological well-being and mental health. Bauer and colleagues have shown that people who prioritize intrinsic motivations in their life stories—motivations that spring from inner desires for personal fulfillment rather than extrinsic goals of status and social acceptance—tend to score higher on measures of subjective well-being than do individuals whose life stories show fewer themes of intrinsic motivation (e.g., Bauer, McAdams, & Sakaeda, 2005). Happiness and well-being have also been associated with life stories that show positive resolution of life conflicts (e.g., King & Hicks, 2006).

Researchers also have identified a form of life narration that appears to be strongly linked to depression and low levels of psychological well-being. In a *contamination sequence*, the narrator describes a scene that begins with joy, excitement, or some other highly positive emotional state but turns suddenly and irrevocably negative (McAdams, Diamond, de St. Aubin, & Mansfield, 1997). The bad outcome of the scene undoes, contaminates, or ruins all the good that preceded it. Adler, Kissel, and McAdams (2006) coded lengthy life-narrative interviews told by midlife adults for evidence of contamination imagery. They also coded the same accounts for the depressogenic attributional style—ascribing negative events to stable and global causes—a way of thinking and narrating that is linked to depressive symptoms. The number of contamination sequences identified in the autobiographical texts was a stronger predictor or self-reported depression than was depressogentic attributional style (Adler et al., 2006).

Life stories are both influenced by personality variables, such as traits and motives, and are part and parcel of personality itself. McAdams and Pals (2006) have developed a broad conceptual model that divides personality into three separate levels or domains (see also, Singer, 2005). Level 1 includes broad *dispositional traits*, such as those encompassed in the well-known Big Five trait taxonomy (extraversion, neuroticism, conscientiousness, agreeableness, and openness to experience; McCrae & Costa, 1990). Accounting for broad consistencies in behavior and thought across situations and over time, dispositional traits sketch an outline of psychological individuality. Level 2 includes *characteristic adaptations*—motives, goals, domain-specific strategies, values, interests, schemas, and a wide assortment of more specific personality constructs, contextualized in developmental time, social place, and/or social role. These adaptations fill in many of the details of psychological individuality. Level 3 consists of integrative *life stories* that comprise narrative identity. These stories speak to the overall meaning of a person's life. Personality, then, can be seen as a person's unique and evolving patterning of *traits*, *adaptations*, and *narratives* set in time and culture.

Social and cultural factors have an impact on all three levels of personality. Culture has a modest impact on the development of dispositional traits by providing rules and norms for the display of trait-related behavior. For example, high levels of extraversion may be expressed in very different ways in, say, New York City and Kyoto, Japan. Culture has a stronger impact on the timing and the content of characteristic adaptations. For example, psychologists have uncovered significant differences between collectivist East Asian and more individualistic North American societies with respect to favored values, motives, and goals (Markus & Kitayama, 1991). Culture has its strongest impact, however, on life narratives. Indeed, life narratives may themselves be seen as cultural texts (Rosenwald & Ochberg, 1992). Culture provides people with a menu of images, metaphors, plots, characters, and expected endings regarding how to live a good or worthy life. People pick and choose from the menu, appropriating certain cultural forms and rejecting others as they construct a narrative of the self that captures their lived experience and helps their life make sense (McAdams, 2006). Different cultures allow for varying degrees of innovation in the construction of a narrative identity, but all cultures place limits on what can be told. More importantly, cultures set the full storytelling agenda for lives. They specify the very parameters of story coherence and comprehensibility. In a very real sense, then, every life story is jointly authored by the purported storyteller, him- or herself, and by the cultural milieu within which the story finds its meanings.

## NARRATING SUFFERING, GROWTH, AND SELF-TRANSFORMATION

How do people tell stories of life's defeats, suffering, pain, and loss? The many trials and setbacks that invariably confront people as they move through the adult life course offer the greatest challenges to the construction of a coherent narrative identity. But they also often provide the greatest opportunities. In both life and literature, good stories invariably include danger, suffering, and daunting obstacles to the protagonist's quest (Bruner, 1990). A rapidly growing body of research examines how people narrate negative events in their lives and how these narrations contribute to, or sometimes undermine, psychological health, growth, and development.

When it comes to life storytelling, there are many ways to narrate negative events. Perhaps the most common response is to discount the event in some way. The most extreme examples of discounting fall under the rubrics of repression, denial, and dissociation. Some stories are so bad that they simply cannot be told—cannot be told to others and, in many cases, cannot really be told to the self. Freeman (1993) argues that some traumatic and especially shameful experiences in life cannot be incorporated into narrative identity because the narrator (and perhaps the narrator's audience as well) lacks the world assumptions, cognitive constructs, or experiential categories needed to make sense of the story. Less extreme are examples of what Taylor (1983) called *positive illusions*. People may simply overlook the negative aspects of life events and exaggerate the potentially positive meanings. For example, "I may be sick, but I am not nearly as sick as my good friend's husband"; "God is testing my resolve, and I will rise to the challenge." Bonanno (2004) has shown that many people experience surprisingly little angst and turmoil when stricken with harsh misfortunes in life. People often show *resilience* in the face of adversity, Bonanno maintains. Rather than ruminate over the bad things that happen in their lives, they put it all behind them and move forward. (See also, Lyubomirsky & Dickerhoof, Chapter 13, and Dijkstra, Gibbons, & Buunk, Chapter 11, this volume.)

In many situations, however, people cannot or choose not to discount negative life events. Instead, they try to make meaning out of the suffering they are currently experiencing, or experienced once upon a time. For example, McLean and Thorne (2003) showed that adolescents often report learning lessons and gaining insights from self-defining memories that involve conflict with others. Pals (2006) argues that autobiographical reasoning about negative events ideally involves a two-step process. In the first step the narrator explores the negative experience in depth, thinking long and hard about what the experience feels or felt like, how it came to be, what it may lead to, and what role the negative event may play in one's overall understanding of self. In the second step, the narrator articulates and commits the self to a positive resolution of the event. Pals (2006) warns that one should not pass lightly over the first step. When it comes to narrative identity, Pals suggests, the unexamined life lacks depth and meaning.

Consistent with Pals (2006), a number of studies have shown that exploring negative life events in detail is associated with psychological maturity. For example, King and colleagues have asked people who have faced daunting life challenges to tell stories of "what might have been," had their lives developed in either a more positive or more expected direction (see King & Hicks, 2006, for an overview). In one study mothers of infants with Down syndrome reflected upon what their lives might have been like had they given birth to babies not affected by the syndrome. Those mothers who were able to articulate detailed and thoughtful accounts, suggesting a great deal of exploration and meaning making in their processing of this negative life event, tended to score higher on Loevinger's (1976) measure of ego development than did mothers who discounted what might have been (King, Scollon, Ramsey, & Williams, 2000). In other studies, King and colleagues examined life narrative accounts from women who had been divorced after many years of marriage and from gay and lesbian adults who reflected on what might have been had they been straight (King & Raspin, 2004; King & Smith, 2005). In both studies psychological maturity was associated with greater personal exploration in narrative accounts, and greater exploration predicted increases in maturity in a 2-year follow-up.

The second step in making narrative sense of negative life events involves constructing a positive meaning or resolution (Pals, 2006). This can be done in many ways. The narrator may derive a particular lesson from the event (e.g., "I learned that I should never criticize my mother") or a more general insight about life (e.g., "I realized how important it is to cherish every moment") (McLean & Thorne, 2003). The narrator may show how the negative event ultimately made it possible for very positive events to occur later, on or how it turned the person's life in a positive direction (McAdams, Reynolds, Lewis, Patten, & Bowman, 2001). The positive turn in life may involve a move toward activities that are of deep intrinsic interest to the person, serving to reconnect the person to what he or she feels to be the "true" or authentic self (Bauer et al., 2005). Or the positive turn may enhance intimacy and consolidate social relationships (King & Smith, 2005). When narrators are able to derive positive or redemptive meanings from negative life events, they may feel that they have now fully worked through the event and attained a sense of narrative closure.

Numerous studies have shown that deriving positive meanings from negative events is associated with life satisfaction and indicators of emotional well-being (e.g., King & Hicks, 2006; McAdams et al., 2001). Finding positive meanings in negative events, furthermore, is the central theme that runs through McAdams's (2006) conception of *the redemptive self*. In a series of nomothetic and case-based studies conducted over the past 15 years, McAdams and colleagues have consistently found that midlife American adults who score especially high on self-report measures of generativity—suggesting a strong commitment to promoting the well-being of future generations and improving the world in which they live (Erikson, 1963)—tend to see their own lives as narratives of redemption. Compared to their less generative American counterparts, highly generative adults tend to construct life stories that feature redemption sequences in which the protagonist is delivered from suffering to an enhanced status or state.

Beyond redemption sequences themselves, highly generative American adults are also more likely than their less generative peers to construct life stories in which the protagonist (1) enjoys a special advantage or blessing early in life, (2) expresses sensitivity to the suffering of others or societal injustice as a child, (3) establishes a clear and strong value system in adolescence that remains a source of unwavering conviction through the adult years, (4) experiences significant conflicts between desires for agency/power and communion/love, and (5) seeks to achieve goals to benefit society in the future. Taken together, these themes articulate a general script or narrative prototype that many highly generative American adults employ to make sense of their own lives. With its moral mandate to give back in gratitude for early blessings received, with its unwavering conviction regarding the goodness and truth of one's quest, and with the confidence that the story instills regarding the possibility that bad things can be overcome, the redemptive self serves to support a life committed to making a positive difference in the world. This is a good story to have, or to make, if one wishes to leave a positive mark on the world for generations to come.

At the same time, the redemptive self may say as much about American culture and tradition as it does about the highly generative American adults who tend to tell this kind of story about their lives. The life-story themes expressed by highly generative American adults recapture and couch in a psychological language especially cherished, as well as hotly contested, ideas in American cultural history—ideas that appear prominently in spiritual accounts of the 17th-century Puritans, Benjamin Franklin's 18th-century autobiography, slave narratives and Horatio Alger stories from the 19th century, and the literatures of self-help and American entrepreneurship from more recent times (McAdams, 2006). Evolving from the Puritans to Emerson to Oprah, the redemptive self has morphed into many different storied forms in the past 300 years as Americans have sought to narrate their lives as redemptive tales of atonement, emancipation, recovery, self-fulfillment, and upward social mobility. The stories speak of heroic individual protagonists—the *chosen people*—whose *manifest destiny* is to make a positive difference in a dangerous world, even when the world does not wish to be redeemed. The stories translate a deep and abiding script of American exceptionalism into the many contemporary narratives of success, recovery, development, liberation, and self-actualization that so pervade American popular discourse, talk shows, therapy sessions, sermons, and commencement speeches. It is as if especially generative American adults, whose lives are dedicated to making the world a better place for future generations, are, for better and sometimes worse, the most ardent narrators of a general life story format as American as apple pie and the Super Bowl.

## CLINICAL IMPLICATIONS: NARRATIVES AND THERAPY

Psychotherapy is a redemptive enterprise. Through therapy, people work to transform suffering into well-being, convert confusion into coherence, and edit their self-stories in order to open up new possibilities for being. In modern American culture, therapy has come to represent the obvious place for revising the self (Cushman, 1995), and regardless of the specific content of treatment or the therapeutic orientation of the clinician, the work of therapy can easily be understood in narrative terms.

In recent years psychotherapists and counselors have developed new approaches that make the work of editing and revising one's personal stories the explicit focus of treatment. For example, White and Epston (1990) encourage clients to externalize their problems, objectifying them and personifying them as entities distinct from the self, with whom they are currently in a difficult relationship. They contend that this practice fosters a sense of authorship of one's own life story and empowers clients to reauthor these stories in ways that are more conducive to psychological well-being. This process of editing and revising is undertaken both literally, through the use of letter writing (between client and therapist, between client and important others, and between client and personified problems) throughout treatment, and ultimately at the level of narrative identity.

Others have also explicitly incorporated narrative techniques into the therapist's toolbox. For example, Angus, Levitt, and Hardtke (1999) developed a taxonomy of narrative processes that occur in the therapeutic context. They identified examples of clients who adopted one of three different modes: *external* (telling stories about a life event), *internal* (providing a descriptive elaboration of subjective experiences of an event), and *reflexive* (reflecting, interpreting, or analyzing an event or one's subjective experiences of the event). The authors developed an empirical and reliable coding system for these three narrative processes and suggested that a client's distinctive pattern of shifts between processes has important implications for therapy, because such shifts may signal emotional distress or disrupt the coherence of the treatment.

Psychotherapy can thus be understood as a fundamentally narrative endeavor—one in which clients and therapists use stories as tools and seek to revise and edit the problematic stories of episodes that have been incorporated into the client's narrative identity. The precise mechanisms whereby therapy works in this context could be many—from giving clients a safe arena wherein they can simply talk about experiences they have avoided talking about in the past to providing opportunities for making narrative sense of difficult experiences and integrating them into one's evolving sense of self. Furthermore, the experience of going to therapy is itself an episode that is likely to be reconstructed later and thus influence narrative identity. Indeed, in a study of women's life stories, Lieblich (2004) found that her participants quite often spontaneously mentioned their experiences in therapy and tended to point to these experiences as key areas of their personality development. If identity is comprised of the collection of self-relevant stories one constructs about oneself, stories about therapy may be especially important. In a classic book on psychotherapy, Jerome Frank wrote that weaving the "myth" of the therapeutic experience is vital to the individual's continued well-being once treatment has ended (1961, p. 327). This sentiment was echoed by Spence (1982) when he wrote that the therapeutic narrative "may also maintain its structure over time and enable the patient to better retain what he [*sic*] learned during the analysis" (p. 270). So, in addition to being good candidates for incorporation into narrative identity, stories about therapy serve a fundamental role in the development and maintenance of therapeutic gains.

Researchers have begun to focus on the types of stories clients tell about their experiences in therapy and the relationship between these stories and important dimensions of psychological functioning, such as subjective well-being and ego development. Adler and

McAdams (2007) collected therapy stories from a diverse group of adults who had recently ended treatment. They found that individuals who were high in psychological well-being (compared to those low) tended to recall their therapy experience as the story of a victorious battle from the past. In this kind of story, a personal problem rises from obscurity to become (temporarily) a fierce antagonist, only to be defeated once and for all by a reenergized self. In contrast, those adults high in ego development (compared to those low) tended to recall their therapy experience as one chapter in an ongoing narrative of self-development. In this kind of story, the self continues to face new problems over time, but the central therapeutic relationship facilitates the individual's journey of ongoing growth.

Crafting the story of one's experience in therapy is a challenging task. Certain life experiences are relatively easy to narrate and fit smoothly into the person's ongoing story of self. Events such as leaving one's parents' home, getting a job, and pregnancy are milestones that occur in many people's lives, and most people are familiar with common cultural stories about these types of occasions. By contrast, other experiences pose a significant challenge to successful narration. They may be unexpected or difficult and are rarely found in people's imagined future scripts. When these events do occur, they resist easy incorporation into one's narrative identity, for the individual is posed with the often daunting task of constructing a story about them in order to render them meaningful. The experience of having been in psychotherapy is a good example of one of these particularly challenging episodes. Yet, as explained above, it may be vitally important to craft a coherent narrative of one's psychotherapy experience in order to maintain the gains from treatment. Adler, Wagner, and McAdams (2007) found that individuals who were high in ego development (compared to those low) told more coherent stories about their experiences in therapy. This finding suggests that high levels of ego development may provide narrators with the kind of sophisticated frameworks for meaning making that are especially well-suited for the important task of making good sense of the psychotherapy experience. It should be noted, however, that ego development is typically positively associated with measures of intelligence, though at modest levels. It would not be surprising to learn that IQ correlates with the coherence of narrative accounts. At the same time, the significant association between ego development and narrative coherence found in Adler et al. (2007) still held after controlling for educational level and a measure of verbal fluency, both themselves typically associated with intelligence.

The accumulated body of theory and research on narrative identity and psychotherapy has produced several avenues for influencing the work of psychotherapists. First and foremost, the narrative perspective provides a new way for therapists to understand the therapy process. Regardless of the specific theoretical orientation one adopts or the unique therapeutic techniques employed, therapy can be understood as essentially a narrative endeavor. Indeed, whether a therapist is using the tools of exposure therapy to help a client overcome a specific fear of flying or bringing the insight and interpretation of psychodynamic perspectives to help a client understand his or her lifelong relational patterns, both of these interventions seek to help the client come to a new way of understanding the self—to tell a new story about his or her life. Second, the narrative perspective reminds therapists that there is a broad range of potential outcomes for successful therapy, not all of which can be quantified with typical questionnaire-based measures. Elliott and James (1989) lamented that psychotherapy outcome research and practice "may dwell excessively on client perceptions of symptom relief, at the expense of other changes important to clients" (p. 456). Indeed, narratives tap into clients' continual experience of self, and as such, they should not be regarded as simply an isolated cognitive phenomenon or as a straightforward byproduct of recovery (Lysaker, Lancaster, & Lysaker, 2003). This narrative reformulation of the therapeutic enterprise provides a richer and more personal conception of the client as an individual and encourages treating the whole person (e.g., Singer, 2005).

Third, the narrative perspective puts a new set of tools at the clinician's disposal. The development of explicitly narrative therapies has expanded the range of interventions therapists can undertake to modify clients' self-stories. In addition, basic research on narrative identity has produced a growing list of toxic narrative patterns, such as contamination sequences and incoherent plots, as well as beneficial ways of constructing personal stories, such as redemption sequences and positive closure. These patterns provide obvious sources of intervention for therapists as they become aware of their clients' narrative styles and encourage them to adopt different patterns.

Finally, the "storying" of the therapeutic experience itself may be vitally important for clients. Different ways of narrating therapy are related to different constellations of psychological functioning once treatment has ended (e.g., Adler & McAdams, 2007). Psychotherapists should be aware that their clients are in a constant process of constructing stories about their experiences in therapy and that they will carry these stories with them after termination. Thus, therapists may want to talk with their clients about what types of stories they are crafting about the therapy itself and help shape these nascent narratives into stories that will promote health and well-being for years to come.

## REFERENCES

Ackerman, S., Zuroff, D., & Moscowitz, D. S. (2000). Generativity in midlife and young adults: Links to agency, communion, and well-being. *International Journal of Aging and Human Development*, *50*, 17–41.

Adler, J., Kissel, E., & McAdams, D. P. (2006). Emerging from the CAVE: Attributional style and the narrative study of identity in midlife adults. *Cognitive Therapy and Research*, *30*(1), 39–51.

Adler, J. M., & McAdams, D. P. (2007). Telling stories about therapy: Ego development, well-being, and the therapeutic relationship. In R. Josselson, D. P. McAdams, & A. Lieblich (Eds.), *The meaning of others: Narrative studies of relationships* (pp. 213–236). Washington, DC: American Psychological Association.

Adler, J. M., Wagner, J. W., & McAdams, D. P. (2007). Personality and the coherence of psychotherapy narratives. *Journal of Research in Personality*, *41*, 1179–1198.

Angus, L. E., Levitt, H., & Hardtke, K. (1999). The Narrative Process Coding System: Research applications and implications for psychotherapy practice. *Journal of Clinical Psychology*, *55*(10), 1255–1270.

Angus, L. E., & McLeod, J. (2004). Toward an integrative framework for understanding the role of narrative in the psychotherapy process. In L. E. Angus & J. McLeod (Eds.), *The handbook of narrative and psychotherapy: Practice, theory, and research* (pp. 367–374). Thousand Oaks, CA: Sage.

Bakan, D. (1966). *The duality of human existence*. Boston: Beacon Press.

Bauer, J. J., McAdams, D. P., & Sakaeda, A. R. (2005). Interpreting the good life: Growth memories in the lives of mature, happy people. *Journal of Personality and Social Psychology*, *88*, 203–217.

Bonanno, G. A. (2004). Loss, trauma, and human resilience: Have we underestimated the human capacity to thrive after extremely aversive events? *American Psychologist*, *59*, 20–28.

Bruner, J. S. (1990). *Acts of mind*. Cambridge, MA: Harvard University Press.

Conway, M. A., & Pleydell-Pearce, C. W. (2000). The construction of autobiographical memories in the self-memory system. *Psychological Review*, *107*, 261–288.

Cushman, P. (1995). *Constructing the self, constructing America: A cultural history of psychotherapy*. Cambridge, MA: Perseus.

Elliott, R., & James, E. (1989). Varieties of client experience in psychotherapy: An analysis of the literature. *Clinical Psychology Review*, *9*(4), 443–467.

Epstein, S. (1973). The self-concept revisited: Or a theory of a theory. *American Psychologist*, *28*, 404–416.

Erikson, E. H. (1958). *Young man Luther.* New York: Norton.

Erikson, E. H. (1963). *Childhood and society* (2nd ed.). New York: Norton.

Frank, J. D. (1961). *Persuasion and healing: A comprehensive study of psychotherapy.* Baltimore, MD: Johns Hopkins University Press.

Freeman, M. (1993). *Rewriting the self.* London: Routledge.

Giddens, A. (1991). *Modernity and self-identity: Self and society in late modern age.* Stanford, CA: Stanford University Press.

Habermas, T., & Bluck, S. (2000). Getting a life: The emergence of the life story in adolescence. *Psychological Bulletin*, *126*, 748–769.

Josselson, R., & Lieblich, A. (Eds.). (1993). *The narrative study of lives*. Thousand Oaks, CA: Sage.

Kelly, G. (1955). *The psychology of personal constructs*. New York: Norton.

King, L. A., & Hicks, J. A. (2006). Narrating the self in the past and future: Implications for maturity. *Research in Human Development*, *3*, 121–138.

King, L. A., & Raspin, C. (2004). Lost and found possible selves: Subjective well-being and ego development in divorced women. *Journal of Personality*, *72*(3), 603–632.

King, L. A., Scollon, C. K., Ramsey, C., & Williams, T. (2000). Stories of life transition: Subjective well-being and ego development in parents of children with Down syndrome. *Journal of Research in Personality*, *34*, 509–536.

King, L. A., & Smith, S. N. (2005). Happy, mature, and gay: Intimacy, power, and difficult times in coming out stories. *Journal of Research in Personality*, *39*, 278–298.

Lieblich, A. (2004). The place of psychotherapy in the life stories of women in households without men. In A. Lieblich, D. P. McAdams, & R. Josselson (Eds.), *Healing plots: The narrative basis of psychotherapy* (pp. 171–188). Washington, DC: American Psychological Association.

Lieblich, A., McAdams, D. P., & Josselson, R. (Eds.). (2004). *Healing plots: The narrative basis of psychotherapy*. Washington, DC: American Psychological Association.

Loevinger, J. (1976). *Ego development*. San Francisco: Jossey-Bass.

Lysaker, P. H., Lancaster, R. S., & Lysaker, J. T. (2003). Narrative transformation as an outcome in the psychotherapy of schizophrenia. *Psychology and Psychotherapy: Theory, Research and Practice*, *76*(3), 285–299.

Markus, H., & Kitayama, S. (1991). Culture and the self: Implications for cognition, emotion, and motivation. *Psychological Review*, *98*, 224–253.

McAdams, D. P. (1982). Experiences of intimacy and power: Relationships between social motives and autobiographical memory. *Journal of Personality and Social Psychology*, *42*, 292–302.

McAdams, D. P. (1985). *Power, intimacy, and the life story*. New York: Guilford Press.

McAdams, D. P. (1993). *The stories we live by*. New York: Morrow.

McAdams, D. P. (2001). The psychology of life stories. *Review of General Psychology*, *5*, 100–122.

McAdams, D. P. (2006). *The redemptive self.* New York: Oxford University Press.

McAdams, D. P., Anyidoho, N. A., Brown, C., Huang, Y. T., Kaplan, B., & Machado, M. A. (2004). Traits and stories: Links between dispositional and narrative features of personality. *Journal of Personality*, *72*, 761–783.

McAdams, D. P., Booth, L., & Selvik, R. (1981). Religious identity among students at a private college: Social motives, ego stage, and development. *Merrill–Palmer Quarterly*, *27*, 219–239.

McAdams, D. P., Diamond, A., de St. Aubin, E., & Mansfield, E. D. (1997). Stories of commitment:

The psychosocial construction of generative lives. *Journal of Personality and Social Psychology, 72*, 678–694.

McAdams, D. P., & Pals, J. L. (2006). A new Big Five: Fundamental principles for an integrative science of personality. *American Psychologist, 61*, 204–217.

McAdams, D. P., Reynolds, J., Lewis, M., Patten, A., & Bowman, P. J. (2001). When bad things turn good and good things turn bad: Sequences of redemption and contamination in life narrative, and their relation to psychosocial adaptation in midlife adults and in students. *Personality and Social Psychology Bulletin, 27*, 472–483.

McCrae, R. R., & Costa, P. T., Jr. (1990). *Personality in adulthood.* New York: Guilford Press.

McLean, K. C., & Thorne, A. (2003). Late adolescents' self-defining memories about relationships. *Developmental Psychology, 39*, 635–645.

Pals, J. L. (2006). Authoring a second chance in life: Emotion and transformational processing within narrative identity. *Research in Human Development, 3*, 101–120.

Pasupathi, M., & Mansour, E. (2006). Adult age differences in autobiographical reasoning in narratives. *Developmental Psychology, 42*, 798–808.

Piaget, J. (1970). *Genetic epistemology.* New York: Columbia University Press.

Rosenwald, G. C., & Ochberg, R. L. (Eds.). (1992). *Storied lives: The cultural politics of self-understanding.* New Haven, CT: Yale University Press.

Rubin, D. C. (2006). The basic-systems model of episodic memory. *Perspectives in Psychological Science, 1*, 277–311.

Singer, J. A. (2005). *Personality and psychotherapy: Treating the whole person.* New York: Guilford Press.

Singer, J. A., & Salovey, P. (1993). *The remembered self.* New York: Free Press.

Spence, D. P. (1982). *Narrative truth and historical truth: Meaning and interpretation in psychoanalysis.* New York: Norton.

Taylor, S. E. (1983). Adjustment to threatening events: A theory of cognitive adaptation. *American Psychologist, 38*, 624–630.

Tomkins, S. S. (1979). Script theory. In H. E. Howe, Jr. & R. A. Dienstbier (Eds.), *Nebraska symposium on motivation* (Vol. 26, pp. 201–236). Lincoln, NE: University of Nebraska Press.

White, M., & Epston, M. (1990). *Narrative means to therapeutic ends.* New York: Norton.

Woike, B. A., Gersekovich, I., Piorkowski, R., & Polo, M. (1999). The role of motives in the content and structure of autobiographical memory. *Journal of Personality and Social Psychology, 76*, 600–612.

# 4 Social Psychology of the Stigma of Mental Illness

## *Public and Self-Stigma Models*

Patrick W. Corrigan
Jonathon E. Larson
Sachiko A. Kuwabara

Mental illness is a complex phenomenon that cuts into human lives like a double-edged sword. On one side, illness and medication side effects negatively impact emotions, cognitive abilities, memory, problem-solving skills, decision-making abilities, social skills, interpersonal communication, and other domains of functioning. On the other, mental illness leads to public and self-stigma that interfere with opportunities to attain and maintain life goals. Complete intervention requires addressing both sides of the equation. This chapter focuses on the latter issue: the impact of stigma. In our work we have distinguished public stigma, the negative attitudes and behaviors of the general population toward individuals with serious mental illnesses (e.g., schizophrenia, bipolar disorder, major depression), from self-stigma, the negative consequences of internalizing stigma. We end the chapter with an extensive review of strategies that might diminish types of stigma and their effects. This discussion is partly based on the research literature on social attitudes and services approaches to understanding mental illness and its treatments.

### TYPES OF STIGMA

*Stigma* is a multileveled term alternately representing the cues or marks that *signal* stereotypes and prejudice, and the rubric representing the *overall* stereotypical and prejudicial process. The word *stigma* is used herein to represent the overall process. Current models of mental illness stigma are described as cognitive-behavioral constructs (Crocker, Major, & Steele, 1998; Major & O'Brien, 2005) and are illustrated in Figure 4.1. *Marks* are the cues that signal cognitive-behavioral processes. Being labeled with a mental illness is the first step in the stigma process. Stereotypes are the cognitive products that emerge from the cue or mark; they provide social knowledge structures that efficiently categorize information about social groups (Hilton & von Hippel, 1996; Judd & Park, 1996; Krueger, 1996). They are considered *social* because they represent collectively agreed-upon notions of specific groups; these ideas are *efficient* because they allow people to quickly generate impressions and expectations of individuals belonging to the stereotyped group (Hamilton & Sherman, 1994).

*Prejudice* comprises the endorsement of a stereotype and an emotional response (Devine, 1989; Hilton & von Hippel, 1996; Krueger, 1996). Just because individuals are aware of stereotypes does not necessarily mean they endorse them (Jussim, Nelson, Manis, & Soffin, 1995). Through this evaluative process, prejudicial attitudes typically lead to negative viewpoints about the target group (Allport, 1954/1979; Eagly & Chaiken, 1993). *Discrimination* is the behavioral result of prejudice (e.g., deciding not to hire someone because he or she is a member of a negatively stereotyped group).

## Public Stigma

Many people who have been labeled "mentally ill" face the prejudice and discrimination associated with a "spoiled identity" (Goffman, 1963). The general population demonstrates public stigma through negative reactions to people with severe mental illness. As outlined in Figure 4.1 and consistent with our structural model, public stigma consists of stereotypes,

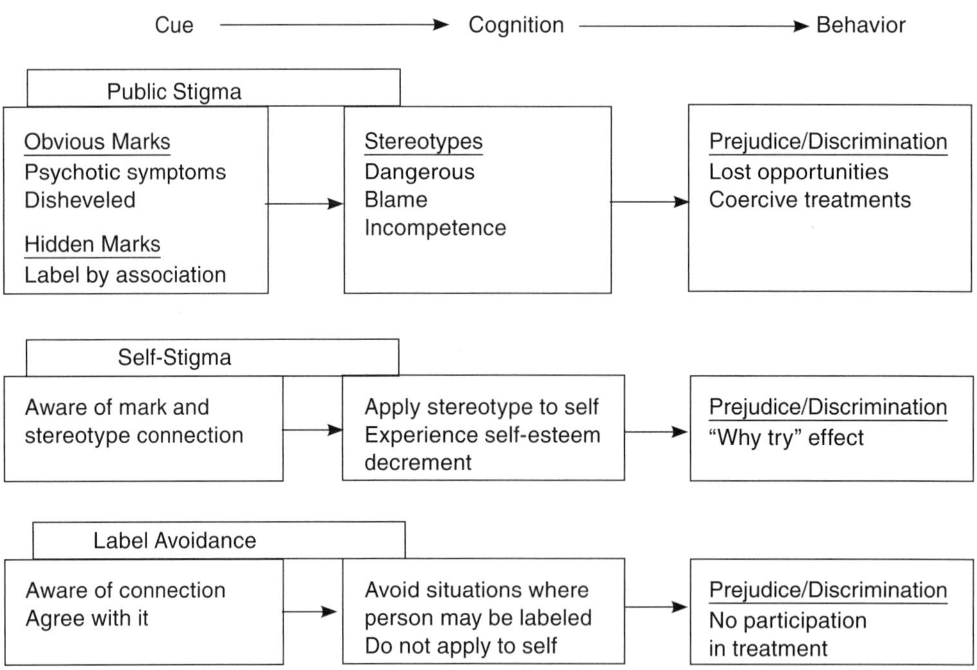


**FIGURE 4.1.** The three types of mental illness stigma.

prejudice, and discrimination. Obvious marks lead to stereotypes; such marks may include psychotic behavior, inappropriate appearance, or asocial interactions (Penn & Martin, 1998). Labels embody an alternative mark, and some people labeled *mentally ill* may be tagged with stereotypes. Labels are conferred directly when a person's mental illness status is publicly discussed (Corrigan, Watson, & Barr, 2006) or indirectly through association; for example, a person is seen exiting a psychiatrist's office. Although subtler than obvious marks, labels may be just as potent in impact (Link, 1982). Three kinds of stereotypes are common for mental illness (Brockington, Hall, Levings, & Murphy, 1993): *dangerousness*—people with mental illness are unpredictable, which leads to concerns about violence; *blame*—people with mental illness lack personal integrity and hence are responsible for their mental illness; and *incompetence*—people with mental illness are unlikely to be successful in work or independent housing goals.

Stigma includes marks and stereotypes that lead to prejudice and discrimination. Prejudice yields anger, fear, blame, and other emotional responses toward individuals with mental illness (Corrigan, 2000). Discrimination diminishes the quality of life of individuals with mental illness. Stigma may rob individuals of important life opportunities, including gainful employment, safe and comfortable housing, relationships, community functions, and educational opportunities (Corrigan & Kleinlein, 2005, Farina & Felner, 1973; Farina, Thaw, Lovern, & Mangone, 1974; Page, 1995). Examples of these effects may occur in two ways. First, individuals labeled with mental illness find it difficult to achieve their important life goals because of discriminating practices endorsed by employers, landlords, and other groups (Brockington et al., 1993; Madianos, Madianou, Vlachonikolis, & Stefanis, 1987). Second, health care systems withhold appropriate medical services from individuals due to stigma (Desai, Rosenheck, Druss, & Perlin, 2002; Druss & Rosenheck, 1997). Specifically, individuals with mental illness receive fewer insurance benefits and medical services than the general public, and insurance plans provide fewer mental health benefits than physical health services (Druss, Allen, & Bruce, 1998; Druss & Rosenheck, 1998).

## Self-Stigma

Some people internalize public stigma, harming themselves in ways that culminate in negative cognitive and behavioral outcomes; see Figure 4.1 (Corrigan & Watson, 2002; Sirey et al., 2001). A study by Link, Cullen, Frank, and Wozniak (1987) showed that the negative effects of self-stigma on psychological well-being can endure even when psychiatric symptoms have remitted because of treatment. Self-stigma may also interfere with the pursuit of such rehabilitation goals as living independently and obtaining competitive work (Wahl, 1999). Link (1982) defined a primary form of self-stigma in terms of perceived stereotypes. Link and others (1987) argued that people with mental illnesses who internalize stereotypes about mental illness experience a loss of self-esteem and self-efficacy (Markowitz, 1998; Ritsher & Phelan, 2004). Some people labeled with mental illnesses and living in a culture with prevailing stereotypes about these illnesses may automatically anticipate and internalize attitudes that reflect devaluation.

Four factors comprise the perception of the mark and subsequent stereotype that comprise self-stigma (see Figure 4.1) (Corrigan et al., 2006; Watson, Corrigan, Larson, & Sells, 2007). These are called the three A's plus the personal impact of self-stigma. The first two A's overlap with the *awareness* and *agreement* factors in Link's model of perceived stigma. First, is the person *aware* of the link between the marks of mental illness and corresponding stereotypes? Research suggests that many individuals with mental illness report being aware of these stereotypes (Bowden, Schoenfeld, & Adams, 1980; Kahn, Obstfeld, & Heiman, 1979; Shurka, 1983; Wright, Gronfein, & Owens, 2000). Second, if they are aware of stereotypes, do they *agree* with them? Up to this point, stereotypes have not been internalized and hence yield no self-stigma effects. Third, are the recognized and agreed-upon stereotypes *applied* to oneself? After agreeing with the stereotype, individuals *apply* the stereotype to themselves, leading to reduced self-efficacy and self-esteem. For example, "I have a mental illness, which must be my fault, and I won't be successful." This stereotype leads to self-discrimination, in which individuals engage in behaviors related to the stereotype application. For example, "I have a mental illness and I won't be able to succeed, so I'm not going to look for a job." In this example, self-discrimination leads to the behavior of avoiding the pursuit of employment. Some individuals engage in self-discrimination, leading to behaviors that negatively impact the pursuit of goals, whereas others either ignore or positively address the self-stigma process through personal coping skills (Corrigan et al., 2006; Watson et al., 2007). Self-discrimination and the accompanying reduction in self-efficacy and self-esteem lead to the "why try" effect, which undermines confidence in achieving life goals such as getting a job, living independently, and developing meaningful relationships (Corrigan, Larson, & Kuwabara, in press). Examples of "why try" include, "Why should I try to get work? Someone like me is not able to handle a job!" "Why should I try to live on my own? Someone like me is not worthy of such goals!" (Vogel, Wade, & Haake, 2006; Rosenfield & Neese-Todd, 1993).

## Label Avoidance

Stigma can also harm a third group; those who do not yet have a mental illness history and who avoid mental health care in order to remain unmarked (Corrigan, 2004). Personal decisions like these occur despite ample research showing that psychiatric symptoms, psychological distress, and life disabilities caused by many mental illnesses may be significantly remedied by a variety of psychopharmacological and psychosocial treatments (see the special sections on evidence-based treatments in *Psychiatric Services*, Vol. 52—Bond et al., 2001; Mellman et al., 2001; Phillips et al., 2001). Unfortunately, research also suggests that many people who meet criteria for treatment and who are likely to improve after participation, either opt not to seek services or fail to fully adhere to treatments once they are prescribed. Results from the Epidemiologic Catchment Area (ECA) study show that only 60% of people with schizophrenia participate in treatment (Reiger, Narrow, Rae, & Manderscheid, 1993). The National Comorbidity Survey (NCS), on the epidemiology of adult psychopathologies showed people with serious mental illness are no more likely to participate in treatment than people with minor disorders (Kessler et al., 2001). Less than 40% of the 6.2% of respondents with serious mental illness in the previous year received stable treatment. The NCS follow-up, completed in 2003, yielded similar sobering implications; many people who might benefit from services do not participate in them (Wang et al., 2005).

Several variables might explain the disconnect between available treatments and personal need. Unequal distribution of mental health services across racial and socioeconomic communities is one example. However, other people choose not to pursue mental health services because they want to avoid a "mental patient" label leading to prejudice and discrimination. Some support for the relationship between stigma and participation in mental health care services was provided by the epidemiological studies discussed above. Results from the NCS suggest several beliefs that might sway people from treatment (Kessler et al., 2001). These include concerns about what others might think and the desire to solve one's own problems. Using the Scale of Perceived Stigma (Link, Cullen, Struening, Shrout, & Dohrenwend, 1989), a 20-item scale that represents beliefs about the devaluation and discrimination directed toward persons with mental illness, Sirey and colleagues (2001) found a direct relationship between stigmatizing attitudes, as perceived by people with a mental illness, and treatment adherence. Scores on the scale were associated with whether research participants were compliant with their antidepressant medication regimen 3 months later. Hence, perceptions of, and identification with, existing stereotypes about mental illness can hinder persons from getting mental health assistance, the absence of which may make their lives unnecessarily more difficult. These correlational findings may suggest alternatively that people who fail to adhere to their medication regimen are bothered by stigma more than people who use antidepressants. Future research is needed to sort out the direction of this association.

Label avoidance is different from the kinds of experiences found in public or self-stigma. Public stigma is what the population does to the *group* by endorsing and implementing the stereotypes, prejudice, and discrimination that comprise mental illness stigma. Self-stigma is what people within the group do to themselves. Label avoidance is dodging the group altogether in order to escape the negative effects of public and self-stigma. People avoiding the label are aware of the stereotype and may even agree with it. However, they are strongly inclined to not apply the label to themselves and seek to avoid any group that will lead to this mark.

## Stigma, Psychiatric Symptoms, and the Disabilities of Mental Illness

Many of the assumptions of our stigma model are based on social psychological research on other discriminated groups, including persons of color and women (Major & O'Brien, 2005). There are, however, two distinctive characteristics of people with mental illness that moderate the direct application of these theories to psychiatric stigma. First, unlike other stigmatized groups, diminished self-esteem and self-efficacy are intrinsic to definitions of some specific mental illnesses such as depression (American Psychiatric Association, 1994; Millon, 1981). Problems with self-esteem and self-efficacy may arise directly from mental illness, not secondarily from the stigma experienced by the group. Hence, investigators need to develop research strategies that distinguish the problems of self-esteem and self-efficacy resulting from mental illness versus problems that are caused by stigma alone. One way to do this is to determine whether diminished self-esteem varies with the waxing and waning of dysphoria, thereby suggesting that a depressive process, and not self-stigma, accounts for the decrements in self-worth.

Second, serious mental illnesses such as schizophrenia and bipolar disorder include problems with such psychological variables as social skills (Pratt, Mueser, Smith, & Lu, 2005) and social cognition (Corrigan, Mueser, Bond, Drake, & Solomon, 2008; Penn, Corrigan, Bentall, Racenstein, & Newman, 1997). These dysfunctions are likely to influence factors that affect public and self-stigma. For example, individuals with limitations in social cognition may not understand the ramifications of the prejudice and discrimination that comprise mental illness stigma. Advocates need to consider these variables when crafting antistigma strategies. Advocates must also avoid falling into the trap of characterizing all people with mental illness similarly by recognizing that they comprise a heterogeneous group.

One last question about symptoms and disabilities to consider (Corrigan et al., 2008) is whether or not what we call discrimination is a normal response to the odd and threatening behaviors of people with severe mental illnesses. The research of Link and colleagues (Link et al., 1987, 1989; Link & Phelan, 2001) suggests that some of the stigmatizing responses to severe mental illnesses are indeed reasonable reactions to the symptoms and disabilities of these diseases. However, they have also shown that prejudice and stereotypes account for public reactions after the reasonable reactions are parsed out. Additional research indicated that public members are more likely to engage in prejudice and discrimination when they overgeneralize negative characteristics about a subgroup of people (Hewstone & Lord, 1998).

## STRATEGIES THAT CHALLENGE STIGMA

Descriptive and explanatory research on mental illness stigma is only the first step in understanding and addressing stereotypes, prejudice, and discrimination. Advocates already know that stigma is prominent and pernicious; they want to learn effective ways to challenge and erase its effects. Research and development models have evolved somewhat separately when examining strategies that reduce the stigma of public versus self-stigma. Hence, change models are explained in the remainder of the chapter in terms of these two overarching constructs. Research on effectively addressing stigma related to label avoidance is comparatively limited and thus only briefly reviewed here.

### Challenging Public Stigma

A review of the social psychological literature research identified three approaches as diminishing the impact of public stigma experienced by people with mental illness: protest, education, and contact (Corrigan & Penn, 1999). Groups *protest* inaccurate and hostile representations of mental illness as a way to challenge the stigmas they represent. These efforts send two messages. To the media: STOP reporting inaccurate representations of mental illness. To the public: STOP believing negative views about mental illness. This kind of message is frequently given in a lecture with the speaker presenting disrespectful images of mental illness (e.g., the movie *Psycho* perpetuates the notion that people with mental illness are dangerous). With this kind of presentation in tow, people are encouraged to suppress "bad" thoughts about mental illness.

Unfortunately, protest seems to have a limited effect on public prejudice. Instead, research suggests that protest might actually lead to a rebound, such that people are more likely to endorse stigmatizing attitudes about mental illness (Ottati, Bodenhausen, & Newman, 2005; Wenzlaff & Wegner, 2000). For example, Macrae, Bodenhausen, Milne, and Jetten (1994) showed that attitudes about a publically disrespected group such as skinheads actually increased when research subjects were instructed to suppress negative viewpoints about this group. Research participants who were instructed to stifle negative thoughts about an indexed group actually worsened subsequently in their attitudes toward this group.

Suppression effects were less flagrant in a study on mental illness stigma. A negative effect per se was not found. Instead, in one study (Corrigan et al., 2001) in which protest was compared against other forms of stigma change (education and contact, described below), the other approaches were shown to yield positive gains, whereas no such effects were found for protest. In fact, challenging stigma due to protest led to slightly lower stigmatizing scores in this condition compared to those in the no-intervention control group.

Largely anecdotal evidence suggests, however, that protest campaigns have been effective in getting stigmatizing images of mental illness withdrawn from the media (Wahl, 1995). In this regard, protest may be a way to limit discriminatory behavior of people who intentionally or unintentionally endorse prejudice. Consider, for example, what happened to ABC's show *Wonderland* in 2000, which in the first episode depicted a person with mental illness shooting at several police officers and stabbing a pregnant psychiatrist in the abdomen with a hypodermic needle. In response to a coordinated effort, advocates forced the network to cut the show after only a few episodes. In like manner, theaters, newspapers, and other media may be less likely to distribute a stigmatizing product when experiencing the disapproval of protest from people with mental illnesses and their families. This reality suggests that "economic protest" might have a significant impact on the news and entertainment media. Nevertheless, research is needed to explore these effects.

### *Stigma and Education*

Education involves challenging the myths of mental illness (e.g., people with mental illness are incapable of being productive members of the work world) with facts (many people who receive vocational rehabilitation for psychiatric disability achieve employment goals) (Bond et al., 2001). Evidence generally shows that people with a better understanding of mental illness are less likely to endorse stigma and less likely to discriminate (Brockington et al., 1993; Link & Cullen, 1986; Link et al., 1987; Roman & Floyd, 1981). Education programs do produce short-term improvements in attitudes (Holmes, Corrigan, Williams, Canar, & Kubiak, 1999; Keane, 1991; Morrison & Teta, 1980; Penn, Guynan, Daily, & Spaulding, 1994; Penn, Kommana, Mansfield, & Link, 1999; Tanaka, Ogawa, Inadomi, Kikuchi, & Ohta, 2003). However, research suggests that the impact of education programs might be limited. Research on the immediate effects of educational programs found that these kinds of programs produce small reductions in the stigma of mental illness (Corrigan et al., 2001). These positive effects, however, returned to baseline when 2-week follow-up measures were examined (Corrigan et al., 2002).

A benefit of pursuing antistigma goals via education is exportability. Developing educational materials, including curricula and videotaped testimonials, and dispersing them to the public at large can be a relatively easy task. The Center for Mental Health Services (CMHS) in the Substance Abuse and Mental Health Services Administration, for example, provides a website with information about education programs that attempt to address mental illness stigma. Through their "Elimination of Barriers Initiative (EBI)," CMHS and its contractors put together a package of antistigma educational services: a kick-off town meeting in participating states and a portfolio of radio, television, and print public services announcements (cf. Corrigan & Gelb, 2006). Evaluations have shown that EBI has been widely disseminated (Troust, personal communication, September 9, 2005). Of particular note is the distribution of a public service announcement (PSA)—called "Mental Health: It's Part of Our Lives"—to more than 7,200 broadcast and cable outlets that represent a viewership of more than 150 million people. Numbers like these clearly show the breadth of dissemination possible with education programs, especially PSAs. However, research on the impact of PSAs proffer different demands than those reviewed thus far vis-à-vis social psychological models. Assessments of PSAs need to examine penetration and outcome variables. Penetration is sometimes framed as the number of people in a viewership who recall seeing the PSA as part of its normal distribution. In other words, out of the 150 million conceivable people, how many recall actually viewing this PSA during normal television viewing. Exposure of a PSA is not sufficient; it needs to stand out among typical TV fare for its impact to be realized.

### *Challenging Stigma through Contact*

Contact is the third public approach to addressing stigma. Members of the public who interact with people who have mental illness are less likely to endorse stigmatizing beliefs and more likely to endorse positive statements about the group (Couture & Penn, 2003). Typical of research in this area is comparison of contact with antistigma programs such as education; these studies are done using randomized conditions. One study showed that those who were randomly assigned to a contact condition experienced significantly greater reduction in stigmatizing attitudes than did people who were assigned to an education-only condition (Corrigan et al., 2001). A second study showed that the effects of contact on stigmatizing beliefs were significantly better than education and control conditions (Corrigan et al., 2002). This effect was evident regardless of the content of the conditions; in the latter study, research participants were randomized to contact and education effects that varied in content (on whether people with mental illness are responsible for their disabilities or that people with mental illness are dangerous). Contact was shown to yield better effects, whether blame or dangerousness was the discussed topic. The impact of contact has been validated in two additional randomized controlled trials (Corrigan, Larson, Sells, Niessen, & Watson, 2007; Reinke, Corrigan, Leonhard, Lundin, & Kubiak, 2004).

Altering attitudes seem to maintain over time for contact interventions but not for education interventions. Follow-up evaluations showed that improvements at posttest were still observed (Corrigan et al., 2002). Finally, there is some evidence suggesting that contact leads to positive behavioral change when compared to control or education conditions. One study (Corrigan et al., 2002) showed that financial support for the National Alliance on Mental Illness (NAMI), a nationally known advocacy group, increased significantly after contact. In this study, research participants were told, upon receiving $10 for their work, that they could donate any or all this money to NAMI. Research participants in the contact group donated more money than those in education or control groups.

Researchers have tested several variables that enhance contact effects. Contact yields better outcomes when the person with mental illness interacts with a targeted group as peers (Pettigrew, 2000). In addition, contacts with individuals in respected positions (physician or a minister) with mental illness reduces public stigma. Contact is more effective when the person with mental illness actually interacts with a targeted group on a shared task (Desforges et al., 1991). One example of this kind of joint effort is collaboration between people with and without mental illness working on an antistigma program for people with mental illness. Finally, contact effects are enhanced when the person with mental illness has the social support of those in power in the specific group (Watson & Corrigan, 2005). For example, a pastor can introduce the person as someone that is providing an important message for the congregation. This kind of presentation avoids "back alley" experiences (i.e., the person is proverbially sneaked in the back door because the message is unimportant and, perhaps, even embarrassing).

Despite the promise of contact, it has its limitations, especially in terms of exportability. The greatest limitation of contact is that it requires individuals to have the courage to "come out of the closet" to tell their stories to one group at a time. Some interventions have attempted to address limitations of contact strategies. Videos of contact conditions (of a person talking about his or her mental health) have been shown to yield better outcomes than a videotaped education session (Corrigan et al., 2007). Moreover , NAMI provides In Our Own Voice, a consumer-based antistigma program in which participants tell their story about illness and recovery; preliminary research has shown significant reductions in stigmatizing beliefs for program participants (Wood & Wahl, 2006).

As the research thus far has shown, one contact yields positive outcomes. Hence, multiple contacts yield even better effects. People with mental illness who "come out" yield positive effects in multiple settings over multiple times. How big is this potential group? Epidemiological research suggests that people with serious mental illness may represent one in five in the general population (Kessler et al., 2005). Many of these people are "in the closet" about their illness in order to avoid the label and associated stigma. If even a fraction of these people came out, the impact of contact would be large (Couture & Penn, 2006). This point is more fully developed in the next section on self-stigma strategies.

Lessons can be learned about coming out in other communities. Research shows, for example, that the gay and lesbian community increases benefits by coming out both as individuals and as a group (Beals & Peplau, 2001; Cass, 1979; Corrigan et al., in press; Rosario, Hunter, Maguen, Gwadz, & Smith, 2001). By coming out as individuals, gay men and lesbians demonstrated reduced self-stigma. By coming out as groups, the gay community demonstrated success in reducing public discrimination related to employment, housing, and personal rights. In like manner, the community of people with mental illness may experience fewer problems when they come out in mass.

### *Targeting Stigma*

Individual approaches to public stigma strategies are more effective when targeting specific groups such as police officers, employers, landlords, health care providers, teachers, and ministers. The logic of a target-specific approach is all the more compelling when compared to the alternative—a generic effort to change the attitudes of the population as a whole. In terms of the latter, consider a video with the message that "mental illness affects 20% of the citizenry and hence is neither rare nor bizarre." This kind of mass appeal suffers because it is not particularly meaningful to the populace as a whole. It is unclear who exactly is supposed to take note of this message. Moreover, the expected products of these efforts are fuzzy; it does not specify exactly how people should change, given the highlighted stereotypes and prejudice. People might think, "Okay, so 20% of the population may be mentally ill in their lifetime. Now, what should I do about it?"

A targeted approach that focuses on changing specific discriminatory behaviors of specific groups lends itself to the practical approach outlined in Table 4.1. First, antistigma programs target powerful groups—e.g., employers, landlords, criminal justice professionals, policymakers, and the media—that make important decisions about the resources and

**TABLE 4.1. Targeted Model of Stigma Change**

| Targets | Discriminatory behavior | Attitudes |
|---|---|---|
| Employers | • Fail to hire<br>• No reasonable accommodation | • Dangerousness<br>• Incompetence |
| Landlords | • Fail to lease<br>• No reasonable accommodation | • Dangerousness<br>• Irresponsibility |
| Criminal justice professionals | • Unnecessarily coercive<br>• Fail to use mental health services | • Dangerousness<br>• Responsibility/blame |
| Policymakers | • Insufficient resource allocation<br>• Unfriendly interpretation of regulations | • Dangerousness<br>• Responsibility/blame |
| The media | • Perpetuation and dissemination of stigmatizing images | • Dangerousness<br>• Responsibility/blame<br>• Incompetence<br>• Irresponsibility |

opportunities available to persons with mental illness. Individuals acting out these power roles are significantly influenced by institutional and organizational factors (Link & Phelan, 2001; Oliver, 1992; Pincus, 1999; Scott, 1995) and may be more likely to rely on stereotypes about a group than are persons in less powerful roles (Fiske, 1993). Thus, for each group, antistigma programs identify the discriminatory behavior and corresponding attitudes they would like to change. For example, antistigma programs might address employers' unwillingness to hire persons with mental illness. Corresponding problematic attitudes might relate to beliefs in the incompetence and dangerousness to other employees posed by people with mental illness.

Once target group behaviors and attitudes are identified, the most appropriate strategy for stigma change can be selected. Although the effect of protest on attitudes is unclear, it seems to be useful for eliminating undesirable behaviors such as negative images in the media and discriminatory housing and labor practices. Education appears to improve attitudes on a short-term basis and can be implemented relatively inexpensively. Contact appears to be the most promising strategy, especially when it is structured to include "optimal" interactions. Ultimately, antistigma campaigns may employ a combination of strategies to address the problematic attitudes and behaviors of a particular group.

## Diminishing Self-Stigma

Some people internalize the stigma experience. Strategies to reduce self-stigma provide means of attenuating the impact of this experience. Three specific strategies useful for reducing self-stigma are reviewed here: programs that directly enhance empowerment; the empowerment of decisions to disclose one's psychiatric history; and cognitive reframing of the negative self-statements that result from stigma.

### *Empowerment and Anti-Stigma Programs*

The loss of self-esteem and self-efficacy caused by self-stigma is viewed as anchoring one end of a continuum with personal empowerment at the other end (McCubbin & Cohen, 1996;

Rappaport, 1987; Speer, Jackson, & Peterson, 2001). People who believe they have control over their treatment, in particular, and their lives, in general, are less likely to be plagued by self-stigma. Several elements of program design and treatment decisions enhance empowerment and decrease self-stigma (Rogers, Chamberlin, Ellison, & Crean, 1997; Stein & Test, 1980). First, state-of-the-art services are collaborative, with patients and practitioners as partners, rather than paternalistic with professionals telling patients what to do. In collaborative exchanges, individuals and practitioners view each other as peers and work together to understand the illness and develop a treatment plan; this gives people control over an important part of their life. A related element of treatment that diminishes self-stigma is consumer satisfaction; people with mental illness experience empowerment when programs are based on their feedback rather than when they exclude consumer involvement (Corrigan & Calabrese, 2005).

Coaching-based psychosocial services also facilitate empowerment. Coaches provide services and support that help people experience success in various important settings: work, housing, education, and health (Becker & Drake, 2003). Impact on empowerment further increases when peers with psychiatric illness actually provide coaching services (Mowbray, Moxley, & Collins, 1998). Individuals offering services and overcoming mental illness describe personal success stories that provide inspiration (Solomon & Draine, 2001). People with mental illness offer a special experience and critical viewpoint that enhances the quality of care. These individuals gain empowerment when they develop programs and provide services to assist others with recovery goals.

### *Disclosing One's Mental Illness*

The stigma of mental illness is largely hidden. The public frequently does not know whether specific individuals meet the criteria for mental illness. As individuals experience mental illness and the corresponding threats of stigma, they need to decide whether to disclose their illness history (Cain, 1991; Corrigan & Matthews, 2003). As suggested earlier in the chapter, several costs may result from disclosing. People risk the disapproval of peers, bosses, coworkers, neighbors, and community members. Disapproval may result in termination or a decrease in one's job role, being overlooked for opportunities with neighbors, and being excluded in community functions. Moreover, people who disclose may experience more stress because they are worrying what others think of them (Corrigan & Lundin, 2001).

There are, however, significant benefits to disclosing (Besner & Spungin, 1995). People who disclose typically feel better about themselves because the sense of shame that accompanies being "in the closet" disappears. Being in the closet impedes access to peers with similar experiences; these peers can help the person address stigma and learn strategies to accomplish life goals. Through disclosure, those people with similar mental health experiences who might provide support emerge (Beals & Peplau, 2001). Disclosing also decreases the general prejudice against the community of people with mental illness (Corrigan et al., 2007).

"Coming out" about a stigmatized characteristic or status can be represented on a continuum (Herold, 1995; Thampanichawat, 1999). Telling some people about mental illness does not necessarily mean everyone in the community knows about the disclosure. Separate and independent social spheres in which to disclose may include work settings, family situations, and community functions. People may opt to tell peers in one setting but not another (Bradmiller, 1997). Moreover, coming out is not an unequivocal decision. There are different ways in which individuals can approach disclosure (Herman, 1993). They may selectively let people know about their experience by approaching those individuals who seem open-minded to general issues related to mental illness. Alternately, they may let everyone know about their mental illness. This does not mean blatantly proclaiming one's experience with mental illness, but it does means no longer hiding one's experience with mental illness. Factors influencing decisions to disclose are complex and reflect the benefits and costs discussed previously. Individuals disclosing should make these decisions for themselves.

### *Cognitive Reframing*

Cognitive reframing provides a mechanism with which to change negative self-thoughts related to stigmatizing statements. When self-stigmatizing, people internalize self-statements representing hurtful stereotypes. "All people with mental illness are lazy" is a negative bias. "I must be lazy" is the result of applying the stereotype to oneself. These self-statements may lead to low self-esteem—"I must be a bad person because I am lazy"—and diminished self-efficacy—"A lazy person like me is not capable of finding and keeping a job." Cognitive reframing and related approaches may help the person to manage these self-statements.

Cognitive reframing involves teaching the stigmatized person to identify and challenge harmful self-statements. Kingdon and Turkington (1991, 1994) expanded cognitive therapy of psychosis beyond addressing specific symptoms to include the person's catastrophic interpretation of his or her symptoms and the stigma attached to mental illness generally. Noting that psychotic symptoms represent points on a continuum of functioning, researchers attempt to "normalize" the symptoms of therapy participants by comparing their symptoms to everyday kinds of experiences. Both uncontrolled research (Kingdon & Turkington, 1991) and randomized trials (Garety, Fowler, & Kuipers, 2000; Kingdon & Turkington, 1994) have supported the utility of this approach. With a waiting-list trial, Knight, Wykes, and Hayward (2006) demonstrated that cognitive-behavioral therapy positively influenced self-esteem and self-stigma for individuals with schizophrenia.

How might self-stigma of this kind actually be diminished? People who self-stigmatize may challenge their own prejudicial beliefs by asking whether friends and acquaintances agree with this statement: "Do you think I am lazy or in some other way bad because I have a mental illness?" This process is even more effective if the person with stigma picks a life mentor and asks him or her about the self-statement (Corrigan & Calabrese, 2005). Life mentors may include spiritual leaders or senior family members. Once individuals learn to challenge the internalized stereotype, they may develop a counterstereotype that may diminish the effects of future self-stigma. "I am not lazy! Despite my disabilities, I am working as much as possible."

## Reducing Label Avoidance

Research on understanding and reducing label avoidance is not as well developed as research on public stigma and self-stigma. Research suggests, however, that antistigma strategies for the public should also reduce the concerns of people who are contemplating treatment but are worried about the risks of being labeled as having a mental illness. Hence, contact with people who have mental illness may influence a person's decision about the pursuit of treatment. Education may also challenge myths about mental illness that interfere with care seeking or treatment participation. Reducing label avoidance and its effects needs to be at the center of future research on stigma reduction.

## SUMMARY

This chapter described the complex phenomena and negative impact of stigma on the lives of individuals with severe mental illness. Several important points emerged from this discussion. Public stigma, self-stigma, and label avoidance rob individuals of important life opportunities. Society commonly reacts to the label of mental illness with fear and disgust, which lead to reduced contact and minimized occasions for life growth for the labeled person. Public stigma and self-stigma consist of stereotypes (negative beliefs), prejudice (agreement with beliefs), and discrimination (behavior in response to beliefs). Three approaches were identified as diminishing aspects of the public stigma experienced by people with mental illness: protest, education, and contact. Three specific strategies were also identified as useful for self-stigma: empowering programs, choosing to disclose, and cognitive reframing. These models provide frameworks for the ongoing development of antistigma programs championed by advocates. These approaches also provide direction for ongoing research on stigma and stigma change. Stigma is best influenced only through a marriage of advocates and investigators.

## REFERENCES

Allport, G. W. (1979). *The nature of prejudice.* Reading, MA: Addison-Wesley. (Original work published 1954)

American Psychiatric Association. (1994). *Diagnostic and statistical manual of mental disorders* (4th ed.). Washington, DC: Author.

Beals, K. P., & Peplau, L. A. (2001). Social involvement, disclosure of sexual orientation, and the quality of lesbian relationships. *Psychology of Women Quarterly, 25,* 10–19.

Becker, D. R., & Drake, R. E. (2003). *A working life for people with severe mental illness.* New York: Oxford University Press.

Besner, H. F., & Spungin, C. I. (1995). *Gay and lesbian students: Understanding their needs.* Philadelphia: Taylor & Francis.

Bond, G. R., Becker, D. R., Drake, R. E., Rapp, C. A., Meisler, N., Lehman, A. F., et al. (2001). Implementing supported employment as an evidence-based practice. *Psychiatric Services, 52,* 313–322.

Bowden, C. L., Schoenfeld, L. S., & Adams, R. L. (1980). Mental health attitudes and treatment expectations as treatment variables. *Journal of Clinical Psychology, 36,* 653–657.

Bradmiller, M. A. (1997). *Consumer models of long-term mental illness.* Unpublished doctoral dissertation, University of Maryland College Park, College Park, MD.

Brockington, I. F., Hall, P., Levings, J., & Murphy, C. (1993). The community's tolerance of the mentally ill. *British Journal of Psychiatry, 162,* 93–99.

Cain, R. (1991). Stigma management and gay identity development. *Social Work, 36,* 67–73.

Cass, V. C. (1979). Homosexual identity formation: A theoretical model. *Journal of Homosexuality, 4,* 219–235.

Corrigan, P. W. (2000). Mental health stigma as social attribution: Implications for research methods and attitude change. *Clinical Psychology: Science and Practice, 7,* 48–67.

Corrigan, P. W. (2004). Target-specific stigma change: A strategy for impacting mental illness stigma. *Psychiatric Rehabilitation Journal, 28,* 113–121.

Corrigan, P. W., & Calabrese, J. D. (2005). Strategies for assessing and diminishing self-stigma. In P. W. Corrigan (Ed.), *On the stigma of mental illness: Practical strategies for research and social change* (pp. 239–256). Washington, DC: American Psychological Association Press.

Corrigan, P. W., & Gelb, B. (2006). Three programs that use mass approaches to challenge the stigma of mental illness. *Psychiatric Services, 57*, 393–398.

Corrigan, P. W., & Kleinlein, P. (2005). The impact of mental illness stigma. In P. W. Corrigan (Ed.), *On the stigma of mental illness: Practical strategies for research and social change* (pp. 11–44). Washington, DC: American Psychological Association.

Corrigan, P. W., Larson, J. E., Hautamaki, J., Matthews, A., Kuwabara, S., & Oshaughnessy, J. (in press). What lessons do coming out as gay or lesbian have for stigmatized health conditions? *Community Mental Health Journal.*

Corrigan, P. W., Larson, J. E., & Kuwabara, S. K. (in press). Self-stigma and the why try effect. *Community Mental Health Journal.*

Corrigan, P. W., Larson, J. E., Sells, M., Niessen, N., & Watson, A. C. (2007). Will filmed presentations of education and contact diminish mental illness stigma? *Community Mental Health Journal, 43*(2), 171–181.

Corrigan, P. W., & Lundin, R. (2001). *Don't call me nuts: Coping with the stigma of mental illness.* Tinley Park, IL: Recovery Press.

Corrigan, P. W., & Matthews, A. K. (2003). Stigma and disclosure: Implication for coming out of the closet. *Journal of Mental Health, 12*(3), 235–248.

Corrigan, P. W., Mueser, K. T., Bond, G. R., Drake, R. E., & Solomon, P. (2008). *Principles and practice of psychiatric rehabilitation: An empirical approach.* New York: Guilford Press.

Corrigan, P. W., & Penn D. L. (1999). Lessons from social psychology on discrediting psychiatric stigma. *American Psychologist, 54*, 765–776.

Corrigan, P. W., River, L., Lundin, R. K., Penn, D. L., Uphoff-Wasowski, K., Campion, J., et al. (2001). Three strategies for changing attributions about severe mental illness. *Schizophrenia Bulletin, 27*(2), 187–195.

Corrigan, P. W., Rowan, D., Green, A., Lundin, R., River, P., Uphoff-Wasowski, K., et al. (2002). Challenging two mental illness stigmas: Personal responsibility and dangerousness. *Schizophrenia Bulletin, 28*, 293–310.

Corrigan, P. W., & Watson, A. C. (2002). The paradox of self-stigma and mental illness. *Clinical Psychology: Science and Practice, 9*, 35–53.

Corrigan, P. W., Watson, A. C., & Barr, L. (2006). The self-stigma of mental illness: Implications for self-esteem and self efficacy. *Journal of Social and Clinical Psychology, 25*, 875–884.

Couture, S. M., & Penn, D. L. (2003). Interpersonal contact and the stigma of mental illness: A review of the literature. *Journal of Mental Health, 12*(3), 291–305.

Couture, S. M., & Penn, D. L. (2006). The functional significance of social cognition in schizophrenia: A review. *Schizophrenia Bulletin, 32*(Suppl. 1), S44–S63.

Crocker, J., Major, B., & Steele, C. (1998). Social stigma. In D. Gilbert, S. T. Fiske, & G. Lindzey (Eds.), *The handbook of social psychology* (4th ed., pp. 504–553). New York: McGraw-Hill.

Desai, M. M., Rosenheck, R. A., Druss, B. G., & Perlin, J. B. (2002). Mental disorders and quality of care among postacute myocardial infarction outpatients. *Journal of Nervous and Mental Disease, 190*, 51–53.

Desforges, D. M., Lord, C. G., Ramsey, S. L., Mason, J. A., Van Leeuwen, M. D., West, S. C., et al. (1991). Effects of structured cooperative contact on changing negative attitudes toward stigmatized social groups. *Journal of Personality and Social Psychology, 60*, 531–544.

Devine, P. G. (1989). Stereotypes and prejudice: Their automatic and controlled components. *Journal of Personality and Social Psychology, 56*(1), 5–18.

Druss, B. G., Allen, H. M. J., & Bruce, M. L. (1998). Physical health, depressive symptoms, and managed care enrollment. *American Journal of Psychiatry, 155*, 878–882.

Druss, B. G., & Rosenheck, R. (1997). Use of medical services by veterans with mental disorders. *Psychosomatics, 38*, 451–458.

Druss, B. G., & Rosenheck, R. (1998). Mental disorders and access to medical care in the United States. *American Journal of Psychiatry, 155*, 1775–1777.

Eagly, A., & Chaiken, S. (1993). *The social psychology of attitudes*. Ft. Worth, TX: Harcourt, Brace Jovanovich.

Farina, A., & Felner, R. D. (1973). Employment interviewer reactions to former mental patients. *Journal of Abnormal Psychology, 82*(2), 268–272.

Farina, A., Thaw, J., Lovern, J., & Mangone, D. (1974). People's reactions to a former mental patient moving to their neighborhood. *Journal of Community Psychology, 2*, 108–112.

Fiske, S. T. (1993). Controlling other people: The impact of power on stereotyping. *American Psychologist, 48*, 621–628.

Garety, P. A., Fowler, D., & Kuipers, E. (2000). Cognitive-behavioral therapy for medication-resistant symptoms. *Schizophrenia Bulletin, 26*(1), 73–86.

Goffman, E. (1963). *Stigma: Notes on the management of spoiled identity*. Englewood Cliffs, NJ: Prentice-Hall.

Hamilton, D. L., & Sherman, J. W. (1994). Stereotypes. In R. S. Wyer & T. K. Srull (Eds.), *Handbook of social cognition* (Vol. 2, 2nd ed., pp. 1–68). Hillsdale, NJ: Erlbaum.

Herman, J. L. (1993). *Trauma and recovery*. New York: Basic Books.

Herold, K. P. P. (1995). *The effects of an interviewee's self-disclosure and disability on selected perceptions and attitudes of interviewers*. Unpublished doctoral dissertation, University of Southern Mississippi, Hattiesburg, MS.

Hewstone, M., & Lord, C. G. (1998). Changing intergroup cognitions and intergroup behavior: The role of typicality. In C. Sedikes, J. Schopler, & C. A. Insko (Eds.), *Intergroup cognition and intergroup behavior* (pp. 367–392). Mahwah, NJ: Erlbaum.

Hilton, J. L., & von Hippel, W. (1996). Stereotypes. *Annual Review of Psychology, 47*, 237–271.

Holmes, E., Corrigan, P. W., Williams, P., Canar, J., & Kubiak, M. A. (1999). Changing attitudes about schizophrenia. *Schizophrenia Bulletin, 25*, 447–456.

Judd, C. M., & Park, B. (1996). Definition and assessment of accuracy in social stereotypes. *Psychological Review, 100*(1), 109–128.

Jussim, L., Nelson, T. E., Manis, M., & Soffin, S. (1995). Prejudice, stereotypes, and labeling effects: Sources of bias in person perception. *Journal of Personality and Social Psychology, 68*, 228–246.

Kahn, M. W., Obstfeld, L., & Heiman, E. (1979). Staff conceptions of patients' attitudes toward mental disorder and hospitalization as compared to patients' and staff's actual attitudes. *Journal of Clinical Psychology, 35*, 415–420.

Keane, C. (1991). Socioenvironmental determinants of community formation. *Environment and Behavior, 23*, 27–46.

Kessler, R. C., Berglund, P. A., Bruce, M. L., Koch, R., Laska, E. M., Leaf, P. J., et al. (2001). The prevalence and correlates of untreated serious mental illness. *Health Services Research, 36*, 987–1007.

Kessler, R. C., Demler, O., Frank, R. G., Olfson, M., Pincus, H. A., Walters, E. E., et al. (2005). Prevalence and treatment of mental disorders, 1990 to 2003. *New England Journal of Medicine, 352*(24), 2515–2523.

Kingdon, D., & Turkington, D. (1991). The use of cognitive behavior therapy with a normalizing rationale in schizophrenia: A preliminary report. *Journal of Nervous and Mental Disease, 179*, 207–211.

Kingdon, D., & Turkington, D. (1994). *Cognitive-behavioral therapy of schizophrenia*. New York: Guilford Press.

Knight, M. T. D., Wykes, T., & Hayward, P. (2006). Group treatment of perceived stigma and self-esteem in schizophrenia: A waiting list trial. *Behavioural and Cognitive Psychotherapy, 34*, 305–318.

Krueger, J. (1996). Personal beliefs and cultural stereotypes about racial characteristics. *Journal of Personality and Social Psychology, 71*, 536–548.

Link, B. G. (1982). Mental patient status, work and income: An examination of the effects of a psychiatric label. *American Sociological Review*, *47*, 202–215.

Link, B. G., & Cullen, F. T. (1986). Contact with the mentally ill and perceptions of how dangerous they are. *Journal of Health and Social Behavior*, *27*, 289–302.

Link, B. G., Cullen, F. T., Frank, J., & Wozniak, J. (1987). The social rejection of former mental patients: Understanding why labels matter. *American Journal of Sociology*, *92*, 1461–1500.

Link, B. G., Cullen, F. T., Struening, E. L., Shrout, P. E., & Dohrenwend, B. (1989). A modified labeling theory approach to mental disorders: An empirical assessment. *American Sociological Review*, *54*, 400–423.

Link, B. G., & Phelan, J. C. (2001). Conceptualizing stigma. *Annual Review of Sociology*, *27*, 363–385.

Macrae, C. N., Bodenhausen, G. V., Milne, A. B., & Jetten, J. (1994). Out of mind but back in sight: Stereotypes on the rebound. *Journal of Personality and Social Psychology*, *67*, 808–817.

Madianos, M., Madianou, D., Vlachonikolis, J., & Stefanis, C. (1987). Attitudes towards mental illness in the Athens area: Implications for community mental health intervention. *Acta Psychiatrica Scandinavica*, *75*(2), 158–165.

Major, B., & O'Brien, L. T. (2005). The social psychology of stigma. *Annual Review of Psychology*, *46*, 393–421.

Markowitz, F. E. (1998). The effects of stigma on the psychological well-being and life satisfaction of persons with mental illness. *Journal of Health and Social Behavior*, *39*, 335–347.

McCubbin, M., & Cohen, D. (1996). Extremely unbalanced: Interest divergence and power disparities between clients and psychiatry. *International Journal of Law and Psychiatry*, *19*, 1–25.

Mellman, T. A., Miller, A. L., Weissman, E. M., Crimson, M. L., Essock, S. M., & Marder, S. R. (2001). Evidence-based pharmacological treatment for people with severe mental illness: A focus on guidelines and algorithms. *Psychiatric Services*, *52*, 619–625.

Millon, T. (1981). *Millon Clinical Multiaxial Inventory–II*. Minneapolis: National Computer Systems.

Morrison, J. K., & Teta, D. C. (1980). Reducing students' fear of mental illness by means of seminar-induced belief change. *Journal of Clinical Psychology*, *36*, 275–276.

Mowbray, C. T., Moxley, D. P., & Collins, M. E. (1998). Consumer as mental health provider: First-person accounts of benefits and limitations. *Journal of Behavioral Health Services and Research*, *25*(4), 397–412.

Oliver, C. (1992). The antecedents of deinstitutionalization. *Organization Studies*, *13*, 563–588.

Ottati, V., Bodenhausen, G., & Newman, L. (2005). Social psychological models of mental illness stigma. In P. W. Corrigan (Ed.), *On the stigma of mental illness: Practical strategies for research and social change* (pp. 99–128). Washington, DC: American Psychological Association.

Page, S. (1995). Effects of the mental illness label in 1993: Acceptance and rejection in the community. *Journal of Health and Social Policy*, *7*, 61–68.

Penn, D. L., Corrigan, P. W., Bentall, R. P., Racenstein, J. M., & Newman, L. (1997). Social cognition in schizophrenia. *Psychological Bulletin*, *121*, 114–132.

Penn, D. L., Guynan, K., Daily, T., & Spaulding, E. (1994). Dispelling the stigma of schizophrenia: What sort of information is best? *Schizophrenia Bulletin*, *20*, 567–578.

Penn, D. L., Kommana, S., Mansfield, M., & Link, B. G. (1999). Dispelling the stigma of schizophrenia: II. The impact of information on dangerousness. *Schizophrenia Bulletin*, *25*, 437–446.

Penn, D. L., & Martin, J. (1998). The stigma of severe mental illness: Some potential solutions for a recalcitrant problem. *Psychiatric Quarterly*, *69*, 235–247.

Pettigrew, T. F. (2000). Systematizing the predictors of prejudice. In D. Sears, J. Sidanius, & L. Bobo (Eds.), *Racialized politics: The debate about racism in America*. Chicago: University of Chicago Press.

Phillips, S., Burns, B., Edgar, E., Mueser, K., Jenkins, K., Rosenheck, R., et al. (2001). Moving assertive community treatment into standard practice. *Psychiatric Services*, *52*, 771–779.

Pincus, F. L. (1999). From individual to structural discrimination. In F. L. Pincus & H. J. Ehrlich (Eds.), *Race and ethnic conflict: contending views on prejudice, discrimination, and ethnoviolence* (pp. 120–124). Boulder, CO: Westview Press.

Pratt, S., Mueser, K., Smith, T., & Lu, W. (2005). Self-efficacy and psychosocial functioning in schizophrenia: A mediational analysis. *Schizophrenia Research, 78*(2–3), 187–197.

Rappaport, J. (1987). Terms of empowerment/exemplars of prevention: Toward a theory for community psychology. *American Journal of Community Psychology, 15*(2), 121–148.

Reiger, D. A., Narrow, W. E., Rae, D. S., & Manderscheid, R. W. (1993). The de facto U.S. mental and addictive disorders service system: Epidemiologic Catchment Area prospective 1-year prevalence rates of disorders and services. *Archives of General Psychiatry, 50*, 85–94.

Reinke, R. R., Corrigan, P. W., Leonhard, C., Lundin, R. K., & Kubiak, M. A. (2004). Examining two aspects of contact on the stigma of mental illness. *Journal of Clinical and Social Psychology, 23*(3), 377–389.

Ritsher, J. B., & Phelan, J. (2004). Internalized stigma predicts erosion of morale among psychiatric outpatients. *Psychiatry Research, 129*, 257–265.

Rogers, E. S., Chamberlin, J., Ellison, M., & Crean, T. (1997). A consumer-constructed scale to measure empowerment. *Psychiatric Services, 48*, 1042–1047.

Roman, P., & Floyd, H. (1981). Social acceptance of psychiatric illness and psychiatric treatment. *Social Psychiatry, 16*, 21–29.

Rosario, M., Hunter, J., Maguen, S., Gwadz, M., & Smith, R. (2001). The coming-out process and its adaptational and health-related associations among gay, lesbian, and bisexual youths: Stipulation and exploration of a model. *American Journal of Community Psychology, 29*, 113–160.

Rosenfield, S., & Neese-Todd, S. (1993). Why model programs work: Factors predicting the subjective quality of life of the chronic mentally ill. *Hospital and Community Psychiatry, 44*, 76–78.

Scott, R. W. (1995). *Institutions and organizations*. Thousand Oaks, CA: Sage.

Shurka, E. (1983). The evaluation of ex-mental patients by other ex-mental patients. *International Journal of Social Psychiatry, 29*, 286–291.

Sirey, J., Bruce, M. L., Alexopoulos, G. S., Perlick, D., Friedman, S. J., & Meyers, B. S. (2001). Perceived stigma and patient-rated severity of illness as predictors of antidepressant drug adherence. *Psychiatric Services, 52*, 1615–1620.

Solomon, P., & Draine, J. (2001). The state of knowledge of the effectiveness of consumer provided services. *Psychiatric Rehabilitation Journal, 25*(1), 20–28.

Speer, P. W., Jackson, C. B., & Peterson, N. A. (2001). The relationship between social cohesion and empowerment: Support and new implications for theory. *Health, Education, and Behavior, 28*(6), 716–732.

Stein, L. I., & Test, M. A. (1980). Alternative to mental hospital treatment: I. Conceptual model, treatment program, and clinical evaluation. *Archives of General Psychiatry, 37*, 392–397.

Tanaka, G., Ogawa, T., Inadomi, H., Kikuchi, Y., & Ohta, Y. (2003). Effects of an educational program on public attitudes towards mental illness. *Psychiatry Clinical Neuroscience, 57*, 595–602.

Thampanichawat, W. (1999). *Thai mothers living with HIV infection in urban areas*. Unpublished doctoral dissertation, University of Washington, Seattle.

Vogel, D. L., Wade, N. G., & Haake, S. (2006). Measuring the self-stigma associated with seeking psychological help. *Journal of Counseling Psychology, 53*, 325–337.

Wahl, O. F. (1995). *Media madness: Public images of mental illness*. New Brunswick, NJ: Rutgers University Press.

Wahl, O. F. (1999). *Telling is risky business: Mental health consumers confront stigma*. New Brunswick, NJ: Rutgers University Press.

Wang, P. S., Lane, M., Olfson, M., Pincus, H. A., Wells, K. B., & Kessler, R. C. (2005). Twelve-month use of mental health services in the United States: Results from the National Comorbidity Survey replication. *Archives of General Psychiatry, 62*, 629–640.

Watson, A. C., & Corrigan, P. W. (2005). Challenging public stigma: A targeted approach. In P. W. Corrigan (Ed.), *On the stigma of mental illness: Implications for research and social change.* Washington, DC: American Psychological Association.

Watson, A. C., Corrigan, P. W., Larson, J. E., & Sells, M. (2007). Self-stigma in people with mental illness. *Schizophrenia Bulletin, 33*, 1312–1318.

Wenzlaff, R. M., & Wegner, D. M. (2000). Thought suppression. In S. T. Fiske (Ed.), *Annual review of psychology* (Vol. 51, pp. 59–91). Palo Alto, CA: Annual Reviews.

Wood, A. L., & Wahl, O. F. (2006). Evaluating the effectiveness of a consumer-provided mental health recovery education presentation. *Psychiatric Rehabilitation Journal, 30*(1), 46–53.

Wright, E. R., Gronfein, W. P., & Owens, T. J. (2000). Deinstitutionalization, social rejection, and the self-esteem of former mental patients. *Journal of Health Social Behavior, 41*, 68–90.

# Self-Regulation

# 5 Self-Regulatory Strength and Psychological Adjustment

## *Implications of the Limited Resource Model of Self-Regulation*

Celeste E. Doerr
Roy F. Baumeister

The ability to self-regulate is arguably one of humans' most crucial evolutionary adaptations. Self-regulation is often defined as the capacity to adapt the self as necessary to bring the self into accord with the environment (e.g., Rothbaum, Weisz, & Snyder, 1982; Tangney, Baumeister, & Boone, 2004). The human capacity for self-regulation affects our ability to conceive and implement plans for the future, to interact in constructive ways with other members of the species, and to care effectively for our own needs and those of our offspring. Because it empowers us to overcome selfish impulses for the sake of living in society, self-regulation has been called the "master virtue" (Baumeister & Exline, 1999, p. 1165). Thus, the capacity for self-regulation is of great benefit to human survival and social organization.

However, the benefits of self-regulation for individual psychological adjustment have not always been clearly understood by psychologists. Excesses of self-regulation have even been blamed, historically, for some forms of psychological maladjustment. Freud's (1908) characterization of the obstinate, withholding, anal-retentive personality implicates self-regulation, as do some more modern conceptions of clinical disorders, such as obsessive–compulsive disorder (OCD) and anorexia nervosa (Tangney et al., 2004). Somewhat conversely, current social psychological theory holds that high and effective self-regulation is universally advantageous to psychological adjustment.

## COMPONENTS OF SELF-REGULATION

In order for any self-regulating system, whether human or electronic, to produce effective self-regulation, at least three ingredients are necessary (e.g., Baumeister & Heatherton, 1996, 2004; Baumeister, Heatherton, & Tice, 1993; Carver & Scheier, 1982, 1998). First, there must be some *standards* indicating what is right, correct, or desirable. These may take the form of ideals, goals, or other specifications of desirable states. For example, a competitive runner might determine that he or she would be more likely to win an upcoming race by running 30 seconds faster each mile. Second, *monitoring* must occur. Comparisons are made between the current state or situation and the desired outcome dictated by the standard. The runner would likely measure and record the time for each mile and compare his or her performance to the goal. Finally, there must be a *capacity for change* to bring the current state in line with the standards. The runner must be physically capable of running faster than he or she does already.

The human self-regulation system differs from electronic systems in that a fourth ingredient is necessary, that is, *motivation*. Our runner might have the clear standard of running each mile 30 seconds faster, compare each mile's time to the goal, and be capable of improving. However, if he or she cares vehemently about watching television and very little about winning races, few miles will be run, few comparisons made, and little improvement attained. Thus, if motivation is lacking, effective self-regulation is unlikely to occur.

As with motivation, deficiencies or misjudgments related to the other three ingredients can lead to self-regulatory errors or failure (Baumeister & Heatherton, 1996, 2004; Baumeister et al., 1993). Appropriate levels of all four ingredients are necessary for self-regulation. When there are problems with standards, monitoring, or the capacity for change, the self-regulatory process breaks down and failures occur.

Standards must be clear, consistent, and appropriate. If standards are lacking, there will be no reference state against which to compare one's current state. The ability to monitor one's state and alter it toward a more desirable state will be impaired. Ambiguous or conflicting standards can also hinder self-regulation. Inner conflicts about competing standards impede attempts at action and undermine self-regulatory success (Baumeister & Heatherton, 1996; Emmons & King, 1988; Van Hook & Higgins, 1988). Similarly, having standards that are excessively or insufficiently ambitious can prevent effective self-regulation by making exertions seem futile or unnecessary (Baumeister & Heatherton, 1996; Heatherton & Ambady, 1993).

Monitoring must be both consistent and accurate to promote self-regulation (Baumeister & Heatherton, 1996). Many self-regulatory failures can be attributed to lapses in monitoring. For example, binge eating among dieters tends to occur when self-monitoring is interrupted (e.g., Heatherton & Baumeister, 1991; Polivy, 1976). The failure to accurately assess discrepancies between current and desired states can also result in self-regulatory failure (Baumeister & Heatherton, 1996). Authentic judgment of the current state of affairs supports efforts to align that state with one's standards. Some heavy drinkers, for instance, recognize their own problem drinking patterns and the need for controls when asked to simply monitor their alcohol consumption (Agostinelli, Floyd, Grube, Woodall, & Miller, 2004).

Finally, the capacity for change is vital to self-regulatory success. This refers not only to the ability to bring about behaviors intended to reach a desired goal, but also to the potential for enacting and sustaining self-regulatory efforts. Self-regulation relies upon a limited resource that can become exhausted with use (e.g., Baumeister, Bratslavsky, Muraven, &

Tice, 1998; Baumeister, Gailliot, & Tice, 2009; Muraven, Tice, & Baumeister, 1998; Vohs & Heatherton, 2000). Efforts to self-regulate, such as by suppressing unwanted thoughts or controlling emotional responses to a film, can diminish people's subsequent capacity for self-regulation on other tasks (Muraven et al., 1998).

## A LIMITED RESOURCE

A growing body of evidence suggests that the capacity for self-regulation is likely to be a limited resource (e.g., Muraven & Baumeister, 2000). This may help explain why the human capacity for self-control remains partial and indeed far less than might seem ideal, despite adaptive benefits that would lead one to predict that natural selection would have endowed humans with enormous self-regulatory powers rather than leaving the glass half full. All else being equal, strong self-regulatory powers should improve fitness and reproductive success—but if self-regulation is psychologically and biologically expensive, then each increment in self-regulation must be balanced against the increased cost.

Evidence that the capacity for self-regulation is a limited resource can be found in studies indicating that exertions of self-regulation result in a temporary reduction in one's capacity for further self-regulation. These findings suggest that some limited resource is consumed by the first act, thereby leaving less available for the second task.

The exhaustion of self-regulatory resources, termed *ego depletion*, occurs across an array of behaviors that are conceptually and functionally unrelated. Exercising self-regulation in one domain is likely to result in subsequent difficulties with self-regulation in other domains, as when dieters return from a long day of work and find that they are unable to resist the temptation to get into the ice cream. This type of research indicates that ego depletion represents the exhaustion of a single resource that is shared by all self-regulatory processes, across domains, rather than a problem that is relevant only to certain types of self-control. Put another way, the capacity for self-regulation appears to be domain general.

In one demonstration of ego depletion, Baumeister et al. (1998, Experiment 1) presented hungry participants with a stack of tempting chocolate chip cookies and a bowl of radishes. One group of participants was permitted to indulge in eating the cookies, whereas another group was instructed to avoid eating cookies and instead to eat radishes. A control group was not presented with the cookies or the radishes. Participants were then asked to work on a set of frustrating, unsolvable geometric puzzles, and the experimenters measured persistence at this task. Although restraining one's eating and persisting at puzzles should logically call for different sets of skills and motivations, the eating manipulation affected participants' puzzle persistence. Those participants who saw the cookies but ate the radishes subsequently gave up on the puzzle task sooner than participants who either ate cookies or were not exposed to food at all. Thus, regulating their eating decreased participants' ability to self-regulate in response to the frustrating puzzles.

Ego depletion, therefore, can occur as a result of deliberate acts of self-control over impulses, such as the impulse to eat tasty cookies and not radishes. It can also occur as a result of volitional acts that do not appear to directly involve the self-regulation of impulses. Baumeister et al. (1998, Experiment 2) found that participants who chose to make a counterattitudinal speech showed signs of ego depletion on a later self-regulation task. The experiment included three conditions in which the speech was either counterattitudinal or proattitudinal and the degree to which participants chose to make the speech was either high or low. A control condition was included, in which participants completed the self-regulation task, but were not asked to make a speech first. Participants who chose to make the counterattitudinal speech persisted less than control-group participants at solving frustrating geometric puzzles. However, participants who were instructed to make the counterattitudinal speech, without an element of choice, persisted as long as control-group participants. Participants who chose to make the counterattitudinal speech might have been expected to have a subsequent decrement in self-regulation due to cognitive dissonance (e.g., Festinger & Carlsmith, 1959; see especially, Linder, Cooper, & Jones, 1967). However, participants who chose to make the proattitudinal speech also showed signs of ego depletion on the self-regulation task. For participants in this experiment, it appears to have been the mere act of making a choice, not the nature of the choice itself, that resulted in ego depletion. (No one actually gave the speech, so the depletion cannot be explained on the basis of the difficulty of public speaking.) Self-regulation, therefore, relies upon a resource that is necessary to acts of conscious choice and that is expendable.

Additional studies by Vohs et al. (2008) have confirmed that making choices depletes the same resource as self-regulation. People who made a series of choices were found to be lower subsequently in their capacity for self-control than people who thought about the same issues but did not choose. The various studies in that investigation had participants make decisions about consumer products, about their psychology course materials and future courses, and about future wedding gifts they would like to receive. Making choices, as opposed to merely thinking about the options, led to significant decrements on various measures of self-control, including persistence in the face of failure, holding one's hand in ice water, and drinking a healthful but bad-tasting beverage.

Human willpower might be conceived as purely psychological—an issue of mind over matter. However, recent research indicates that the nature of self-regulatory resources might be biological, at least in part. The brain and body depend on glucose for fuel. Glucose deficits are associated with deficiencies in self-control (Gailliot & Baumeister, 2006). Gailliot et al. (2007) concluded that there is a relationship between self-regulatory strength and blood glucose levels. They found that participants' blood glucose levels decreased after completion of a self-regulatory task and that the lower participants' glucose levels were, the worse they performed at self-regulation. In an experiment that tested whether glucose could boost regulation, participants were given lemonade drinks that were either made with table sugar (containing glucose) or an artificial sweetener, and then they were instructed to complete a self-regulatory task. Participants who received the glucose drinks showed less evidence of ego depletion than participants who received the artificially sweetened drinks. Although the authors hesitate to identify glucose as the sole component of self-regulatory resources (Baumeister et al., 2009; Gailliot et al., 2007), the likening of self-regulatory resources to an energy source is more than metaphorical. Self-regulation likely requires the same energy source as other psychological and physiological functions.

## SELF-REGULATION FAILURES

The self-regulatory energy resource is a necessary, but not sufficient, ingredient for effective self-regulation. Failures of self-regulation can occur due to shortfalls in self-regulatory strength. They can also be caused by insufficiencies in standards, monitoring, or motivation. Self-regulatory failure takes one of two forms: *underregulation* or *misregulation* (Baumeister & Heatherton, 1996, 2004; Carver & Scheier, 1982, 1998). When self-regulatory strength is insufficient to meet situational demands, *underregulation* can occur. In underregulation, people fail to expend adequate energy to meet self-regulatory demands. Underregulation can also occur when standards, monitoring, or motivation is faulty or lacking. For example, holding standards that are too low, failing to monitor how well one's current state matches those standards, or lacking motivation can all result in a failure to devote enough resources to regulation.

Problems with any of the ingredients of self-regulation can also result in *misregulation*, which differs from underregulation in that sufficient energy is expended, but it is spent in ways that are misguided or otherwise ineffective for meeting self-regulatory goals (Baumeister & Heatherton, 1996, 2004). Having standards for controlling things that cannot practically be brought under one's control can result in misregulation. For example, mood states are unlikely to be altered by willpower alone, and attempts to directly alter one's emotional state are likely to fail or backfire (Baumeister & Heatherton, 1996). Holding sets of mutually incompatible standards can also result in misregulation. In fact, attempting to enact new and emotionally difficult self-regulatory measures while maintaining existing standards for one's mood state is a common cause of self-regulatory failure (Baumeister & Heatherton, 1996; Tice & Bratslavsky, 2000).

Excessively high self-control has sometimes been thought to be deleterious. People might fail to discontinue self-regulation when the situation no longer calls for it, or they might prioritize self-regulatory goals at the expense of life's normal and beneficial pleasures (Block, 2002; Block & Block, 1980; Letzring, Block, & Funder, 2005). In the past, these problems have been characterized as overregulation. However, more recently, unyieldingly high self-regulation has been conceptualized as self-regulatory rigidity, a form of misregulation (Tangney et al., 2004). When self-regulation is rigid, adequate self-regulatory strength is available, but it is directed toward inappropriate standards, monitoring, or motivation. Effective self-regulation, by comparison, is flexible. It includes the ability to monitor and moderate self-regulatory efforts.

## GOOD SELF-REGULATION AND PSYCHOLOGICAL WELL-BEING

Despite the energy expenditure it requires to initiate, maintain, and adjust to the situation, self-regulation appears to be a worthwhile enterprise for individuals. Social psychological research consistently supports the notion that effective self-regulation is good for psychological adjustment. There are numerous correlations between self-regulation and various indicators of adjustment. People who possess high levels of self-regulation report greater subjective happiness (Letzring et al., 2005), higher and stabler levels of self-esteem (Tangney et al., 2004), and more productive strategies for dealing with anger and provocation (Baumeister et al., 2009; DeWall, Baumeister, Stillman, & Gailliot, 2005; Tangney et al., 2004) than those who are low in self-regulation.

Additionally, self-regulation is negatively related to markers of a variety of psychological disorders, including eating disorders, alcoholism, somatization, obsessive–compulsive patterns, depression, anxiety, and psychoticism (Tangney et al., 2004). So, people who have a high capacity for self-regulation seem to be happier and to experience greater psychosocial adjustment than people with who are low in self-regulation.

Good self-regulation certainly helps people enact beneficial behaviors, such as studying and saving money, and to avoid maladaptive behaviors such as overeating, overspending, and abusing alcohol or other substances (e.g., Baumeister & Heatherton, 1996; Tangney et al., 2004). The ability to self-regulate might also support good psychological adjustment by enabling people to adjust their emotional and cognitive responses to potentially troubling situations. Emotional regulation is a special case of self-regulation in which individuals monitor their internal psychological responses and attempt to adjust them to meet their standards for how one ought to respond (Tice & Bratslavsky, 2000). Because emotional regulation can entail replacing one emotion with a different, incompatible one, it resembles other forms of self-regulation and is likely to draw upon limited self-regulatory resources.

There is evidence that people who have good self-regulatory skills are less likely than others to wallow in personal distress and more likely to experience guilt rather than shame in response to interpersonal conflicts (Leith & Baumeister, 1998; Tangney et al., 2004). Guilt in response to one's own undesirable actions, as opposed to shame, can have beneficial interpersonal and motivational consequences (e.g., Baumeister, Stillwell, & Heatherton, 1994; Tangney, 1991, 1995; Van Hook & Higgins, 1988), whereas proneness to shame is related to symptoms of psychopathology and a depressogenic attributional style (Tangney, Wagner, & Gramzow, 1992). Individuals who are high in self-regulation have less anger and better methods of managing anger (DeWall et al., 2005; Tangney et al., 2004) than people who lack self-regulatory skills. Thus, high self-regulatory ability seems to relate to a constellation of interpersonally and intrapersonally adaptive emotional patterns.

## SELF-REGULATION AND PSYCHOLOGICAL PROBLEMS

Some psychological disorders are unambiguously related to self-regulation. Difficulties in controlling impulsive behaviors or prioritizing long-term well-being over immediate gratification serve as diagnostic criteria for a number of psychological problems categorized in the *Diagnostic and Statistical Manual of Mental Disorders* (4th ed., American Psychiatric Association, 1994), such as impulse control disorders and substance-related disorders (Strayhorn, 2001; Tangney et al., 2004). A sense of deficient control over one's eating is a diagnostic hallmark of bulimia nervosa (American Psychiatric Association, 1994; Strayhorn, 2001), and people who are low in self-control are more prone than high self-regulators to experience symptoms of impulse control disorders, alcohol abuse, and bulimia (Tangney et al., 2004).

It is somewhat less clear why self-regulation corresponds with symptoms of disorders that are not typically associated with impulse control deficiencies. Self-regulation is negatively related to markers of depression, anxiety, and phobic anxiety (Tangney et al., 2004). The relationship between self-control and emotional responses suggests a mechanism by which self-regulation failures might be related to such psychological problems. Clinical models of psychological distress involving depression and anxiety address emotional regulation as a key element of both etiology and treatment (e.g., Aldea & Rice, 2006; Greenberg, 2004; Greenberg & Safran, 1989). Emotional regulation is a subclass of more general self-regulatory skills (Tice & Bratslavsky, 2000) that depend upon a single, limited resource

(Baumeister et al., 1998; Baumeister et al., 2009; Muraven et al., 1998). Therefore, problems with emotion regulation are likely to accompany more general self-regulatory deficits.

Self-regulation failures due to misregulation are also likely to promote psychological problems. Failure to live up one's standards can result in emotional distress (e.g., Higgins, 1987; Scheier & Carver, 1982). Lasting discrepancies between one's standards and one's actual state are associated with chronic and clinically relevant emotional symptoms (e.g., Scott & O'Hara, 1993; Strauman, 1989). Holding chronically unrealistic standards, then, is likely to produce lasting forms of emotional discomfort.

Misregulation due to competition between incompatible standards is certainly implicated in disorders involving impulse control. Often, people indulge their impulses in order to maintain the standards they set for their emotional states (Tice & Bratslavsky, 2000; Tice, Bratslavsky, & Baumeister, 2001). People who are affected by substance-related disorders and disorders related to impulse control often use alcohol, other drugs, and addictive behaviors to improve their moods (e.g., Dickerson, 1991; Sayette, 1993).

Similarly, people who experience compulsions associated with OCD often engage in compulsive behaviors for the sake of relieving anxiety (American Psychiatric Association, 1994). These behaviors represent strategies for regulating anxiety that are momentarily effective but are ineffective in the long run. Traditionally, OCD has been conceptualized as a problem of overregulation. Certainly, people who are affected by it behave in ways that seem to require impressive self-regulation, such as repeated, perfectionistic organization of their belongings. If OCD involved excesses of regulation, one would expect to observe a curvilinear relationship between self-regulation and markers for this disorder, with individuals who possess unusually high levels of self-regulation being more likely than others to report symptoms (Tangney et al., 2004). On the contrary, better self-regulation at all levels is associated with fewer symptoms, as measured by the Symptom Checklist–90 (SCL-90; Derogatis, Lipman, & Covi, 1973). The linearity of this relationship suggests that OCD is more likely to involve misregulation than overregulation.

Although self-regulation is likely to affect psychological adjustment and pathology, the reverse is also true (Strayhorn, 2001; Tangney et al., 2004). The relationship between self-regulation and psychological well-being is bidirectional. Self-regulation relies upon a limited resource that is also used up in making conscious choices (Baumeister et al., 1998; Vohs et al., 2008), engaging in effortful thinking (Schmeichel, Vohs, & Baumeister, 2003), controlling thought (Gailliot, Schmeichel, & Baumeister, 2006; Muraven et al., 1998), and maintaining desired mood states (Tice & Bratslavsky, 2000). Managing undesirable feelings and intrusive thoughts or impulses is likely to seriously diminish self-regulatory resources (Strayhorn, 2001; Tangney et al., 2004). Muraven et al. (1998) showed that suppressing either forbidden emotions (Study 1) or thoughts (Study 2, Study 3) produces ego depletion. Of particular relevance to clinical applications, the authors found that participants who tried to avoid thinking about a white bear were later unable to successfully regulate their emotional expression. It is likely that controlling one's emotions would also reduce success at avoiding unwanted thoughts, because emotional regulation and regulation of thoughts are two specific applications of self-regulation.

Merely coping with threatening thoughts, in the absence of any explicit goal to suppress them, can also impair self-regulation. In a series of studies testing the relationship between mortality salience and self-control, Gailliot et al. (2006) had participants write about death or a negatively valenced control topic before performing one of a variety of self-regulatory tasks. After writing about the thoughts and feelings associated with their own deaths, participants showed impaired controlled processing, analytical reasoning, and persistence, relative to those who wrote about a control topic.

Psychological problems might also produce patterns of misregulation. Competition between behavioral standards, such as avoiding addictive substances, and goals for emotional states, such as avoiding negative moods, might thwart attempts to control substance intake, impulses, or compulsions (Strayhorn, 2001; Tice & Bratslavsky, 2000). A person who is abstaining from addictive substances or behaviors can experience immediate, negative mood effects. Indulging in addictive drugs or other risky behaviors may hold the promise of feeling better in the short run, and this appeal may outweigh any rational calculation of increased danger in the long run.

The reciprocal relationship between self-regulation and psychological adjustment and pathology might present a difficult paradox for people who are trying to cope with and recover from clinical disorders. It also poses a potentially frustrating conundrum for clinicians (Strayhorn, 2001).

## IMPROVING SELF-REGULATION

Some clinical interventions target self-regulation directly. For example, one component of emotion coaching is the development of emotion regulation skills (Greenberg, 2002, 2004). Mindfulness treatments, utilizing deliberate focusing of awareness on emotional states along with breathing techniques, have been used to treat some anxiety disorders and help prevent relapse in depression (Greenberg, 2004).

Other treatment approaches do not specifically seek to alter self-control, but they depend upon it implicitly in order to be carried out. For example, physical exercise is sometimes recommended for people with depression (Lawlor & Hopkins, 2001), but maintaining an exercise regimen is a self-regulatory challenge that even many nondepressed individuals fail to meet. All interventions rely on self-regulation, to some degree, for their success. Behavioral interventions are unlikely to be effective if a client is unwilling or unable to devote self-regulatory resources toward changing his or her behavior. The most effective intervention will not be very helpful if it is simply too burdensome to carry out (Strayhorn, 2001). Even keeping an appointment or swallowing a pill requires some degree of self-regulatory effort.

Fortunately, people's capacity to self-regulate can be improved (e.g., Muraven & Baumeister, 2000; Muraven et al., 1999). That is, although self-regulatory strength is a limited resource, it is not a fixed commodity. Self-regulation has been compared to a muscle, in that it relies upon a limited source of energy that can be exhausted in the short term but strengthened over time through use (Muraven & Baumeister, 2000; Muraven et al., 1998). So, although specific attempts at self-regulation can result in ego depletion, persistent practice can produce gains in self-regulatory strength over time. Moreover, these gains appear to increase general powers of self-control, rather than just producing improvement in some specific skill or knowledge.

A growing body of research supports the contention that exercising self-control produces long-term improvements in self-regulatory strength (for a review, see Baumeister, Gailliot, DeWall, & Oaten, 2006). In an experiment by Muraven et al. (1999), participants completed a measure of their baseline susceptibility to ego depletion in an initial laboratory session. Participants were then instructed to return to the laboratory in 2 weeks for a second session. Some participants were given self-control exercises to practice in the interim, such as maintaining good posture at all times or improving their moods as consistently as possible. Other participants were given no exercises to complete. When participants returned to the lab 2 weeks later, those who had been given practice in self-control were less susceptible to ego depletion than participants who had not been practicing. It is important to note that the laboratory measures bore no discernible resemblance to the home exercises, because this confirms that the improvements take the form of strengthening the core ability for self-control, rather than improving skill in one particular kind of behavior.

A recent longitudinal study by Oaten and Cheng (2006) indicated that self-regulatory improvements in one domain can enhance self-regulation overall. The authors reasoned that the demands of academic examinations could undermine self-regulatory success in domains unrelated to school. They were interested in determining whether an academic-related self-control intervention would decrease students' self-regulatory failures in a number of domains unrelated to academic performance. Participants' self-regulation during exam time was compared to their baseline reports and to measures administered to another group of participants that was placed on a waiting list for the intervention. The authors found that the self-control intervention improved participants' performance on a challenging visual tracking task that was administered during academic exam week. In addition, during their exam week, participants reported fewer self-control failures. They were better able to regulate their smoking, alcohol, and caffeine consumption, self-care behaviors, and eating than those who did not receive the intervention. Again, these generalizing improvements suggest an increase in strength rather than a gain in specific skills.

Oaten and Cheng (2006) acknowledged that they sacrificed some experimental control in order to examine real-world behaviors over time. Nonetheless, taken together with the previous findings of Muraven et al. (1999), their work contributes to the emergent consensus regarding the development and training of self-regulatory capacity. Self-regulation can be improved through practice, such that individuals can develop a resistance to the ego-depleting effects of self-regulating. Furthermore, consistently practicing self-regulation in one domain seems to produce relatively long-term improvements in people's overall abilities to self-regulate (Muraven et al., 1999).

## CONCLUSIONS

Good self-regulation supports psychological adjustment, whereas poor self-regulation is related to, and probably contributes to, a variety of psychological problems and maladjustment patterns. Much of the extant research on self-regulation and psychological adjustment is correlational. The literature relating self-regulation to psychological adjustment would benefit from contributions involving experimental designs. Whereas it would be ethically unacceptable to use manipulations resulting in long-term self-regulatory deficits in order to prove that these deficits result in heightened pathology, research using interventions for increasing regulatory abilities has demonstrated that self-regulation can be improved and that practice in one area of self-control can result in broad self-regulatory gains. Because self-regulation correlates with indicators of psychological adjustment, it is possible that gains in self-regulation would benefit adjustment. We have not, however, found any studies that measured indicators of adjustment or psychological symptoms as a function of self-control training.

The current analysis is based entirely on research that was conducted with nonclinical populations. Theoretically, the mechanisms underlying self-regulation are not limited to nonclinical populations. However, it remains to be determined whether individual differences in self-regulation relate to psychological symptoms in the same way for people who are affected by psychological disorders as they do for the nonclinical participants in past studies. Knowing the patterns of self-regulatory capabilities associated with specific disorders would likely be of help to clinicians, as well as beneficial to self-regulation research and theory. Knowing whether people in the clinical population differ from others in self-regulatory strength or the effectiveness of their self-regulatory efforts would likely inform options for interventions. It would also improve understanding of the long-term consequences of problems with self-regulation.

In particular, it would be helpful to know how different types of self-regulatory failures relate to different forms of psychological symptoms in clinical populations. Underregulation has historically received substantial attention. Misregulation has been related to impulse control and substance-related disorders. However, misregulation might also contribute to the etiology and perpetuation of psychological symptoms. Currently, little empirical information exists regarding the role of misregulation in psychological problems that do not involve impulse control or addiction.

Psychological adjustment probably has a reciprocal relationship to self-regulation, such that psychological problems are likely to impair the ability to self-regulate. Because of this, clinicians are faced with the dilemma of developing and implementing interventions for people whose self-regulatory capacity might be taxed already. It would likely be useful to clinicians to be able to ascertain the self-regulatory strengths and weaknesses of individual clients. Having information about people's self-regulatory capacity would likely inform efforts toward interventions; scales exist for measuring self-regulatory strength (e.g., Letzring et al., 2005; Tangney et al., 2004). It might be even more advantageous to have tools for assessing patterns of potential weaknesses related to standards, monitoring, capacity for change, and motivation, the four elements of self-regulatory success. Such an assessment would allow the development of self-regulation profiles that could be used to indicate the need for self-control interventions.

The relationship between self-regulation and psychological adjustment is bidirectional and complex. Nonetheless, social and clinical psychology alike have much to gain from its continued study. Both subfields would benefit from (1) continued inquiry regarding the clinical relevance of specific forms of self-regulatory failure, (2) the development of tools for assessing patterns of self-regulatory ability, and (3) the provision of effective self-regulation interventions. Moreover, ongoing self-regulation research has the potential to support people in their efforts to maintain psychological adjustment and avoid the personal, social, and psychological pratfalls of poor self-control.

## REFERENCES

Agostinelli, G., Floyd, T. E., Grube, J. W., Woodall, G., & Miller, J. H. (2004). Alcohol problem recognition as a function of own and others' perceived drinking. *Addictive Behaviors*, *29*, 143–157.

Aldea, M. R., & Rice, K. G. (2006). The role of emotional dysregulation in perfectionism and psychological distress. *Journal of Counseling Psychology*, *53*, 498–510.

American Psychiatric Association. (1994). *Diagnostic and statistical manual of mental disorders* (4th ed.). Washington, DC: Author.

Baumeister, R. F., Bratslavsky, E., Muraven, M., & Tice, D. M. (1998). Ego depletion: Is the active self a limited resource? *Journal of Personality and Social Psychology*, *74*, 1252–1265.

Baumeister, R. F., & Exline, J. J. (1999). Virtue, personality, and social relations: Self-control as the moral muscle. *Journal of Personality*, *67*(6), 1165–1194.

Baumeister, R. F., Gailliot, M. T., De Wall, C. N., & Oaten, M. (2006). Self-regulation and personality: How interventions increase regulatory success, and how depletion moderates the effects of traits on behavior. *Journal of Personality*, *74*(6), 1773–1801.

Baumeister, R. F., Gailliot, M. T., & Tice, D. M. (2009). Free willpower: A limited resource theory of volition, choice, and self-regulation. In E. Morsella, J. A. Bargh, & P. M. Gollwitzer (Eds.), *The Oxford handbook of human action*. New York: Oxford University Press.

Baumeister, R. F., & Heatherton, T. F. (1996). Self-regulation failure: An overview *Psychological Inquiry*, *7*, 1–15.

Baumeister, R. F., & Heatherton, T. F. (2004). Self-regulation failure: An overview. In R. M. Kowalski & M. R. Leary (Eds.), *The interface of social and clinical psychology: Key readings* (pp. 51–69). New York: Psychology Press.

Baumeister, R. F., Heatherton, T. F., & Tice, D. M. (1993). When ego threats lead to self-regulation failure: Negative consequences of high self-esteem. *Journal of Personality and Social Psychology*, *64*, 141–156.

Baumeister, R. F., Stillwell, A. M., & Heatherton, T. F. (1994). Guilt: An interpersonal approach. *Psychological Bulletin*, *115*, 243–267.

Block, J. H. (2002). *Personality as an affect-processing system*. Mahwah, NJ: Erlbaum.

Block, J. H., & Block, J. (1980). The role of ego-control and ego-resiliency in the organization of behavior. In W. A. Collins (Ed.), *Development of cognition, affect, and social relations: The Minnesota symposia on child psychology* (Vol. 13, pp. 39–101). Hillsdale, NJ: Erlbaum.

Carver, C. S., & Scheier, M. F. (1982). Control theory: A useful conceptual framework for personality–social, clinical, and health psychology. *Psychological Bulletin*, *92*, 111–135.

Carver, C. S., & Scheier, M. F. (1998). *On the self-regulation of behavior*. New York: Cambridge University Press.

Derogatis, L. R., Lipman, R. S., & Covi, L. (1973). The SCL-90: An outpatient psychiatric rating scale. *Psychopharmacology Bulletin*, *9*, 13–28.

DeWall, C. N., Baumeister, R. F., Stillman, T. F., & Gailliot, M. T. (2005). Violence restrained: Effects of self-regulation and its depletion on aggression. *Journal of Experimental Social Psychology*, *43*, 62–76.

Dickerson, M. (1991). Internal and external determinants of persistent gambling: Implications for treatment. In N. Heather, W. R. Miller, & J. Greeley (Eds.), *Self control and the addictive behaviors* (pp. 317–338). Botany, Australia: Macmillan.

Emmons, L. A., & King, R. A. (1988). Conflict among personal strivings: Immediate and long-term implications for psychological and physical well-being. *Journal of Personality and Social Psychology*, *54*, 1040–1058.

Festinger, L., & Carlsmith, J. M. (1959). Cognitive consequences of forced compliance. *Journal of Abnormal and Social Psychology*, *58*, 203–210.

Freud, S. (1908). Character and anal eroticism. In J. Strachey (Ed.), *The standard edition of the complete psychological works of Sigmund Freud* (pp. 167–175). London: Hogarth Press.

Gailliot, M. T., & Baumeister, R. F. (2007). The physiology of willpower: Linking blood glucose to self-control. *Personality and Social Psychology Review*, *11*, 303–327.

Gailliot, M. T., Baumeister, R. F., DeWall, C. N., Maner, J. K., Plant, E. A., Tice, D. M., et al. (2007). Self-control relies on glucose as a limited energy source: Willpower is more than a metaphor. *Journal of Personality and Social Psychology*, *92*, 325–336.

Gailliot, M. T., Schmeichel, B. J., & Baumeister, R. F. (2006). Self-regulatory processes defend against the threat of death: Effects of self-control depletion and trait self-control on thoughts and fears of dying. *Journal of Personality and Social Psychology, 91*, 49–62.

Greenberg, L. S. (2002). *Emotion-focused therapy: Coaching clients to work through their feelings.* Washington, DC: American Psychological Association.

Greenberg, L. S. (2004). Emotion-focused therapy. *Clinical Psychology and Psychotherapy, 11*, 3–16.

Greenberg, L. S., & Safran, J. D. (1989). Emotion in psychotherapy. *American Psychologist, 44*, 19–29.

Heatherton, T. F., & Ambady, N. (1993). Self-esteem, self-prediction, and living up to commitments. In R. F. Baumeister (Ed.), *Self-esteem: The puzzle of low self-regard* (pp. 131–145). New York: Plenum Press.

Heatherton, T. F., & Baumeister, R. F. (1991). Binge eating as escape from self-awareness. *Psychological Bulletin, 110*, 86–108.

Higgins, E. T. (1987). Self-discrepancy: A theory relating self and affect. *Psychological Review, 94*, 319–340.

Lawlor, D. A., & Hopkins, S. W. (2001). The effectiveness as exercise as an intervention in the management of depression: Systematic review and meta-regression analysis of randomized controlled trials. *British Medical Journal, 322*, 763–766.

Leith, K. P., & Baumeister, R. F. (1998). Empathy, shame, guilt, and narratives of interpersonal conflicts: Guilt-prone people are better at perspective-taking. *Journal of Personality, 66*, 1–37.

Letzring, T. D., Block, J., & Funder, D. C. (2005). Ego-control and ego-resiliency: Generalization of self-report scales based on personality descriptions from acquaintances, clinicians, and the self. *Journal of Research in Personality, 39*, 395–422.

Linder, D. E., Cooper, J., & Jones, E. E. (1967). Decision freedom as a determinant of the role of incentive magnitude in attitude change. *Journal of Personality and Social Psychology, 6*, 245–254.

Muraven, M., & Baumeister, R. F. (2000). Self-regulation and depletion of limited resources: Does self-control resemble a muscle? *Psychological Bulletin, 126*, 247–259.

Muraven, M., Baumeister, R. F., & Tice, D. M. (1999). Longitudinal improvement of self-regulation through practice: Building self-control strength through repeated exercise. *Journal of Social Psychology, 139*, 446–457.

Muraven, M., Tice, D. M., & Baumeister, R. F. (1998). Self-control as a limited resource: Regulatory depletion patterns. *Journal of Personality and Social Psychology, 74*, 774–789.

Oaten, M., & Cheng, K. (2006). Improved self-control: The benefits of a regular program of academic study. *Basic and Applied Social Psychology, 28*, 1–16.

Polivy, J. (1976). Perception of calories and regulation of intake in restrained and unrestrained subjects. *Addictive Behaviors, 1*, 237–243.

Rothbaum, F., Weisz, J. R., & Snyder, S. S. (1982). Changing the world and changing the self: A two-process model of perceived control. *Journal of Personality and Social Psychology, 42*, 5–37.

Sayette, M. A. (1993). An appraisal-disruption model of alcohol's effectiveness on stress responses in social drinkers. *Psychological Bulletin, 114*, 459–476.

Scheier, M. F., & Carver, C. S. (1982). Cognition, affect, and self-regulation. In M. S. Clark & S. T. Fiske (Eds.), *Affect and cognition: The seventeenth annual Carnegie Symposium on cognition* (pp. 157–183). Hillsdale, NJ: Erlbaum.

Schmeichel, B. J., Vohs, K. D., & Baumeister, R. F. (2003). Intellectual performance and ego depletion: Role of the self in logical reasoning and other information processing. *Journal of Personality and Social Psychology, 85*, 33–46.

Scott, L., & O'Hara, M. W. (1993). Self-discrepancies in clinically anxious and depressed university students. *Journal of Abnormal Psychology, 102*, 282–287.

Strauman, T. J. (1989). Self-discrepancies in clinical depression and social phobia: Cognitive structures that underlie emotional disorders? *Journal of Abnormal Psychology, 98*, 14–22.

Strayhorn, J. M. (2001). Self control: Theory and research. *Journal of the American Academy of Child and Adolescent Psychiatry, 41*, 7–16.

Tangney, J. P. (1991). Moral affect: The good, the bad, and the ugly. *Journal of Personality and Social Psychology, 61*, 598–607.

Tangney, J. P. (1995). Recent advances in the empirical study of shame and guilt. *American Behavioral Scientist, 38*, 1132–1145.

Tangney, J. P., Baumeister, R. F., & Boone, A. L. (2004). High self-control predicts good adjustment, less pathology, better grades, and interpersonal success. *Journal of Personality, 72*, 271–322.

Tangney, J. P., Wagner, P., & Gramzow, R. (1992). Proneness to shame, proneness to guilt, and psychopathology. *Journal of Abnormal Psychology, 101*, 469–478.

Tice, D. M., & Bratslavsky, E. (2000). Giving in to feel good: The place of emotion regulation in the context of general self-control. *Psychological Inquiry, 11*, 149–159.

Tice, D. M., Bratslavsky, E., & Baumeister, R. F. (2001). Emotional distress regulation takes precedence over impulse control: If you feel bad, do it! *Journal of Personality and Social Psychology, 80*, 53–67.

Van Hook, E., & Higgins, E. T. (1988). Self-related problems beyond the self-concept: Motivational consequences of discrepant self-guides. *Journal of Personality and Social Psychology, 55*, 625–633.

Vohs, K. D., Baumeister, R. F., Schmeichel, B. J., Twenge, J. M., Nelson, N. M., & Tice, D. M. (2008). Making choices impairs subsequent self-control: A limited-resource account of decision making, self-regulation, and active initiative. *Journal of Personality and Social Psychology, 94*, 883–898.

Vohs, K. D., & Heatherton, T. F. (2000). Self-regulatory failure: A resource-depletion approach. *Psychological Science, 11*, 249–254.

# 6 Self-Regulation and Psychopathology

## *Toward an Integrative Perspective*

Timothy J. Strauman
Megan C. McCrudden
Neil P. Jones

The nature and consequences of human behavior cannot be fully understood without taking into account the many ways in which people try to control their own thoughts, emotions, and behaviors. All organisms have multiple layers of mechanisms for behavior regulation, but the complexity of those mechanisms is most evident in humans. The concept of *self-regulation* refers to the processes by which people initiate, maintain, and control their own thoughts, behaviors, or emotions, with the goal of producing a desired outcome or avoiding an undesired outcome (Carver & Scheier, 1990; Karoly, 1993). Self-regulatory processes can be identified at both psychological and physiological levels, and consistent with the complexity of its component mechanisms, self-regulation is both reflexive/mechanistic and intentional/agentic (Bandura, 2001). It is precisely this complexity that makes self-regulation research so challenging, and at the same time, so important to our understanding of adaptive and maladaptive functioning.

Human behavior shares much of the genomic, neural, and physiological bases of animal behavior. However, human beings also purposefully regulate behaviors, thoughts, and emotions to achieve desired goals, to bring behavior in line with internal or external standards, and to function effectively in the social world (Posner & Rothbart, 2000). These capabilities evolved to allow us to deal with challenges and opportunities that arise in our physical and social environments, but they also render us more vulnerable to a range of significant health problems, including psychological disorders such as depression and anxiety (Leary & Buttermore, 2003).

Although humans have a remarkable capacity for effective self-regulation, self-regulatory dysfunction is implicated when people overeat, fail to control their temper, succumb to ethical lapses, procrastinate, and underachieve. Self-regulation failure is at the core of health problems such as obesity, eating disorders, cardiovascular disease, smoking, and substance abuse (Ryan, Kuhl, & Deci, 1997). Problems in self-regulation can arise in connection with people's efforts to eat healthfully, exercise, practice safe sex, follow medical regimens, and drive safely (Bonin, McCreary, & Sadava, 2000; Polivy, Herman, & McFarlane, 1994; Sayette, Martin, Wertz, Shiffman, & Perrott, 2001). Evidence also suggests that domestic violence, child abuse, and sexual assault arise from the inability to control anger and aggressive urges. In each case, dysfunction of psychological mechanisms for self-regulation interacts with regulatory mechanisms at other levels to initiate and maintain disorders (Barkley, 2001).

In this chapter we describe a general framework in which different manifestations of psychopathology can be conceptualized as dysfunctions in one or more mechanisms of self-regulation. Our framework is based on the assertion that *self-regulation constitutes a critical locus for the proximal influence on motivation, cognition, emotion, and behavior of more distal factors such as temperament, socialization history, physiology, and the physical and social environment* (Karoly, 1999; Strauman, 2002). Furthermore, we propose that social psychological theories of self-regulation are ideal platforms from which to integrate the study of self-regulation across traditional disciplines. We begin by identifying multiple levels of analysis relevant to the study of self-regulation, while acknowledging that no current theory has yet been integrated with those complementary levels of analysis. We then highlight several influential theories of self-regulation that have been applied extensively to the study of psychopathology and have been linked with physiological processes. We briefly review the role of self-regulation in a set of psychological disorders that represents important public health problems both nationally and internationally. In the final section we discuss salient conceptual and empirical issues that will arise as behavioral researchers move toward more integrative perspectives on self-regulatory dysfunction and vulnerability to emotional disorders.

## THEORIES AND LEVELS OF ANALYSIS

### Levels of Analysis in Self-Regulation

Although most behavioral scientists studying self-regulation have focused their research primarily at a single (i.e., psychological) level of analysis, human self-regulation occurs simultaneously at multiple interacting levels. Thus, a range of regulatory factors must be considered, including genetic/genomic processes; neurophysiology (particularly executive and emotional/motivational processes); psychological processes (cognitive, motivational, and emotional); and interpersonal, social, and cultural factors that elicit, facilitate, or impede people's efforts to self-regulate. It is important to recognize from the outset that the psychological processes by which self-regulation is made possible are themselves linked bidirectionally with physiological and social processes critical to the disorders of interest.

Theories of self-regulation are among the most influential and most extensively validated models in behavioral science. Although different theories make unique predictions, all of them are intended to explain how perceived progress, or lack of progress, toward goals influences motivation, cognition, affect, and behavior (Carver, 2004). The current interest in self-regulation among psychologists stemmed from work on delay of gratification (Mischel, 1966; Mischel & Moore, 1973) as well as from discrepancy reduction and cybernetic models of self-evaluation (Carver & Scheier, 1981; Higgins, 1987). Self-regulation research has examined the nature of internal guides to behavior (e.g., goals, values, life tasks, personal strivings), factors that enhance and diminish people's ability to self-regulate, the automaticity of regulatory processes, strategies for behavioral control, and individual differences in the capacity to self-regulate (see Cantor & Kihlstrom, 1987; Emmons & King, 1988; Higgins, Roney, Crowe, & Hymes, 1994; Shah & Higgins, 2001).

Although psychological mechanisms for self-regulation operate "within the head" of the individual, so to speak, social psychologists have long recognized that people's capacity for self-regulation is tied to their relationships and to the cultural context in which they live. For example, our views of which behavioral impulses must be controlled (as well as how to control them) are strongly determined by social factors, and motivation to regulate behavior is often facilitated by a desire to conform to other people's standards (Higgins, Strauman, & Klein, 1987). People often enlist others to assist in their self-regulatory efforts, and belonging to groups composed of individuals who are struggling with similar self-regulation failures (such as Alcoholics Anonymous or domestic violence groups) can be of substantial benefit. Even when others are not present, people often imagine potential reactions of friends, family members, neighbors, or coworkers as they try to control undesired impulses. The essence of social psychology—that is, the effect of the real or implied presence of others on behavior—can be readily identified within the self-regulation literature (Hoyle, Kernis, Leary, & Baldwin, 1999).

Cognitive and behavioral neuroscientists also have been engaged in studying mechanisms for self-regulation, typically focusing on neural processes that underlie so-called "executive functions" critical for successful self-regulation (Lewis & Todd, 2007). Processes such as selective attention, attentional switching, sustained attention, memory, emotional control, choice, self-reflection, and decision making all have been implicated in goal pursuit and behavior regulation, intentional as well as automatic. Much of this work has confirmed the primary role of the prefrontal and frontal cortices in executive functions (Stuss & Levine, 2002). For instance, damage to the ventromedial–orbitofrontal cortex results in disinhibition, failure to consider long-term consequences of one's behavior, lapses in decision making, an inability to behave in ways that one knows are morally correct, and an inability to use other people's social cues to regulate one's own behavior (Blair & Cipolotti, 2000; Damasio, Tranel, & Damasio, 1990; Stuss & Alexander, 2000). Furthermore, the prefrontal and frontal cortices are involved in representing goals, initiating action, and maintaining ongoing behavior, and these brain regions also have been implicated in addictions (Volkow & Fowler, 2000). Other areas of the brain, including the anterior cingulate cortex, the hypothalamus, and the amygdala, are involved in regulatory processes. Experimental data have been supplemented by case studies from neuropsychiatry that have examined patients who have lost self-regulatory capacities (e.g., Hart, Schwartz, & Mayer, 1999). Similarly, computational models of brain function have been developed to describe the dynamic neural basis of self-regulation (Cooper & Shallice, 2000). Finally, a complementary approach to self-regulation can be found in the emerging field of neuroeconomics (e.g., Glimcher & Kanwisher, 2006), which seeks to understand how models of choice and economic behavior inform descriptions of brain mechanisms of behavioral control, and vice versa.

Functional neuroimaging studies, in turn, implicate the importance of neurotransmitter systems in both voluntary and involuntary mechanisms of self-regulation (Depue & Collins, 1999). For instance, it is now well documented that modulation of fast neurotransmission by monoamines is critically involved in numerous physiological functions and psychopathological conditions (Gainetdinov & Caron, 2003). Transporters for neurotransmitters such as dopamine, serotonin, and norepinephrine are established targets of many psychoactive drugs, and data regarding the impact of cognitive and behavioral phenomena on neurotransmitter availability and transport are becoming available (e.g., Dunlop & Nemeroff, 2007). Furthermore, emerging developmental research linking behavioral, functional neuroimaging, and neurophysiological measures of self-regulatory processes (e.g., Viding, Williamson, & Hariri, 2006) offers intriguing glimpses of interactions among the processes underlying human self-regulation.

Perhaps the broadest biobehavioral perspective on self-regulation to emerge over the past two decades focuses on bidirectional pathways of influence between genomic processes and behavior (Moffitt, Caspi, & Rutter, 2005). Although phenotypic differences between genetically identical organisms have long been observed, only recently have behavioral variables been examined systematically as potential consequences of, and/or explanations for, these differences. It has already been hypothesized for a number of disorders that during specific phases of development, variations in environment and/or behavior can trigger or suppress gene expression. The proliferating number of examples in which behavioral self-regulation leads to epigenetic differences between monozygotic twins over the life course (e.g., Fraga et al., 2005) indicates that genomic processes must be included within a truly comprehensive science of self-regulation (Hariri, Drabant, & Weinberger, 2006). For example, a relatively frequent single-nucleotide polymorphism in the catechol-*O*-methyltransferase (*COMT*) gene has been shown to influence dopamine neurotransmission and, in turn, to have implications for cognitive, motivational, and affective processes regulated by the orbital frontal cortex (OFC). Drabant et al. (2006) examined the role of the *COMT* genotype as a predictor of individual differences in affect regulation and associated patterns of brain activation. Using a within-subject functional magnetic resonance imaging (fMRI) experimental design based on a perceptual task that involved matching angry and fearful facial expressions, Drabant et al. observed that heritable variation in dopaminergic neurotransmission associated with the *COMT* genotype impacted the functional reactivity of frontal and limbic circuitry implicated in the regulation of emotional arousal.

## Models of Self-Regulation as a Proximal Locus for Dysfunction and Psychopathology

Social psychologists have not focused extensively on the physiology of self-regulation. However, several of the most influential social psychological models of self-regulation have been linked conceptually and empirically with both psychopathology and physiology, particularly in terms of mechanisms underlying goal activation and pursuit.

### *Control Theory*

Control theory (Carver & Scheier, 1981, 1990, 1998, 1999) is a model of the psychological processes that occur when a person is engaged in intentional behavior. The theory states that goals guide human behavior through a process referred to as a *feedback loop* (Miller,

Galanter, & Pribram, 1960). Shifts in attention away from the external environment inward toward the self engage the process of self-regulation. Several factors, including individual differences in attention, physiological arousal, moods, and difficulties in goal attainment, are responsible for shifts in attention from external cues in the environment to the self (Carver & Scheier, 1981; Karoly, 1993). With increased self-focus, a person's current self-regulatory status becomes more salient; this state (i.e., making or not making progress toward a desired end state) is then compared to the standard or goal (i.e., the *reference value*) relevant to that behavior. This comparison process can result in the detection of discrepancy or congruency between the actual behavior and the reference value. The detection of congruency results in no change in the ongoing behavior (output) until the goal is attained. Alternately, the detection of a discrepancy between current behavior and a reference value results in different actions, depending on whether the relevant goal is framed in terms of approach (a negative feedback loop) or avoidance (a positive feedback loop).

A *negative* feedback loop refers to an attempt to modify behavior in such a way as to minimize an existing discrepancy by approaching a desired goal. For example, a student receives a failing grade on his or her midterm exam, which is discrepant with his or her goal of getting an "A" in the course. The student may realize that he or she is more likely to attain this goal by studying harder and seeking help from other students prior to taking the final exam. After receiving his or her final exam grade the student then evaluates his or her current standing in the course to determine if he or she has accomplished the goal. This self-evaluation may result in further attempts to regulate his or her behavior toward the goal, such as asking for extra credit options, or he or she may decide to disengage from the feedback loop by accepting a lower grade. A *positive* feedback loop refers to the attempt to modify behavior in such a way as to avoid a congruency between current behavior and a negative goal (an "antigoal"). In this case, the desired action is to increase the distance away from some undesired outcome. According to Carver and Scheier (1999), trying to avoid an undesired outcome often leads to approaching a desired outcome. For example, trying to avoid showing one's true emotions while talking to a friend may result in approaching topics of conversation that will not elicit the emotions you are trying to mask.

Control theory postulates that goals are organized hierarchically (cf. Shah & Kruglanski, 2000), meaning that goals are specified at different levels of abstraction from the most abstract and general to the more concrete and specific (Powers, 1973). At the highest level are *systems* concepts, which refer to constructs such as an idealized sense of self. This sense of self may be comprised of several *principles*, such as "Be intelligent." To enact these principles, *programs* of behavior may exist, for example, "Study hard." In turn, in order to enact programs, individuals may use specific *sequences* of action, such as, "Open book and begin reading." Control theory postulates that goals at higher levels of abstraction provide reference values for feedback loops at lower levels in the system. This organization of goals implies that the further up the hierarchy, the more abstract the goal and the more likely it constitutes a core aspect of the self. Another implication of this structure is that the importance of reference values at the low end of the hierarchy depends on the degree to which their attainment facilitates discrepancy reduction at higher levels.

A significant contribution of control theory to the understanding of self-regulation is the explanation provided for the generation of positive and negative affect. The theory states that affect is the result of a parallel system that evaluates the status of the behavioral feedback loop that has been engaged. This metamonitoring process evaluates the perceived rate of discrepancy reduction against an active goal or standard. Carver and Scheier (1990) postulate that the output from the metamonitoring process manifests in two forms, the first being a sense of expectancy (optimism or doubt) and the second being affect per se (positive or negative). The metamonitoring process for negative feedback loops generates positive affect when progress toward a goal occurs at a rate greater than the standard. Alternately, negative affect is generated when (1) no progress toward attaining the goal occurs, (2) progress toward a goal occurs at a rate slower than the standard, or (3) the discrepancy in the behavioral loop becomes magnified. Control theory postulates that affect generated from positive feedback loops occurs in a similar manner. In positive feedback loops, positive emotion occurs when progress away from an undesired goal occurs at a rate greater than the standard. Alternately, negative affect is generated when (1) no progress toward avoiding the undesired outcome is made, (2) progress away from the undesired goal is slower than expected, or (3) the discrepancy in the behavioral loop is reduced.

Carver and Scheier (1990) articulated specific forms of affect resulting from discrepancy-reducing (approach system) versus discrepancy-enlarging (avoidance system) feedback loops. Specifically, they postulated that in discrepancy-reducing loops, the quality of affect produced ranges on a continuum from elation/joy, when discrepancy reduction occurs at a rate greater than expected, to depression when no discrepancy-reduction occurs or when it occurs at a rate slower than expected. Alternately, affect from discrepancy-enlarging feedback loops ranges on a continuum from relief, when the discrepancy is enlarged at a rate greater than expected, to anxiety when the rate of discrepancy enlargement is slower than expected or the discrepancy is reduced. The assertion that positive and negative affect are generated as a function of the rate of discrepancy reduction or enlargement is supported by a number of studies (e.g., Brunstein, 1993; King, Richards, & Stemmerich, 1998; Lawrence, Carver, & Scheier, 2002).

The relevance of control theory for the study of psychopathology can be illustrated by examining its predictions regarding the affective consequences of difficulties with goal attainment. The theory postulates that when a goal impediment is encountered (signaling a decrease in the perceived rate of progress), an individual will periodically step outside of engaging in the behavior to evaluate the likelihood of attainment. If the assessment yields a low expectancy of success, then the individual may disengage from goal pursuit. Carver and Scheier (1999) postulate that the negative affect generated by doubt and an inability to make progress toward the goal, combined with an inability to disengage from the goal, can lead to distress, which may in turn culminate in a clinically diagnosable mood or anxiety disorder (e.g., Carver, Lawrence, & Scheier, 1999; Hyland, 1987; Johnson & Carver, 2006).

### *Self-Discrepancy Theory*

Self-discrepancy theory (SDT; Higgins, 1987) is a model of self and affect that proposes that different relations between a person's representations of his or her actual behaviors and attributes (the *actual self*) and personally significant goals or standards (*self-guides*) have different motivational and emotional consequences. SDT postulates different domains of self, including the actual self, the ideal self, and the ought self. Patterns of relations between these self-state representations serve to indicate an individual's progress toward personal goals. The *actual self* is a representation of the attributes that an individual believes he or she actually possesses. The *ideal self* is a representation of the attributes that an individual ideally would like to possess (his or her hopes, wishes, or aspirations). The *ought self* is a representation of the attributes that an individual believes it is his or her obligation or duty to possess. SDT also postulates different *standpoints* on the self, including the individual's own standpoint as well as those of significant others (as perceived by the individual).

According to the theory, discrepancies between the actual self and particular self-guides lead to distinct negative emotional states. The self-guide involved in a particular self-discrepancy could represent either the individual's own standpoint or that of a significant other. An actual-self/ideal-self discrepancy is hypothesized to lead to dejection-related emotions (e.g., sadness, disappointment) because such a perceived discrepancy signifies a failure to attain a hoped-for state. In contrast, an actual-self/ought-self discrepancy is hypothesized to lead to agitation-related emotions (e.g., anxiety, worry, guilt) because such a perceived discrepancy signifies a failure to live up to one's responsibilities or obligations. Although the predicted correlations between specific self-discrepancies and particular affective states are not always found (e.g., Tangney, Niedenthal, Covert, & Barlow, 1998), the theory's predictions have received consistent support in experimental studies (e.g., Higgins, 1999). Many of these studies have used the Selves Questionnaire (SQ; Higgins, Bond, Klein, & Strauman, 1986) to assess self-discrepancy. In brief, the SQ is a free-response measure that asks participants to list attributes that describe their actual self, their ideal self, and their ought self. Congruencies and discrepancies are identified between actual self and the ideal and ought selves respectively, and actual/ideal (AI) as well as actual/ought (AO) discrepancy scores are calculated for each individual.

Many experimental studies of self-discrepancy have used a "priming" technique in which each participant is incidentally exposed to his or her own ideal or ought guides (as identified from a structured interview administered in a previous session). The participant's self-guides are coded as congruent or discrepant with the actual self (i.e., "the kind of person you believe you actually are"). The priming attributes used in these experimental studies are positively valenced (e.g., "intelligent," "successful," "attractive," and "popular"). When participants are exposed to these attributes, specific negative motivational and emotional states result, even though the attributes are literally positive. According to SDT, it is the self-regulatory significance of these stimuli that accounts for their motivational and emotional impact (Higgins, 1997).

The concept of self-discrepancy has been shown to be conceptually and empirically distinct from related concepts such as mastery, self-esteem, and self-efficacy (Förster, Grant, Idson, & Higgins, 2001). The predictions of SDT regarding the affective consequences of self-evaluation have important clinical implications. The theory asserts that the negative affect produced by discrepancies initially triggers self-regulatory processes aimed at reducing the discrepancies. However, when individuals are unable to reduce discrepancy, they experience more intense and prolonged distress, which, in turn, increases their vulnerability to disorders such as depression, generalized anxiety, and eating disorders (Fairbrother & Moretti, 1998; Harrison, 2001; Scott & O'Hara, 1993; Strauman, 1989, 1992; Weilage & Hope, 1999).

Studies using self-discrepancy theory have provided evidence that the consequences of negative self-evaluation include physiological changes. There is much evidence that, in general, discrepancies between the actual self and some desired end state are painful and motivating, which is consistent with a number of classic and contemporary theories in personality and social psychology. Studies of self-discrepancy theory, in particular, have found specific effects of self-discrepancies on a broad range of physiological indices. Strauman and Higgins

(1987) observed that changes in skin conductance and heart rate were discriminantly linked with momentary priming of actual–ideal versus actual–ought discrepancies. Strauman, Lemieux, and Coe (1993) used a similar priming procedure in a sample of anxious and dysphoric college students and found that activation of self-discrepancies induced acute changes in plasma cortisol levels as well as natural killer cell cytotoxicity. More recently, Strauman, Coe, Woods, Schneider, and Kwapil (2004) observed that priming of self-discrepancies and self-congruencies had opposite effects on natural killer cell cytotoxicity, which also varied as a function of whether the individual was characterized by high versus low levels of self-discrepancy.

### *Regulatory Focus Theory*

Regulatory focus theory (RFT; Higgins, 1997, 1998) builds upon self-discrepancy theory to provide a more general psychological model of the cognitive and motivational processes involved in approaching desired end states. Self-regulation theories and biological models (e.g., Carver & Scheier, 1990, 1998) have treated "approaching reward" and "approaching nonpunishment" as equivalent. In contrast, RFT distinguishes between self-regulation with respect to a promotion focus versus a prevention focus.

*Promotion-focused* self-regulation represents a concern with advancement, growth, and accomplishment based on nurturance needs, strong ideals (e.g., strong aspirations, hopes for oneself), and situations that are framed in terms of the presence or absence of positive outcomes (gain/nongain). Promotion-focused self-regulation involves sensitivity to the presence or absence of positive outcomes, approach as a strategy for attaining desired end states, and an eagerness for advancement and gains (i.e., maximizing attainment, ensuring against missed opportunities for attainment) as a means of pursuing personal goals—a motivational orientation that can be described as "making good things happen."

In contrast, *prevention-focused* self-regulation represents a concern with protection, safety, and responsibility based on security needs, strong oughts (i.e., a strong sense of one's duties and responsibilities), and situations framed in terms of the presence or absence of negative outcomes (loss/nonloss). Prevention-focused self-regulation involves a sensitivity to the presence or absence of negative outcomes, avoidance as a strategy for attaining desired end states, and vigilance to ensure safety and nonloss (i.e., vigilance against making mistakes and ensuring against committing the error of producing them) as a means of pursuing goals—a motivational orientation that can be described as "keeping bad things from happening."

RFT proposes that individuals differ in their chronic promotion or prevention focus. Such differences may arise from variation in the quality of parental involvement during childhood (Manian, Papadakis, Strauman, & Essex, 2006). A parental history of protection and using punishment as discipline induces a strong sense of one's duties and responsibilities and concern with safety and security (i.e., a prevention focus). Parenting characterized by encouraging accomplishments and withdrawing love as discipline induces strong aspirations and hopes for oneself and concerns with accomplishments and advancement (i.e., a promotion focus).

RFT postulates that successful self-regulation (i.e., congruency or match with ideal self-guide) in a promotion focus results in the presence of positive outcomes and the experience of cheerfulness-related emotions (e.g., happiness). In contrast, unsuccessful self-regulation (mismatch with ideal self-guide) in a promotion focus results in the absence of positive outcomes and the experience of dejection-related emotions. Successful self-regulation in a prevention focus (i.e., congruency with the ought self-guide) results in the absence of a negative outcome and the experience of quiescence-related emotions (e.g., relief or contentment). In contrast, unsuccessful self-regulation in a prevention focus (i.e., a mismatch with the ought self-guide) results in the presence of a negative outcome and the experience of agitation-related emotions (e.g., anxiety). Higgins and Spiegel (2004) summarized the body of evidence in support of these predictions.

Studies of mood and anxiety disorders have begun to incorporate a regulatory focus perspective. Strauman's (2002) model of vulnerability to depression proposes that individuals experiencing chronic failure to attain promotion goals are especially vulnerable to mood disorder. Based on that model, Strauman and his colleagues (2006) developed a brief psychotherapy for depression, *self-system therapy*. This intervention was more efficacious than standard cognitive therapy for a subset of depressed individuals characterized by chronic failure to make progress toward promotion goals. Miller and Markman (2007) tested predictions of RFT in a sample of distressed undergraduates and observed that, as expected, a promotion focus was negatively associated with symptoms of hopelessness depression.

Most recently, studies using neuroimaging techniques to examine the brain correlates of social cognition have tested predictions of RFT. Eddington, Dolcos, Cabeza, Krishnan, and Strauman (2007) observed that incidental priming of promotion goals was associated with activation in the left orbital cortex. Similarly, Cunningham, Raye, and Johnson (2005) reported that individual differences in regulatory focus predicted activation patterns in the amygdala, anterior cingulate, and extrastriate cortex in response to good/bad judgments using a standard stimulus set. These studies provide a basis for extending RFT, as a general psychological model, to incorporate neurophysiological mechanisms of self-regulation.

## REPRESENTATIVE FINDINGS

In this section we summarize findings linking psychological processes in self-regulation (specifically SDT and RFT) with psychopathology. Our summary examines four common problems: depression, anxiety disorders, eating disorders/body image, and substance abuse. The reviews are brief of necessity, but we refer the reader to broader summaries that consider self-regulatory cognition as a risk factor for a range of disorders (e.g., Bardone-Cone et al., 2007; Barry, Naus, & Rehm, 2006; Johnson, 2005; Lee & Shafran, 2004; Stravynski, Bond, & Amado, 2004).

### Depression

Social psychology has a distinguished history of contributing both conceptually and empirically to our understanding of depression. Self-regulation theories, in particular, have proven their value in guiding research on both the etiology and treatment of depression, beginning in the 1970s when the study of psychopathology was transitioning from psychoanalytic to biological and cognitive approaches. Akiskal and McKinney (1973), foreshadowing contemporary efforts to develop integrative models of major depressive disorder (MDD), proposed that depression was a functional disorder that represented a "final common pathway" resulting from a broad range of distal contributory causal factors. They suggested that the core of depression was the loss of motivation to respond effectively to cues for reward, and that this loss simultaneously affected neurotransmitter systems, motivation, and behavior. Acknowledging that vulnerability to MDD had a genetic basis and that repeated episodes of depression caused permanent changes in the central nervous system (CNS), they argued that depression resulted from perceived failure to attain personally desired outcomes. Akiskal and McKinney's view of the core of depression—loss of motivation to respond effectively to cues for reward—is consistent with a self-regulation approach as well as with neurophysiological models of depression (e.g., Mayberg, 2003).

Following the tripartite model of Clark, Watson, and Mineka (1994; see also Watson, 2005), Strauman (2002) proposed a self-regulation model of depression with these components:

- MDD is characterized by failure of cognitive–motivational mechanisms for strategic approach ("making good things happen") resulting from chronic self-perceived failure in goal pursuit.
- Certain symptoms associated with MDD (e.g., dysphoric mood, anhedonia, decreased libido/energy, hopelessness) reflect the hypoactive state of psychological and physiological mechanisms for strategic approach.
- Symptoms shared by MDD and generalized anxiety disorder (GAD), such as guilt, worry, rumination, and physiological arousal, reflect dysregulation of the cognitive and motivational mechanisms for strategic avoidance ("keeping bad things from happening").

This model implies a fundamental distinction between biobehavioral and social cognitive mechanisms of goal pursuit—both of which are likely to be involved in depression. Specifically, whereas the behavioral activation and inhibition systems underlie spatiotemporal approach and avoidance in response to evolutionarily shaped cues for reward and punishment, social cognitive mechanisms for self-regulation are primarily strategic in nature and operate to link representations of goals with behaviors that increase the likelihood of goal attainment.

Considerable research supports the prediction that AI discrepancy is discriminantly associated with depression, whereas AO discrepancy is discriminantly associated with anxiety (e.g., Strauman, 1989, 1992). These discriminant patterns of associations have been observed in both dysphoric and clinically diagnosed samples (e.g., Fairbrother & Moretti, 1998; Scott & O'Hara, 1993). The presence of chronic self-discrepancy increases the likelihood that the individual will experience repeated bouts of negative affect, which, in combination with other factors, increases risk for depression. To the extent that the individual experiences chronic failure to attain a promotion (ideal) goal, having that goal activated incidentally could create a "chain reaction" of negative self-evaluation and resultant negative affect, even without the conscious participation or awareness of the individual.

These findings linking actual–ideal discrepancy with depressive symptomatology have been replicated and extended over the past decade. Bruch, Rivet, and Laurenti (2000) reported that AI discrepancy was consistently associated with depressive affect and symptoms of depression. Roelofs et al. (2007) found that AI discrepancy and individual differences in rumination combined to predict susceptibility to depressive symptoms. In a similar study of adolescent girls, Papadakis, Prince, Jones, and Strauman (2006) observed that whereas

AI discrepancy predicted depression, teenage girls characterized by high levels of both AI discrepancy and tendencies to ruminate reported the severest depressive symptoms. Bentall, Kinderman, and Manson (2005) extended this model to bipolar disorder, finding that bipolar patients in a depressed phase manifested substantial AI discrepancy, whereas bipolar patients in a hypomanic or manic phase manifested high levels of AI consistency. In a study of depression among adults who had suffered traumatic brain injuries, Cantor et al. (2005) found that those individuals with high levels of AI discrepancy reported greater depression and associated distress. Miller and Markman (2007) tested the predictions of Strauman's (2002) self-regulation model of depression and observed that loss of promotion focus predicted vulnerability to symptoms of hopelessness depression.

### Anxiety Disorders

SDT predicts that perceived inconsistency between the actual self and an ought guide will lead to agitated affect, and that chronic actual–ought inconsistency will be associated with symptoms of anxiety disorders. Early studies based on SDT reported associations between AO discrepancy and anxious affect (e.g., Higgins, Klein, & Strauman, 1985; Higgins et al., 1986; Strauman & Higgins, 1987, 1988). Over the next decade, other studies likewise reported that AO discrepancy was discriminantly associated with anxious affect and symptoms, whereas AI discrepancy (as discussed above) was associated with dysphoric affect and depressive symptoms. Scott and O'Hara (1993) found that clinically anxious individuals had higher levels of AO discrepancy than either clinically depressed individuals or controls. Katz and Farrow (2000) found a discriminant association between AO discrepancy and anxiety in young adult women. Using both correlational and experimental designs, Strauman (1989, 1992) also found the predicted discriminant associations linking AO discrepancy with anxiety and AI discrepancy with depression.

Other investigators reported less consistent findings linking AO discrepancy with anxiety, suggesting that in contrast to the association between AI discrepancy and depression, the role of self-discrepancy in anxiety was more likely to involve mediator and moderator variables (e.g., Rodebaugh & Donahue, 2007; Tangney et al., 1998). In response, Higgins (1999) suggested that research identifying the conditions under which self-discrepancies do and do not lead to distress would be useful. A number of investigators have contributed such findings. For example, Carver et al. (1999) found evidence for an interaction between the undesired self and the ought self that potentially alters the association between AO discrepancy and agitation-related affect. Specifically, among individuals who perceived themselves as being at a considerable distance from their undesired self, a statistically significant and discriminant association between AO discrepancy and anxious affect was found. However, for those who perceived their actual self as closer to their undesired self, the AO–anxiety correlation was nonsignificant, whereas there was a clear association between actual-self–feared-self congruence and anxiety. Heppen and Ogilvie (2003) used a different method to assess self-discrepancy and observed patterns of associations between AI and AO self-discrepancy and dysphoric and anxious affect that parallel the findings of Carver et al. (1999), suggesting the relevance of both the ought self and the feared self for vulnerability to anxiety.

Other studies similarly suggest that the role of ought guides within the process of self-regulation is complex. For example, there is evidence that the contributions of AO discrepancy to anxiety disorders may differ as a function of the type of anxiety. Strauman (1989) and Weilage and Hope (1999) found an association of discrepancy between the actual self and an individual's ought guides from the perspective of significant others and social anxiety. Amico, Bruch, Haase, and Sturmer (2004) replicated this pattern but noted that it was particularly significant for individuals with high levels of trait shyness. Similarly, recent investigations have found interactions between self-discrepancy and individual difference variables in predicting anxious and dysphoric affect. Moscovitch, Hofmann, and Litz (2005) reported that the link between AO discrepancy and social anxiety was stronger for women. Gonnerman, Lavine, and Huff (2000) found that individuals characterized by high levels of trait self-monitoring manifested larger associations of AO and AI discrepancy to anxious versus depressive symptoms, respectively, relative to those low in trait self-monitoring. Similarly, Fromson (2006) reported that individuals with high levels of public as well as private self-consciousness showed stronger associations between self-discrepancy and distress than individuals with low self-consciousness, particularly for AO discrepancy and anxiety.

### Eating Disorders and Body Image

SDT's emphasis on the motivational and affective consequences of discrepancy versus congruency of the actual and ideal selves provides a useful framework for exploring how dissatisfaction with body image is associated with risk for eating disorders. Strauman, Vookles, Berenstein, Chaiken, and Higgins (1991) were among the first to apply SDT to problems with body image and eating. They found that AI discrepancy was associated with body shape dissatisfaction, independent of actual body mass or number of appearance-related self-beliefs. AI discrepancy also related to bulimic behaviors, whereas AO discrepancy was associated with anorexic-related attitudes and behaviors. Snyder (1997) also found that AI discrepancies were linked to bulimic symptoms and to dissatisfaction with body shape.

Other investigators have broadened this research. Forston and Stanton (1992) reported that AO discrepancy was a better predictor of bulimic behaviors than was AI discrepancy. Szymanski and Cash (1995) found that both ideal and ought discrepancies (whether from the standpoint of self or significant other) were moderately associated with eating disturbance. It should be noted that Cash and Szymanski as well as Forston and Stanton assessed self-discrepancy specific to physical appearance, whereas Strauman and Glenberg (1994) observed that general AI discrepancy was more strongly associated with body dissatisfaction than appearance-specific AI discrepancy. For instance, in the Cash and Szymanski study, subjects were asked to rate 11 different physical attributes according to actual, ideal, and ought selves, both from their own and from another's perspective. Similarly, in a meta-analytic review, Cash and Deagle (1997) noted that measures of self-evaluation (e.g., AI discrepancies) yielded larger effect sizes and distinguished more reliably between women with and without eating disorders as well as between anorexic and bulimic groups than did measures of estimated body size. They concluded that the magnitude of the AI discrepancy, particularly as related to self-perceived physical attributes, was conceptually and empirically related to body dissatisfaction and eating disturbances.

Applications of SDT to the study of body dissatisfaction and eating disorders have expanded into both the social and clinical literatures. Harrison (2001) demonstrated that exposure to thin-ideal media activated self-discrepancies in vulnerable individuals, predicting dissatisfaction with appearance. Interestingly, she observed that exposure to thin-rewarded portrayals activated AI discrepancy, whereas exposure to fat-punished portrayals activated

AO discrepancies. In a prospective follow-up study, Harrison and Hefner (2006) observed that television viewing of thin-ideal content predicted disordered eating as well as a thinner postpubescent body image and body ideal 1 year later. Bessenoff (2006) found that highly self-discrepant women exposed to thin-ideal media images verbalized more negative evaluations of their appearance than low-self-discrepant women. Veale, Kinderman, Riley, and Lambrou (2003) found that individuals with body dysmorphic disorder displayed higher ideal and should (their term for *ought*) appearance-related self-discrepancies compared to both a psychiatric control group and a normal control group. Both kinds of studies hold the potential to guide the development of interventions to alleviate and prevent eating disorders (Wonderlich et al., 2008).

### Substance Abuse

Theories of alcohol and substance abuse have examined the role of self-regulation as a risk factor for initiation as well as maintenance of substance use (Tarter, 2002). Much of this research has considered self-regulatory processes from the perspective of behavioral self-control and beliefs about normative behaviors (e.g., Gibbons et al., 2004); however, over the past decade a number of investigators have applied SDT to study risk for substance abuse. Using a modified version of the SQ, Avants, Singer and Margolin (1993–1994) investigated the association between self-discrepancy and addiction. They found that cocaine users had greater AI discrepancy and more negative self-descriptors among their actual-self beliefs than either opiate addicts (who were maintained on methadone) or nonusers. Consistent with the SDT literature, cocaine users also reported more depressive symptoms than nonusers. Furthermore, the cocaine users reported that they were more vulnerable to drug use when depressed.

Some researchers have theorized that self-discrepancy is also related to alcohol use and abuse. According to Banaji and Steele (1989), alcohol may disinhibit self-evaluative conflicts such that when an important dimension of self-concept is cued, alcohol inflates self-evaluation by impairing access to inhibiting or contrary information—that is, "alcohol myopia" (Steele & Josephs, 1990) may temporarily reduce self-discrepancy. Banaji and Steele suggested that alcohol's role in reducing the conflict caused by self-discrepancy means that chronic self-discrepancies may increase risk for alcohol abuse. Wolfe and Maisto (2000) examined the impact of self-discrepancy and discrepancy salience on alcohol consumption among college students. They observed a complex set of interactions between magnitude of self-discrepancy and salience of discrepancy, suggesting that although alcohol use is not likely to be motivated primarily by the desire for discrepancy reduction, it offers an "escape from aversive self-awareness" (Heatherton & Baumeister, 1991) that reinforces its use particularly in situations of real or implied social comparison. In a follow-up study, however, Wolfe and Maisto (2007) found that alcohol intoxication did not produce substantial changes in body self-discrepancy among female undergraduates who had a history of dieting and bingeing behavior. Although these studies show limited support for Banaji and Steele's theory, a rigorous evaluation of the relationship between alcohol abuse and self-discrepancy remains to be conducted.

Translational studies applying SDT to the prevention of alcohol and substance use likewise have begun to appear. Drawing upon the aforementioned findings of Avants and colleagues (1993–1994), Avants, Margolin, and Singer (1994) developed and tested a brief cognitive intervention based on SDT to reduce AI discrepancy and increase perceived discrepancy between actual-self and addict behaviors. In turn, the intervention developed by Avants and colleagues provided a conceptual and practical basis for the development of self-system therapy (Strauman et al., 2006), which applied both SDT and RFT to the treatment of depression. Barnett, Far, Mauss, and Miller (1996) created a values clarification intervention for college students that was intended to reduce students' perception of alcohol use norms and expectancies of their peers and to increase the salience of personal standards for behavior. These investigators observed that changes in norm estimates predicted changes in subsequent alcohol use.

## ISSUES FOR INTEGRATION

In order to investigate whether and how psychological processes of self-regulation contribute to psychopathology within a more comprehensive and integrative perspective, a number of conceptual and methodological issues must be considered. Foremost among these issues is the complex question of *dys*function: That is, what accounts for the transformation (either quantitative or qualitative, abrupt or gradual) from effective to ineffective self-regulation, particularly insofar as such dysregulation has profound consequences for our biology? We propose that self-regulatory psychological processes interact with mechanisms at related levels of analysis in the etiology and maintenance of psychological disorders. We refer to SDT and RFT to illustrate the kinds of issues that arise for investigators seeking to translate theories of self-regulation into models for the emergence and persistence of psychopathology.

### Antecedent, Correlate, or Consequence?

The rise of cognitive psychology and cognitive neuroscience over the last 50 years triggered a reexamination of the nature of psychological causality among philosophers of science as well as behavioral scientists. These issues are particularly vexing for theories of psychopathology, which in principle can locate critical causal influences at any of a number of levels of analysis (Bolton & Hill, 2004). For present purposes, the critical question to be considered is this: What do theories of self-regulation imply about the status of psychological mechanisms as contributory factors to psychopathology, particularly when such disorders are viewed as biological as well as psychological?

Although not a theory of psychopathology, SDT clearly implies a causal direction. Activation of a self-discrepancy is hypothesized to induce a specific negative state encompassing motivation, affect, physiology, and behavior. There is strong evidence for these predictions, particularly from priming studies in which "downstream" consequences of activating self-discrepancies have been observed using measures of peripheral psychophysiology (Strauman & Higgins, 1987), stress hormones (Strauman et al., 1993), immune function (Strauman et al., 2004), and brain activation (Eddington et al., 2007). Likewise, a substantial body of evidence supports the predictions of control theory and its derivatives regarding the affective and motivational consequences of goal pursuit failure (e.g., Mansell, 2005; Vancouver, 2005).

Since ethical and practical concerns preclude designing research attempting to induce psychopathology (e.g., a depressive episode) in vulnerable individuals, evidence for the chronic impact of self-discrepancy comes primarily from retrospective and prospective longitudinal studies. For example, Strauman (1992) observed that individuals manifesting high levels of AI versus AO discrepancy reported more depressive versus anxious symptoms, respectively, 4 months later. In a follow-up assessment 3 years later, the same discriminant predictive patterns emerged (Strauman, 1996). Studies of SDT and control theory in samples diagnosed with MDD and/or anxiety disorders have been primarily cross-sectional (e.g., Johnson, Turner, & Iwata, 2003; Scott & O'Hara, 1993), though they too have been consistent with the theory's predictions. Not surprisingly, there also is evidence that depression can increase the accessibility of self-discrepancies (Strauman & Kolden, 1997), and that successful treatment for depression can reduce the accessibility and/or magnitude of self-discrepancy (Strauman et al., 2001).

Investigators have begun to explore integrative models in which self-regulatory processes are viewed as both contributing to, and being altered by, the onset of psychological disorders (e.g., Karoly, 1999; Little, 2006), but we are not aware of any truly comprehensive model for any single disorder. Of course, such a model likely represents an ideal that any single theory should not be expected to attain. Nonetheless, without an integration across theories of self-regulation to consider how psychological processes influence, and are influenced by, processes at nearby levels, our understanding of psychopathology will remain inherently limited. In particular, we will be vulnerable to simplistic explanations that elevate one level of analysis to primary causal status and relegate others to consequences or epiphenomena. (For distinct critiques of this unfortunate trend, see Nelson et al., 2002; Post & Weiss, 2002.)

### Self-Regulatory Failure: Degenerative versus Catastrophic

Social psychological theories of self-regulation such as control theory and SDT, which were intended to model basic psychological processes, typically are silent on a particular issue of critical importance to the study of psychology: How does dysfunction of the mechanisms underlying self-regulation lead to disorders (here using depression as an example)? Although there is a healthy debate in the literature regarding whether disorders such as MDD and GAD are extremes on a continuum or are discrete states, there is no debate that not everyone with, for example, high levels of self-discrepancy becomes severely dysphoric or anxious. This question, of course, is a more specific version of the ubiquitous challenge for all theories of psychopathology. Logically speaking, at least two different pathways linking self-regulatory failure with the onset of a depressive episode can be hypothesized: a gradual, "degenerative" course or an abrupt, "catastrophic" one. The degenerative course is consistent with a downward spiral of perceived failure in goal pursuit, culminating over time in a generalized state in which the perceived likelihood of a positive outcome is zero (Carver, 1998). The catastrophic course has been conceptualized in association with major negative life events (Paykel, 2003) but could likewise be related to less traumatic events that signal failure in pursuit of a goal with which an individual's self-worth is too strongly identified or upon which his or her self-regulatory orientation is primarily based (Showers, Abramson, & Hogan, 1998). Patients' experiences of the onset of depression have been described both ways (Blatt, 2004), and the presumed heterogeneity of depression itself suggests that translation of self-regulation theories to account for the onset of depression will require testing of multiple hypothetical sequences of causal events.

A self-regulation model of depression could account for both degenerative and catastrophic onsets of disorder (Strauman, 2002). The former course has been discussed from the perspective of a number of self-regulatory models, including control theory, SDT, and RFT. The latter course is not intuitively obvious from a self-regulation perspective, but one potential model would involve individual differences in strength of orientation to promotion goals (Manian et al., 2006). For example, individuals with a strong orientation toward promotion goals might be vulnerable to depression under the following circumstances: (1) an individual with a history of success in attaining personal goals experiences failure in pursuit of a particularly important goal; (2) because of his or her overall self-regulatory orientation and the importance of the particular goal, he or she is unable to discontinue pursuit of that goal and unable to substitute another goal; (3) because of his or her history of success in goal pursuit, the individual has not developed robust coping strategies to help him or her deal more effectively with goal blockages. Even though the goal pursuit failure might not appear to be catastrophic from another person's perspective, under such circumstances the failure might be sufficiently disruptive to become depressogenic.

## Moderating and Mediating Processes

Current theories of self-regulation provide robust and thoughtful accounts of how individuals pursue personal goals and the kinds of motivational and emotional states that they experience when they see themselves as attaining, or failing to attain, such goals. However, as noted above, these theories themselves do not articulate comprehensively how the experience of *acute* emotional distress following failure to attain important goals becomes the *chronic* emotional distress characteristic of mood and anxiety disorders. Since only a subset of individuals experiencing chronic difficulties attaining goals ever becomes depressed, there are likely to be other factors (psychological, biological, etc.) that determine whether a particular individual responds adaptively in the face of continued failure feedback or becomes mired in a downward spiral of negative self-evaluation, doubt, and distress.

One psychological candidate for such a factor is maladaptive repetitive thought, also known as *rumination*. The tendency to engage in specific types of ruminative thought in response to goal blockage predicts the likelihood of self-regulatory failure (Carver & Scheier, 1990). Martin and Tesser (1996) proposed a theory of rumination, which they defined as a "class of conscious thoughts that revolve around a common instrumental theme and that recur in the absence of immediate environmental demands requiring the thoughts" (p. 7). They posited that rumination is instigated by a failure to make progress toward a desired goal, and that attaining or disengaging from the blocked goal will terminate the ruminative process. However, directing thoughts away from the distressing content or reducing negative affect associated with the goal blockage is likely to only temporarily halt the process, because the continual cueing of goal-related thoughts by features of the social environment make continued distraction difficult. An unfavorable assessment of the expectancy of succeeding at goal-directed action instigates the process of rumination, especially if the blocked goal is central to the self (Carver, 2007).

Nolen-Hoeksema has studied rumination as a coping mechanism in depression (e.g., Nolen-Hoeksema, 2000). She defines ruminative as coping "behaviors or thoughts that focus an individual's attention [on] the possible causes and consequences of that mood" (Nolen-Hoeksema, Morrow, & Fredrickson, 1993, p. 20). In this account, rumination is not instigated by a self-regulatory failure but is instead a maladaptive response to dysphoric mood.

Indeed, dysphoric individuals who ruminate demonstrate lower problem solving and less ability to generate effective solutions to interpersonal problems when compared to nondysphoric and dysphoric individuals who use distraction (Lyubomirsky, Tucker, Caldwell, & Berg, 1999).

These findings could be integrated within the self-regulatory perspective taken by Martin and Tesser (1996) to create a more elaborated theory of how acute failure feedback (which everyone experiences) becomes transformed over time into chronic failure feedback (which many people experience) and ultimately into a clinically depressed state (which most people receiving failure feedback do *not* experience). In the ongoing process of self-regulation, the individual evaluates his or her progress by monitoring the magnitude of perceived discrepancy between actual behavior and a particular goal or standard (Higgins, 1987, 1997) and the perceived rate of discrepancy reduction or enlargement (Carver & Scheier, 1990). Specifically, when using promotion-related strategies (Higgins, 1997) as a means of self-regulating behavior, dysphoric emotions occur when the individual detects a discrepancy and subsequently concludes that insufficient progress is being made. The intensity of the emotional discomfort resulting from this monitoring process is directly related to the magnitude, accessibility, and contextual relevance of the detected self-discrepancy, as well as the centrality of the discrepancy to a person's self-concept. A large self-discrepancy which is highly accessible, contextually relevant, and central to a person's self-concept is associated with more intense negative affect.

The monitoring also generates an expectancy (optimism or doubt) that influences subsequent motivation (Carver & Scheier, 1990). Under conditions that signal difficulties in goal attainment, a sense of optimism or doubt is generated that causes the person to initially respond by increasing the degree of persistence and effort of the initial instrumental behavior (Martin & Tesser, 1996). Detection of a large discrepancy generates doubt, whereas detection of a small discrepancy generates optimism that determines the degree of effort placed into repeating the instrumental behavior (a form of self-efficacy belief). At this stage, the evaluation that insufficient progress is being made causes the individual to disengage from the initial instrumental behavior to engage in a full evaluation of the likelihood of success (Carver & Scheier, 1998). In parallel with the expectancy evaluation, an individual may engage in problem solving: defining and representing the problem mentally, developing a solution strategy, organizing current knowledge about the problem, and allocating mental and physical resources needed to solve the problem (Pretz, Naples, & Sternberg, 2003). Problem solving may entail attempts to specify alternate pathways that lead to attainment of the higher-order goal, redefining the goal at lower level of specification or engaging in a process of redefining the self.

Combining this cognitive perspective on self-evaluation with the affective and motivational mechanisms proposed in RFT suggests that a particular sequence of events would be discriminantly associated with depression. Over time, the repeated inability to attain promotion goals could result in disengagement from attempts to pursue them; that is, a discontinuation of active pursuit of concerns related to advancement and growth (Kasch, Rottenberg, Arnow, & Gotlib, 2002). Furthermore, appraising maladaptive rumination as aversive and dangerous could create a prevention goal of stopping the rumination, causing a paradoxical increase in prevention concerns. As individuals enter a prevention-focused state, the strategic inclination to use vigilance to monitor for potential mistakes may generate a need to continue searching the environment for ways to reduce the discrepancy or understand why they keep failing. Paradoxically, this vigilance also would make a person more likely to confront cues associated with existing discrepancies related to both promotion and prevention concerns that trigger further maladaptive rumination (Wenzlaff & Wegner, 2000).

## Approach and Avoidance: Biobehavioral and Social Cognitive Perspectives

Psychologists have long conceptualized differences among people in terms of the kinds of goals they pursue and their characteristic ways of pursuing them. Austin and Vancouver (1996) defined goals as internal representations of desired states and identified approach and avoidance goals as among the most important classes of goals. Two levels of analysis currently dominate the study of individual differences in approach and avoidance: biobehavioral and social cognitive (Ryan et al., 1997). The *biobehavioral* level emphasizes constructs reflecting early-appearing, stable, individual differences derived from underlying biological systems. Biobehavioral theories of individual differences postulate brain–behavior systems that mediate goal-directed approach and avoidance behaviors (Carver & White, 1994; Depue & Collins, 1999; Fowles, 1994; Watson, Wiese, Vaidya, & Tellegen, 1999). These systems are major influences on approach and avoidance behaviors and on responsiveness to reward and threat cues (Clark, Watson, & Mineka, 1994).

The *social cognitive* perspective (e.g., Bandura, 1986; Mischel, 1990) emphasizes knowledge structures that function in reciprocal interaction with the social environment (Cervone, 2000). A number of social cognitive models for individual differences in approach and avoidance have appeared (e.g., Carver & Scheier, 1998; Elliot & Thrash, 2002). Despite the extensive literatures on individual differences in biobehavioral and social-cognitive systems mediating approach and avoidance goal pursuit, it remains unclear whether the two levels of analysis are manifestations of common underlying mechanisms or are distinct (Carver, Sutton, & Scheier, 2000; Caspi, 2000; Cervone, 2000; Elliot & Thrash, 2002). Developing integrative models that could account for the independent and interactive influences of biobehavioral and social cognitive mechanisms for self-regulation will be essential for our understanding of psychopathology. We offer some preliminary observations and suggestions toward that end.

Brain–behavior systems are biobehavioral constructs denoting characteristic patterns of activity in the CNS that underlie behavioral, motivational, and affective responses to classes of stimuli (Fowles, 1994; Kling & Steklis, 1976; LeDoux, 2000). A consensus has emerged regarding systems underlying approach–avoidance motivation and associated goal-directed behavior (Gable, Reis, & Elliot, 2003). These constructs originated in the animal literature but have been assimilated into models of human temperament, motivation, and affect (Watson et al., 1999).

The *behavioral activation system* (BAS; Fowles, 1994), also called the behavioral approach system (Gray, 1990) or the behavioral facilitation system (Depue & Iacono 1989), is hypothesized to underlie approach motivation and behavior in the presence of cues for reward. Motivational states related to approach or reward, energetic arousal, and positive affect, as well as personality traits such as extraversion, impulsivity, novelty seeking, and positive affectivity, all have been linked to the BAS (Revelle, 1995). Depression has been linked with hypoactivity in the BAS (e.g., John & Gross, 2007). The *behavioral inhibition system* (BIS; Fowles, 1994; Gray, 1990) is a brain–behavior system hypothesized to underlie avoidance motivation and behavior in the presence of cues for threat. The BIS is postulated to underlie sensitivity to cues for punishment, nonreward, and novelty, as well as to innate fear stimuli. Activation of the BIS is postulated to lead to behavioral inhibition, an increment in tense arousal, and increased attention in order to avoid negative or painful outcomes (Revelle, 1995). Neuroticism is understood to reflect chronic levels of BIS activity, and negative affect and state anxiety are presumed to be state markers of BIS activation (Arnett & Newman, 2000).

Although BAS and BIS imply differential states of physiological activation, individual differences in BAS and BIS strength are typically measured via questionnaire, and the construct validity of BAS and BIS, as measured via self-report, is well established (MacAndrew & Steele, 1991; Carver & White, 1994; Gable et al., 2003; Watson et al., 1999). The personality dimensions of extraversion and neuroticism are conceptualized as behavioral manifestations of individual differences in BAS and BIS strength, respectively. Questionnaire measurement of individual differences in BAS–BIS strength is valid and reliable even after controlling for response biases common in self-report instruments (Elliot & Thrash, 2002). Social cognitive models of goal-directed behavior assign primary causal status to goal representations that develop and function in reciprocal interaction with the social environment (Cervone, 2000). Social cognitive models of approach and avoidance behavior are typically described as "top-down" theories of self-regulation—a conceptualization that distinguishes such models from BAS and BIS, which historically have been viewed as "bottom-up" processes driven primarily by evolutionarily determined stimuli (Carver & Scheier, 1998).

What potential similarities and differences between BAS–BIS and social cognitive mechanisms for goal pursuit might be most salient for understanding psychopathology? Certainly both kinds of systems serve the adaptive functions of maximizing positive outcomes while minimizing negative outcomes. One potential distinction involves the motivational impetus that the different mechanisms convey. Whereas BAS and BIS presumably evolved to support *spatiotemporal* approach and avoidance (i.e., literally moving toward or away from external stimuli), social cognitive mechanisms are better characterized as facilitating *strategic* approach and avoidance (i.e., "bringing about" or "preventing"). In RFT, for example, the strategic inclinations associated with promotion and prevention can be conceptualized in signal detection terms (Tanner & Swets, 1954). Individuals with a chronic or situationally induced promotion focus are motivated to ensure "hits" (gains) and to ensure against errors of omission or "misses" (nongains). Individuals with a chronic or situationally induced prevention focus are motivated to ensure "correct rejections" (nonlosses) and to ensure against errors of commission or "false alarms" (losses). Similarly, in control theory higher-order goals are typically abstract, general, and strategic rather than concrete or situation-specific.

Another potentially important distinction involves the kinds of stimuli to which the different mechanisms may be "tuned" to respond. From a biobehavioral perspective, variability in neurally based sensitivities to nomothetically defined stimulus classes provides the cross-situational consistency that is the hallmark of individual differences (Gable et al., 2003; McCrae & Costa, 1997). BAS and BIS, as motivational systems, are organized around a basic set of salient stimuli (e.g., food, sex, predators) and affective states (Fowles, 1994). In contrast, social cognitive models presume that goal representations serve as primary organizing principles for goal pursuit (Cantor & Zirkel, 1990; Carver & Scheier, 2000). As such, salient stimuli are individually variable, contextually embedded, often symbolic, and subject to well-documented cognitive and motivational influences on social construct accessibility (Higgins, 1990).

Neither level of analysis provides a sufficient account of approach and avoidance behavior in either healthy or clinically diagnosed populations (Carver & Scheier, 2000; Depue & Collins, 1999; Mischel, 1990). Individual differences in BAS–BIS strength reliably predict behavior aggregated across situations, but typically manifest only modest associations with behaviors within specific situations (Kagan, 2003). Goal construct activation reliably predicts behavior in particular situations, but goals appear to be more variable over time than temperament-based personality traits (Caspi, 2000). Furthermore, both spatiotemporal and strategic approach–avoidance mechanisms are highly adaptive (Cacioppo, Berntson, Sheridan, & McClintock, 2000).

Our research group has proposed that although BAS and BIS have had a major impact on theories of motivation and emotion, a biobehavioral systems model does not provide a sufficient explanation for psychopathology (Strauman, 2002; Tomarken & Keener, 1998). For example, such a model is silent regarding the role of perceived failure in goal pursuit for vulnerability to depression, and so cannot provide a complete explanation of why certain people become depressed in certain circumstances (Strauman, 2002). Instead, we propose that the motivational systems for pursuit of approach and avoidance goals in humans might be reconceptualized as *self–brain–behavior systems*, encompassing the psychological, neurobiological, and behavioral processes that enable the pursuit of personal goals (Strauman, 2002; Vieth, Strauman, Kolden, Woods, & Klein, 2003).

The potential implications of an integrative self–brain–behavior systems view are intriguing. For example, consider the notion that human psychological capabilities evolved in response to an increasingly complex social environment (Leary & Buttermore, 2003). One likely evolutionary pressure would be for motivational systems to acquire the capacity to monitor the individual's status in reference to others upon whom he or she depends for survival (Posner & Rothbart, 2000). In developmental terms, children must learn to behave in ways that maintain the nurturance and security they require from caregivers (Kochanska, 1995). If the approach and avoidance systems operate in service of maximizing positive outcomes and minimizing negative outcomes, respectively, then to be effective those systems must be capable of self-representation and self-evaluation within the social context, and higher-level representational, monitoring, and evaluative functions must be integral parts of each system.

Furthermore, if self-regulatory cognition is integral to the approach and avoidance systems, then the systems must be fundamentally different in humans than in animals. For instance, most animals have a restricted repertoire of approach goals and a limited set of strategies for achieving those goals; for such organisms, it is accurate to describe the positive-outcome motivational system as an "approach" system. In contrast, the kinds of positive outcomes that humans pursue can be as mundane as sating one's hunger or as abstract as achieving world peace. For many of the goals that people pursue, there is no literal or spatiotemporal "moving toward"; rather, the strategies people use instantiate a different sense of approach, that is, "setting about." The use of the terms *promotion* and *prevention* in RFT was intended, in part, to signify this latter conceptualization of motivation and goal pursuit.

Finally, a self–brain–behavior perspective on self-regulation permits generation of novel hypotheses regarding how various psychological and biological processes are functionally associated—both under normal circumstances and as typically adaptive systems begin to malfunction. This perspective allows us to study psychopathology within a framework that acknowledges the complex processes contributing to the onset and maintenance of disorders and offers a number of potential advantages. First, the insights of existing theories are translatable into self-regulation terms. For example, hopelessness, the core construct in Abramson et al.'s (2002) model of depression, can be conceptualized as a state in which the perceived probability of a positive outcome in approach-based (promotion-oriented) goal pursuit is zero (Cornette et al., 2009). Second, a self-regulation perspective can account for correlations across different components of motivational systems, such as associated changes in hedonic capacity, self-representation, approach motivation, interpersonal effectiveness, and hypothalamic–pituitary–adrenal (HPA) axis function following an experience of failure. Third, a self–brain–behavior perspective addresses the concern that the experience of loss or failure is frequently in the eye of the beholder and therefore only predictable based on the goals and beliefs that a particular individual possesses.

## CONCLUSION: TOWARD AN INTEGRATIVE PERSPECTIVE ON SELF-REGULATION AND PSYCHOPATHOLOGY

Psychopathology poses an enormous public health burden, with untold personal suffering and incalculable economic impact. At a time when extramural research funding trends have moved away from an emphasis on psychosocial factors to a more molecular view, social psychologists must reassert the essential contributions of their unique level of analysis. Likewise, given the unfortunate tendency for contemporary research in psychopathology and treatment to take a reductionistic neurobiological perspective, it has never been more important for the public interest that psychopathology research take seriously the models and data that social psychology has to offer. Ironically, as theories of psychopathology evolve to become more complex and dimensional and less strictly categorical, they increasingly draw situational factors into the diagnostic equation. Psychopathology does not lie solely under the skin, in the brain, or in each individual's unique past; it also is manifest in reactivity to ordinary and extraordinary circumstances, in how people are differentially exposed to pathogenic situations, and in tendencies to engage in activities that do not fit well with an individuals' underlying proclivities (Caspi, 2000). All of these contributory factors, we believe, can be seen as operating through the proximal influence of self-regulatory neurobiological and psychological processes.

One need only look at emerging data documenting the efficacy (and cost-effectiveness) of brief psychological interventions for depression and other disorders to be encouraged about the future applicability of self-regulation research to the treatment and prevention of psychopathology. For instance, not only is cognitive therapy (CT) as efficacious as antidepressant medication for mild, moderate, and even severe depression (DeRubeis et al., 2005), but CT outperforms medication in preventing relapse and recurrence (Hollon, Thase, & Markowitz, 2002). Furthermore, depressed individuals often manifest increasing resistance to subsequent trials of antidepressant medication, but no such resistance has been observed for CT. In turn, the mechanisms of action hypothesized to mediate the efficacy of CT can be understood in self-regulation terms (Strauman et al., 2001). In addition, a recently developed brief therapy for depression drawing on RFT, self-system therapy, has been shown to be as efficacious as standard CT and may be differentially effective for a subset of depressed individuals manifesting poor promotion goal pursuit capacities (Strauman et al., 2006).

Substantial evidence in favor of a more integrative, multilevel perspective on self-regulation currently exists. There are promising data from a number of disciplines, and our intent in this chapter has been to suggest how conceptual models might be developed in an explicit effort to study the mechanisms of self-regulation more comprehensively. We offer one final observation: the need for investigators in each field to examine their assumptions (often implicit) regarding what causes psychopathology if truly new, integrative models are to be realized. Kendler (2005) proposed the adoption of a multilevel perspective on psychopathology that acknowledged the reality of both *brain → mind* and *mind → brain* causal processes in the pathogenesis of mental disorders. Moreover, Kendler called for the widespread adoption of *explanatory pluralism*, in which investigators focusing on particular levels of analysis are more forthright about the importance of complementary levels and more ambitious in their efforts to collaborate in cross-level studies. As this volume illustrates, social psychology in general—and the study of self-regulation and goal pursuit more specifically—deserve a place at the table among contributors to a better understanding of psychopathology.

## REFERENCES

Abramson, L. Y., Alloy, L. B., Hankin, B. L., Haeffel, G. J., MacCoon, D. G., & Gibb, B. E. (2002). Cognitive vulnerability–stress models of depression in a self-regulatory psychobiological context. In I. H. Gotlib & C. L. Hammen (Eds.), *Handbook of depression* (pp. 268–294). New York: Guilford Press.

Akiskal, H. S., & McKinney, W. T. (1973). Depressive disorders: Toward a unified hypothesis. *Science*, *182*, 20–29.

Amico, K. R., Bruch, M. A., Haase, R. F., & Sturmer, P. J. (2004). Trait shyness, actual–ought self-discrepancy, and discomfort in social interaction. *Personality and Individual Differences*, *36*, 1597–1610.

Arnett, P. A., & Newman, J. P. (2000). Gray's three-arousal model: An empirical investigation. *Personality and Individual Differences*, *28*, 1171–1189.

Austin, J. T., & Vancouver, J. B. (1996). Goal constructs in psychology: Structure, process, and content. *Psychological Bulletin*, *120*(3), 338–375.

Avants, S. K., Margolin, A., & Singer, J. L. (1994). Self-reevaluation therapy: A cognitive intervention for the chemically dependent patient. *Psychology of Addictive Behaviors*, *8*(4), 214–222.

Avants, S. K., Singer, J. L., & Margolin, A. (1993–1994). Self-representations and negative affect in cocaine-dependent individuals. *Imagination, Cognition, and Personality*, *13*(1), 3–24.

Banaji, M. R., & Steele, C. M. (1989). The social cognition of alcohol use. *Social Cognition*, *7*, 137–151.

Bandura, A. (1986). *Social foundations of thought and action: A social cognitive theory*. Englewood Cliffs, NJ: Prentice-Hall.

Bandura, A. (2001). Social cognitive theory: An agentic perspective. *Annual Review of Psychology*, *52*, 1–26.

Bardone-Cone, A. M., Wonderlich, S. A., Frost, R. O., Bulik, C. M., Mitchell, J. E., Uppala, S., et al. (2007). Perfectionism and eating disorders: Current status and future directions. *Clinical Psychology Review*, *27*, 384–405.

Barkley, R. A. (2001). The executive functions and self-regulation: An evolutionary neuropsychological perspective. *Neuropsychology Review*, *11*, 1–25.

Barnett, L. A., Far, J. M., Mauss, A. L., & Miller, J. A. (1996). Changing perceptions of peer norms as a drinking reduction program for college students. *Journal of Alcohol and Drug Education*, *41*(2), 39–62.

Barry, E. S., Naus, M. J., & Rehm, L. P. (2006). Depression, implicit memory, and self: A revised memory model of emotion. *Clinical Psychology Review*, *26*, 719–745.

Bentall, R. P., Kinderman, P., & Manson, K. (2005). Self-discrepancies in bipolar disorder: Comparison of manic, depressed, remitted and normal participants. *British Journal of Clinical Psychology*, *44*, 457–473.

Bessenoff, G. R. (2006). Can the media affect us? Social comparison, self-discrepancy, and the thin ideal. *Psychology of Women Quarterly*, *30*, 239–251.

Blair, R., & Cipolotti, L. (2000). Impaired social response reversal: A case of acquired sociopathy. *Brain*, *123*, 1122–1141.

Blatt, S. J. (2004). *Experiences of depression: Theoretical, clinical, and research perspectives*. Washington, DC: American Psychological Association.

Bolton, D., & Hill, J. (2004). *Mind, meaning, and mental disorder: The nature of causal explanation in psychology and psychiatry* (2nd ed.). New York: Oxford University Press.

Bonin, M. F., McCreary, D. R., & Sadava, S. W. (2000). Problem drinking behavior in two community-based samples of adults: Influence of gender, coping, loneliness, and depression. *Psychology of Addictive Behaviors*, *14*, 151–161.

Bruch, M. A., Rivet, K. M., & Laurenti, H. J. (2000). Type of self-discrepancy and relationships to components of the tripartite model of emotional distress. *Personality and Individual Differences*, *29*, 37–44.

Brunstein, J. C. (1993). Personal goals and subjective well-being: A longitudinal study. *Journal of Personality and Social Psychology*, *65*, 1061–1070.

Cacioppo, J., Berntson, G. G., Sheridan, J. F., & McClintock, M. K. (2000). Multilevel integrative analyses of human behavior: Social neuroscience and the complementing nature of social and biological approaches. *Psychological Bulletin*, *126*, 829–843.

Cantor, J. B., Ashman, T. A., Schwartz, M. E., Gordon, W. A., Hibbard, M. R., Brown, M., et al. (2005). The role of self-discrepancy theory in understanding post-traumatic brain injury affective disorders: A pilot study. *Journal of Head Trauma Rehabilitation*, *20*(6), 527–543.

Cantor, N., & Kihlstrom, J. F. (1987). *Personality and social intelligence*. Englewood Cliffs, NJ: Prentice-Hall.

Cantor, N., & Zirkel, S. (1990). Personality, cognition, and purposive behavior. In L. A. Pervin (Ed.), *Handbook of personality: Theory and research* (pp. 135–164). Hillsdale, NJ: Erlbaum.

Carver, C. S. (1998). Generalization, adverse events, and development of depressive symptoms. *Journal of Personality*, *66*(4), 607–619.

Carver, C. S. (2004). Self-regulation of action and affect. In R. F. Baumeister & K. D. Vohs (Eds.), *Handbook of self-regulation: Research, theory, and applications* (pp. 13–39). New York: Guilford Press.

Carver, C. S. (2007). Stress, coping, and health. In H. S. Friedman & R. C. Silver (Eds.), *Foundations of health psychology* (pp. 117–144). New York: Oxford University Press.

Carver, C. S., Lawrence, J. W., & Scheier, M. F. (1999). Self-discrepancies and affect: Incorporating the role of feared selves. *Personality and Social Psychology Bulletin*, *25*, 783–792.

Carver, C. S., & Scheier, M. R. (1981). *Attention and self-regulation: A control theory approach to human behavior.* New York: Springer-Verlag.

Carver, C. S., & Scheier, M. R. (1990). Origins and functions of positive and negative affect: A control-process view. *Psychological Review*, *97*, 19–35.

Carver, C. S., & Scheier, M. R. (1998). *On the self-regulation of behavior.* New York: Cambridge University Press.

Carver, C. S., & Scheier, M. R. (1999). Themes and issues in the self-regulation of behavior. In R. S. Wyer, Jr. (Ed.), *Advances in social cognition* (pp. 1–105). Mahwah, NJ: Erlbaum.

Carver, C. S., & Scheier, M. F. (2000). On the structure of behavioral self-regulation. In M. Boekaerts,

P. R. Pintrich, & M. Zeidner (Eds.), *Handbook of self-regulation* (pp. 41–84). New York: Cambridge University Press.

Carver, C. S., Sutton, S. K., & Scheier, M. F. (2000). Action, emotion, and personality: Emerging conceptual integration. *Personality and Social Psychology Bulletin, 26*, 741–751.

Carver, C. S., & White, T. L. (1994). Behavioral inhibition, behavioral activation, and affective responses to impending reward and punishment: The BIS/BAS Scales. *Journal of Personality and Social Psychology, 67*, 319–333.

Cash, T. F., & Deagle, E. A. (1997). The nature and extent of body-image disturbances in anorexia nervosa and bulimia nervosa: A meta-analysis. *International Journal of Eating Disorders, 22*, 107–125.

Caspi, A. (2000). The child is father of the man: Personality continuities from childhood to adulthood. *Journal of Personality and Social Psychology, 78*, 158–172.

Cervone, D. (2000). Evolutionary psychology and explanation in personality psychology. *American Behavioral Scientist, 43*, 1001–1014.

Clark, L. A., Watson, D., & Mineka, S. (1994). Temperament, personality, and the mood and anxiety disorders. *Journal of Personality and Social Psychology, 54*, 296–308.

Cooper, R., & Shallice, T. (2000). Contention scheduling and the control of routine activities. *Cognitive Neuropsychology, 17*, 297–338.

Cornette, M. M., Strauman, T. J., Abramson, L. Y., & Busch, A. M. (2009). Self-discrepancy and suicidal ideation. *Cognition and Emotion, 23*, 504–527.

Cunningham, W. A., Raye, C. L., & Johnson, M. K. (2005). Neural correlates of evaluation associated with promotion and prevention regulatory focus. *Cognitive, Affective, and Behavioral Neuroscience, 5*, 202–211.

Damasio, A. R., Tranel, D., & Damasio, H. (1990). Individuals with sociopathic behavior caused by frontal damage fail to respond automatically to social stimuli. *Behavioral Brain Research, 41*, 81–94.

Depue, R. A., & Collins, P. (1999). Neurobiology of the structure of personality: Dopamine, facilitation of incentive motivation, and extraversion. *Behavioral and Brain Sciences, 22*, 491–569.

Depue, R. A., & Iacono, W. (1989). Neurobehavioral aspects of affective disorders. *Annual Review of Psychology, 40*, 457–492.

DeRubeis, R. J., Hollon, S. D., Amsterdam, J. D., Shelton, R. C., Young, P. R., Salomon, R. M., et al. (2005). Cognitive therapy versus medications in the treatment of moderate to severe depression. *Archives of General Psychiatry, 62*, 409–416.

Drabant, E. M., Hariri, A. R., Meyer-Lindenberg, A., Munoz, K. E., Mattay, V. S., Kolachana, B. S., et al. (2006). Catechol-O-methyltransferase val$^{158}$met genotype and neural mechanisms related to affective arousal and regulation. *Archives of General Psychiatry, 63*, 1396–1406.

Dunlop, B. W., & Nemeroff, C. B. (2007). The role of dopamine in the pathophysiology of depression. *Archives of General Psychiatry, 64*, 327–337.

Eddington, K. M., Dolcos, F., Cabeza, R., Krishnan, K. R. R., & Strauman, T. J. (2007). Neural correlates of promotion and prevention goal activation: An fMRI study using an idiographic approach. *Journal of Cognitive Neuroscience, 19*, 1152–1162.

Elliot, A. J., & Thrash, T. M. (2002). Approach–avoidance motivation in personality: Approach and avoidance temperaments and goals. *Journal of Personality and Social Psychology, 82*, 804–818.

Emmons, R. A., & King, L. A. (1988). Conflict among personal strivings: Immediate and long-term implications for psychological and physical well-being. *Journal of Personality and Social Psychology, 48*, 1040–1048.

Fairbrother, N., & Moretti, M. (1998). Sociotropy, autonomy, and self-discrepancy: Status in depressed, remitted depressed, and control participants. *Cognitive Therapy and Research, 22*, 279–297.

Förster, J., Grant, H., Idson, L. C., & Higgins, E. T. (2001). Success/failure feedback, expectancies, and approach/avoidance motivation: How regulatory focus moderates classic relations. *Journal of Experimental Social Psychology, 37*, 253–260.

Forston, M. T., & Stanton, A. L. (1992). Self-discrepancy theory as a framework for understanding bulimic symptomatology and associated distress. *Journal of Social and Clinical Psychology, 11*(2), 103–118.

Fowles, D. C. (1994). A motivational theory of psychopathology. In W. Spaulding (Ed.), *Integrative views of motivation, cognition, and emotion. Nebraska symposium on motivation, Vol. 41* (pp. 181–238). Lincoln: University of Nebraska Press.

Fraga, M. F., Ballestar, E., Paz, M. F., Ropero, S., Setien, F., Ballestar, M. L., et al. (2005). Epigenetic differences arise during the lifetime of monozygotic twins. *Proceedings of the National Academy of Sciences, 102*, 10604–10609.

Fromson, P. M. (2006). Self-discrepancies and negative affect: The moderating roles of private and public self-consciousness. *Social Behavior and Personality, 34*(4), 333–350.

Gable, S. L., Reis, H. T., & Elliot, A. J. (2003). Evidence for bivariate systems: An empirical test of appetition and aversion across domains. *Journal of Research in Personality, 37*, 349–372.

Gainetdinov, R. R., & Caron, M. G. (2003). Monoamine transporters: From genes to behavior. *Annual Review of Pharmacology and Toxicology, 43*, 261–284.

Gibbons, F. X., Gerrard, M., Vande Lune, L. S., Wills, T. A., Brody, G., & Conger, R. D. (2004). Context and cognitions: Environmental risk, social influence, and adolescent substance use. *Personality and Social Psychology Bulletin, 30*(8), 1048–1061.

Glimcher, P. W., & Kanwisher, N. (2006). Cognitive neuroscience: Editorial overview. *Current Opinion in Neurobiology, 16*, 127–129.

Gonnerman, M. E., Jr., Lavine, H., & Huff, J. (2000). The relationship between self-discrepancies and affective states: The moderating roles of self-monitoring and standpoints on the self. *Personality and Social Psychology Bulletin, 26*(7), 810–819.

Gray, J. A. (1990). Brain systems that mediate both emotion and cognition. *Cognition and Emotion, 4*, 269–288.

Hariri, A. R., Drabant, E. M., & Weinberger, D. R. (2006). Imaging genetics: Perspectives from studies of genetically driven variation in serotonin function and corticolimbic affective processing. *Biological Psychiatry, 59*, 888–897.

Harrison, K. (2001). Ourselves, our bodies: Thin-ideal media, self-discrepancies, and eating disorder symptomatology in adolescents. *Journal of Social and Clinical Psychology, 20*, 289–323.

Harrison, K., & Hefner, V. (2006). Media exposure, current and future body ideals, and disordered eating among preadolescent girls: A longitudinal panel study. *Journal of Youth and Adolescence, 35*(2), 153–163.

Hart, T., Schwartz, M. F., & Mayer, N. (1999). Executive function: Some current theories and their applications. In N. R. Varney & R. J. Roberts (Eds.), *The evaluation and treatment of mild traumatic brain injury* (pp. 133–148). Mahwah, NJ: Erlbaum.

Heatherton, T. F., & Baumeister, R. F. (1991). Binge eating as escape from self-awareness. *Psychological Bulletin, 110*(1), 86–108.

Heppen, J. B., & Ogilvie, D. M. (2003). Predicting affect from global self-discrepancies: The dual role of the undesired self. *Journal of Social and Clinical Psychology, 22*(4), 347–368.

Higgins, E. T. (1987). Self-discrepancy: A theory relating self and affect. *Psychological Review, 94*, 319–340.

Higgins, E. T. (1990). Personality, social psychology, and person-situation relations: Standards and knowledge activation as a common language. In L. A. Pervin (Ed.), *Handbook of personality: Theory and research* (pp. 301–338). New York: Guilford Press.

Higgins, E. T. (1997). Beyond pleasure and pain. *American Psychologist, 52*, 1280–1300.

Higgins, E. T. (1998). Promotion and prevention: Regulatory focus as a motivational principle. In M. P. Zanna (Ed.), *Advances in experimental social psychology* (Vol. 30, pp. 1–46). New York: Academic Press.

Higgins, E. T. (1999). When do self-discrepancies have specific relations to emotions? The second-generation question of Tangney, Niedenthal, Covert, and Barlow (1998). *Journal of Personality and Social Psychology, 77*, 1313–1317.

Higgins, E. T., Bond, R., Klein, R., & Strauman, T. J. (1986). Self-discrepancies and emotional vulnerability: How magnitude, type and accessibility of discrepancy influence affect. *Journal of Personality and Social Psychology*, *51*, 5–15.

Higgins, E. T., Klein, R., & Strauman, T. J. (1985). Self-concept discrepancy theory: A psychological model for distinguishing among aspects of depression and anxiety. *Social Cognition*, *3*(1), 51–76.

Higgins, E. T., Roney, C., Crowe, E., & Hymes, C. (1994). Ideal versus ought predilections for approach and avoidance: Distinct self-regulatory systems. *Journal of Personality and Social Psychology*, *66*, 276–286.

Higgins, E. T., & Spiegel, S. (2004). Promotion and prevention strategies for self-regulation: A motivated cognition perspective. In R. F. Baumeister & K. D. Vohs (Eds.), *Handbook of self-regulation: Research, theory, and applications* (pp. 171–187). New York: Guilford Press.

Higgins, E. T., Strauman, T. J., & Klein, R. (1987). Self-discrepancies: Distinguishing among self-states, self-state conflicts, and emotional vulnerabilities. In K. Yardley & T. Honess (Eds.), *Self and identity: Psychosocial perspectives* (pp. 130–155). New York: Wiley.

Hollon, S. D., Thase, M. E., & Markowitz, J. C. (2002). Treatment and prevention of depression. *Psychological Science in the Public Interest*, *3*, 39–77.

Hoyle, R. H., Kernis, M. H., Leary, M. R., & Baldwin, M. W. (1999). *Selfhood: Identity, esteem, regulation*. Boulder, CO: Westview Press.

Hyland, M. E. (1987). Control theory interpretation of psychological mechanism of depression: Comparison and integration of several theories. *Psychological Bulletin*, *102*, 109–121.

John, O. P., & Gross, J. J. (2007). Individual differences in emotion regulation. In J. J. Gross (Ed.), *Handbook of emotion regulation* (pp. 351–372). New York: Guilford Press.

Johnson, S. L. (2005). Mania and dysregulation in goal pursuit: A review. *Clinical Psychology Review*, *25*, 241–262.

Johnson, S. L., & Carver, C. S. (2006). Extreme goal setting and vulnerability to mania among undiagnosed young adults. *Cognitive Therapy and Research*, *30*, 377–395.

Johnson, S. L., Turner, R. J., & Iwata, N. (2003). BIS/BAS levels and psychiatric disorder: An epidemiological study. *Journal of Psychopathology and Behavioral Assessment*, *25*(1), 25–36.

Kagan, J. (2003). Biology, context, and developmental inquiry. *Annual Review of Psychology*, *54*, 1–23.

Karoly, P. (1993). Mechanisms of self-regulation: A systems view. *Annual Review of Psychology*, *44*, 23–52.

Karoly, P. (1999). A goal systems self-regulatory perspective on personality, psychopathology, and change. *Review of General Psychology*, *3*, 264–291.

Kasch, K. L., Rottenberg, J., Arnow, B. A., & Gotlib, I. H. (2002). Behavioral activation and inhibition systems and the severity and course of depression. *Journal of Abnormal Psychology*, *111*, 589–597.

Katz, J., & Farrow, S. (2000). Discrepant self-views and young women's sexual and emotional adjustment. *Sex Roles*, *42*(9/10), 781–805.

Kendler, K. S. (2005). Toward a philosophical structure for psychiatry. *American Journal of Psychiatry*, *162*, 433–440.

King, L. A., Richards, J. H., & Stemmerich, E. (1998). Daily goals, life goals, and worst fears: Means, ends, and subjective well-being. *Journal of Personality*, *66*, 713–744.

Kling, A., & Steklis, H. D. (1976). A neural substrate for affiliative behavior in nonhuman primates. *Brain, Behavior and Evolution*, *13*, 216–238.

Kochanska, G. (1995). Children's temperament, mothers' discipline, and security of attachment: Multiple pathways to emerging internalization. *Child Development*, *66*, 597–615.

Lawrence, J. W., Carver, C. S., & Scheier, M. F. (2002). Velocity toward goal attainment in immediate experience as a determinant of affect. *Journal of Applied Social Psychology*, *32*, 788–802.

Leary, M. R., & Buttermore, N. R. (2003). The evolution of the human self: Tracing the natural history of self-awareness. *Journal for the Theory of Social Behaviour*, *33*, 365–404.

LeDoux, J. E. (2000). Emotion circuits in the brain. *Annual Review of Neuroscience*, *23*, 155–184.

Lee, M., & Shafran, R. (2004). Information processing biases in eating disorders. *Clinical Psychology Review*, *24*, 215–238.

Lewis, M. D., & Todd, R. M. (2007). The self-regulating brain: Cortical-subcortical feedback and the development of intelligent action. *Cognitive Development*, *22*, 406–430.

Little, B. R. (2006). Personality science and self-regulation: Personal projects as integrative units. *Applied Psychology: An International Review*, *55*(3), 419–427.

Lyubomirsky, S., Tucker, K. L., Caldwell, N. D., & Berg, K. (1999). Why ruminators are poor problem solvers: Clues from the phenomenology of dysphoric rumination. *Journal of Personality and Social Psychology*, *77*, 1041–1060.

MacAndrew, C., & Steele, T. (1991). Gray's behavioral inhibition system: A psychometric examination. *Personality and Individual Differences*, *12*, 157–171.

Manian, N., Papadakis, A. A., Strauman, T. J., & Essex, M. J. (2006). The development of children's ideal and ought self-guides: The influence of parenting on individual differences in guide strength. *Journal of Personality*, *74*, 1619–1645.

Mansell, W. (2005). Control theory and psychopathology: An integrative approach. *Psychology and Psychotherapy: Theory, Research, and Practice*, *78*, 141–178.

Martin, L., & Tesser, A. (1996). Some ruminative thoughts. In R. S. Wyer (Eds.), *Advances in Social Cognition* (Vol. 9., pp. 1–48). Hillsdale, NJ: Erlbaum.

Mayberg, H. S. (2003). Modulating dysfunctional limbic-cortical circuits in depression: Towards development of brain-based algorithms for diagnosis and optimised treatment. *British Medical Bulletin*, *65*, 193–207.

McCrae, R. R., & Costa, P. T., Jr. (1997). Personality trait structure as a human universal. *American Psychologist*, *52*, 509–516.

Miller, A. K., & Markman, K. D. (2007). Depression, regulatory focus, and motivation. *Personality and Individual Differences*, *43*, 427–436.

Miller, G. A., Galanter, E., & Pribram, K. H. (1960). *Plans and the structure of behavior.* New York: Holt, Rinehart & Winston.

Mischel, W. (1966). Theory and research on the antecedents of self-imposed delay of reward. In B. A. Maher (Ed.), *Progress in experimental personality research* (Vol. 3, pp. 85–131). New York: Academic Press.

Mischel, W. (1990). Personality dispositions revisited and revised: A view after three decades. In L. Pervin (Ed.), *Handbook of personality: Theory and research* (pp. 111–134). New York: Guilford Press.

Mischel W., & Moore, B. (1973). Effects of attention to symbolically presented rewards on self-control. *Journal of Personality and Social Psychology*, *28*, 172–179.

Moffitt, T. E., Caspi, A., & Rutter, R. (2005). Strategy for investigating interactions between measured genes and measured environments. *Archives of General Psychiatry*, *62*, 473–485.

Moscovitch, D. A., Hofmann, S. G., & Litz, B. T. (2005). The impact of self-construals on social anxiety: A gender-specific interaction. *Personality and Individual Differences*, *38*, 659–672.

Nelson, C. A., Bloom, F. E., Cameron, J. L., Amaral, D., Dahl, R. E., & Pine, D. (2002). An integrative, multidisciplinary approach to the study of brain–behavior relations in the context of typical and atypical development. *Development and Psychopathology*, *14*, 499–520.

Nolen-Hoeksema, S. (2000). The role of rumination in depressive disorders and mixed anxiety/depressive symptoms. *Journal of Abnormal Psychology*, *109*, 504–511.

Nolen-Hoeksema, S., Morrow, J., & Fredrickson, B. L. (1993). Response styles and the duration of episodes of depressed mood. *Journal of Abnormal Psychology*, *102*, 20–28.

Papadakis, A. A., Prince, R. P., Jones, N. P., & Strauman, T. J. (2006). Self-regulation, rumination, and vulnerability to depression in adolescent girls. *Development and Psychopathology*, *18*, 815–829.

Paykel, E. C. (2003). Life events and affective disorders. *Acta Psychiatrica Scandinavica*, *108*(418), 61–66.

Polivy, J., Herman, C. P., & McFarlane, T. (1994). Effects of anxiety on eating: Does palatability moderate distress-induced overeating in dieters? *Journal of Abnormal Psychology*, *103*, 505–510.

Posner, M. I., & Rothbart, M. K. (2000). Developing mechanisms of self-regulation. *Development and Psychopathology*, *12*, 427–441.

Post, R. M., & Weiss, S. R. B. (2002). Psychological complexity: Barriers to its integration into the neurobiology of major psychiatric disorders. *Development and Psychopathology*, *14*, 635–651.

Powers, W. T. (1973). *Behavior: The control of perception*. Chicago: Aldine.

Pretz, J. E., Naples, A. J., & Sternberg, R. J. (2003). Recognizing, defining, and representing problems. In J. E. Davidson & R. J. Sternberg (Eds.), *The psychology of problem solving* (pp. 3–30). New York: Cambridge University Press.

Revelle, W. (1995). Personality processes. *Annual Review of Psychology*, *46*, 295–328.

Rodebaugh, T. L., & Donahue, K. L. (2007). Could you be more specific, please: Self-discrepancies, affect, and variation in specificity and relevance. *Journal of Clinical Psychology*, *63*(12), 1193–1207.

Roelofs, J., Papageorgiou, C., Gerber, R. D., Huibers, M., Peeters, F., & Arntz, A. (2007). On the links between self-discrepancies, rumination, metacognitions, and symptoms of depression in undergraduates. *Behaviour Research and Therapy*, *45*, 1295–1305.

Ryan, R. M., Kuhl, J., & Deci, E. L. (1997). Nature and autonomy: An organizational view of social and neurobiological aspects of self-regulation in behavior and development. *Development and Psychopathology*, *9*, 701–728.

Sayette, M. A., Martin, C. S., Wertz, J. M., Shiffman, S., & Perrott, M. A. (2001). A multidimensional analysis of cue-elicited craving in heavy smokers and tobacco chippers. *Addiction*, *96*, 1419–1432.

Scott, L., & O'Hara, M. W. (1993). Self-discrepancies in clinically anxious and depressed university students. *Journal of Abnormal Psychology*, *102*, 282–287.

Shah, J. Y., & Higgins, E. T. (2001). Regulatory concerns and appraisal efficiency: The general impact of promotion and prevention. *Journal of Personality and Social Psychology*, *80*, 693–705.

Shah, J. Y., & Kruglanski, A. W. (2000). Aspects of goal networks: Implications for self-regulation. In M. Boekaerts, P. R. Pintrich, & M. Zeidner (Eds.), *Handbook of self-regulation* (pp. 41–84). San Diego, CA: Academic Press.

Showers, C. J., Abramson, L. Y., & Hogan, M. E. (1998). The dynamic self: How the content and structure of the self-concept change with mood. *Journal of Personality and Social Psychology*, *75*(2), 478–493.

Snyder, R. (1997). Self-discrepancy theory, standards for body evaluation, and eating disorder symptomatology among college women. *Women and Health*, *26*, 69–84.

Steele, C. M., & Josephs, R. A. (1990). Alcohol myopia: Its prized and dangerous effects. *American Psychologist*, *45*, 921–933.

Strauman, T. J. (1989). Self-discrepancies in clinical depression and social phobia: Cognitive structures that underlie emotional disorders? *Journal of Abnormal Psychology*, *98*, 14–22.

Strauman, T. J. (1992). Self-guides, autobiographical memory, and anxiety and dysphoria: Toward a cognitive model of vulnerability to emotional distress. *Journal of Abnormal Psychology*, *101*, 87–95.

Strauman, T. J. (1996). Stability within the self: A longitudinal study of the structural implications of self-discrepancy theory. *Journal of Personality and Social Psychology*, *71*, 1142–1153.

Strauman, T. J. (2002). Self-regulation and depression. *Self and Identity*, *1*, 151–157.

Strauman, T. J., Coe, C. L., Woods, T., Schneider, K., & Kwapil, L. (2004). Self-regulatory cognition and immune reactivity: Idiographic success and failure feedback effects on the natural killer cell. *Brain, Behavior, and Immunity*, *18*, 544–554.

Strauman, T. J., & Glenberg, A. M. (1994). Self-concept and body-image disturbance: Which self-beliefs predict body size overestimation? *Cognitive Research and Therapy*, *18*, 105–125.

Strauman, T. J., & Higgins, E. T. (1987). Automatic activation of self-discrepancies and emotional syndromes: When cognitive structures influence affect. *Journal of Personality and Social Psychology*, *53*, 1004–1014.

Strauman, T. J., & Higgins, E. T. (1988). Self-discrepancies as predictors of vulnerability to different syndromes of chronic emotional distress. *Journal of Personality, 56*, 685–707.

Strauman, T. J., & Kolden, G. G. (1997). The self in depression: Research trends and clinical implications. *In Session, 3*, 5–21.

Strauman, T. J., Kolden, G., Davis, N., Stromquist, V., Kwapil, L., & Heerey, E. (2001). The effects of treatments for depression on failure in self-regulation. *Cognitive Therapy and Research, 25*, 693–712.

Strauman, T. J., Lemieux, A., & Coe, C. (1993). Self-discrepancies and natural killer cell activity: The influence of individual differences in self-regulation on stress physiology. *Journal of Personality and Social Psychology, 64*, 1042–1052.

Strauman, T. J., Vieth, A. Z., Merrill, K. A., Kolden, G. G., Woods, T. E., Klein, M. H., et al. (2006). Self-system therapy as an intervention for self-regulatory dysfunction in depression: A randomized comparison with cognitive therapy. *Journal of Consulting and Clinical Psychology, 74*, 367–376.

Strauman, T. J., Vookles, J., Berenstein, V., Chaiken, S., & Higgins, E. T. (1991). Self-discrepancies and vulnerability to body dissatisfaction and disordered eating. *Journal of Personality and Social Psychology, 61*, 946–956.

Stravynski, A., Bond, S., & Amado, D. (2004). Cognitive causes of social phobia: A critical appraisal. *Clinical Psychology Review, 24*, 421–440.

Stuss, D. T., & Alexander, M. P. (2000). The anatomical basis of affective behavior, emotion and self-awareness: A specific role of the right frontal lobe. In G. Hatano, N. Okada, & H. Tanabe (Eds.), *Affective minds: The 13th Toyota conference* (pp. 13–25). Shizuoke, Japan: Elsevier Science.

Stuss, D. T., & Levine, B. (2002). Adult clinical neuropsychology: Lessons from studies of the frontal lobes. *Annual Review of Psychology, 53*, 401–433.

Szymanski, M. L., & Cash, T. F. (1995). Body-image disturbances and self-discrepancy theory: Expansion of the body-image ideals questionnaire. *Journal of Social and Clinical Psychology, 14*, 134–146.

Tangney, J. P., Niedenthal, P. M., Covert, M. V., & Barlow, D. H. (1998). Are shame and guilt related to distinct self-discrepancies? A test of Higgins's (1987) hypotheses. *Journal of Personality and Social Psychology, 75*, 256–268.

Tanner, W. P., Jr., & Swets, J. A. (1954). A decision making-theory of visual detection. *Psychological Review, 61*, 401–409.

Tarter, R. E. (2002). Etiology of adolescent substance abuse: A developmental perspective. *American Journal on Addictions, 11*, 171–191.

Tomarken, A. J., & Keener, A. D. (1998). Frontal brain asymmetry and depression: A self-regulatory perspective. *Cognition and Emotion, 12*(3), 387–420.

Vancouver, J. B. (2005). The depth of history and explanations as benefit and bane for psychological control theories. *Journal of Applied Psychology, 90*(1), 38–52.

Veale, D., Kinderman, P., Riley, S., & Lambrou, C. (2003). Self-discrepancy in body dysmorphic disorder. *British Journal of Clinical Psychology, 42*, 157–169.

Viding, E., Williamson, D. E., & Hariri, A. R. (2006). Developmental imaging genetics: Challenges and promises for translational research. *Development and Psychopathology, 18*, 877–892.

Vieth, A., Strauman, T. J., Kolden, G., Woods, T., & Klein, M. H. (2003). Self-System Therapy: A theory-based psychotherapy for depression. *Clinical Psychology: Science and Practice, 10*, 245–268.

Volkow, N. D., & Fowler, J. S. (2000). Addiction, a disease of compulsion and drive: Involvement of the orbitofrontal cortex. *Cerebral Cortex, 10*, 318–325.

Watson, D. (2005). Rethinking the mood and anxiety disorders: A quantitative hierarchical model for DSM-V. *Journal of Abnormal Psychology, 114*, 522–536.

Watson, D., Wiese, D., Vaidya, J., & Tellegen, A. (1999). The two general activation systems of affect:

Structural findings, evolutionary considerations, and psychobiological evidence. *Journal of Personality and Social Psychology*, *76*, 820–838.

Weilage, M., & Hope, D. A. (1999). Self-discrepancy in social phobia and dysthymia. *Cognitive Therapy and Research*, *23*, 637–650.

Wenzlaff, R. M., & Wegner, D. M. (2000). Thought suppression. In S. T. Fiske (Ed.), *Annual review of psychology* (Vol. 51, pp. 59–91). Palo Alto, CA: Annual Reviews.

Wolfe, W. L., & Maisto, S. A. (2000). The effect of self-discrepancy and discrepancy salience on alcohol consumption. *Addictive Behaviors*, *25*(2), 283–288.

Wolfe, W. L., & Maisto, S. A. (2007). The effect of alcohol on body size discrepancy and self-awareness in young women. *Psychology of Addictive Behaviors*, *32*, 2340–2344.

Wonderlich, S. A., Engel, S. G., Peterson, C. B., Robinson, M., Crosby, R. D., Mitchell, J. E., et al. (2008). Examining the conceptual model of integrative cognitive-affective therapy for BN: Two assessment studies. *International Journal of Eating Disorders*, *41*, 748–754.

# 7 Strategies of Setting and Implementing Goals

## *Mental Contrasting and Implementation Intentions*

Gabriele Oettingen
Peter M. Gollwitzer

When Viktor Frankl (1959/1984) reflected on how to master the challenges of life, in his case the horrendous task of living through a concentration camp, he found the following answer:

> It did not really matter what we expected from life, but rather what life expected from us. We needed to stop asking about the meaning of life, and instead to think of ourselves as those who were being questioned by life—daily and hourly. Our answer must consist, not in talk and meditation, but in right action and in right conduct. Life ultimately means taking the responsibility to find the right answer to its problems and to fulfill the tasks which it constantly sets for each individual. (p. 122)

Frankl seems to suggest that taking charge of one's actions is the way to master the challenges of daily life. But how can people take charge of their actions? In the present chapter, we suggest an effective way of taking charge of one's actions: self-regulating one's goal pursuits.

Research on the psychology of goals suggests that successful goal pursuit hinges on solving two sequential tasks: goal setting and goal implementation. The distinction between the setting and the implementing of goals was originally emphasized by Kurt Lewin (1926; Lewin, Dembo, Festinger, & Sears, 1944). This distinction turns out to be very useful for understanding the many new findings produced by the recent upsurge of research on goals (Bargh, Gollwitzer, & Oettingen, 2010; Oettingen & Gollwitzer, 2001), and thus we use it to organize the present chapter. We first discuss research on the self-regulation of setting goals, and then turn to findings on the self-regulation of implementing set goals. Finally, we propose a self-regulation-enhancing intervention that capitalizes on acquiring and using these goal setting and goal implementation strategies.

## SETTING GOALS

If people want to achieve their goals, they need to set goals framed in a way that maximizes their attainment. Framing one's goals in terms of promoting positive outcomes versus preventing negative outcomes (promotion vs. prevention goals; Higgins, 1997) facilitates goal attainment, as does attempting to acquire competence rather than demonstrate the possession of competence (learning vs. performance goals; Dweck, 1999; Dweck & Elliot-Moskwa, Chapter 8, this volume), and anticipating internal rewards rather than external rewards (intrinsic vs. extrinsic goals; Ryan & Deci, 2001). That is, promotion, learning, and intrinsic goals are commonly attained more successfully than prevention, performance, and extrinsic goals. The precision with which the desired future outcome is explicated also influences success in goal attainment. For example, goals with a proximal versus a distal time frame (Bandura & Schunk, 1981) are more likely to be achieved, and goals with specific rather than vague standards (e.g., "I will do my best") lead to better performances (Locke & Latham, 1990).

It is also useful to set goals to which one can strongly commit because such goals (intentions) have a better chance of being attained (Ajzen, 1991; meta-analysis by Webb & Sheeran, 2006). Strong goal commitments are based on the belief that a given goal is both highly desirable and feasible (Ajzen, 1991; Atkinson, 1957; Bandura, 1997; Gollwitzer, 1990; Klinger, 1975; Locke & Latham, 1990). *Desirability* comprises the summarized beliefs about the pleasantness of expected short-term and long-term consequences of goal attainment (Heckhausen, 1977). *Feasibility* is defined as expectations that future events and actions will occur (Gollwitzer, 1990). Prominent examples include expectations of whether one can execute a behavior necessary for realizing a specific outcome (i.e., self-efficacy expectations; Bandura, 1977, 1997; Maddux, 1999), expectations that a behavior will lead to a specified outcome (i.e., outcome expectations; Bandura, 1977; instrumentality beliefs; Vroom, 1964), and judgments about the general likelihood of a certain outcome (i.e., general expectations; Oettingen & Mayer, 2002). It is important to recognize, however, that perceiving a desirable goal as feasible does not guarantee strong goal commitment yet.

### Effective Goal Setting: The Self-Regulation Strategy of Mental Contrasting

The model of *fantasy realization* differentiates three modes of self-regulatory thought: mental contrasting, indulging, and dwelling (Oettingen, 2000; Oettingen, Pak, & Schnetter, 2001). It proposes that mentally contrasting a desired future with the reality that impedes its realization will create expectancy-dependent goal commitments. Specifically, in *mental contrasting*, people imagine the attainment of a desired future (e.g., becoming a clinical psychologist; giving a good talk) and then reflect on the present reality that stands in the way of attaining the desired future (e.g., high competition for the qualified programs; evaluation anxiety). The conjoint elaboration of the future and the present reality makes both simultaneously accessible and links them together in the sense that the reality stands in the way of realizing the desired future. Mental contrasting helps people to make up their mind about whether to commit to the goal of realizing the future by scrutinizing the feasibility of reaching the goal. When feasibility (expectations of success) is high, people commit strongly to attaining the goal; when feasibility is low, they form a weak goal commitment or none at all. In other words, mental contrasting makes a person sensitive to the question of which goals are reachable, and it gets people to go for reachable goals and keep clear of unreachable ones. This strategy ultimately should protect personal resources (time, energy, and money), as people will not show any engagement in the face of unreachable goals, but will engage without restraint in the face of reachable goals.

In line with Newell and Simon's (1972) theory of problem solving, fantasy realization theory envisages people who want to achieve an imagined positive future as facing the problem of wanting something and needing to engage in actions that they can perform to attain the desired outcome (p. 72). Accordingly, the objective problem space (defined as the objective task demands posed by the environment) entails both the desired future and the impediments to getting there. If the subjective problem space (defined as the internal subjective representation of the problem at hand) matches the objective problem space, people will recognize that they need to act on the status quo in order to arrive at the desired future. Therefore, the perceived feasibility (expectations of success) of attaining the desired future should determine people's commitment to attaining the desired future.

However, if the subjective problem space entails only part of the objective problem space (either only the positive future or only the negative status quo), people will fail to recognize that they need to act on the status quo in order to arrive at the desired future. Accordingly, goal commitments stemming from focusing only on a positive future or focusing only on a negative reality (i.e., indulging or dwelling) should fail to be expectancy-dependent. That is, the level of goal commitment reflects the a priori commitment that people hold with respect to the issue at hand, regardless of whether their expectations of success are high or low (Oettingen et al., 2001).

In sum, only mental contrasting, not one-sided elaborations of either the future or the reality adjusts goal commitments to people's expectations of success. That is, indulging and dwelling are less effective in protecting people's resources than is mental contrasting; individuals who indulge and dwell show a medium level of engagement even when no engagement (in the case of low expectations of success) or full engagement (in the case of high expectations of success) would be the resource-efficient strategy.

One might argue that the model of fantasy realization resembles cybernetic theories such as the test–operate–test–exit model (TOTE; Miller, Galanter, & Pribram, 1960), the theory of the control of perception (Powers, 1973), or its spin-off, the self-regulatory control-process model (Carver & Scheier, 1990). These feedback loop models share with fantasy realization theory their focus on the control of behavior or perception. However, in contrast to fantasy realization theory, the cybernetic models assume that a discrepancy between feedback (given state) and a set standard (ideal state) is discovered by a comparator and thus leads to attempts to reduce the discovered discrepancy. Fantasy realization theory specifies strategies that differentially influence whether people will use their fantasies about a desired future to build smart (expectancy-dependent) goal commitments. Elaborating the desired future and seeing the reality as a potential obstacle leads to smart (selective) goal commitment. One-sided thinking will lead to uniform, moderate goal commitment. That is, fantasy realization theory pertains to vague fantasies about the future and not to a set standard, it refers to anticipating potential obstacles and not to experienced feedback, and it assumes a link between future and obstacle, and not a comparator. In addition, it specifies modes of thought that divert a person from discrepancy reduction despite existing discrepancies. In short, feedback, standard, and comparator—the central variables in the feedback loop models—do not play a role in fantasy realization theory, which specifies the strategies that people can use to create goal commitments that are either based or not based on their expectations of success (see also, Oettingen & Kappes, 2009).

Fantasy realization theory may also be associated with the concept of possible selves (Markus & Nurius, 1986; Oyserman & Markus, 1990)—that is, individuals' ideas of what they might become, what they would like to become, and what they are afraid of becoming. Possible selves are the cognitive components of hopes, expectations, fears, goals, and threats, and they work as incentives for behavior. Fantasy realization theory shares with the concept its focus on thinking about the future. In contrast to the omnibus concept of possible selves, however, fantasy realization theory focuses on the processes that turn vague ideas about future selves either into binding goal commitments based on a person's expectations of success or into half-hearted goal commitments that are oblivious to the person's perceived chances of success.

## Empirical Evidence

A multitude of studies have tested the effects of mental contrasting, indulging, and dwelling on goal commitment and goal striving (i.e., goal pursuit; Oettingen, 2000; Oettingen et al., 2001). For example, in one study, freshmen enrolled in a vocational school for computer programming (Oettingen et al., 2001, Study 4) first indicated their expectations of excelling in mathematics. Then they named aspects that they associated with excelling in mathematics (e.g., feelings of pride, increasing job prospects) and impediments to excelling (e.g., being distracted, feeling lazy). Subsequently, three experimental conditions were established to correspond with the three modes of thought. In the mental contrasting condition, participants had to elaborate in writing two positive aspects of the future and two aspects of reality, in alternating order, beginning with a positive aspect of the future. Participants in the indulging condition were asked to elaborate four positive aspects of the future. In the dwelling condition, they instead elaborated four negative aspects of reality. As a dependent variable, participants indicated how energized they felt with respect to excelling in mathematics (e.g., how active, eventful, energetic). Further, 2 weeks after the experiment, participants' teachers reported how much effort each student had invested for the last 2 weeks and provided each student with a grade for that time period.

As predicted, only in the mental contrasting group did the students feel energized, exert effort, and earn grades in accord with their expectations: Those with high expectations of success felt the most energized, invested the most effort, and received the highest course grades, while those with low expectations of success felt the least energized, invested the least effort, and received the lowest course grades. To the contrary, participants in the indulging and dwelling conditions felt moderately energized, exerted moderate effort, and received moderate grades independent of their expectations of success.

A variety of studies pertaining to different life domains have replicated this pattern of results. For example, experiments pertained to studying abroad (Oettingen et al., 2001,

Study 2) and acquiring a second language (Oettingen et al., 2000, Study 1); to giving and receiving help (Oettingen, Mayer, Stephens, & Brinkmann, in press), getting to know an attractive stranger (Oettingen, 2000, Study 1), finding a balance between work and family life (Oettingen, 2000, Study 2), and improving oneself (Oettingen, Mayer, Thorpe, Janetzke, & Lorenz, 2005, Study 1), to smoking reduction (Oettingen, Mayer, & Thorpe, in press) as well as to various idiosyncratic interpersonal and personal wishes of great importance (Oettingen et al., 2001, Studies 1 and 3). Further, goal commitment and goal striving were assessed by cognitive (e.g., making plans), affective (e.g., feeling responsible for the wished-for ending), motivational (e.g., feeling energized), and behavioral indicators (e.g., invested effort and achievements). Indicators were measured via self-report or observations and either directly after the experiment or weeks later. In all of these studies the same pattern of results appeared: Given high expectations of success, participants in the mental contrasting group showed the strongest goal commitment and goal striving; given low expectations, people showed the least goal commitment and goal striving. Participants who indulged in positive images about the future or who dwelled on negative images of reality showed moderate commitment regardless of their expectations of success.

The outcomes of mental contrasting do not occur as a result of changes in expectations (feasibility) or incentive value (desirability), but rather as a result of the mode of self-regulatory thought, aligning commitment with expectations (Oettingen et al., 2001, 2009). Furthermore, the effects of mental contrasting depend on the person perceiving that the present reality is standing in the way of realizing the future. When engaging in mental contrasting, individuals first elaborate a desired future and establish it as their reference point, and then elaborate aspects of the present reality, thereby perceiving the negative aspects as obstacles standing in the way of attaining the future. Reversing this order (i.e., reverse contrasting), by first elaborating the negative reality and then elaborating the desired future, conceals seeing present reality as an obstacle to fantasy realization and thus fails to elicit goal commitment congruent with expectations of success (Oettingen et al., 2001, Study 3). The studies presented next explore the underlying motivational and cognitive processes responsible for the reported effects of mental contrasting and provide neurological data substantiating and extending the theoretical principles.

## Mechanisms of Mental Contrasting

### *Energization*

Locke and Latham (2002) identify feelings of energization as critical to promoting goal-directed behavior. They contend that commitment to realizing a desired future is linked to an energizing function, also referred to as *activity incitement* (Brunstein & Gollwitzer, 1996). For example, desired futures that prove more challenging to achieve (e.g., high school students practicing the Scholastic Aptitude Test [SAT], setting their sights on beating their personal score) give rise to greater effort than less challenging desired futures (e.g., high school students practicing the SAT, setting their sights on achieving their usual score; Locke & Latham, 2002). Energization was hypothesized and found to mediate the effects of mental contrasting on fostering selective goal pursuit (i.e., goal setting and goal striving) as measured by persistence as well as subjective and objective quality of performance (Oettingen et al., 2009). Specifically, economics students were informed that they were to deliver a speech in front of a video camera to help with the development of a measure of professional skills. Participants were randomly assigned to either a mental contrasting or an indulging condition. As dependent variables, the students indicated their initial feelings of energization (e.g., "How energized do you feel when you think about giving your talk?"), and they were asked to rate their actual performance. Persistence of goal pursuit was indicated by the length of each participant's presentation, and quality of goal pursuit was assessed via independent raters' evaluations of the quality of the videotape content (Oettingen et al., 2009, Study 2).

Consistent with previous mental contrasting studies, individuals in the mental contrasting group, but not those in the indulging condition, evidenced a strong link between perceived expectations of success and goal pursuit as measured by subjective self-evaluations of performance and objective ratings of the videotaped presentations. Moreover, feelings of energization not only showed the same pattern of results as the goal pursuit variables but they also mediated the relation between expectations of success and both objective and subjective presentation quality in the mental contrasting condition. Physiological data, as measured by systolic blood pressure, showed the same pattern of results (Oettingen et al., 2009, Study 1). Cardiovascular responses such as systolic blood pressure are considered reliable indicators of physiological arousal states and effort mobilization (Gendolla & Wright, 2005; Wright & Kirby, 2001).

### *Planning for Upcoming Hindrances*

Failing to prepare and plan for hindrances one could encounter on the way toward achieving a desired future compromises one's chances of success (Gollwitzer, 1990). Since mental contrasting leads individuals to view the negative aspects of the present reality as obstacles to the attainment of a desired future, high-expectancy mental-contrasting individuals may readily prepare for potential impediments by planning in advance how to tackle them. Specifically, high-expectancy mental contrasting individuals should spontaneously form *if ... then ...* plans shown to be highly effective facilitators of goal striving in a host of domains (meta-analysis by Gollwitzer & Sheeran, 2006). Moreover, because these plans emerge during mental contrasting (Oettingen et al., 2001, Study 1; Oettingen et al., 2005, Study 2), they qualify as a cognitive mechanism responsible for the effects of mental contrasting on goal attainment. To test this assumption, Oettingen and Stephens (2009) had students mentally contrast, indulge, dwell, or reverse contrast regarding an interpersonal concern. Thereafter, participants answered questions assessing their commitment to resolving their goals (e.g., putting effort into achieving their goals).

To assess the mediating variable for this study, two independent raters content-analyzed participants' elaborations of the negative aspects of the reality in the mental contrasting, dwelling, and reverse contrasting conditions to assess the number of *if ... then ...* plans (e.g., "*If* I come home feeling overworked, *then* I will still spend at least half an hour with [my partner]"). A significant benefit of this content-analysis method is its ability to capture participants' plan formation during the process of mental contrasting versus noncontrasting thought (i.e., dwelling and reverse contrasting). As in the previously described studies on the mediating variable of energization, *if ... then ...* plans showed the same pattern of results as the dependent variables, and in the mental contrasting condition *if ... then ...* plans mediated the relation between expectations and goal commitment. Thus, when people engage in mental contrasting and have high expectations of success, they consider a course of action toward goal attainment and make plans to overcome anticipated obstacles. Such planning, in turn, facilitates goal commitment and goal striving.

### *Neural Correlates*

Mental contrasting (as opposed to indulging) is a cognitively demanding task that requires individuals to look into the future, past, and present to form goal commitments (i.e., intentions) in line with their expectations. Therefore, mental contrasting should be associated with greater activity in brain regions linked to working memory processes. Because mental contrasting effects are based on mentally placing the present negative reality in the way of the desired future, it also should lead to greater activity in brain areas associated with episodic memory. Elaborations in mental contrasting should recruit memories of relevant obstacles that were experienced in the past as well as relevant memories about past successes and failures in trying to overcome them. Further, mental contrasting should be linked to heightened activity in brain regions that are related to vividly imagining events. Because the mental contrasting procedure demands switching back and forth from positive images about a desired future to images of impeding obstacles, images of both the desired future and obstacles should become particularly vivid and crystallized. Finally, mental contrasting should lead to greater activity in brain regions that are related to holding intentions and action preparation, because mental contrasting leads to the formation of strong goal commitment, given that relevant expectations of success are high.

Indeed, a study using continuous magnetoencephalography (MEG), a brain imaging technique that measures magnetic fields produced by electrical activity in the brain (Achtziger, Fehr, Oettingen, Gollwitzer, & Rockstroh, 2009), showed that mental contrasting and indulging are two distinct mental activities. Specifically, as compared to indulging and resting, mental contrasting went along with heightened activity in brain regions responsible for working memory and intention formation, suggesting that mental contrasting directs attention toward critical information, such as positioning the present, negative reality in the way of the desired future. Moreover, mental contrasting heightened activity in regions responsible for episodic memory and vivid mental imagery, suggesting that mental contrasting is rooted in the retrieval of past personal events, as well as the processing of complex stimuli, such as reexperiencing past incidents. In contrast, indulging relies less on episodic memory processes. Indulging in a positive future primarily entails loose associations between aspects of the not-yet-experienced desired positive future rather than the mental exploration of past experiences (Oettingen, 2000; Oettingen et al., 2001). Furthermore, mental contrasting requires a critical look at both the desired future and the negative reality, and thus evokes more vivid images than does indulging which did not differ from resting. Future studies should investigate the mental activities in dwelling and reverse contrasting. We expect that these two self-regulatory strategies will differ from mental contrasting and show similar patterns to indulging and resting.

Going beyond prior research, these findings suggest that certain conditions must be met in order for mental contrasting to be most effective. For example, because mental contrasting taxes working memory, people should not be able to perform it effectively when cognitive resources are blocked by dual-task activities (e.g., being occupied by demanding cognitive tasks, coping with interpersonal stressors, extreme fatigue, or physical frailty and pain). Moreover, because mental contrasting is based on the effective retrieval of relevant obstacles experienced in the past, it should be particularly effective for people who have carefully encoded past experiences with obstacles and thus can easily and accurately retrieve them from memory. Vividly depicted in the present MEG study is the cognitive complexity of mental contrasting.

### Summary

Findings supporting the model of fantasy realization show that perceiving the future as desirable (positive attitude or high incentive value) and feasible (e.g., high expectation of success) are only the prerequisites for the emergence of strong goal commitments. To create strong goal commitments, people need to translate these positive attitudes and high expectations into binding goals, a process that is facilitated by mentally contrasting the positive future with the negative present reality. Such mental contrasting has been found to produce expectancy-dependent goal commitments in widely different life domains (e.g., interpersonal, achievement, and health). It is based on the motivational process of energization and the cognitive process of *if ... then ...* planning when translating expectations into goal commitment and subsequent striving, and it has been linked to brain activity typical of purposeful problem solving based on one's past experiences and performance history.

## IMPLEMENTING SET GOALS

Kurt Lewin's distinction between goal setting and goal striving reminds us that goal attainment may not be secured solely by forming strong goal commitments and framing the goals at hand in an appropriate manner. There is the second issue of implementing a chosen goal (i.e., goal striving), and one wonders what people can do to enhance their chances of being successful at this phase of goal pursuit. The answer seems to be the following: People need to prepare themselves so that their chances of overcoming the major difficulties of goal implementation are kept high. But what are these difficulties or problems? At least four problems stand out: getting started with goal pursuit, staying on track, calling a halt to futile goal striving, and not overextending oneself. For all of these problems, the self-regulation strategy of forming implementation intentions has been shown to be beneficial.

### Implementation Intentions: Planning Goal Implementation in Advance

To form an implementation intention (i.e., make an *if ... then ...* plan; Gollwitzer, 1993, 1999), one needs to identify a future goal-relevant situational cue and a related planned response to that cue. Whereas goal intentions merely specify desired end states ("I want to achieve goal *X*!"), implementation intentions in the format "If situation *Y* arises, then I will initiate behavior *Z*!" additionally specify when, where, and how a person intends to pursue a goal. Implementation intentions thus delegate control over the initiation of the intended goal-directed behavior to a specified opportunity by creating a strong link between a situational cue and a goal-directed response. For example, a person who has the goal to eat more healthily can form the implementation intention "When I'm at my favorite restaurant and the waiter asks me for my order, then I'll request a vegetarian meal!" Implementation intentions have been found to help people close the gap between initial goal setting and actually meeting their goals. Indeed, a recent meta-analysis involving over 8,000 participants in 94 independent studies revealed a medium-to-large effect size ($d = 0.65$; Cohen, 1992) of implementation intentions on goal achievement, on top of the effects of mere goal intentions (Gollwitzer & Sheeran, 2006). As goal intentions by themselves already have a facilitating effect on behavior enactment (Webb & Sheeran, 2006), the size of the implementation intention effect is remarkable.

### *How Do Implementation Intention Effects Come About?*

The mental links created by implementation intentions facilitate goal attainment on the basis of psychological processes that relate to both the anticipated situation (specified in the *if* part of the plan) and the intended behavior (specified in the *then* part of the plan). Because forming an implementation intention implies the selection of a critical future situation, the mental representation of this situation becomes highly activated and hence more accessible (Gollwitzer, 1999). This heightened accessibility of the *if* part of the plan has been observed in several studies (e.g., Aarts, Dijksterhuis, & Midden, 1999; Parks-Stamm, Gollwitzer, & Oettingen, 2007; Webb & Sheeran, 2007, 2008). This accessibility persists over time until the plan is enacted or the respective goal is achieved or dismissed. The heightened activation of the critical situation helps people to easily recall the specified situation, and it leads to swift allocation of attention when the situation arises.

Implementation intentions also forge a strong association between the specified opportunity and the specified response (Webb & Sheeran, 2007, 2008). The upshot of these strong links is that, once the critical cue is encountered, the initiation of the goal-directed response specified in the *then* component of the implementation intention exhibits features of automaticity, including immediacy, efficiency, and redundancy of conscious intent. When people have formed an implementation intention, they can act in situ without having to deliberate on when and how they should act. Evidence that *if . . . then . . .* planners act quickly (Gollwitzer & Brandstätter, 1997, Experiment 3), deal effectively with cognitive demands (Brandstätter, Lengfelder, & Gollwitzer, 2001), and do not need to consciously intend to act in the critical moment (Bayer, Achtziger, Gollwitzer, & Moskowitz, 2009; Sheeran, Webb, & Gollwitzer, 2005, Study 2) is consistent with this idea.

These component processes of implementation intentions (enhanced cue accessibility, automation of responding) mean that *if . . . then . . .* planning enables people to see and seize good opportunities to move toward their goals. Fashioning an *if . . . then . . .* plan *strategically automates* goal striving (Gollwitzer & Schaal, 1998); people intentionally make *if . . . then . . .* plans that delegate control of goal-directed behavior to preselected situational cues with the explicit purpose of reaching their goals. That is, automatic action initiation achieved by implementation intentions originates from a conscious act of will rather than practice (i.e., exerting the critical behavior in the critical situation repeatedly and consistently).

### *Implementation Intentions and Overcoming Problems of Goal Implementation*

Given these special features of action control by implementation intentions, one wonders whether people benefit from forming implementation intentions when they are confronted with the four central problems of goal implementation named above. Numerous studies suggest that problems of *getting started* on one's goals can be solved effectively by forming implementation intentions. For instance, Gollwitzer and Brandstätter (1997, Study 2) analyzed a goal intention (i.e., writing a report about how the participants spent Christmas Eve) that had to be performed at a time when people are commonly busy with other things (i.e., during the subsequent 2 days, which are family holidays in Europe). Still, research participants who had furnished their goal intention with an implementation intention that specified when, where, and how they wanted to get started on this project were about three times as likely to actually write the report than mere goal intention participants. Similarly, Oettingen, Hönig, and Gollwitzer (2000, Study 3) observed that implementation intentions helped students to act on their task goals (i.e., performing math homework) on time (e.g., at 10 A.M. in the morning of every Wednesday over the next 4 weeks).

Other studies have examined the ability of implementation intentions to foster a willingness to strive toward goals involving behaviors that are somewhat unpleasant to perform. For instance, goals to perform regular breast examinations (Orbell, Hodgkins, & Sheeran, 1997) or cervical cancer screenings (Sheeran & Orbell, 2000), to resume functional activity after joint replacement surgery (Orbell & Sheeran, 2000), to eat a low-fat diet (Armitage, 2004), to recycle (Holland, Aarts, & Langendam, 2006), and to engage in physical exercise (Milne, Orbell, & Sheeran, 2002) were all more readily acted upon when people had developed implementation intentions—even though there was an initial reluctance to execute these behaviors. Moreover, implementation intentions were associated with goal attainment in domains where it is easy to forget to act (e.g., regular intake of vitamin pills; Sheeran & Orbell, 1999; the signing of worksheets by the elderly; Chasteen, Park, & Schwarz, 2001).

Many goals cannot be accomplished by simple, discrete, one-shot actions but require that people continue to strive for the goal over an extended period of time. Such *staying on track* may become very difficult when certain internal stimuli (e.g., being anxious, tired, overburdened) or external stimuli (e.g., temptations, distractions) interfere with and potentially derail ongoing goal striving. Implementation intentions can suppress the negative influence of interferences from outside the person (Gollwitzer & Schaal, 1998). For instance, if a person wants to avoid being unfriendly to a friend who is known to make outrageous requests, he or she can form suppression-oriented implementation intentions, such as: "If my friend approaches me with an outrageous request, then I will not respond in an unfriendly manner!" The *then* component of suppression-oriented implementation intentions does not have to be worded in terms of not showing the critical behavior; it may alternatively specify an antagonistic behavior (" . . . , then I will respond in a friendly manner!") or focus on ignoring the critical cue (" . . . , then I'll ignore her request!").

Suppression-oriented implementation intentions can also be used to shield ongoing goal striving from disruptive inner states. Achtziger, Gollwitzer, and Sheeran (2008) report two field experiments concerned with dieting (Study 1) and athletic goals (Study 2), in which goals were shielded by suppression implementation intentions geared toward controlling potentially interfering inner states (i.e., cravings for junk food in Study 1, and disruptive thoughts, feelings, and physiological states in Study 2).

An alternative way of using implementation intentions to protect ongoing goal striving from derailment is to form *if . . . then . . .* plans geared toward stabilizing the ongoing goal pursuit at hand (Bayer, Gollwitzer, & Achtziger, 2010). Using again the example of a person who is approached by her friend with an outrageous request, let us assume that he or she is also tired or irritated and thus particularly likely to respond in an unfriendly manner. If he or she has stipulated in advance in an implementation intention how he or she will converse with the friend, the interaction may come off as planned, and being tired or irritated should fail to affect the person's behavior toward her friend.

In a negotiation study Trötschel and Gollwitzer (2007) explored whether spelling out one's goal striving via implementation intentions makes goal striving less vulnerable not only to internal interferences but also to external ones. They found that loss-framed negotiation settings failed to produce the typical negative effects on fair and cooperative negotiation outcomes (i.e., when the commodities to be shared are framed in terms of losses rather than gains, negotiators typically behave more competitively and produce inferior joint profits). In Trötschel and Gollwitzer's studies, negotiators who had furnished the goal intention to be cooperative (i.e., "I want to cooperate with my counterpart!") with *if . . . then . . .* plans that spelled out in advance how they wanted to achieve this goal (i.e., "If I receive a proposal, then I'll make a cooperative counterproposal!") no longer evidenced negative effects of loss framing. Negotiators in the loss-framed negotiation setting who had clear cooperative goal intentions now achieved the same high performance in joint profits as was observed with negotiators in the gain-frame control group.

The self-regulatory problem of *calling a halt* to a futile goal striving (i.e., disengaging from a chosen but noninstrumental means or from a chosen goal that has become unfeasible or undesirable) can also be ameliorated by forming implementation intentions. People often fail to readily disengage from chosen means and goals that turn out to be faulty because of a strong self-justification motive (i.e., we tend to adhere to the irrational belief that decisions we have made deliberately must be good; Brockner, 1992). Such escalation effects (e.g., sticking with a chosen means or goal even if negative feedback on goal progress mounts) are reduced effectively, however, by the use of implementation intentions. These *if . . . then . . .* plans only have to specify receiving negative feedback as the critical cue in the *if* component and switching to available alternative means or goals as the appropriate response in the *then* component (Henderson, Gollwitzer, & Oettingen, 2007).

Finally, the assumption that implementation intentions subject behavior to the direct control of situational cues (Gollwitzer, 1993) implies that the person does not have to exert deliberate effort. As a consequence, the self should not become depleted (Muraven & Baumeister, 2000; see also Doerr & Baumeister, Chapter 5, this volume) when task performance is regulated by implementation intentions, and thus for individuals using implementation intentions, *not overextending* themselves should become easier. Indeed, even using different ego-depletion paradigms, research participants who used implementation intentions to self-regulate in one task did not show reduced self-regulatory capacity in a subsequent task. Whether the initial self-regulation task was controlling emotions while watching a humorous movie (Gollwitzer & Bayer, 2000) or performing a Stroop task (Webb & Sheeran, 2003, Study 1), implementation intentions successfully preserved self-regulatory resources as demonstrated by greater persistence on subsequent difficult tasks.

### *Using Implementation Intentions to Support Therapeutic Goals*

Bayer and Gollwitzer (2007) combatted dysfunctional beliefs in difficult academic tasks (e.g., taking the Raven intelligence test). Even when people start taking a test with high self-efficacy beliefs, encountering a difficult test item may lead to weakened self-efficacy for subsequent test items. To counter such *lowered self-efficacy*, Bayer and Gollwitzer (2007) asked participants to bolster their goal intentions to perform well ("I will correctly solve as many test items as possible!") with implementation intentions specifying a self-efficacy strengthening response ("And if I start a new test item, then I'll tell myself: I can solve it!").

Participants in the implementation intention condition performed better than those in the mere goal intention to perform well condition; they also performed better than participants in a further condition where a self-efficacy strengthening goal intention had to be formed ("I will tell myself: I can do these test items!").

Recent research also has explored whether adding implementation intentions to emotion regulation goals make these goals more effective (Schweiger Gallo, Keil, McCulloch, Rockstroh, & Gollwitzer, 2009). In one study, the control of fear in people with spider phobias was analyzed. Based on Gross's (2002) distinction between response-focused versus antecedent-focused emotion regulation strategies, implementation intention participants were asked to furnish their goal to not get frightened when spider pictures were presented with either a response-focused implementation intention ("If a see a spider, then I will stay calm and relaxed") or an antecedent-focused implementation intention ("If I see a spider, then I'll ignore it"). As compared to mere goal intention participants, implementation intention participants showed weaker fear responses to the presented spider pictures no matter whether they had formed a response-focused or an antecedent-focused implementation intention. Actually, participants using implementation intentions managed to control their fear to the low level that was observed with control participants who had no fear of spiders at all. In a final study using dense-array electroencephalography, the effectiveness of *ignore* implementation intentions for the control of fear in participants with spider phobias was replicated, and the obtained electrocortical correlates revealed that those participants who bolstered their goal intention with an *ignore* implementation intention showed significantly reduced early activity in the visual cortex in response to spider slides, as reflected in a smaller P1 (assessed at 120 milliseconds [ms] after the spider pictures were presented). This finding suggests that implementation intentions indeed lead to strategic automation of the specified goal-directed response (in the present case, an *ignore* response) when the critical cue (in the present case, a spider picture) is encountered, as conscious effortful action initiation is known to take longer than 120 ms (i.e., at least 300 ms).

Finally, implementation intentions have also been found to be effective in helping people overcome bad habits (e.g., unhealthy eating habits; Verplanken & Faes, 1999). This comes as no surprise, as Cohen, Bayer, Jaudas, and Gollwitzer (2008, Study 2) observed that implementation intentions can control even the Simon effect (Lu & Proctor, 1995), which is based on the following ingrained response: Stimuli presented on the left side of a person are commonly dealt with by using the left arm, whereas stimuli presented on the right side are responded to by the right arm. In the Simon task, classification responses that are incongruent (i.e., the critical stimulus and the critical response are located at different sides to the person's position) commonly take longer response times than classification responses that are congruent (i.e., the stimulus and the response are on the same side). Cohen et al. (2008) found that the effect of spatial location on classification responses for cues that had been specified in the *if* part of implementation intentions was abolished.

### *Moderators of Implementation Intention Effects*

There are various moderators of the effects of implementation intentions on goal attainment pertaining to characteristics of the superordinate goal (e.g., intrinsic interest, Koestner, Lekes, Powers, & Chicoine, 2002; strength of commitment and activation state, Sheeran et al., 2005), the implementation intention itself (e.g., commitment to the *if . . . then . . .*

plan; Gollwitzer, 1999), and characteristics of the individual. Implementation intentions have been found to be also useful for individuals with poor self-regulatory abilities, such as people with schizophrenia, substance abuse disorders (Brandstätter et al., 2001, Studies 1 & 2), and frontal lobe damage (Lengfelder & Gollwitzer, 2001). Benefits are also found for children with attention-deficit/hyperactivity disorder (ADHD) who are known to have difficulties with tasks that require response inhibition (e.g., go/no-go tasks). For example, the response inhibition performance in the presence of stop signals can be improved in children with ADHD by having form them implementation intentions (Gawrilow & Gollwitzer, 2008). This improved response inhibition is reflected in electrocortical data as well (Paul et al., 2007). Typically, the P300 component (i.e., an event related potential, ERP, recorded at a latency of 300 milliseconds) evoked by no-go stimuli has greater amplitude than the P300 evoked by go stimuli. This difference is less pronounced in children with ADHD. Paul et al. (2007) found that *if* ... *then* ... plans improved response inhibition and increased the P300 difference (no-go/go) in children with ADHD.

### Summary

Implementation intentions help people to cope more effectively with the major problems of goal striving: getting started, staying on track, calling a halt, and not overextending oneself. In a conscious act of will ("If situation *X* arises, then I will show behavior *Y*!"), people link an anticipated critical internal or external cue to a goal-directed response. The latter then becomes automatically triggered in the presence of the critical cue. Implementation intentions can be used to facilitate the attainment of all kinds of difficult goals, including therapeutic goals such as changing expectations (self-efficacy) and overcoming fears or bad habits. They also seem to work for those groups of people who are known to have difficulties with action control (e.g., children with ADHD).

## AN INTERVENTION TO ENHANCE A PERSON'S SELF-REGULATORY SKILLS: COMBINING MENTAL CONTRASTING WITH IMPLEMENTATION INTENTIONS

A variety of theories view enhanced self-regulation as an important goal of psychotherapy, although different theories have different terms for the concept. Psychodynamic approaches refer to enhanced self-regulation as character development, Adlerians call it lifestyle modification, behaviorists talk of acquiring an adaptive social repertoire, and psychologists adhering to the humanist tradition talk of a fully functioning person (see Karoly & Anderson, 2000). When Viktor Frankl (1959/1984) explicates that "life ultimately means taking the responsibility to find the right answer to its problems and to fulfill the tasks which it constantly sets for each individual," he seems to agree that effective self-regulation is a desirable therapeutic outcome.

How can psychotherapies help people achieve effective self-regulation? In recent research we explored whether it is possible to construct an intervention that teaches people to use, on their own, an integrated combination of mental contrasting and forming implementation intentions in order to become more effective self-regulators in their goal setting and goal striving. This intervention—called MCII, for *m*ental *c*ontrasting and *i*mplementation intentions—was tested in a first study that used MCII integrated into a standard therapy for patients with chronic back pain. In a second study middle-age women were taught MCII as a metacognitive strategy to be applied in everyday life to enhance health-promoting behavior (i.e., exercising regularly). Finally, in a third study MCII was taught, again as a metacognitive strategy, this time to help students cope with the stresses of college life. To assess the implications of the MCII intervention for personality development, broader variables such as changes in self-discipline and self-esteem were the dependent variables.

In all of these studies, the MCII combination enhanced goal pursuit. For implementation intentions to be effective, strong goal commitments must be in place (Sheeran et al., 2005, Study 1), and mental contrasting creates such strong commitments. Additionally, mental contrasting guarantees the identification of obstacles to goal attainment. These obstacles may then be addressed with *if* ... *then* ... plans by specifying critical situations in the *if* component that are linked to instrumental goal-directed responses in the *then* component. Moreover, mental contrasting increases a person's readiness to make *if* ... *then* ... plans (Oettingen et al., 2001, 2009). Accordingly, an intervention such as MCII, which explicitly suggests forming *if* ... *then* ... plans after mental contrasting can capitalize on these effects.

## MCII as a Strategy to Reach a Specific Therapeutic Goal

A first study testing these ideas focused on improving mobility in a clinical sample of patients with chronic back pain. A great challenge facing many physical therapists who work with such patients is motivating them to exercise. One obstacle to successful rehabilitation is that pain sufferers anticipate pain in any activity-related situation and thus tend to avoid activity altogether. A second obstacle is patients' beliefs that passive treatments (e.g., surgery, massage) are the most effective or only avenue for pain control. Patients who hope that such "passive" treatments will eliminate their pain are less likely to learn how they themselves can effectively self-manage and overcome their pain (Vlaeyen & Linton, 2000), a difficult, yet necessary, step for successful rehabilitation. Because long-term behavior change in the form of physical activity is necessary for these patients to recover and improve their quality of life, and because long-term behavior often fails to be maintained over time (Marcus et al., 2000), a supplementary MCII intervention should be useful.

Christiansen, Oettingen, Dahme, and Klinger (in press) recruited outpatients with chronic back pain from a rehabilitation center in Germany. Participants were randomly assigned to either a control group (i.e., standard outpatient back pain program) or an intervention group (i.e., standard program plus MCII intervention). The standard program entailed 3–4 weeks of treatment, including elements of cognitive-behavior therapy, individualized information seminars (e.g., relaxation techniques, handling stress), medical care and psychological consultation, physical therapy, and exercise. The MCII intervention consisted of two half-hour sessions. In the first session, participants mentally contrasted positive aspects of improved exercise (e.g., feeling fitter, joining the family walk on Sunday) with obstacles standing in the way of improved exercise (e.g., fear that the pain will worsen, feeling shy to ask family members to slow down). During the second session, participants formed *if* ... *then* ... plans after identifying behaviors in response to the obstacles generated in the first session (e.g., "If I get anxious that my pain will increase, then I will assure myself that I can only benefit from exercise"; "If I feel shy to talk to my family on Sunday during the walk, I will ask my children to walk ahead and wait for me in the coffee place"). Dependent variables were physical strength and appropriate lifting behavior (i.e., "handling load" of the functional capacity evaluation [FCE]; Gouttebarge, Wind, Kuijer, & Frings-Dresen, 2004; and a bicycle ergometer test) and pain severity. The measures were taken at preintervention, 10 days postintervention, and 3 months postintervention.

The standard treatment + MCII intervention improved physical mobility in patients with chronic back pain more than the standard treatment only as observed 10 days and 3 months after the intervention, and as assessed by subjective and objective measures. These effects were independent of participants' reported pain, which did not significantly differ between conditions during and after treatment. The MCII intervention proved to be time- and cost-effective in that it consisted of only two sessions for a total of 1 hour. Other short-term psychological interventions for patients with chronic back pain take at least 4–6 hours (e.g., Linton & Nordin, 2006; for review, see the findings of the "Cochrane Back Group": Ostelo et al., 2006).

## MCII as a Metacognitive Strategy for Everyday Life

In recent years psychologists have begun to analyze metacognitive knowledge in such areas as decision making and memory (e.g., Bless & Forgas, 2000; Koriat & Goldsmith, 1996; Metcalfe & Shimamura, 1994; Nelson & Narens, 1994). For example, children (especially those with little metacognitive knowledge) improve their memory performance if told about clustering and rehearsal techniques (Schneider, Borkowski, Kurtz, & Kerwin, 1986). The use of metacognitive knowledge should be particularly important for effective goal pursuit. For example, teaching people that intelligence is malleable should lead them to take on learning goals (rather than performance goals) that, in turn, foster effort in the face of setbacks (Dweck & Elliot-Moskwa, Chapter 8, this volume). In addition, teaching people to mentally contrast desirable and feasible future outcomes with respective realities should help people form binding goal commitments. Finally, teaching people to make *if* ... *then* ... plans (implementation intentions) should automate the initiation of goal-directed responses and thus facilitate the attainment of these goals. To date, however, most interventions tell people to strive for an a priori defined goal (e.g., weight control, Stice, Shaw, & Marti, 2006; alcohol control, Lock, 2004; forgiveness, Harris et al., 2006; see also, Christiansen et al., in press, described above). In such interventions, participants are asked to engage in goal-directed thoughts, feelings, and actions that are targeted specifically at attaining a given predefined desired outcome; they are not encouraged to use these same strategies to set and strive for their goals in general.

However, in everyday life, people commonly wish to attain a multitude of different outcomes varying in domains. Therefore, people should benefit from metacognitive knowledge about strategies that are content free and that involve prioritizing and planning goal pursuit in advance. Indeed, a recent study shows that mental contrasting can be successfully taught and used as a metacognitive strategy (Oettingen, Mayer, & Brinkmann, 2010). German personnel managers who were taught to mentally contrast self-identified unsettling but controllable everyday concerns reported better time management, more ease of decision making, and more effective project completion, as compared to a control group (control participants were merely asked to think positively about their everyday concerns). The next two studies tested whether MCII could also be taught as a metacognitive strategy.

### *Effects on Health Behavior in Middle-Age Professional Women*

Middle-age women were recruited to take part in a study focusing on healthy lifestyles (Stadler, Oettingen, & Gollwitzer, 2009). Participants were randomly assigned to either an information-only control group or a MCII intervention group. In the information-only control group, women learned about the benefits of regular exercise. In the MCII group, participants received the same information and additionally learned the MCII technique. Participants learned the mental contrasting strategy with respect to the goal of exercising regularly (e.g., going for a run three times week), and then were instructed to form three implementation intentions regarding an obstacle standing in the way of exercising (e.g., feeling too tired in the evening to go for a run) in the form of *if . . . then . . .* statements: one to overcome the obstacle generated by mental contrasting (e.g., "If I feel exhausted when I get home from work tonight, then I will put on my running shoes and go for a jog in the neighborhood"), one to prevent this obstacle (e.g., "If I hear the clock chime five o'clock, then I will pack my things and leave the office to go for a run"), and one identifying a good opportunity to act (e.g., "If the sun is shining, then I will go for a 30-minute jog in the park"). Participants were then told to apply this MCII procedure to the concern of more exercise whenever possible in the weeks to come. Participants were free to choose whatever form of exercise they wanted to engage in, and they were encouraged to identify obstacles that were personally most relevant.

Participants maintained daily behavioral diaries to keep track of the amount of time they exercised every day. Overall, the MCII technique enhanced exercise more than the information intervention immediately after the intervention, and this effect remained stable for 4, 8, and 16 weeks after the intervention. Participants in the MCII group exercised nearly twice as much—that is, 1 hour more per week—than participants in the information-only control group. Thus, using the MCII technique was effective for both initial success and long-term maintenance of improving exercise behavior.

### *Increasing Self-Discipline and Self-Esteem in College Students*

Given that MCII as a metacognitive strategy improves self-regulation of a variety of goals, we have examined its effects on broader variables of personality development: self-discipline and self-esteem. In line with the conceptualization of self-discipline (self-control) by Tangney, Baumeister, and Boone (2004), we identified its key components: time management, project completion, and a feeling of being on top of things. In addition, as MCII should foster strong goal commitment and successful goal completion in a variety of areas, we hypothesized that our MCII intervention might even affect people's self-esteem. As highlighted by William James (1890), self-esteem rises and falls as a function of aspirations and successes. The effect of mental contrasting—a better match between the subjective likelihood of attaining one's goals and commitment to them—should bring commitments in line with objective competence, and using implementation intentions to pursue goals should provide frequent success. Both of these outcomes should raise self-esteem.

Undergraduate participants were assigned either to a MCII intervention group or to a control group (Oettingen, Barry, Guttenberg, & Gollwitzer, 2010). In the MCII intervention group, participants first learned how to use the mental contrasting strategy, then learned how to form implementation intentions by identifying the behavior necessary to overcome or circumvent an obstacle (e.g., a noisy roommate as an obstacle to studying effectively for an upcoming test) generated during mental contrasting. To do so, participants imagined a desired outcome and a potential obstacle in vivid detail, then created three *if ... then ...* statements focusing on overcoming the obstacle (e.g., "If my roommate starts to get noisy again tonight, then I will talk to her about her behavior"), preventing the obstacle (e.g., "If see my roommate at lunch, then I will ask her to turn the music down this evening"), and on planning to approach the desired outcome (e.g., "If I pass a drugstore on the way home, then I will buy myself a pair of earplugs"). Students practiced using the MCII procedure with the help of the experimenter so that they could perform the strategy on their own regarding a multitude of everyday concerns over the course of 1 week.

Participants rated self-discipline and self-esteem at two time points: immediately before the intervention, and once again 1 week after the intervention. The MCII intervention directly enhanced MCII participants' reports of self-discipline and their self-esteem, in comparison to control-group participants (who failed to show any improvements) over a mere 1-week period. The effects of the MCII intervention were not moderated by any other measured variables (e.g., sex, age, school year, depression, perceived stress, life satisfaction, troublesome events, college life satisfaction, self-efficacy). Presumably, MCII empowered individuals with self-regulatory skills helping them commit to more feasible goals and helping them to effectively achieve these goals. Thus, this powerful yet simple combination of strategies helped the college students to recognize and realize their potential and feel a sense of self-discipline and self-esteem in their everyday lives.

### Summary

The combination of mental contrasting and forming implementation intentions can be used to help people meet specific behavioral goals (e.g., mobility goals in patients with back pain) or, when taught as a meta-cognitive strategy, to meet goals in general (e.g., exercising more regularly or coping with college life). It even influenced outcomes related to personality development, such as self-discipline and self-esteem. Furthermore, as the intervention studies include samples from the United States and Germany, from young adults to middle-age individuals, and from diverse domains ranging from professional and academic realms to improved health behavior, it seems evident that mental contrasting with implementation intentions (MCII) can be ubiquitously applied to help people manage the challenges of life.

## CONCLUSION

Beginning with Viktor Frankl's observation that meaning in life may originate from action more than talk and meditation, we have reviewed research on the self-regulation of goal pursuit. It seems important that people selectively set goals that are desirable and feasible, and then strive for them in an effective manner. For both of these tasks of goal pursuit there exist effective self-regulatory strategies: mental contrasting for goal setting and forming implementation intentions for goal striving. Importantly, a mental contrasting with implementation intentions (MCII) intervention can be used to teach people the combined use of these two strategies to meet short-term as well as long term goals. The effectiveness of the MCII intervention suggests that people can take charge of their everyday life and personal development by effective self-regulation of their goal pursuits.

## REFERENCES

Aarts, H., Dijksterhuis, A. P., & Midden, C. (1999). To plan or not to plan? Goal achievement of interrupting the performance of mundane behaviors. *European Journal of Social Psychology, 29*, 971–979.

Achtziger, A., Fehr, T., Oettingen, G., Gollwitzer, P. M., & Rockstroh, B. (2009). Strategies of intention formation are reflected in continuous MEG activity. *Social Neuroscience, 4*, 11–27.

Achtziger, A., Gollwitzer, P. M., & Sheeran, P. (2008). Implementation intentions and shielding goal striving from unwanted thoughts and feelings. *Personality and Social Psychology Bulletin, 34*, 381–393.

Ajzen, I. (1991). The theory of planned behavior. *Organizational Behavior and Human Decision Processes, 50*, 179–211.

Armitage, C. J. (2004). Evidence that implementation intentions reduce dietary fat intake: A randomized trial. *Health Psychology, 23*, 319–323.

Atkinson, J. W. (1957). Motivational determinants of risk-taking behavior. *Psychological Review, 64*, 359–372.

Bandura, A. (1977). Self-efficacy: Toward a unifying theory of behavioral change. *Psychological Review, 84*, 191–215.

Bandura, A. (1997). *Self-efficacy: The exercise of control.* New York: Freeman.

Bandura, A., & Schunk, D. H. (1981). Cultivating competence, self-efficacy, and intrinsic interest through proximal self-motivation. *Journal of Personality and Social Psychology, 41*, 586–598.

Bargh, J. A., Gollwitzer, P. M., & Oettingen, G. (2010). Motivation. In S. T. Fiske, D. T. Gilbert, & G. Lindzay (Eds.), *Handbook of social psychology* (Vol. 1, pp. 268–316, 5th ed.). New York: Wiley.

Bayer, U. C., Achtziger, A., Gollwitzer, P. M., & Moskowitz, G. (2009). Responding to subliminal cues: Do if-then plans facilitate action initiation without conscious intent? *Social Cognition, 27*, 183–201.

Bayer, U. C., & Gollwitzer, P. M. (2007). Boosting scholastic test scores by willpower: The role of implementation intentions. *Self and Identity, 6*, 1–19.

Bayer, U. C., Gollwitzer, P. M., & Achtziger, A. (2010). Staying on track: Planned goal striving is protected from disruptive internal states. *Journal of Experimental Social Psychology, 46*, 505–514.

Bless, H., & Forgas, J. P. (Eds.). (2000). *The message within: The role of subjective experience in social cognition and behavior.* New York: Psychology Press.

Brandstätter, V., Lengfelder, A., & Gollwitzer, P. M. (2001). Implementation intentions and efficient action initiation. *Journal of Personality and Social Psychology, 81*, 946–960.

Brockner, J. (1992). The escalation of commitment to a failing course of action: Toward theoretical progress. *Academy of Management Review, 17*, 39–61.

Brunstein, J. C., & Gollwitzer, P. M. (1996). Effects of failure on subsequent performance: The importance of self-defining goals. *Journal of Personality and Social Psychology, 70*, 395–407.

Carver, C. S., & Scheier, M. F. (1990). Origins and functions of positive and negative affect: A control-process view. *Psychological Review, 97*, 19–35.

Chasteen, A. L., Park, D. C., & Schwarz, N. (2001). Implementation intentions and facilitation of prospective memory. *Psychological Science, 12*, 457–461.

Christiansen, S., Oettingen, G., Dahme, B., & Klinger, R. (in press). A short goal-pursuit intervention to improve physical capacity: A randomized clinical trial in chronic back pain patients. *Pain.*

Cohen, A.-L., Bayer, U. C., Jaudas, A., & Gollwitzer, P. M. (2008). Self-regulatory strategy and executive control: Implementation intentions modulate task switching and Simon task performance. *Psychological Research, 72*, 12–26.

Cohen, J. (1992). A power primer. *Psychological Bulletin, 112*, 155–159.

Dweck, C. S. (1999). *Self-theories: Their role in motivation, personality, and development.* Philadelphia: Psychology Press.

Frankl, V. E. (1984). *Man's search for meaning*. New York: Washington Square Press. (Original work published 1959)

Gawrilow, C., & & Gollwitzer, P. M. (2008). Implementation intentions facilitate response inhibition in ADHD children. *Cognitive Therapy and Research*, *32*, 261–280.

Gendolla, G. H. E., & Wright, R. A. (2005). Motivation in social settings studies of effort-related cardiovascular arousal. In J. P. Forgas, K. D. Williams, & S. M. Laham (Eds.), *Social motivation: Conscious and unconscious processes* (pp. 71–90). New York: Cambridge University Press.

Gollwitzer, P. M. (1990). Action phases and mind-sets. In E. T. Higgins & R. M. Sorrentino (Eds.), *Handbook of motivation and cognition: Foundations of social behavior* (pp. 53–92). New York: Guilford Press.

Gollwitzer, P. M. (1993). Goal achievement: The role of intentions. *European Review of Social Psychology*, *4*, 141–185.

Gollwitzer, P. M. (1999). Implementation intentions: Strong effects of simple plans. *American Psychologist*, *54*, 493–503.

Gollwitzer, P. M., & Bayer, U. C. (2000, October). *Becoming a better person without changing the self*. Paper presented at the annual meeting of the Society of Experimental Social Psychology, Atlanta, Georgia.

Gollwitzer, P. M., & Brandstätter, V. (1997). Implementation intentions and effective goal pursuit. *Journal of Personality and Social Psychology*, *73*, 186–199.

Gollwitzer, P. M., & Schaal, B. (1998). Metacognition in action: The importance of implementation intentions. *Personality and Social Psychology Review*, *2*, 124–136.

Gollwitzer, P. M., & Sheeran, P. (2006). Implementation intentions and goal achievement: A meta-analysis of effects and processes. *Advances in Experimental Social Psychology*, *38*, 69–119.

Gouttebarge, V., Wind, H., Kuijer, P. P. F. M., & Frings-Dresen, M. H. W. (2004). Reliability and validity of functional capacity evaluation methods: A systematic review with reference to Blankenship system, Ergos work simulator, Ergo-Kit and Isernhagen work system. *International Archives of Occupational and Environmental Health*, *77*, 527–537.

Gross, J. J. (2002). Emotion regulation: Affective, cognitive, and social consequences. *Psychophysiology*, *39*, 281–291.

Harris, A. H. S., Luskin, F., Norman, S. B., Standard, S., Bruning, J., Evans, S., et al. (2006). Effects of a group forgiveness intervention on forgiveness, perceived stress, and trait-anger. *Journal of Clinical Psychology*, *62*, 715–733.

Heckhausen, H. (1977). Achievement motivation and its constructs: A cognitive model. *Motivation and Emotion*, *1*, 283–329.

Henderson, M. D., Gollwitzer, P. M., & Oettingen, G. (2007). Implementation intentions and disengagement from a failing course of action. *Journal of Behavioral Decision Making*, *20*, 81–102.

Higgins, E. T. (1997). Beyond pleasure and pain. *American Psychologist*, *52*, 1280–1300.

Holland, R. W., Aarts, H., & Langendam, D. (2006). Breaking and creating habits on the working floor: A field experiment on the power of implementation intentions. *Journal of Experimental Social Psychology*, *42*, 776–783.

James, W. (1890). *Principles of psychology* (Vol. 1). New York: Holt.

Karoly, P., & Anderson, C. W. (2000). The long and short of psychological change: Toward a goal-centered understanding of treatment and durability and adaptive success. In C. R. Snyder & R. E. Ingram (Eds.), *Handbook of psychological change* (pp. 154–176). New York: Wiley.

Klinger, E. (1975). Consequences of commitment to and disengagement from incentives. *Psychological Review*, *82*, 1–25.

Koestner, R., Lekes, N., Powers, T. A., & Chicoine, E. (2002). Attaining personal goals: Self-concordance plus implementation intentions equals success. *Journal of Personality and Social Psychology*, *83*, 231–244.

Koriat, A., & Goldsmith, M. (1996). Monitoring and control processes in the strategic regulation of memory accuracy. *Psychological Review*, *103*, 490–517.

Lengfelder, A., & Gollwitzer, P. M. (2001). Reflective and reflexive action control in frontal lobe patients. *Neuropsychology*, *15*, 80–100.

Lewin, K. (1926). Vorsatz, Wille, und Bedürfnis [*Intention, will, and need*]. *Psychologische Forschung*, *7*, 330–385.

Lewin, K., Dembo, T., Festinger, L., & Sears, P. S. (1944). Level of aspiration. In J. McHunt (Ed.), *Personality and the behavioral disorders* (Vol. 1, pp. 333–378). New York: Ronald Press.

Linton, S. J., & Nordin, E. (2006). A 5-year follow-up evaluation of the health and economic consequences of an early cognitive behavioral intervention for back pain: A randomized, controlled trial. *Spine*, *31*, 853–858.

Lock, C. A. (2004). Screening and brief alcohol interventions: What, why, who, where and when? A review of the literature. *Journal of Substance Use*, 9, 91–101.

Locke, E. A., & Latham, G. P. (1990). *A theory of goal setting and task performance*. Englewood Cliffs, NJ: Prentice-Hall.

Locke, E. A., & Latham, G. P. (2002). Building a practically useful theory of goal setting and task motivation: A 35-year odyssey. *American Psychologist*, *57*, 705–717.

Lu, C.-H., & Proctor, R. W. (1995). The influence of irrelevant information on performance: A review of Simon and spatial Stroop effects. *Psychonomic Bulletin and Review*, 2, 174–207.

Maddux, J. E. (1999). Expectancies and the social cognitive perspective: Basic principles, processes, and variables. In I. Kirsch (Ed.), *How expectancies shape behavior* (pp. 17–40). Washington, DC: American Psychological Association.

Marcus, B. H., Dubbert, P. M., Forsyth, L. H., McKenzie, T. L., Stone, E. J., Dunn, A. L., et al. (2000). Physical activity behavior change: Issues in adoption and maintenance. *Health Psychology*, *19*, 32–41.

Markus, H., & Nurius, P. (1986). Possible selves. *American Psychologist*, *41*, 954–969.

Metcalfe, J., & Shimamura, A. P. (Eds.). (1994). *Metacognition: Knowing about knowing*. Cambridge, MA: MIT Press.

Miller, G. A., Galanter, E., & Pribram, K. H. (1960). *Plans and the structure of behavior*. New York: Holt, Rinehart & Winston.

Milne, S., Orbell, S., & Sheeran, P. (2002). Combining motivational and volitional interventions to promote exercise participation: Protection motivation theory and implementation intentions. *British Journal of Health Psychology*, 7, 163–184.

Muraven, M., & Baumeister, R. F. (2000). Self-regulation and depletion of limited resources: Does self-control resemble a muscle? *Psychological Bulletin*, *126*, 247–259.

Nelson, T. O., & Narens, L. (1994). *Why investigate metacognition?* Cambridge, MA: MIT Press.

Newell, A., & Simon, H. A. (1972). *Human problem solving*. Oxford, UK: Prentice-Hall.

Oettingen, G. (2000). Expectancy effects on behavior depend on self-regulatory thought. *Social Cognition*, *18*, 101–129.

Oettingen, G., Barry, H., Guttenberg, K., & Gollwitzer, P. M. (2010). *Improving self-discipline and self-esteem: A mental contrasting with implementation intentions intervention*. Manuscript submitted for publication.

Oettingen, G., & Gollwitzer, P. M. (2001). Goal setting and goal striving. In A. Tesser & N. Schwarz (Eds.), *Intraindividual process. Vol. I. Blackwell Handbook in Social Psychology* (pp. 329–347). Oxford, UK: Blackwell.

Oettingen, G., Hönig, G., & Gollwitzer, P. M. (2000). Effective self-regulation of goal attainment. *International Journal of Educational Research*, *33*, 705–732.

Oettingen, G., & Kappes, A. (2009). Mental contrasting of the future and reality to master negative feedback. In K. D. Markman, W. M. P. Klein, & J. A. Suhr (Eds.), *Handbook of imagination and mental simulation* (pp. 395–412). New York: Psychology Press.

Oettingen, G., & Mayer, D. (2002). The motivating function of thinking about the future: Expectations versus fantasies. *Journal of Personality and Social Psychology*, *83*, 1198–1212.

Oettingen, G., Mayer, D., & Brinkmann, B. (2010). *Mental contrasting of future and reality: Managing the demands of everyday life in health care professionals.* Manuscript under review.

Oettingen, G., Mayer, D., Sevincer, A. T., Stephens, E. J., Pak, H., & Hagenah, M. (2009). Mental contrasting and goal commitment: The mediating role of energization. *Personality and Social Psychology Bulletin, 35*, 608–622.

Oettingen, G., Mayer, D., Stephens, M. E. J., & Brinkmann, B. (in press). Mental contrasting and the self-regulation of helping relations. *Social Cognition.*

Oettingen, G., Mayer, D., & Thorpe, J. (in press). Self-regulation of commitment to reduce cigarette consumption: Mental contrasting of future and reality. *Psychology and Health.*

Oettingen, G., Mayer, D., Thorpe, J. S., Janetzke, H., & Lorenz, S. (2005). Turning fantasies about positive and negative futures into self-improvement goals. *Motivation and Emotion, 29*, 237–267.

Oettingen, G., Pak, H., & Schnetter, K. (2001). Self-regulation of goal-setting: Turning free fantasies about the future into binding goals. *Journal of Personality and Social Psychology, 80*, 736–753.

Oettingen, G., & Stephens, E. J. (2009). Fantasies and motivationally intelligent goal setting. In G. B. Moskowitz & H. Grant (Eds.), *The psychology of goals* (pp. 153–178). New York: Guilford Press.

Orbell, S., Hodgkins, S., & Sheeran, P. (1997). Implementation intentions and the theory of planned behavior. *Personality and Social Psychology Bulletin, 23*, 945–954.

Orbell, S., & Sheeran, P. (2000). Motivational and volitional processes in action initiation: A field study of the role of implementation intentions. *Journal of Applied Social Psychology, 30*, 780–797.

Ostelo, R. W., van Tulder, M. W., Vlaeyen, J. W., Linton, S. J., Morley, S. J., & Assendelft, W. J. (2005). Behavioural treatment for chronic low-back pain. Cochrane Database Syst Rev.: CD002014.

Oyserman, D., & Markus, H. R. (1990). Possible selves and delinquency. *Journal of Personality and Social Psychology, 59*, 112–125.

Parks-Stamm, E. J., Gollwitzer, P. M., & Oettingen, G. (2007). Action control by implementation intentions: Effective cue detection and efficient response initiation. *Social Cognition, 25*, 248–266.

Paul, I., Gawrilow, C., Zech, F., Gollwitzer, P. M., Rockstroh, B., Odenthal, G., et al. (2007). If-then planning modulates the P300 in children with attention deficit hyperactivity disorder. *NeuroReport, 18*, 653–657.

Powers, W. T. (1973). *Behavior: The control of perception.* New York: Aldine/DeGruyter.

Ryan, R. M., & Deci, E. L. (2001). On happiness and human potential: A review of research on hedonic and eudaimonic well-being. *Annual Review of Psychology, 52*, 141–166.

Schneider, W., Borkowski, J. G., Kurtz, B. E., & Kerwin, K. (1986). Metamemory and motivation: A comparison of strategy use and performance in German and American children. *Journal of Cross-Cultural Psychology, 17*, 315–336.

Schweiger Gallo, I., Keil, A., McCulloch, K. C., Rockstroh, B., & Gollwitzer, P. M. (2009). Strategic automatization of emotion control. *Journal of Personality and Social Psychology, 96*, 11–31.

Sheeran, P., & Orbell, S. (1999). Implementation intentions and repeated behavior: Augmenting the predictive validity of the theory of planned behavior. *European Journal of Social Psychology, 29*, 349–369.

Sheeran, P., Webb, T. L., & Gollwitzer, P. M. (2005). The interplay between goal intentions and implementation intentions. *Personality and Social Psychology Bulletin, 31*, 87–98.

Stadler, G., Oettingen, G., & Gollwitzer, P. M. (2009). Physical activity in women. Effects of a self-regulation intervention. *American Journal of Preventive Medicine, 36*, 29–34.

Stice, E., Shaw, H., & Marti, C. N. (2006). A meta-analytic review of obesity prevention programs for children and adolescents: The skinny on interventions that work. *Psychological Bulletin, 132*, 667–691.

Tangney, J. P., Baumeister, R. F., & Boone, A. L. (2004). High self-control predicts good adjustment, less pathology, better grades, and interpersonal success. *Journal of Personality, 72*, 271–322.

Trötschel, R., & Gollwitzer, P. M. (2007). Implementation intentions and the willful pursuit of goals in negotiations. *Journal of Experimental Social Psychology, 43*, 519–598.

Verplanken, B., & Faes, S. (1999). Good intentions, had habits, and effects of forming implementation intentions on healthy eating. *European Journal of Social Psychology*, *29*, 591–604.

Vlaeyen, J. W., & Linton, S. J. (2000). Fear-avoidance and its consequences in chronic musculoskeletal pain: A state of the art. *Pain*, *85*, 317–332.

Vroom, V. H. (1964). *Work and motivation*. Oxford, UK: Wiley.

Webb, T. L., & Sheeran, P. (2003). Can implementation intentions help to overcome ego-depletion? *Journal of Experimental Social Psychology*, *39*, 279–286.

Webb, T. L., & Sheeran, P. (2006). Does changing behavioral intentions engender behavior change? A meta-analysis of the experimental evidence. *Psychological Bulletin*, *132*, 249–268.

Webb, T. L., & Sheeran, P. (2007). How do implementation intentions promote goal attainment? A test of component processes. *Journal of Experimental Social Psychology*, *43*, 295–302.

Webb, T. L., & Sheeran, P. (2008). Mechanisms of implementation intention effects: The role of goal intentions, self-efficacy, and accessibility of plan components. *British Journal of Social Psychology*, *47*, 373–395.

Wright, R. A., & Kirby, L. D. (2001). Effort determination of cardiovascular response: An integrative analysis with applications in social psychology. In M. P. Zanna (Ed.), *Advances in experimental social psychology* (Vol. 33, pp. 255–307). San Diego, CA: Academic Press.

# 8 Self-Theories

## *The Roots of Defensiveness*

Carol S. Dweck
Elaine S. Elliott-Moskwa

> Facts are stubborn things; and whatever may be our wishes, our inclinations, or the dictates of our passion, they cannot alter the state of facts and evidence.
>
> —John Adams (1770)

Although facts *are* stubborn things, people can try to escape from them, and they often do so with alarming success. Defenses serve to keep people away from threatening situations and to ward off or distort threatening information. If overdone, however, defenses can interfere with people's functioning. They can prevent people from having experiences they can learn from and from learning from the experiences they have.

In this chapter we argue that defensiveness, in good measure, can derive from people's self-theories, that is, from assumptions that people make about the fixed versus malleable nature of their personal qualities. We show that when people believe their valued attributes (e.g., intelligence) are fixed, they are strongly motivated to prove to themselves and others that they are well endowed—and they will become defensive in the face of evidence to the contrary. In contrast, when people believe that their valued attributes can be developed, they are more interested in learning and are therefore more open to situations and information, even negative information, that will help them learn.

We review research findings establishing that people with a fixed theory of their attributes engage in far more defensive behavior, at the expense of their learning and success. Their defensive behavior includes avoiding threatening situations (even if they contain valuable learning opportunities), concealing instead of remedying deficiencies, warding off diagnostic information, and selectively attending to flattering information instead of accurate information. We then present research on where self-theories originate and how they can be changed. We end with a proposal that self-theory change be included as a key element in cognitive-behavioral therapies—to change clients' (and therapists') level of defensiveness, to help them welcome new learning experiences, and to enhance their ability to cope with setbacks.

## WHAT ARE SELF-THEORIES AND HOW DO THEY WORK?

### What Are Self-Theories?

We all have many attributes that we care about, be they personality traits, intellectual attributes, artistic skills, or physical abilities. Each of these attributes can be understood in different ways. It may be seen as an endowment or gift that is deeply etched into our natures. Or it may be seen as something that we can develop through effort and education.[1] The latter view does not imply that everyone starts off the same or that anyone can be Einstein; it simply proposes that people can improve over time if they apply themselves. In this sense, talents or gifts are simply starting points, and the trajectory of people's talents depends on how vigorously they dedicate themselves to the task. More and more research, while not denying inborn talents, is showing the role of practice and dedication in the development of talent and even in the development of genius (Bloom, 1985; Ericsson, 1996; Ericsson, Krampe, & Tesch-Romer, 1993; Hayes, 1989; Weisberg, 1986; see also, Dweck, 2008).

In our research we measure the extent to which people believe that a given attribute is fixed or malleable by asking them to agree or disagree with statements such as: "Your intelligence is something very basic about you that you can't really change" (fixed) or "No matter who you are, you can always become substantially more intelligent" (malleable). Or, to assess their self-theories of personality, we ask: "The kind of person you are is something very basic about you and it can't be changed very much" (fixed) or "Everyone, no matter who they are, can significantly change their basic characteristics" (malleable). In general, about 40% of our research participants consistently endorse the fixed view and another 40% consistently endorse the malleable view, with about 20% remaining undecided (Dweck, 1999).

People can have different self-theories in different domains (e.g., intelligence, personality) (Dweck, Chiu, & Hong, 1995), and self-theories are, in general, fairly stable over time (Robins & Pals, 2002). However, despite the stability of self-theories when left to themselves, they can be changed with targeted interventions. These interventions can be temporary influences (as in short-term experiments, e.g., Nussbaum & Dweck, 2008) or relatively longer-term ones (as in systematic workshops, e.g., Aronson, Fried, & Good, 2002; Blackwell, Trzesniewski, & Dweck, 2007). In either case, the effects on motivation, behavior, and performance can be dramatic.

### How Do Self-Theories Work?

How can changing one belief have such a dramatic impact? This is the case because the fixed and malleable self-theories create entirely different psychological frameworks, in which the same things can have completely different, even opposite, meanings (Molden & Dweck, 2006). Let us take the example of intelligence.

People who hold a fixed theory of intelligence are always measuring their intelligence because they are never sure *at what level* it is fixed. They readily view mistakes, setbacks, and failures as meaning that their intelligence is lacking, because if their intelligence were great enough, they would not have run into these problems (Blackwell et al., 2007; Robins & Pals, 2002). Even effort has a negative meaning (Blackwell et al., 2007; Hong, Chiu, Dweck, Lin, & Wan, 1999). Many people with a fixed theory believe that if they had sufficiently high ability, they would not have to exert much effort. Indeed, they erroneously believe that all things come easily to people who have true ability. Thus people who hold a fixed theory of intelligence often believe that being intelligent is critically important but also see many danger signals that raise doubts about their own intelligence. This is why defensive maneuvers become necessary (Dweck, 2002).

People who hold a malleable theory of intelligence value intellectual ability but view it as something they can develop further if their present level is not up to the job. Thus they can stop worrying about how much they have at any given moment and instead focus on learning. In this framework, challenges are welcomed rather than seen as threatening (Blackwell et al., 2007; Robins & Pals, 2002; see also, Mueller & Dweck, 1998). Mistakes and setbacks are a natural and potentially informative part of learning. And effort, rather than being something that undermines ability, is seen as something that powers ability and helps it increase over time. When people are open to learning in this way, defensiveness becomes less necessary and less desirable because avoiding challenging or threatening situations can limit learning, as can hiding from or distorting negative feedback.

There is considerable research evidence that people with the fixed theory engage in more defensive behavior and in so doing deny themselves opportunities to learn, grow, and succeed in intellectual, social, and business-related endeavors.

## LOOK COMPETENT AT ALL COSTS

Much of what we argue springs from the basic finding that people with different self-theories value different goals; specifically, those with a fixed theory value looking smart (a "performance goal"), whereas people with a malleable theory value "learning goals."

Robins and Pals (2002) followed several hundred students over their college years, measuring their theories of intelligence and their goals. Those with a fixed theory were far less likely than those with a malleable theory to endorse the statement "The knowledge I gain in school is more important than the grades I receive." Similarly, Blackwell et al. (2007) studied several hundred students who were making the transition to junior high school. They, too, measured students' theories of intelligence and assessed their goals and values. They found that students with a fixed view were significantly less likely to endorse items that emphasized learning over looking smart, such as "I like school work that I'll learn from even if I make a lot of mistakes," "I like school work best when it makes me think hard," or "An important reason why I do my school work is because I like to learn new things" (see also Mangels, Butterfield, Lamb, Good, & Dweck, 2006).

Mueller and Dweck (1998) praised students in ways that transmitted a fixed or a malleable theory of intelligence, and then gave them a choice of problems to work on next. (It is important to note that none of the manipulations we discuss affected participants' *confidence* in their abilities. Thus if those given a malleable theory of ability choose harder tasks, it is not because they had higher regard for their skills.) Some of the choices offered represented performance goals that focused on looking smart (e.g., "I'd like problems that I'm pretty good at, so I can show that I'm smart"), whereas another choice represented a learning goal that emphasized the development of ability over looking good (e.g., "I'd like problems that I'll learn a lot from, even if I won't look so smart"). Across three studies, the clear majority of the students in the fixed intelligence condition chose the performance goal, making sure they would look smart. In contrast, the overwhelming majority of those in the malleable intelligence condition chose the challenging learning goal.

The fixed versus malleable distinction can also apply to the social domain. Beer (2002) studied people's self-theories about social skills and shyness. She first assessed whether participants believed that shyness is a fixed quality or one that can be changed by asking them to agree or disagree with statements such as "I have a certain level of shyness, and it is something that I can't do much about." They were then given a choice with respect to an upcoming social interaction that would be videotaped: Did they want to engage in an interaction in which they would learn new and useful social skills, although they might appear awkward on the videotape? Or did they want to be paired with someone who was even less skilled than they were so that their social skills would look good to others? Eighty-eight percent of the participants with a malleable theory chose the social interaction task they could learn from, but only a little more than half (53%) of those with the fixed theory so chose. This means that almost half of the latter chose to forego a learning opportunity in favor of looking better than a highly unskilled person.

Kray and Haselhuhn (2007) examined the impact of people's theories about negotiation ability on their negotiation goals and their performance on negotiation tasks. In one study, after teaching participants a fixed or malleable theory of negotiation skills, they gave them a choice of negotiation tasks:

Performance Goal Task: "This type of task involves problems of different levels. Some are hard, some are easier. If you pick this type of task, although you won't learn new negotiation skills, it will really demonstrate to the experimenter what you can do as a negotiator."

Learning Goal Task: "This type of task involves learning several new negotiation skills. Although you'll probably make a bunch of mistakes, get a little confused, and maybe feel a little dumb at times, eventually you'll learn some useful negotiation skills."

In line with previous results, those taught the malleable theory displayed a very strong desire for the learning-oriented task, whereas those taught the fixed theory did not. As before, almost half of those in the fixed theory condition chose the performance goal task instead of the learning goal task.

We now move to the question of whether the desire to look smart versus learn promotes defensive behavior.

## DON'T ADMIT MISTAKES OR REVEAL DEFICIENCIES

Despite people's fondest desires to appear competent, there are inevitably times when they have or reveal inadequacies. What happens then? Clearly, over the long run their best bet is to confront and remedy the deficiencies rather than to hide them and thus perpetuate them.

Hong et al. (1999) caught freshmen as they were signing up for their first semester courses at the University of Hong Kong. At that university, everything (books, lectures, papers, and exams) is in English, but not all students are proficient in English when they arrive. Hong et al. had measured students' theories of intelligence and obtained their English proficiency scores and now gave them an option. They reminded the students that English proficiency was critical for their academic success and then asked them how likely they would be to take a highly effective remedial English course if it were offered. Among the students with low English proficiency, those with a malleable theory of intelligence were highly enthusiastic about the offering. However, those with the fixed theory were lukewarm; that is, they were not very inclined to take the course. This suggests that they might choose to put their college success in jeopardy rather than reveal their deficiency.

### If You Do Reveal Deficiencies, Then Run from or Hide Them

When students with a malleable theory experience failure, they tend to confront it and take steps to learn what they do not know so that they can be successful again. However, if one thinks that the failure indicates a lack of ability that cannot be remedied, then one must take other, more circuitous, steps. Thus, students with a fixed theory try to escape from the arena, lie about their failure, or distort their beliefs.

Blackwell et al. (2007) followed students across their transition to junior high school and found that when students confronted a failure (e.g., on the first test in a new course), those with the malleable theory reported that they would work harder and find new study strategies. However, those with the fixed theory were significantly more likely than those with the malleable theory to say that they would study *less*, would try never to take a course in that area again, and would consider cheating on the next test. They were saying, in effect, that they would flee rather than fight (or they would fight unfairly).

Nussbaum and Dweck (2008) gave engineering students a three-part test that was said to tap three different facets of basic engineering skills. After the test, students were told that they had scored very well on two parts but poorly on the third. They were then given the choice to take a tutorial on one of the three skills areas and to retake the test in that area—which would determine their final score in the study. Students who had been taught the malleable theory overwhelmingly chose to take the tutorial in their weak area. However, students taught the fixed theory far more often chose to take the tutorial that went over material they already knew in one of their strong areas. They chose to shore up their view of themselves, not by improving their skills, but by fleeing the negative information and immersing themselves in the positive.

Expecting prejudicial treatment can make people defensive, and protecting themselves is often warranted. However, as with many defensive behaviors, by doing so people can rob themselves of important opportunities. In a study by London, Downey, and Dweck (2006), African American college students received critical feedback on an essay from an arrogant white professor. They received this feedback online and were then given the chance to meet with the professor in person to follow up on the feedback and revise their essay. Students with a malleable theory of intelligence were significantly more likely to rate this as a learning opportunity, and significantly more likely to elect to avail themselves of the chance to follow up. It was not that they failed to detect the arrogance of the professor, as the word *arrogant* entered into many of their free descriptions of the professor. They simply were not going to let that deprive them of the education they were there to receive. Those with a fixed theory of their intelligence were highly dismissive of the professor, thought he was prejudiced against them, and sought to protect themselves from further evaluation (but also further learning).

There are other ways to escape from negative feedback: One can lie about it. In Mueller and Dweck (1998), described above, students were praised in ways that influenced their theories of intelligence. They then were given some extremely difficult problems to work on, and most of them did quite poorly. Later, they were asked to (anonymously) report their scores on those problems to an unknown peer in another school. Almost 40% of the students in the fixed theory condition *lied* about their scores, and always in the favorable direction. Only 13% of those in the malleable theory condition lied. This finding suggests that when students believe that their intelligence is fixed they cannot reveal a deficiency—even to unknown others and perhaps even to themselves. This is another way of hiding from, rather than ameliorating, a deficiency.

Similar processes can also operate in relationships. Kammrath and Dweck (2006) studied how people coped with conflict in their close relationships. First, they measured people's belief in the malleability of human attributes (e.g., "Everyone is a certain kind of person and there is not much that can be done to really change that" versus. "Everyone, no matter who they are, can significantly change their basic characteristics"). In two studies they then assessed the strategies people typically used when they encountered a conflict in their romantic relationship. Those with a malleable theory, significantly more than those with the fixed view, used a strategy called "voice." That is, they more often tried to voice the issue to their partner in an effort to reach a mutually satisfactory resolution ("I openly discussed the situation with my partner," "I tried to work with my partner to find a solution to the problem," and "I tried to bring my concerns out into the open so that the issue could be resolved in the best possible way"). This strategy follows from the belief that people can be influenced. In addition, the more serious the conflict was, the more they used this strategy.

Those with the fixed theory were not only less likely to use the voicing strategy of direct problem solving, they were more likely to accept silently the partner and the problem (e.g., "I accepted his faults and didn't try to change him," "I tried to accept the situation and move on," and "I learned to live with it"). The more serious the conflict, the *less* likely they were to use the voicing strategy and directly address the conflict. Because they believed that people cannot change, their decision was to grin and bear it. One would imagine that in order to stay in a relationship in which one does not broach serious conflict, a goodly amount of defensive distortion may often need to take place. When this fails, the alternative may simply be to leave the relationship (see Knee, Patrick, Vietor, & Neighbors, 2004). As with other kinds of tasks, when people do not believe in change, the choices that remain may often involve mental or physical escape from problems.[2]

## DO THESE DEFENSIVE STRATEGIES WORK?

All of the defensive strategies outlines above are designed to shore up fixed theorists' sense of competence. Do they work?

## Managing Self-Esteem

The research we have discussed concerns how people manage their self-esteem in the face of setbacks, but we have not as yet discussed it in this way. Nussbaum and Dweck (2008) examined this question directly. First, they gave college students scientific articles to read that in previous research had been shown to induce different self-theories (fixed versus malleable). They then gave students a reading comprehension test that was said to measure a very basic component of intelligence. However, due to the difficulty of the test, students performed very poorly. Both students with fixed theories and those with malleable theories showed a sharp decrease in their state self-esteem, that is, in their current feelings of competence in the area.

Next, they were given the opportunity to examine the scores and strategies of either students who had performed worse than they had or students who had performed better than they had. Students in the malleable intelligence group mostly examined the scores and strategies of students who had done better than they had done, presumably to learn from them and shore up their skills. Moreover, the more that they made this choice, the more their self-esteem recovered. In contrast, students in the fixed intelligence group examined mainly the scores and strategies of students who had done *worse* than they had, and the more they did this the more their self-esteem recovered! Even though they had chosen to view very few useful strategies, they now said they felt highly confident about their abilities in the area. These findings suggest that when people have a fixed view of their ability and that ability is discredited, their best option, as they see it, may be to distort the data to put themselves in a favorable light rather than to try to remedy the ability deficit.

## Defensively Ensuring a Sense of High Competence

Research has shown that people tend to be overconfident about their abilities and performance across a wide variety of tasks (Dunning, 2005; Ehrlinger & Dunning, 2003). Ehrlinger and Dweck (2008) showed that this effect was almost entirely due to people with a fixed theory. Indeed those with a malleable theory had fairly accurate views of their ability and performance.

Ehrlinger and Dweck then probed *how* the overconfidence of the fixed theorists came about. They did this by monitoring participants' attention as they (the participants) reviewed their work on a task that contained a mixture of quite difficult problems and easier problems. In reviewing their work, those with a fixed theory of their intelligence dwelled on the easier problems and gave short shrift to the harder ones. In other words, because they needed to think well of their permanent ability, those with the fixed theory focused on flattering information (problems they could readily do) and neglected the harder problems from which they could learn. As in past research, those with the malleable theory, who were oriented toward learning, were more open to all kinds of information. Interestingly, in a later study, when people were *required* to attend to the difficult problems, the overconfidence of those with the fixed theory of intelligence disappeared.

Thus, the defensive, self-enhancing strategies work—up to a point. They seem to shore up self-esteem and a sense of competence but at the cost of hiding from the truth. In many of these cases, the truth is simply that one needs to sort out a problem or learn some new things. Left unattended, these problems or skill deficits could accumulate and stand in the way of successfully reaching one's long-term goals.

## EVEN EFFORT IS AN ENEMY

To people who hold a fixed theory, it is not only outright deficiencies that are threatening; effort, too, is an enemy. This is because many people with the fixed theory believe that people with high ability should not need to exert effort to succeed, and conversely that needing effort to succeed means that they do not have high ability (Blackwell et al., 2007; Hong et al., 1999). Since all worthwhile tasks in life require effort at some point, this can be a highly destructive belief. It can lead people to repeatedly flee from tasks or relationships that require effort in favor of ones that do not, or at least ones that do not appear to, at first glance.

If people holding fixed theories have no choice and must remain in a threatening area (e.g., in an academic course or a job), they may resort to that well-known defensive strategy called "self-handicapping" (Rhodewalt, 1994; see Berglas, 1988). Self-handicapping is a strategy whereby people withhold effort before an evaluative task so that their performance on the task will not be diagnostic of their true ability. Examples of self-handicapping include going to a party the night before a test instead of studying, or procrastinating on the preparation of a paper or presentation that is due the next day. Not only is their faith in their ability protected if they fail, but their faith in their ability is boosted if they happen to succeed. In these ways, the fixed theory creates a framework within which threats proliferate and defensive strategies proliferate along with them.

## ACCENTUATE THE POSITIVE, ELIMINATE THE NEGATIVE

As we have shown, a wealth of research supports the idea that people who believe that their qualities are fixed will continually seek strategies that allow them to think of themselves in positive ways. When threatening information comes their way, they often flee from it, even if it is information that they could use to sharpen important skills. In the process, they may manage to convince themselves that their skill level is far higher than it really is, perhaps making it even less likely that they will seek the improvement they need. Within the fixed theory framework, self-deception may become a standard operating procedure because one sees oneself as a finished product, and the product must not be found to be defective.

This is highly reminiscent of Karen Horney's (1950/1991) notion of "fraudulent bookkeeping." Horney argued that some people alter their mental ledgers to keep in the forefront of their minds the data they want to see and believe. The negative information is relegated to the nether regions, hopefully to dwell there and not impinge on their conscious minds. Horney describes the defensive person in this way:

> Like a fraudulent bookkeeper, he goes to any length to maintain the double account; but unlike him, he credits himself only with the favorable one and professes ignorance of the other. I have not yet seen a patient in whom the frank rebellion against reality ... did not strike a familiar chord. (1950/1991, p. 37)

However, as we have seen, this fraudulent bookkeeping comes at a cost, both in terms of the loss of valuable information that could guide learning and growth and, perhaps, in terms of the mental energy required to keep negative information at bay.

## WHERE DO SELF-THEORIES COME FROM?

### Praise

We have studied a number of ways in which self-theories can be communicated, but perhaps the most interesting way is through praise. Mueller and Dweck (1998) and Kamins and Dweck (1999) showed that when children are praised for their underlying traits, such as their intelligence, they adopt a fixed theory. For example, Mueller and Dweck (1998) told one group of students, after a fine performance on a set of IQ test problems, "You must be smart at this." This comment conveyed to students that the evaluator had read a stable trait from their performance. It may also have conveyed that being smart is what students should value above all. In either case, students then showed every symptom of the fixed mindset: a desire to look smart instead of a desire to learn, a tendency to see difficulty as signaling low ability, a sharp drop in motivation after difficulty, and an attempt to conceal the difficulty through lying.

In contrast, students praised for their "process" (e.g., their effort or strategies) adopted more of a malleable theory and remained eager for learning and highly motivated in the wake of difficulty. Moreover, they made few attempts to hide their mistakes.

This research was undertaken at the height of the self-esteem movement, which was advocating frequent praise for children, especially praise for their brains and talents. Indeed, in a survey we took at the time (see Mueller & Dweck, 1998), 85% of parents agreed that you *must* praise your children's intelligence to give them confidence. Yet, we had been studying vulnerability for many years and had seen that students who were focused on their intelligence were the ones who were fragile, not hardy. We thought that focusing students on their intelligence, even in a good way, might breed vulnerability and defensiveness. Our suspicion was correct, and we can only speculate on the effects that such praise, so widely endorsed, has had on the young generations. Many of the students we studied in the 1990s are now in the workforce, and we are hearing much about young workers' inability to take criticism or even feedback without experiencing a blow to their egos (Twenge, 2006). It is disheartening to think that parents and teachers may be creating a cohort of highly defensive individuals in an effort to impart self-esteem.

### Contingent Self-Worth

Carl Rogers (1961/1989) and Karen Horney both suggested that defenses arise when parents are not accepting of their children. Typically, this has been taken to refer to parents who were overly critical or disapproving. However, the results from the Mueller and Dweck (1998) and the Kamins and Dweck (1999) research suggest that children can become defensive when they worry that they cannot live up to their parents' expectations or standards. Praising intelligence or talent may set a standard of performance that children fear they cannot meet. In this sense, it may create in children a sense of contingent self-worth, that is, the idea that they are worthy when they reach that standard but not when they fail to do so (see Burhans & Dweck, 1995; Molden & Dweck, 2000).

A fixed theory may accompany a sense of contingent worth and/or magnify its effects. For example, Niiya, Crocker, and Bartmess (2004) identified college students whose self-esteem was heavily invested in their academic work and monitored them as they reacted to an academic failure. Those who were primed with a fixed theory of intelligence experienced lower self-esteem and higher negative affect after a failure on an academic test, but these negative effects were eliminated for the group in which a malleable theory of intelligence was primed. This study suggests that holding a fixed theory of intelligence goes hand in hand with contingent self-worth—self-worth that falls when people experience setbacks in important areas.

## CHANGING SELF-THEORIES CHANGES DEFENSIVENESS

When people's self-theories are changed, so is their tendency toward defensiveness. Above, we described the study by Hong et al. (1999) in which freshman at the University of Hong Kong were offered an option to take a remedial English course. As you may recall, those with a fixed view of their intelligence were not nearly as enthusiastic about it as students with a malleable view. Hong et al. also conducted a laboratory analogue in which students' self-theories were induced. College students were (temporarily) taught a malleable or a fixed view of intelligence and then given a very difficult intellectual task to perform. Following negative feedback about their performance, they were given the opportunity to take a tutorial before they performed the next trial of the task. Those who were taught the malleable theory were significantly more likely to avail themselves of this tutorial instead of defensively avoiding it (73% took the tutorial, compared to only 13% of those in the fixed intelligence condition). A mediational analysis showed that the greater tendency of those in the malleable intelligence condition to opt for the tutorial stemmed from their far greater emphasis on effort as a factor in their poor performance and hence a factor in the remediation of their performance.

In a similar vein, in the studies by Nussbaum and Dweck (2008) described above, people were taught either a fixed or a malleable theory of intelligence. People in the fixed theory group responded defensively to setbacks. For example, they chose to take a tutorial on something they were already good at rather than on something that needed improvement. They also repaired their self-esteem by examining the scores and strategies of people who had performed worse than they had. In neither case did they address their deficiency. However, people who were taught a malleable theory directly confronted their deficiencies and took steps to repair them.

In a real-world, longer-term intervention, Blackwell et al. (2007) conducted a workshop with seventh graders to promote a malleable theory of intelligence (see also, Good, Aronson, & Inzlicht, 2003). The seventh grade is a time of transition during which many students mentally and emotionally withdraw from school. And indeed the students in this study had been showing sharply declining math grades. Half of the students (the control group) received a wonderful eight-session workshop on study skills. However, we believed that study skills alone would not bring the students to life again. The other half of the students received an eight-session workshop that contained instruction in study skills *and* instruction in a malleable theory of intelligence. In the malleable ability sessions, students were told that the brain is like a muscle and gets stronger with exercise. They also were told that every time they work hard and learn something new, their brains form new connections and that over time these connections make them smarter. In addition, they learned how to apply these lessons to their schoolwork.

Students in the study skills control group continued their downward trajectory in math grades, whereas those in the malleable theory group showed a rapid rebound in grades. Moreover, teachers (blind to condition) singled out three times as many students in the malleable theory workshop (27 vs. 9%) as showing a clear embracing of effort and learning. Thus, removing the issue of fixed ability and substituting the idea of malleable ability appears to allow students to embrace their schoolwork in a more open, undefensive manner.

### Changing Self-Theories Defuses Stereotype Threat

Aronson et al. (2002) showed that changing African American college students' self-theories allowed them to thrive even in the face of stereotype threat (i.e., the perception that people in their school environment held negative stereotypes about their intellectual ability). They taught one group of college students a malleable theory of intelligence. Through a video, discussion, and exercises, they learned of the capacity of the brain to grow with effort and learning. As an additional way to inculcate the idea of expanding ability, students in this group were also asked to teach younger students the malleable theory. This group was then compared to a no-treatment control group and to a comparison group that learned a version of the idea of multiple intelligences (the idea that one should not worry about lacking a particular ability since one might still have high ability in other areas).

By the end of the semester, the African American students in the malleable ability group (but not the other two groups) showed significant improvement in their grades, in their valuing of academics ("Considering all the things that matter to you and make you who you are ... how important is academic achievement?") and in their enjoyment of the educational process (e.g., studying, going to class, taking tests). This improvement occurred even though there was no change whatsoever in their perception of stereotype threat. Students in the malleable intelligence group were just as likely as those in the other groups to agree that "people make judgments about my abilities based on my race" and that "people make judgments about my racial group based on my performances." That is, even though they still believed that they were judged through the lens of stereotypes, they were not held back by these perceptions. Perhaps learning the malleable theory relieved them of the defensiveness that comes with the fear of demonstrating a fixed low ability and released them to value and enjoy their academic work in a nondefensive way.

## A PROPOSAL FOR COGNITIVE-BEHAVIORAL THERAPY

Cognitive-behavioral therapy (CBT) has been documented in approximately 400 outcome studies to be an effective treatment for a wide range of mental health problems. These include, but are not limited to, depression, anxiety, bipolar disorder (in combination with medication), schizophrenia (in combination with medication), eating disorders, body dysmorphic disorder, and borderline personality disorder (see Leahy, 2004, for a review). There is also compelling evidence that therapeutic improvement in CBT is cognitively mediated (Garratt, Ingram, Rand, & Sawalani, 2007; Smits, Rosenfield, McDonald, & Telch, 2006; Wilson, Fairburn, Agras, Walsh, & Kraemer, 2002).

The theoretical rationale of CBT is that people's evaluative thoughts and beliefs are at the heart of much of their misery and maladaptive behavior, and that identifying these thoughts and beliefs and challenging them can help people feel and function better. For example, suppose a bright student becomes depressed every time he or she receives a disappointing grade and thinks, "I'm dumb, I'll never succeed." The cognitive therapist will help the student evaluate the meaning of these events more realistically by, for example, asking questions such as "What is the evidence for and against the idea that you are dumb? How does it help and how does it hurt to say this to yourself? Is there another way of looking at this situation? What is the worst that will happen and how would you deal with it?" The cognitive therapist may also help the student identify underlying beliefs such as "Unless I'm perfect, I will never succeed." The therapist will use a variety of cognitive and behavioral interventions designed to monitor, test, and challenge current thoughts and beliefs and replace them with a more adaptive perspective (e.g., to see the poor grade in the context of other good grades, to understand the possible alternative reasons for obtaining the poor grade, to figure out what to do the next time, and to adopt a more realistic standard for success). However, in most cases, the therapist would not directly try to change the student's self-theory framework from a fixed view to a malleable view.

Self-theories, rooted in the tradition of cognitive mediation, can contribute to cognitive therapy theory and practice. More specifically, the patterns of defensiveness emanating from a fixed self-theory and of openness emanating from a malleable theory can be used to assist cognitive therapists who are treating clients and training other therapists. We focus on three areas in which we believe there may be a productive cross-fertilization of ideas and research: defensiveness and untreated mental health problems, defensiveness and resistance in cognitive therapy, and defensiveness and therapist variables.

## DEFENSIVENESS AND UNTREATED MENTAL HEALTH PROBLEMS

Many people who may benefit from CBT delay initiating contact with providers. Studies supported by the National Institute of Mental Health have documented delays between the onset of symptoms and the seeking of any type of mental health treatment. Some of these delays are decades long, with the median being 10 years and the longest 20 years. The costs of these delays are staggering. Delays lead to an increase in the frequency and severity of episodes and more treatment resistance, and untreated early-onset problems are correlated with a spectrum of difficulties such as academic failure, unemployment, and even violence (see Kessler et al., 2005).

People may delay help seeking for a variety of reasons, including problems with access (e.g., no insurance, lack of facilities; see also, Dearing & Twaragowski, Chapter 21, this volume). Some delays, however, are the result of reluctance to seek professional help. Much has been written about the stigma of mental illness, and many organizations have sought to reach out and educate the public about treatment (National Institute of Mental Health, National Alliance on Mental Illness, American Psychological Association; see also Corrigan, Larson, & Kuwabara, Chapter 4, this volume). These public awareness campaigns seem to have made some difference. For example, education about mood disorders appears to be correlated with a somewhat decreased delay in seeking help (Kessler et al., 2005). People also may be reluctant to seek help because they hold a fixed theory of personality or mental health. A fixed theory may lead people to believe that little can be done to change their mental health status and may heighten the fear that they might be stigmatized as permanently deficient.

With a fixed theory they may also avoid treatment out of concern that therapy might not work and thus confirm that something is *really* wrong with them.

The hypothesis that a fixed theory is associated with reluctance to initiate treatment could be tested initially by measuring beliefs about the fixedness or malleability of personality or mental health and examining its correlation with initiating contact with mental health professionals. In addition, this could also be tested by explicitly teaching a malleable view of personality and mental health in middle or high schools to students and parents and measuring behavioral intentions to seek appropriate resources. Moreover, public health campaigns might incorporate overtly a malleable view of mental health in their ads. For instance, although the National Alliance on Mental Illness has made important contributions to educating the public about mental health problems, its website seems to have embedded, in some of the descriptions of problems, a mix of fixed and malleable educational materials. As an example, the fixed view may be fostered by the following quote from their website: "Mental illnesses are biologically based brain disorders." The website also states that "just as diabetes is a disease of the pancreas, mental illnesses are medical conditions." In contrast, the malleable view seems to be embodied in the following quote from the same website: "Most people diagnosed with a serious mental illness can experience relief from their symptoms by actively participating in an individual treatment plan" and "A key concept is to develop expertise in developing strategies to manage the illness process." Although, no doubt, many have found encouragement and support through this educational website, would framing the information more consistently within a malleable view of mental health motivate even more people to seek available resources? For example, a possible revision of the website might include the following:

> Individuals who have mental health problems sometimes think, "This is who I am. I am a person with a mental illness and this cannot be changed." Mental health problems, however, just like medical conditions like diabetes are modifiable. Just as people with diabetes can change the course of their lives by watching their diet, exercising and taking their medication, people with a mental health problem can change the course of their lives by utilizing the resources available to them. This may involve working with a qualified professional who will collaborate with you to develop new ways of tackling problems that you typically encounter. It may also involve taking medication that will help you to feel better or help you to focus more as you learn new and helpful strategies to face life's challenges. There are many resources available that can be tailored to your individual needs. The first step is to recognize that your mental health condition does not have to define who you are, but that you may define who you are. Although your life may be immensely more challenging with your mental health condition, it can also be immensely more satisfying if you see your mental health as modifiable.

## DEFENSIVENESS AND RESISTANCE DURING COGNITIVE THERAPY

Problems of resistance or defensiveness in CBT are not uncommon, especially among individuals diagnosed with personality disorders. Although the CBT protocol defines the elements of therapy explicitly (Beck, 2005; Beck, Rush, Shaw, & Emery, 1979), even experienced therapists encounter roadblocks in helping clients to adhere to important components of CBT, such as establishing goals for therapy, setting an agenda, monitoring and challenging automatic thoughts, running behavioral experiments to test their beliefs, self-help or homework assignments, and giving the therapist evaluative feedback about the session.

Roadblocks may occur at any point. For example, clients may have difficulty coming up with goals for therapy ("Don't ask me about goals—I don't have goals") or may be reluctant to share their automatic thoughts with the therapist ("I'd rather not share my thoughts about my husband—these are private"). Others will not risk running behavioral experiments designed to test out their maladaptive beliefs and increase their coping skills ("I just can't do that") or repeatedly fail to complete self-help assignments ("I just didn't have the time").

Cognitive and behavioral strategies for dealing with these difficulties include establishing a collaborative relationship with the client, eliciting thoughts and beliefs that are roadblocks to change, teaching self-control strategies, and breaking tasks down into small steps (e.g., Beck, 2005; Leahy, 2001, 2003; Young, Klosko, & Weishaar, 2003).

Implicit in the CBT approach is a malleable view of the client's attributes. Specifically, CBT is a problem-oriented approach that helps the client learn skills and strategies to identify and replace maladaptive thinking and behavior with more adaptive perspectives and behavior. Beck et al. (1979) recommended that "the therapist view his patient as a person who has problems and specific deficits or who holds some irrational beliefs, rather than as a person who is irrational or who has a defective character. ... Such pejorative labeling affects the therapist's and patient's attitude toward the patient. It also implies that the patient is relatively unchangeable and intrinsically defective" (p. 63).

From the perspective of self-theories, the cognitive and behavioral strategies of CBT implicitly help clients shift from a fixed view of their attributes to a malleable view (e.g., view of self as a social failure to view of self as prone to jumping to conclusions in social settings and needing some additional social skills; view of self as a schizophrenic to view of self as a person with schizophrenia whose thoughts, beliefs, and behaviors may exacerbate his or her difficulties). This is not to say that CBT denies the biological correlates of mental health difficulties, but tries to suggest how, given a certain biological predisposition, a person might nevertheless cope and grow.

An explicit protocol teaching clients to view their attributes as malleable versus fixed might increase compliance with the cognitive therapy. CBT is typically structured such that in the initial sessions, the therapist educates the client about the CBT model and what to expect in the course of therapy. Treatment may be enhanced by explicitly teaching a malleable view of self in order to decrease defensiveness and increase compliance with the CBT protocol. For example, the therapist might teach a depressed client to view the depression as malleable by saying the following:

> "Your brain is changeable. You can make new connections. For example, stroke victims can rewire their brains through specific brain exercises and improve their functioning. Likewise, by using CBT you can rewire or reshape your emotional responses to situations. When you are experiencing a depressed mood, your brain tends to go down old pathways. It follows the same road ruts again and again in its interpretation of situations. It is not that you are a depressed person but that currently you have some overused connections that need to be rewired or expanded into a broader network. New connections need to be made. How do you rewire your brain? It takes some effort, practice and risk taking using cognitive therapy. Each time you do a cognitive therapy homework assignment, you are helping your brain to develop these new pathways."

This hypothesis could be experimentally tested by comparing standard CBT with CBT + education about the malleable view. Improvement during CBT also may be correlated with a malleable view. Testing this hypothesis might involve measuring clients' view of their attributes before therapy and correlating this with changes in objective outcome measures.

## DEFENSIVENESS AND THERAPISTS' SELF-THEORIES DURING COGNITIVE THERAPY

CBT requires the therapist to collaborate with clients, some of whom may be quite challenging. For example, clients may behave helplessly, act in a demanding or controlling manner, or appear suspicious or critical. It requires a great deal of effort to persevere and find new strategies with clients who may, for example, resist completing self-help assignments or who may seem locked into maladaptive views and behaviors or who are hopeless or suicidal.

CBT requires the therapist to engage in self-evaluation as well as elicit evaluative feedback from the client, especially when a client seems to be making little progress. This means that the therapist must be open to learning new, evidence-based procedures and to incorporating them into therapy. Sometimes this requires consulting with other mental health professionals. Many have made contributions to defining and elucidating therapist variables that may promote or impede clients' progress in therapy (Beutler, Machado, & Neufeldt, 1994; Saunders, 1999). Therapist's self-theories may be related to their ability to achieve these tasks.

An overview of materials on training CBT therapists indicates that those who teach and mentor CBT therapists seek implicitly to foster a malleable view of psychotherapy skills (Beck et al., 1979.) When faced with difficulty in a session CBT therapists are asked to examine their own automatic thoughts in response to the client (e.g., "I'm a lousy therapist" or "He is a hopeless case"). However, we suggest that it might be beneficial for therapist training programs to incorporate explicit training in the malleable view, that is, in the idea that therapy skills can be developed continually throughout one's career. Evidence can be provided that even the most eminent and well-respected CBT therapists have had to consult with others on difficult cases or have needed and sought to incorporate new evidence-based procedures into their repertoires. Indeed, it should be stressed that seeking help is the sign of a good therapist, not a deficient one. Moreover, therapists in training can be taught that difficult clients, rather than calling the therapist's competence into questions, provide an opportunity to learn new treatment strategies and become a better therapist.

In the same vein, therapists can be explicitly taught a malleable view of clients (see Young et al., 2003). Although the basis of CBT (or any therapy, for that matter) is the idea that clients can be helped to change, some clients may strongly challenge this belief with their helpless, controlling, or critical behavior. As suggested above, rather than becoming discouraged about the client's capacity for change, the therapist can seek and test out new strategies for overcoming the client's defensive behavior.

## CONCLUSION

When people think of themselves in terms of fixed traits—traits that can be judged from their behavior and performance—it gives rise to defensiveness. People who hold fixed theories are apt to flee from or distort information that suggests that they are deficient because they view their deficiencies as permanent. In contrast, when people think of themselves in terms of malleable traits, they are open to challenging experiences that will help them develop their abilities, and they stand ready to confront information about their deficiencies. Further, the malleable view can be taught, and when it is taught, people begin to embrace learning and rebound from setbacks. Indeed, they begin to look more like Carl Rogers' (1961/1989) description of the open individual: "If a person could be fully open to his experience ... every stimulus ... would be freely relayed through the nervous system, without being distorted by any defensive mechanism." Finally, the lessons from self-theory research can be incorporated into cognitive-behavioral therapies to reduce defensiveness on the parts of both clients and therapists.

## NOTES

1. In our technical writing we call the fixed view an *entity theory* and the malleable view an *incremental theory*, and in writing for the lay audience (see, e.g., Dweck, 2006), we have used the terms *fixed mindset* and *growth mindset*. Here we simply refer to the fixed or malleable view/theory.
2. Of course, we do not wish to imply that a partner *will* change or that leaving a relationship is not sometimes the best option. However, we simply wish to point out that direct problem solving is less likely for people with a fixed theory and that premature abandoning of the relationship could result from this tendency.

## REFERENCES


Adams, J. (1770). *Argument in defense of the Soldiers in the Boston Massacre trials.*

Aronson, J., Fried, C., & Good, C. (2002). Reducing the effects of stereotype threat on African American college students by shaping theories of intelligence. *Journal of Experimental Social Psychology, 38*, 113–125.

Beck, A. T., Rush, A. J., Shaw, B. F., & Emery, G. (1979). *Cognitive therapy of depression.* New York: Guilford Press.

Beck, J. S. (2005). *Cognitive therapy for challenging problems: What to do when the basics don't work.* New York: Guilford Press.

Beer, J. S. (2002). Implicit self-theories of shyness. *Journal of Personality and Social Psychology, 83*, 1009–1024.

Berglas, S. (1988). The three faces of self-handicapping: Protective self-presentation, a strategy for self-esteem enhancement, and a character disorder. In R. Hogan (Ed.), *Perspectives in personality* (Vol. 1, pp. 235–270). Greenwich, CN: JAI.

Beutler, L. E., Machado, P. P., & Neufeldt, S. A. (1994). Therapist variables. In A. E. Bergin & S. L. Garfield (Eds.), *Handbook of psychotherapy and behavior change* (pp. 229–269). New York: Wiley.

Blackwell, L. S., Trzesniewski, K., & Dweck, C. S. (2007). Implicit theories of intelligence predict achievement across an adolescent transition: A longitudinal study and an intervention. *Child Development, 78*, 246–263.

Bloom, B. S. (1985). *Developing talent in young people.* New York: Ballentine.

Burhans, K., & Dweck, C. S. (1995). Helplessness in early childhood: The role of contingent worth. *Child Development, 66*, 1719–1738.

Dunning, D. (2005). *Self-insight: Roadblocks and detours on the path to knowing thyself.* New York: Psychology Press.

Dweck, C. S. (1999). *Self-theories: Their role in motivation, personality, and development.* Philadelphia: Psychology Press.

Dweck, C. S. (2002). Beliefs that make smart people dumb. In R. J. Sternberg (Ed.), *Why smart people do stupid things*. New Haven, CT: Yale University Press.

Dweck, C. S. (2006). *Mindset.* New York: Random House.

Dweck, C. S. (2008). Can personality be changed? The role of beliefs in personality and change. *Current Directions in Psychological Science*, *17*, 391–394.

Dweck, C. S., Chiu, C., & Hong, Y. (1995). Implicit theories and their role in judgments and reactions: A world from two perspectives. *Psychological Inquiry*, *6*, 267–285.

Ehrlinger, J., & Dunning, D. (2003). How chronic self-views influence (and potentially mislead) estimates of performance. *Journal of Personality and Social Psychology*, *84*, 5–17.

Ehrlinger, J., & Dweck, C. S. (2008). *Attention and overconfidence: The role of implicit theories.* Unpublished manuscript, Stanford University, Stanford, CA.

Ericsson, K. A. (Ed.). (1996). *The road to excellence: The acquisition of expert performance in the arts and sciences, sports, and games.* Mahwah, NJ: Erlbaum.

Ericsson, K. A., Krampe, R. T., & Tesch-Romer, C. (1993). The role of deliberate practice in expert performance. *Psychological Review*, *100*, 363–406.

Garratt, G., Ingram, R. E., Rand, K. L., & Sawalani, G. (2007). Cognitive processes in cognitive therapy: Evaluation of the mechanisms of change in the treatment of depression. *Clinical Psychology: Science and Practice*, *14*(3), 224–239.

Good, C., Aronson, J., & Inzlicht, M. (2003). Improving adolescents' standardized test performance: An intervention to reduce the effects of stereotype threat. *Journal of Applied Developmental Psychology*, *24*, 645–662.

Hayes, J. R. (1989). Cognitive processes in creativity. In J. Glover, R. Ronning, & C. Reynolds (Eds.), *Handbook of creativity.* New York: Plenum Press.

Hong, Y. Y., Chiu, C., Dweck, C. S., Lin, D., & Wan, W. (1999). Implicit theories, attributions, and coping: A meaning system approach. *Journal of Personality and Social Psychology*, *77*, 588–599.

Horney, K. (1991). *Neurosis and human growth*. New York: Norton. (Original work published 1950)

Kamins, M., & Dweck, C. S. (1999). Person vs. process praise and criticism: Implications for contingent self-worth and coping. *Developmental Psychology*, *35*, 835–847.

Kammrath, L., & Dweck, C. S. (2006). Voicing conflict: Preferred conflict strategies among incremental and entity theorists. *Personality and Social Psychology Bulletin*, *32*, 1497–1508.

Kessler, R. C., Berglund, P., Demler, O., Jin, R., Merikangas, K. R., & Walters, E. E. (2005). Lifetime prevalence and age-of-onset distributions of *DSM-IV* disorders in the National Comorbidity Survey replication. *Archives of General Psychiatry*, *62*, 593–602.

Knee, C. R., Patrick, H., Vietor, N. A., & Neighbors, C. (2004). Implicit theories of relationships: Moderators of the link between conflict and commitment. *Personality and Social Psychology Bulletin*, *30*, 617–628.

Kray, L. J., & Haselhuhn, M. P. (2007). Implicit negotiation beliefs and performance: Experimental and longitudinal evidence. *Journal of Personality and Social Psychology*, *93*, 49–64.

Leahy, R. L. (2001). *Overcoming resistance in cognitive therapy.* New York: Guilford Press.

Leahy, R. L. (2003). *Roadblocks in cognitive-behavioral therapy: Transforming challenges into opportunities for change.* New York: Guilford Press.

Leahy, R. L. (Ed.). (2004). *Contemporary cognitive therapy.* New York: Guilford Press.

London, B., Downey, G., & Dweck, C. S. (2006). *The student's dilemma: Academic engagement in the face of stereotype threat.* Unpublished manuscript, Columbia University, New York.

Mangels, J. A., Butterfield, B., Lamb, J., Good, C. D., & Dweck, C. S. (2006). Why do beliefs about intelligence influence learning success? A social–cognitive–neuroscience model. *Social, Cognitive, and Affective Neuroscience*, *1*, 75–86.

Molden, D. C., & Dweck, C. S. (2000). Meaning and motivation. In C. Sansone & J. Harackiewicz (Eds.), *Intrinsic motivation.* San Diego, CA: Academic Press.

Molden, D. C., & Dweck, C. S. (2006). Finding "meaning" in psychology: A lay theories approach to self-regulation, social perception, and social development. *American Psychologist, 61*, 192–203.

Mueller, C. M., & Dweck, C. S. (1998). Intelligence praise can undermine motivation and performance. *Journal of Personality and Social Psychology, 75*, 33–52.

National Alliance on Mental Illness. Retrieved January 20, 2008, from *www.nami.org/*.

Niiya, Y., Crocker, J., & Bartmess, E. N. (2004). From vulnerability to resilience: Learning orientations buffer contingent self-esteem from failure. *Psychological Science, 15*, 801–805.

Nussbaum, A. D., & Dweck, C. S. (2008). Remediation vs. defensiveness: Implicit theories and self-esteem repair. *Personality and Social Psychology Bulletin, 34*, 599–612.

Rhodewalt, F. (1994). Conceptions of ability, achievement goals, and individual differences in self-handicapping behavior: On the application of implicit theories. *Journal of Personality, 62*, 67–85.

Robins, R. W., & Pals, J. L. (2002). Implicit self-theories in the academic domain: Implications for goal orientation, attributions, affect, and self-esteem change. *Self and Identity, 1*, 313–336.

Rogers, C. (1989). A therapist's view of the good life: The fully functioning person. In H. Kirschenbaum & V. Henderson (Eds.), *The Carl Rogers reader.* New York: Houghton Mifflin. (Original work published 1961)

Saunders, S. M. (1999). Clients' assessment of the affective environment of the psychotherapy session: Relationship to session quality and treatment effectiveness. *Journal of Clinical Psychology, 55*(4), 597–605.

Smits, J. A. J., Rosenfield, D., McDonald, R., & Telch, M. J. (2006). Cognitive mechanisms of social anxiety reduction: An examination of specificity and temporality. *Journal of Consulting and Clinical Psychology, 74*(6), 1203–1212.

Twenge, J. M. (2006). *Generation me.* New York: Free Press.

Weisberg, R. W. (1986). *Creativity: Genius and other myths.* New York: Freeman.

Wilson, G. T., Fairburn, C. C., Agras, W. S., Walsh, B. T., & Kraemer, H. (2002). Cognitive-behavioral therapy for bulimia nervosa: Time course and mechanisms of change. *Journal of Consulting and Clinical Psychology, 70*(2), 267–274.

Young, J., Klosko, J., & Weishaar, M. E. (2003). *Schema therapy: A practitioner's guide.* New York: Guilford Press.

# Interpersonal Processes

# 9 Attachment Theory as a Social–Developmental Psychopathology Framework for the Practice of Psychotherapy

Hal S. Shorey

As a lifespan theory of personality development, attachment theory describes, in a straightforward and parsimonious manner, how initially external social interactions shape the internal structure of personality and thus influence how people characteristically think, feel, and behave across their lifespans (Bowlby, 1969, 1973, 1980, 1988). The theory juxtaposes normal positive development and negative pathological development. In this respect, attachment theory is useful for understanding the development of psychopathology, as well as for helping clinicians conceptualize clients and identify the adaptive processes that can be used to help individuals back onto tracks of optimal functioning.

Capitalizing on more than 20 years of empirical attachment research, clinicians recently have begun to systematically apply the theory to work with children, families, couples, and adult psychotherapy clients. In this spirit, the present chapter aims to move beyond conceptual issues and present clinicians with the latest on clinical assessment and treatment developments.

## HISTORICAL CONTEXT

Attachment theory had its genesis in the works of John Bowlby (1969), a British-trained physician and psychoanalyst who became dissatisfied with psychoanalytic and object relations perspectives, which held that psychopathology originates within children. In contrast, Bowlby (1969) proposed that factors present in the child's external environment (i.e., interactions with parents), not internal drives or fantasies, were the primary forces in personality development and psychopathology.

Bowlby's propositions amounted to nothing less than heresy to those in the British school of psychoanalysis, and his ideas were largely rejected by the psychoanalytic community (for a review of the genesis of attachment theory, see Bretherton, 1992). When psychoanalysis became popular in the United States, it did so without directly incorporating Bowlby's concepts. Owing in large part to Mary Ainsworth's (1973) development of techniques to assess infant attachment styles (Ainsworth, Blehar, Waters, & Wall, 1978), however, attachment theory became a leading social psychology theory of personality development (Davila & Levy, 2006).

One of Ainsworth's colleagues, Mary Main, later extended attachment style assessment to adults through developing a narrative technique (the Adult Attachment Interview [AAI]; George, Kaplan, & Main, 1985/1996). This mode of assessment became the favorite among clinical psychology researchers. Social psychologists, in contrast, developed self-report measures (Bartholomew & Horowitz, 1991; Brennan, Clark, & Shaver, 1998; Hazan & Shaver, 1987) to assess attachment patterns and engaged in ambitious research programs of their own. Much of this social psychology research generated over the past 20 years has profound implications for clinical practice. Thus, attachment theory can truly be said to have come full circle: from a theory rejected by the psychoanalytic community, to a unifying framework for working with clients in clinical and counseling psychology practice.

## THE ATTACHMENT SYSTEM

Drawing on works from the natural sciences, Bowlby (1969, 1988) proposed that young humans, similar to other animals, are biologically predisposed to maintain attachments to groups and more powerful others because maintaining such attachments has basic survival value. The attachment system acts as a homeostatic mechanism that keeps proximity seeking and exploration in balance. When children stray too far from their parents in exploring the environment, anxiety becomes intolerably high and motivates them to reestablish proximity. When children are young, they attain security through seeking real physical contact. As children mature, they build on these early experiences and form internal mental representations of themselves in relation to the parent (termed *working models*). In the event of separation, these working models enable older children to derive "senses" of security without having to actually attain physical proximity.

Working models also allow children to anticipate how others and the environment are likely to respond under various conditions. As such, children can initiate behaviors without always having to rely upon painful trial-and-error learning. Because people tend to behave in ways that elicit reactions from others that are consistent with their expectations (Allen, Coyne, & Huntoon, 1998), attachment working models, and related patterns of thinking, feeling, and behaving, are reinforced throughout the developmental years, carry forward into adulthood, and have profound influences on adjustment and psychopathology (see Batgos & Leadbeater, 1994).

## Optimal Development and Secure Attachment Styles

When parents consistently are available, warm, responsive, and maintain high standards for their children's behaviors, the children typically develop what is termed a *secure attachment style* (Bowlby, 1988). One way that parents maintain consistency of responsiveness is through being sensitively attuned to their children's emotional cues and needs. When parents have such *empathic attunement*, they validate their children's subjective emotional experiences. Empathically attuned parents provide the mirrors through which children learn that what they are feeling corresponds to events in the real external world. When children thus are allowed to experience their authentic emotions, first in direct partnership with the parent (i.e., the parental *holding environment*) and later with representations (i.e., memories and schemas) of the parent, they learn that negative emotions can be tolerated and managed effectively (Bowlby, 1969).

Confident in caregiver availability, secure children are free to focus their energies on exploring their interpersonal and natural environments (see Mikulincer & Shaver, 2003). Having *secure bases* to return to when they meet with inevitable goal blockages or become frightened, these children explore their world in ever-widening circles. Moreover, secure children are increasingly successful in achieving their goals, and they develop hopeful ways of thinking (Bowlby, 1988; Shorey, Snyder, Yang, & Lewin, 2003) as they interact with parents in what is known as a *goal-corrected partnership* (Bowlby, 1969). In this latter respect, when children seek comfort after failures, parents go beyond soothing distress and also provide their children with new strategies to use in successive goal pursuits.

As this process is continually repeated and children begin to internalize their parents' secure base functions (see Bowlby 1969, 1988), they develop the confidence to act autonomously. Accordingly, as they mature through adolescence into adulthood, secure children become increasingly efficacious individuals who believe that (1) they are lovable and worthy of support, (2) others are available and responsive, and (3) the world is a safe and predictable place (see Bowlby, 1969; Brennan et al., 1998).

## Suboptimal Development and Insecure Attachment

When parents, for whatever reason, are not able to provide their children with secure bases, the children will naturally adapt in a way that maximizes their perceptions of security in the parent–child relationship. In this respect, the *insecure attachment styles* that children develop generally are positive adaptations that enable them to cope with adverse environments. The price for these initially positive adaptations is high, however, because resulting deficits in affect regulation and cognitive distortions (e.g., "splitting"; see Kernberg, 1975; Kraemer & Loader, 1995; Lopez, Fuendeling, Thomas, & Sagula, 1997) become maladaptive in later adult contexts.

### *The Anxious/Preoccupied Attachment Style*

When parents are inconsistent (i.e., sometimes available and warm and at other times rejecting and cold), children learn that they cannot take parental security for granted and they become hypervigilant for rejection cues (Bartholomew & Horowitz, 1991). This monitoring acts as an "early warning system" that allows children to adjust their behaviors quickly to avoid potentially painful parental rejections (Main, 1990). Mikulincer and Shaver (2003) conceived of this attentional hypervigilance as a hyperactivation of the attachment system, wherein that part of the homeostatic mechanism that induces anxiety in response to threat, and, by extension, promotes proximity seeking, is stuck in the "on position." Although the goal of this hyperactivation is to ameliorate the child's distressed emotions, this goal never is realized. Children become stuck in chronic states of attachment anxiety, become highly focused on their caregivers, and, by extension, lose touch with their own authentic emotions and values. Because they are highly reactive to the external environment, such individuals are not likely to perceive control over their emotions and are likely to have problems with affect regulation.

This developmental pattern leads to what Ainsworth et al. (1978) labeled the *anxious–ambivalent attachment style.* Anxious–ambivalent children give up a great deal of free exploration, autonomy, and positive self-worth in attempts to attain attachment security—a goal that never is fully realized. As they mature into adulthood, these individuals are likely to be overly dependent on others (Brennan & Shaver, 1998) for problem solving and guidance, their good feelings, and their senses of self-worth. This dependency contributes to their being preoccupied with relationships. Hence, the adult label for this style is *preoccupied* (Bartholomew & Horowitz, 1991).

Preoccupied adults' tend to devalue the self while overvaluing others, which leads them to engage in frequent reassurance seeking. This constant needing of reassurance then sets up the preoccupied individuals for rejection and social failures because these behaviors, accompanied with a high level of emotional reactivity, lead others to feel overwhelmed and resentful. Thus, preoccupied people "pull" for the experience they fear the most—rejection (Bartholomew & Horowitz, 1991). Related to their social failures and high levels of chronic distress, preoccupied individuals evidence much higher levels of psychopathology relative to their securely attached counterparts (see Shorey & Snyder, 2006, for a review of attachment and specific manifestations of psychopathology).

### The Dismissing/Avoidant Attachment Style

In contrast to those with anxious-ambivalent/preoccupied attachment styles, people who develop childhood *avoidant attachment styles* (labeled *dismissing* for adults) regulate their emotions through deactivating the attachment system (Mikulincer & Shaver, 2003). When neediness or negative emotional displays (e.g., crying or expressions of anger) are met consistently with parental rebukes or punishments (Connors, 1997; Main, 1990), children learn to forgo asking parents for attention, comfort, and support. In this case, the child's distress is not ameliorated by the parent, nor can it be tolerated by the child. Thus the only viable way to cope with negative emotions is simply not to experience them.

These children tend to automatically suppress not only the expression, but also the actual experience, of negative emotions. Their physiological reactions to emotionally valenced interpersonal stimuli are just as intense as those of preoccupied persons, but they appear unable to report on their experiences (see Diamond, Hicks, & Otter-Henderson, 2006). This pattern is adaptive because as long as they are able to display neutral or positive affects, the children can avoid parental rejection and maintain proximity. If they become high achievers (e.g., in sports, academics, work), they may even gain parental acceptance and praise because their parents are likely to have high standards for their children's performances (Mayseless, 1996).

Because negative emotions cannot always be suppressed, avoidant children also learn to avoid emotionally charged social interactions—a pattern that quickly generalizes beyond parents to the wider social environment. Intimacy and close interpersonal relationships (peer or romantic) create vulnerability and therefore are avoided. This is not to say that avoidant individuals lack friends. They may even be perceived as popular, particularly since they are likely to be successful in competition and achievement areas. Nevertheless, such people are not likely to share their personal struggles with others and may feel socially isolated (Bartholomew, 1990).

Aside from behavioral avoidance, another way that individuals with this style avoid social threats is by using selective attention to ignore social cues. There is evidence that this attentional mechanism operates automatically, similar to the suppression of emotion. For example, when presented subliminally with social threat cues, dismissing adults have decreased access to cognitive representations of social goals and increased access to representations of achievement goals (Shorey, 2006). Because they do not attend to social threats, dismissing-avoidant individuals are likely to be perceived as confident and self-assured. They grow to view themselves as highly efficacious and self-reliant individuals who simultaneously disavow their needs for interpersonal closeness (Bartholomew, 1990; Connors, 1997; Millon, 1996). Not perceiving their interpersonal styles to be particularly problematic, and suppressing negative emotions, these individuals tend to minimize the reporting of psychological distress and are the least likely of any of the attachment groups to seek psychotherapeutic interventions.

### *Disorganized and Fearful–Avoidant Attachment*

In contrast to those with preoccupied and dismissing attachment styles, children who develop *disorganized* attachment styles are not able to adequately ameliorate distress through hyperactivation or deactivation of the attachment system. The parents of disorganized children often are nonresponsive, frightened, or frightening. Such parents simply are not able to perform their secure-base functions, and there is little that children can do in the way of behavioral or cognitive adaptations to regulate their emotions or gain senses of security (Hesse & Main, 2000).

A paucity of parental responsiveness may occur for various reasons, including the parent's psychopathology (e.g., severe depression) or in situations of domestic violence. When the parent is frightened, she may not be able to soothe her own distress adequately to comfort her frightened child. Similarly, if a parent's emotions are blunted, she will have difficulty being empathically attuned enough to provide adequate reflective functioning (see Carlson, 1998). This deficit is problematic because human infants learn to self-soothe through mirroring and empathic attunement provided by the responsive caregiver. When her baby is distressed, the secure parent is likely to acknowledge this distress with a sympathetic or reflective, pained facial expression. The parent then provides comfort by expressing calming or positive affects, which then are perceived and felt by the infant. Through such sharing of emotional experiences, the caregiver regulates the baby's biological stress responses until the baby learns to do this for him- or herself (Fonagy & Target, 1997; see also de Zulueta, 2006). When this developmental process is circumvented, long-term deficits in the ability to regulate emotions result (see Schore, 2001).

In situations of child abuse, deficits in affect regulation are compounded by the child's inability to predict cause-and-effect relationships and the related failure to develop consistent behavioral response patterns. Abused children find themselves in unsolvable dilemmas wherein the anxiety triggered by the abuse activates the attachment system, which then impels the child to seek proximity to the offending (and anxiety-provoking) parent. Similarly, when they become frightened by events in the environment, such children have no choice but to seek comfort from parents who are just as frightening as that from which they are running. As a result, the children are apt to engage in simultaneous (disorganized) approach-and-avoidance behaviors (Main & Solomon, 1990). In such cases, one source of fear is merely traded for another, and the child's distress is not ameliorated and may even increase.

There is mounting evidence that such early relational experiences and corresponding dysregulation of emotional systems leads to long-term consequences for the young child's neurological organization (Carlson, 1998). In this regard, contemporary theorists propose that severe failures of early attachment relationships, and specifically the abuse and neglect associated with disorganized attachment patterns, are likely to impair the regulatory stress- and coping-related functions of the right brain and limbic system (Bowlby, 1988; Perry, Pollard, Blakley, Baker, & Vigilante, 1995; Schore, 2001; Siegel, 2002). These early distortions in the regulation of emotions and behaviors, as experienced in the parent–child relationship, are likely to lead to later emotional and interpersonal disturbances (Carlson, 1998).

Disorganized children are likely to view themselves as inept, lack social competence, and along with high levels of interpersonal distrust have long-term difficulty attaining their social and achievement goals. Disorganized youth typically become adults with "fearful" attachment styles who avoid closeness because they associate it with pain and injury. At the same time, and in stark contrast to the person with dismissing attachment who does not perceive a need for other people, the fearfully attached person is highly aware of personal vulnerability (Bartholomew, 1990). Fearfully attached individuals are lonely and crave social support, but are too fearful of rejection to take interpersonal risks to gain it. This fear of rejection may prevent them (in childhood or adulthood) from bonding with healthy adults outside of the nuclear family who could provide secure-base functions.

Because of their difficulties in affect regulation and social skills and their inconsistent behaviors/coping strategies, disorganized children and adults with fearful attachment styles are likely to evidence deficits across multiple life areas. Of the four attachment styles, the fearful style is by far associated with the worst mental health outcomes (Brennan & Shaver, 1998). For example, in studying attachment and depression, Murphy and Bates (1997) found that although fearfully attached individuals made up only a small proportion of their overall sample, they represented nearly half of the depressed group.

## CLINICAL APPLICATIONS

Until recently, the role of attachment theory in psychotherapy has been as a conceptual model, with articles and books on "clinical applications" recommending little in the way of specific interventions (Cicchetti, Toth, & Rogosch, 1999). Over the last decade, however, efforts increasingly have focused on developing targeted attachment-based interventions and treatments.

These interventions generally are modeled so as to mimic the natural development of secure attachment styles, with the goal of modifying insecure attachment styles in the direction of security. The treatment approaches differ markedly depending on the age of the target population. For very young, at-risk children, primary interventions (before maladjustment is observed) target the parents' child-rearing behaviors. For older children, attempts to modify already maladaptive working models simultaneously involve working directly with the child as well as with the primary caregiver to modify the parent–child dynamic and interpersonal environments. For adults, interventions focus on deconstructing insecure working models and replacing them with more flexible and adaptive models of self and others.

## Working with Children

### *Assessment*

The assessment of attachment styles in young childhood still is based almost exclusively on Ainsworth et al.'s (1978) Strange Situation Paradigm. In the Strange Situation, children are categorized as having specific attachment styles based on coded observations of how they (1) interact with parents in play and exploration, (2) react to bids for affiliation by a stranger, and (3) react to their parents over a brief separation and reunion.

Ainsworth's securely attached infants acted somewhat distressed when their mothers left, but greeted them eagerly and warmly upon their returns. Anxious–ambivalent infants were distraught and protested when their mothers left; upon their mothers' return, these infants continued to be distressed and protested even though they wanted to be comforted and held. Avoidant infants, in contrast, seemed relatively undisturbed both when their mothers left and returned. The disorganized style identified by Main and Solomon (1990) is characterized by chaotic and conflicted behaviors in response to the Strange Situation task. Such behaviors involve alternating approach and avoidance behaviors, wherein the child may approach the parent upon reunion, only to freeze in a catatonic-like stance, or retreat, only to approach again.

### *Interventions*

Because young children still are in the process of developing and solidifying their attachment working models, it should be possible to promote greater attachment security by effecting environmental changes. Given that the young child's environment consists primarily of the world of the parent, such changes should be facilitated by helping parents modify their parenting practices (Shorey et al., 2003). To date, such interventions have focused on (1) changing parental behaviors to enhance sensitivity, (2) changing parents' own internal working models, (3) providing and enhancing social support for parents, or (4) combining these three approaches to enhance parental mental health and well-being.

Examples of such interventions include Black and Teti's (1997) efforts to change parental sensitivity at a behavioral level by providing mothers with videotaped feedback of interactions with their young children. Interventions to modify the parents' internal attachment-based working models have focused on helping mothers reconstruct their own early relationships with parents so as to free them to create new models in their interactions with their children (Cicchetti et al., 1999; Toth, Rogosch, Manly, & Cicchetti, 2006). Programs to build social supports have provided anxious mothers with experienced mother mentors (Barnett, Blignault, Holmes, Payne, & Parker, 1987). Finally, programs, such as Egeland and Erickson's (1993) STEEP project (Steps Toward Effective, Enjoyable Parenting) have combined social support with sensitivity training with the aim of promoting attachment security in young children.

In their meta-analytic review, Bakermans-Kranenburg, van IJzendoorn, and Juffer (2003) found that the three basic intervention types—behaviorally changing parental sensitivity, modifying parents' working models, and increasing parental social supports—all were effective in increasing parental sensitivity. In comparing effect sizes, however, Bakermans-Kranenburg et al. concluded that interventions with the greatest effects focused on sensitivity specifically, and (1) used written and videotaped sensitivity instruction, (2) used videotaped feedback, (3) were shorter (less than 5 weeks and not more than 16 weeks), (4) were behaviorally focused (e.g., providing holding techniques or carriers for parents to hold their babies close to their chests), and (5) were initiated after the child was older than 6 months (as opposed to starting when infants were younger or prenatally).

Interventions that were more effective in increasing parental sensitivity also were more effective in increasing infant attachment security (although effect sizes were smaller; Bakermans-Kranenburg et al., 2003), thus suggesting a causal relationship between increased parental sensitivity and greater secure child attachment. The interventions that focused on issues other than parental sensitivity were not successful in increasing infant attachment security. Nevertheless, it is more difficult to change attachment security than it is to change parenting behaviors, and recent clinical interventions using combined approaches have yielded success in this area.

In their Circle of Security intervention, Hoffman, Marvin, Cooper, and Powell (2006) used a group format (with individual treatment plans for each parent–child dyad) to change toddlers' and preschoolers' attachment classifications. The intervention's first aim was to establish the group as a secure base for parents to explore their relationships with their children. The intervention then used educational and therapeutic formats to increase parents' (1) sensitivity and understanding of childhood attachment needs, (2) empathic attunement and capacity to provide reflective functioning, (3) empathy for the self and the child in understanding defensive reactions, and (4) awareness of how their own developmental histories and attachment styles affect their behaviors in relation to the child. Although a group format (five to six parents per group) was used, the Circle of Security protocol tailors treatment based on each child's attachment classification as well as the parents' attachment-related behaviors and representations.

Over the course of the 20 weeks of the Circle of Security intervention, 69% of those children originally receiving a disorganized or insecure–other classification changed to a more desirable (organized) attachment classification (secure, avoidant, or anxious ambivalent). Overall, 44% of children initially classified as insecure changed to having a secure attachment classification by the end of the intervention.

In toddler–parent psychotherapy (Cicchetti et al., 1999; Toth et al., 2006), a similar but longer treatment (58 weeks or 45 sessions), clinicians meet with mothers and their toddlers in conjoint therapy sessions. The therapist helps the mother to modify her attachment representations and distorted perceptions and behavior patterns, which are thought to directly affect how she interacts with her child. This working model modification is accomplished by helping the mother become aware of the interpersonal patterns that are observed and providing a corrective emotional experience through empathy, respect, concern, and positive regard. Toddler–parent psychotherapy is effective in changing attachment classifications from insecure to secure and is particularly effective in decreasing rates of disorganized attachment.

For example, Toth et al. (2006) found that 58.8% of treated toddlers originally classified as disorganized changed to a secure classification, compared to 8.0% who changed from disorganized to secure in the control group.

Other researchers also have found that children's insecure attachment styles can be moved in a secure direction by increasing healthy parental behaviors. Dozier, Stovall, Albus, and Bates (2001) found that when children are placed in foster care, their attachment classifications come to resemble those of the foster parent after 3 months in placement. Building on these findings, Becker-Weidman (2006) implemented an attachment-based intervention, dyadic developmental psychotherapy, with adopted and foster-care children ages 6–15 years (mean = 9.4 years). In this intervention therapists strive to modify children's negative working models by working directly and simultaneously with the children and their adoptive/foster caregivers. The primary aim of this intervention is to provide a secure base in treatment and at home through a "contingent collaborative and affectively attuned relationship between therapist and child, between caregiver and child, and between therapist and caregiver" (Becker-Weidman, 2006, p. 148). From this secure base, children can experience many of the processes inherent in normal secure development. The emphasis in working with the child is less on verbal content and more on experiential relearning. Verbal instruction is posited by Becker-Weidman to be ineffective because insecure attachment schemas are often based in traumatic events experienced at preverbal stages of development. Trust, acceptance, and empathic attunement in this intervention, therefore, often are communicated nonverbally through eye contact, tone of voice, touch, and movement.

Dyadic developmental psychotherapy also necessitates a focus on caregivers' attachment styles because insecure styles can interfere with caregivers' abilities to enact secure attachment principles. In a typical session the therapist spends time alone with the parents, instructing them in "attachment parenting methods," and, if needed, helps the parents work through their own insecure attachment issues. In this process, the therapist provides, and thereby models for the parents, the same level of "attuned responsiveness" that is desired for the child. After meeting with the caregiver individually, the therapist typically meets with the caregivers and the child together for 60–90 minutes. Work with the child involves the therapist and parents together (1) being affectively attuned and validating of the child's subjective experience, (2) implementing cognitive-behavioral techniques to help the child make sense of and modify maladaptive behaviors, and (3) facilitating cognitive restructuring of past experiences to increase malleability of relational schemas.

Through parents' use of empathic attunement in a structured environment provided by the therapist, the child can feel safe and remain emotionally engaged while reprocessing distressing emotions associated with past traumas. In this work the child also is repeatedly cycled through the fundamental caregiver–child attachment pattern of (1) sharing emotional experiences, (2) experiencing a breach or separation in the relationship, and (3) reconnecting and realigning caregiver–child emotional states. As these cycles repeat across the course of treatment, just as they do in normal development, the child comes to construct a new working model of the self in relation to others, which then facilitates healthy bonding with caregivers, enabling the secure attachment dynamic to continue after treatment ends.

Becker-Weidman (2006) provided evidence for the efficacy of this 23-week intervention, finding that children in the active treatment group ($n$ = 34) were rated by their adoptive or foster-care parents as having significantly lower levels of attachment disorder and fewer behavior problems after the intervention as compared to a preintervention assessment.

The treatment group also had significantly better outcomes across these same indices than a treatment-as-usual group, which did not show significant improvements in pre- to postintervention assessments.

Because Becker-Weidman's outcome data were based exclusively on caregiver ratings, treatment effects may reflect demand characteristics wherein parents portrayed themselves as successful in the treatment by rating their children as being improved. Nevertheless, the findings are consistent with other research indicating that insecure attachment styles can be modified through sustained disconfirming evidence that contradicts extant working models. These findings also bode well for interventions aimed at modifying working models in adults, because the same principles that guide the childhood interventions also can be implemented with adult psychotherapy clients.

## Working with Adults

### *Treatment Starts with the Therapist*

The quality of the therapeutic alliance, particularly in the early stage of treatment, is an important predictor of treatment outcomes (Horvath & Symonds, 1991; Martin, Garske, & Davis, 2000). From an attachment theory perspective, establishing and sustaining the alliance is predicated on the therapist's ability to provide the client with a secure base from which to explore internal and external environments as well as to experiment with new behaviors acquired in psychotherapy (see Roth & Fonagy, 2005).

It is important for each therapist to begin by considering how his or her attachment style could shape responses to clients, and, by extension, influence the therapeutic alliance and treatment outcomes (Dozier, Cue, & Barnett, 1994). Black, Hardy, Turpin, and Parry (2005) found that therapist attachment styles predicted alliance quality even after controlling for extraversion and neuroticism, with more secure therapists reporting better general therapeutic alliances. Securely attached therapists also achieve better psychotherapy outcomes than insecurely attached therapists (Bruck, Winston, Aderholt, & Muran, 2006). This effectiveness may be the result of the secure therapist's ability to implement open, flexible, and nondefensive approaches in treatment (Dozier & Tyrrell, 1998). Moreover, securely attached therapists should have the skills to handle difficult therapeutic situations (Meyer & Pilkonis, 2001) as well as awareness of what clients are "pulling for" so as to provide noncomplementary responses (Dozier et al., 1994). In this latter respect, Dozier et al. (1994) found that secure clinicians were more responsive to the dependency needs of dismissing clients than to the dependency needs of preoccupied clients.

Although it may not be the result of conscious therapist intentions, therapist–client dissimilarity (Arizmendi, Beutler, Shanfield, Crago, & Hagaman, 1985), particularly in respect to levels of attachment avoidance (Tyrell, Dozier, Teague, & Fallot, 1999), also can promote the delivery of noncomplementary therapist responses and positive treatment outcomes. For example, Tyrell et al. (1999) found that severely disordered clients who were more avoidant had better outcomes with therapists who were less avoidant. Similarly, clients who were less avoidant had better outcomes with therapists who were more avoidant. Therapists who lean toward being more avoidant (i.e., have dismissing attachment styles), however, may find it challenging to remain tolerant, empathic, and connected to "needy," neurotic clients.

Overall, research in this area indicates that insecurely attached therapists tend to reinforce clients' maladaptive working models and recapitulate clients' core conflicts. Dozier et al. (1994) found that in working with preoccupied clients, the more insecure (in relation to attachment) the clinicians were, the more likely they were to respond strongly to clients' pulls to meet dependency needs. Similarly, insecurely attached clinicians reinforced dismissing clients' perceptions of others as superficial and unavailable by responding minimally to these clients' dependency needs. Preoccupied clinicians, in particular, must work to avoid being "pulled in" by clients' emotional experiences and discourses so that they can maintain sufficiently clear interpersonal boundaries to be effective.

Meyer and Pilkonis (2001) proposed that relative to the secure and dismissing style, the preoccupied attachment style is the least desirable in a therapist. These researchers based their conclusion on findings that therapists with preoccupied, relative to secure, attachment styles rated their therapeutic alliances less favorably, reported more problems in the smooth delivery of psychotherapy interventions, and perceived themselves to be less effective in therapy (Black et al., 2005; Meyer & Pilkonis, 2001). An alternative explanation for these findings, however, could be that preoccupied therapists, consistent with their attachment style, simply are more willing than therapists with the other styles to (1) attend to their clients' negative social cues and (2) to self-disclose their therapeutic shortcomings to researchers.

Irrespective of the reasons underlying the aforementioned findings, it is clear that therapists should take stock of their own attachment styles before entering the therapy room. Should clinicians be unclear about their attachment styles, they may wish to engage in one of the assessments described next. Should they find that their insecure styles interfere with their abilities to provide secure bases and corrective experiences for clients, they may wish to find their own secure bases (e.g., in the person of their own therapist or clinical supervisor) from which to explore the significance of their personal attachment working models.

### *Assessment*

Disagreement remains in the contemporary attachment literature as to whether adult attachment should be measured (1) in terms of continuous attachment avoidance and attachment anxiety dimensions (favored by social psychologists) or (2) categorically, according to discrete styles (favored by clinical psychologists). There also is disagreement among the categorical measurement systems regarding the number of attachment style categories, the attachment style labels used, and even the degree of correspondence between similarly labeled styles across measures. These disagreements have resulted in a sometimes confused and disjointed literature. For example, although there is growing consensus that there are four basic adult attachment styles, some published studies (particularly those published prior to 1991) report a three-category typology with labels that correspond to the three original child attachment styles (e.g., secure, avoidant, and anxious). So as not to confuse the reader, however, in the present chapter I used the label *preoccupied* when referring to all results reported for adult anxious attachment styles. Similarly, when studies reported on an adult *avoidant* style, I used the label *dismissing*, even though the reader should be aware that when a three-category typology is used, a certain proportion of those who would be classified as *fearful* in a four-category model will be placed in the avoidant or anxious groups.

The move toward dimensional assessment (i.e., each assessed individual receives a score on his or her level of attachment anxiety and level of attachment avoidance) has lessened this confusion by providing for common language (i.e., reporting on *levels* of attachment avoidance and anxiety). Moreover, dimensional assessment has been found to be superior to the categorical approach from a statistical standpoint (see Shaver, Belsky, & Brennan, 2000). It is my belief, however, that the categorical styles have a descriptive and explanatory utility that is not present in the dimensional approach.

The categorical styles facilitate client conceptualizations by helping the clinician to think about how a specific client is likely to present in therapy and react to other people and various psychotherapeutic interventions. It would be difficult to organize this information only on the basis of orthogonal attachment anxiety and avoidance dimensions because some of the attachment styles involve the interactions of these dimensions (see Figure 9.1). For the secure (low on attachment anxiety and avoidance in Brennan et al.'s [1998] typology), preoccupied (high on attachment anxiety, low on avoidance), and dismissing (low on attachment anxiety, high on avoidance) groups, the continuous dimensions may provide adequate behavioral descriptions. For the fearful style, however, the dimensional descriptions do not adequately capture what happens when a person has high levels of both attachment anxiety and avoidance.

This is one reason that clinical psychologists have favored using the AAI (George et al., 1985/1996) to classify individuals according to styles (the AAI also yields continuous dimensions that do not correspond directly to attachment avoidance and anxiety). The AAI is a clinical interview that codes people's attachment-related narratives of childhood interactions with parents. A similar measurement system, the Adult Attachment Projective (AAP; George & West, 2001), assesses attachment styles based on responses to ambiguous drawings that pull for attachment-related themes. Although they evidence strong clinical utility, the shortcomings of these measures are that they are not in the public domain and they require a substantial investment of time and money to learn to administer and score.

Highly reliable self-report alternatives, in contrast, are available free of charge in the published social psychology literature. These self-report measures can be administered and scored using basic statistical software in the therapy room. One such measure, the Experiences in Close Relationships Scale (ECRS; Brennan et al., 1998), assesses how individuals typically think, feel, and behave in their romantic relationships. It has two subscales that assess the continuous attachment anxiety and avoidance dimensions, or it can be used to derive an attachment classification.

Although the attachment style descriptions provided by the ECRS and other self-report measures are highly similar to those provided by the AAI, the statistical correspondences of the styles across the AAI and self-report measures are only moderate at best (Bartholomew & Horowitz, 1991; Shaver et al., 2000; Simpson, Rholes, Oriña, & Grich, 2002). Thus, I recommend that clinicians use multiple indices before concluding knowledge of a client's attachment style. One index could be the clinician's observations and knowledgeable judgment attained through classes, workshops, or a careful study of the attachment literature. These clinical judgments also could be aided greatly by therapist-reported client rating scales (Westen, Nakash, Thomas, & Bradley, 2006).

The Attachment Prototype Questionnaire (APQ) and the Attachment Questionnaire (AQ; with multi-item scales) were designed for use in ongoing psychotherapy by experienced clinicians (Westen et al., 2006). These resemble narrative approaches (i.e., the AAI) because the clinician must make subtle judgments about patterns of interpersonal behavior and discourse, affect regulation strategies, and the client's representations of self, others, and relationships. Westen et al. (2006) provided evidence for the four-factor structure of the AQ that corresponds to the commonly accepted styles (secure, preoccupied, dismissing, and disorga-

| | | Avoidance<br>Models of Others | |
|---|---|---|---|
| | | Low<br>Positive | High<br>Negative |
| Anxiety<br>Models of Self | Low<br>Positive | *Secure* | *Dismissing* |
| | High<br>Negative | *Preoccupied* | *Fearful* |

**FIGURE 9.1.** Adult attachment styles based on perceptions of self and others (Bartholomew & Horowitz, 1991) and relative levels of attachment avoidance and attachment anxiety (Brennan, Clark, & Shaver, 1998).

nized/fearful). Each client rated on these measures receives a total score for each style, the relative levels of which can be used by the clinician to determine which style is dominant.

Although these measures (APQ and AQ) show great promise, the research on them is in its early stages and correspondences with the AAI and self-report attachment measures have yet to be established. Nevertheless, for those already familiar with attachment theory, these instruments may prove useful as adjuncts to other assessment techniques (McBride, Atkinson, Quilty, & Bagby, 2006).

## Interventions

Attachment-based interventions for adults typically follow Bowlby's (1988) five recommended tasks for psychotherapy: (1) providing clients with a secure base; (2) exploring past attachments; (3) exploring the relationship with the therapist in the here and now; (4) linking past experiences with present ones; and (5) revising internal working models.

These tasks can be seen in Johnson's (1996, 2004) emotionally focused couple therapy, an intervention for couples that conceptualizes marital distress from an attachment theory perspective. The change process involves three stages. Stage 1 involves deescalating negative cycles and increasing emotional engagement by helping partners see how their interactions isolate both of them and lead to attachment injuries. In Stage 2, the therapist helps create tasks and "key bonding events" wherein the spouse whose attachment needs are not being met can ask appropriately, without blame and accusations, for comfort and reassurance. The other more withdrawn spouse then can be assisted by the therapist to respond empathically and demonstrate supportiveness. These events help create more secure attachment bonds by reframing the interpersonal attachment patterns and reprocessing negative emotions. Finally, in Stage 3 attempts are made to generalize changed relational patterns to the couple's daily life. The overall goal of the intervention is to redefine the relationship as a secure base in which distress can be ameliorated, conflicts can be dealt with directly, and challenges in relation to others can be overcome. This intervention has been found to lower marital distress and depressive symptoms and to improve intimacy and marital satisfaction (see Whiffen & Johnson, 1998).

de Zulueta (2006) similarly used attachment theory concepts in developing her treatment for women with posttraumatic stress disorder (PTSD). de Zulueta makes the case that PTSD can be viewed as a disruption of the attachment system. This idea is supported by findings that, relative to individuals who do not report trauma histories, unresolved childhood trauma relates to a higher likelihood of receiving an adult PTSD diagnosis (Stovall-McClough & Cloitre, 2006). In this context, the psychological trauma involves an unexpected and extreme disruption of "affiliative bonds" (see de Zulueta, 2006). To reestablish these affiliative bonds, de Zulueta proposed that it is essential to begin treatment by establishing a secure base. Because establishing the secure base depends on in-depth knowledge of the client, de Zulueta highlighted the need to assess both the client's internal working models and the client's external pattern of social relationships.

de Zulueta (2006) views the assessment process as an intervention in its own right. Consistent with the therapeutic assessment model pioneered by Finn and Tonsager (1997), de Zulueta (2006) emphasized how the assessment and feedback process gives clinicians the opportunity to demonstrate empathic attunement and to be emotionally touched by the world of the client, thus providing the client with a sense of validation and being cared for. As the therapist and client work in partnership to develop a cohesive attachment conceptualization, the secure base takes form and the therapist then can guide the client through exploring his or her experiences. Such exploration includes cognitive restructuring that can be applied either to attachment styles or the effects of trauma and PTSD symptoms.

Gormley (2004), however, suggested that establishing a secure base and therapeutic alliance with women with PTSD is likely to be particularly challenging because such clients have histories of destructive and abusive relationships. These traumatic experiences contribute to the formation of disorganized/fearful attachment styles (Hesse & Main, 2000; Brennan et al., 1998) and to borderline personality disorder (BPD). For these clients, the very act of initiating a therapeutic relationship could result in decreased abilities to tolerate stress and in the dysregulation of emotions (Bowlby, 1988). In order to lower distress and related resistance to treatment, therefore, Gormley (2004) suggested validating the adaptive significance of the client's insecure attachment style. In other words, the therapist can help the client see how current destructive behaviors originated as attempts to get attachment needs met under adverse circumstances in childhood (Gormley, 2004). Gormley (2004) found that such disorganized clients did not respond well to cognitive-behavioral techniques before a sound therapeutic relationship and secure base had been established through interpersonal, emotion-focused treatment (Gormley, 2004).

Transference-based psychotherapy (TFP; Clarkin, Yeomans, & Kernberg, 1999) is one such emotion-focused intervention that has demonstrated effectiveness in the treatment of BPD (see Levy et al., 2006). TFP aims to reduce symptoms and self-destructive behaviors by modifying models of self and others as they manifest in relationship with the therapist. The twice-weekly sessions emphasize the emotionally valenced themes that emerge in the relationship between the client and the therapist in the "here and now." As the client's dominant relational patterns are reenacted and reexperienced in the transference relationship with the therapist, the therapist uses confrontation, clarification, and interpretation to help the client see and restructure faulty models and misperceptions of self and others.

Results from Levy et al.'s (2006) randomized control trial comparing TFP, dialectical behavior therapy (DBT), and psychodynamic supportive psychotherapy (SPT) indicate that clients with BPD treated with TFP, DBT, or SPT show improvements in depression, anxiety, social adjustment, and global functioning. TFP and DBT (but not SPT) were effective in reducing suicidality and anger, but only TFP reduced aggression. Levy et al. examined the mechanisms of change underlying these effects and found that 6 of 21 clients (28.6%), classified as having an insecure attachment style at the beginning of TFP, changed to a secure style over the year of treatment, whereas none of the insecure clients treated with DBT ($n$ = 15) or SPT ($n$ = 21) changed from insecure to secure attachment classifications during this same time period. Levy et al. also found that of the three treatment groups, only TFP increased reflective functioning and coherence of attachment narratives. They concluded that changes in attachment patterns were a primary mechanism responsible for the reported effectiveness of TFP.

Other researchers have examined the interactions of attachment styles and the effectiveness of interpersonal psychotherapy (IPT) and cognitive-behavioral therapy (CBT) for the treatment of major depression (McBride et al., 2006). McBride et al. found that clients' levels of attachment anxiety did not predict outcomes. In contrast, clients who scored higher on attachment avoidance had significantly greater reductions in depressive symptoms with CBT than with IPT. In light of this differential treatment response, scholars increasingly are calling for the consideration of attachment styles, not only in developing interventions, conceptualizing cases, and treatment planning, but also as variables in clinical outcomes research (McBride et al., 2006; Shorey & Snyder, 2006).

## CONCLUSION AND FUTURE DIRECTIONS

Researchers and clinicians increasingly are reaching out to attachment theory for intervention models and treatment options (see Davila & Levy, 2006). Owing to its (1) psychodynamic roots, (2) social basis of personality development, (3) emphasis on the links between cognition, emotions, and behavior, and (4) juxtaposition of positive and negative developmental patterns, attachment theory provides a framework through which clinicians of diverse theoretical orientations can find common ground.

Clinicians could utilize any number of the specialized attachment interventions that I have reviewed in the preceding pages, using the references provided to obtain more detailed treatment information. Learning a specific treatment protocol, however, while certainly worth while, is not necessary to put attachment theory tenets and research findings to good use in the therapy room. In this respect, attachment theory need not supplant existing treatments and can be incorporated into the therapist's favored treatment approach. Incorporating attachment theory will, however, require that therapists remain flexible and open to modifying their existing protocols to suit the needs of clients, based on each client's specific attachment style.

For example, although CBT specifically tailors session content to the individual client, the CBT therapist typically adheres to a well-defined and prescribed structure within each session. The astute clinician, however, will realize that in the initial phase of treatment, this structure may not be maximally beneficial for clients with fearful or preoccupied attachment styles. Gormley (2004) found that clients with these styles are likely to feel invalidated and perceive a lack of care if the therapist begins with a directive or cognitive-behavioral approach. Thus, the cognitive-behavioral therapist may decide to relax session structure in the early phase of treatment. After the client's initial distress is ameliorated and he or she develops trust through being "held" in the secure base of the therapist, the client may become willing to give over perceived control of the therapy session and adhere to the therapist-guided session structure.

On the other end of the spectrum, clients with dismissing attachment styles should benefit maximally when the therapist initially is directive and uses a cognitive-behavioral approach to treatment. This suggestion is supported by McBride et al.'s (2006) findings that depressed individuals with dismissing attachment styles had better outcomes with CBT than with IPT. The interpersonal content and suppressed emotions tapped by interpersonal and psychodynamic therapies may exacerbate distress in dismissing clients and increase the likelihood of early termination. If the therapist begins by using a cognitive-behavioral approach in working on the dismissing client's presenting problem (typically related to themes of achievement), this client may build enough trust in the therapist to risk revealing more interpersonal, emotionally valenced material. This approach mirrors closely Young's (1999) schema approach within CBT, where symptom reduction is facilitated with CBT, and relapse prevention is facilitated by restructuring early relational schema.

The preceding examples should illustrate that, when viewed from an attachment theory lens, the therapist, irrespective of his or her primary treatment model, may choose to take more of what I conceive as a psychodynamic or cognitive-behavioral "stance." The therapist's stance should shift systematically according to clients' attachment styles and the phase of treatment.

Knowledge of attachment theory also should enable clinicians to track themes in sessions and to help clients realize how these themes overlay core (unresolved) conflicts. This work can be advanced by educating clients about attachment dynamics (see Mikulincer & Shaver, 2003) and how their developmental histories contributed to the present attachment style and its cognitive, behavioral, and affective manifestations. This approach can help clients make sense of their experience, lower distress, and reduce resistance to restructuring maladaptive attachment schema.

The client with a preoccupied attachment style, for example, is likely to perceive that if he or she remains vigilant and can understand the fine details of a problem (e.g., social marginalization, abandonment, or rejection), a solution can be found and the problem can be controlled or "fixed." Using the attachment literature as a didactic device, and the client's own experiences as examples, the therapist can gently help the client realize that this approach has rarely worked in solving perceived social problems and actually heightens distress (see Mikulincer & Shaver, 2003).

It is at this point in treatment that many clients ask, "Well, what can I do?" This question signals a new willingness to change and provides an opportunity for the therapist to refocus the preoccupied client on more achievement-oriented life areas (e.g., career, education, sports, and hobbies) that have the potential to increase senses of self-efficacy and worthiness. This shift of attention should lessen the client's problem focus, ameliorate distress, and increase social functioning.

A similar approach can be taken with the dismissing client, who can be helped to see that he or she attains validation and maintains a sense of self-worth almost exclusively through achievement strivings. The therapist should be clear that although distress may be ameliorated when the client gets back on track in achievement areas (e.g., career accomplishment), this improvement is fragile because it depends on continued high achievement. Careful probing by the clinician could help the dismissing client realize that his or her achievement needs are actually social at their core (e.g., for admiration and appreciation) and that such social needs can be attained by directly increasing social (as opposed to exclusively achievement) engagement. In my clinical work with dismissing clients, I have been amazed at their willingness to accept this proposition and by their apparent relief in the increasing realization that they do not have to maintain such high levels of achievement in order to feel good subjectively.

I have included the foregoing clinical descriptions to demonstrate practical ways that attachment theory can be integrated into diverse treatment approaches. Innovative research designs and partnerships among therapists from across schools of psychotherapy, however, will be needed to provide empirical support for such propositions. Outcome research may be particularly challenging because attachment-based interventions are likely to incorporate both psychodynamic and cognitive-behavioral components. This combination will make it difficult to distill the actual mechanisms of change. Nevertheless, psychodynamic and cognitive-behavioral treatment approaches are not at all at odds when viewed from an attachment theory perspective. Rather, these more traditional psychotherapy models can be viewed as different levels of analysis relating to underlying attachment processes and patterns of cognition and behavior. It is my hope that attachment theory will provide a common language that will maximize our common cause of ameliorating clients' distress and getting them back on course of optimal functioning.

## REFERENCES


Ainsworth, M. D. S. (1973). The development of infant–mother attachment. In B. M. Caldwell & H. N. Ricciuti (Eds.), *Review of child development research* (Vol. 3, pp. 1–94). Chicago: University of Chicago Press.

Ainsworth, M. D. S., Blehar, M. C., Waters, E., & Wall, S. (1978). *Patterns of attachment: A psychological study of the Strange Situation.* New York: Basic Books.

Allen, J. G., Coyne, L., & Huntoon, J. (1998). Complex posttraumatic stress disorder in women from a psychometric perspective. *Journal of Personality Assessment, 70*, 277–298.

Arizmendi, T., Beutler, L., Shanfield, S., Crago, M., & Hagaman, R. (1985). Client–therapist value similarity and psychotherapy outcome: A microscopic analysis. *Psychotherapy, 22*, 16–21.

Bakermans-Kranenburg, M. J., van IJzendoorn, M. H., & Juffer, F. (2003). Less is more: Meta-analyses of sensitivity and attachment interventions in early childhood. *Psychological Bulletin, 129*(2), 195–215.

Barnett, B., Blignault, I., Holmes, S., Payne, A., & Parker, G. (1987). Quality of attachment in a sample of 1-year-old Australian children. *Journal of the American Academy of Child and Adolescent Psychiatry, 26*, 303–307.

Bartholomew, K. (1990). Avoidance of intimacy: An attachment perspective. *Journal of Social and Personal Relationships, 7*(2), 147–178.

Bartholomew, K., & Horowitz, L. M. (1991). Attachment styles among young adults: A test of a four-category model. *Journal of Personality and Social Psychology, 61*(2), 226–244.

Batgos, J., & Leadbeater, B. J. (1994). Parental attachment, peer relations, and dysphoria in adolescence. In M. B. Sperling & W. H. Berman (Eds.), *Attachment in adults: Clinical and developmental perspectives* (pp. 155–178). New York: Guilford Press.

Becker-Weidman, A. (2006). Treatment for children with trauma-attachment disorders: Dyadic developmental psychotherapy. *Child and Adolescent Social Work Journal, 23*, 147–171.

Black, M. M., & Teti, L. O. (1997). Promoting mealtime communication between adolescent mothers and their infants through videotape. *Pediatrics, 99*, 432–437.

Black, S., Hardy, G., Turpin, G., & Parry, G. (2005). Self-reported attachment styles and therapeutic orientation of therapists and their relationship with reported general alliance quality and problems in therapy. *Psychology and Psychotherapy: Theory, Research, and Practice, 78*(3), 363–377.

Bowlby, J. (1969). *Attachment and loss: Vol. 1. Attachment.* New York: Basic Books.

Bowlby, J. (1973). *Attachment and loss: Vol. 2. Separation: Anxiety and anger.* New York: Basic Books.

Bowlby, J. (1980). *Attachment and loss: Vol. 3. Loss.* New York: Basic Books.

Bowlby, J. (1988). Developmental psychiatry comes of age. *American Journal of Psychiatry, 145*(1), 1–10.

Brennan, K. A., Clark, C. L., & Shaver, P. R. (1998). Self-report measurement of adult attachment: An integrative overview. In J. A. Simpson & W. S. Rholes (Eds.), *Attachment theory and close relationships* (pp. 46–76). New York: Guilford Press.

Brennan, K. A., & Shaver, P. R. (1998). Attachment styles and personality disorders: Their connections to each other and to parental divorce, parental death, and perceptions of parental caregiving. *Journal of Personality, 66*(5), 835–878.

Bretherton, I. (1992). The origins of attachment theory: John Bowlby and Mary Ainsworth. *Developmental Psychology, 28*(5), 759–775.

Bruck, E., Winston, A., Aderholt, S., & Muran, J. C. (2006). Predictive validity of patient and therapist attachment and introject styles. *American Journal of Psychotherapy, 60*(4), 393–406.

Carlson, E. A. (1998). A prospective longitudinal study of attachment disorganization/disorientation. *Child Development, 69*, 1107–1128.

Cicchetti, D., Toth, S. L., & Rogosch, F. A. (1999). The efficacy of toddler–parent psychotherapy to increase attachment security in offspring of depressed mothers. *Attachment and Human Development, 1*(1), 34–66.

Clarkin, J. F., Yeomans, F., & Kernberg, O. F. (1999). *Psychotherapy of borderline personality disorder: Focusing on object relations.* New York: Wiley.

Connors, M. E. (1997). The renunciation of love: Dismissive attachment and its treatment. *Psychoanalytic Psychology, 14*, 475–493.

Davila, J., & Levy, K. N. (2006). Introduction to the special section on attachment theory and psychotherapy. *Journal of Consulting and Clinical Psychology, 74*(6), 989–993.

de Zulueta, F. (2006). The treatment of psychological trauma from the perspective of attachment research. *Journal of Family Therapy, 28*(4), 334–351.

Diamond, L. M., Hicks, A. M., & Otter-Henderson, K. (2006). Physiological evidence for repressive coping among avoidantly attached adults. *Journal of Social and Personal Relationships, 23*(2), 205–229.

Dozier, M., Cue, K. L., & Barnett, L. (1994). Clinicians as caregivers: Role of attachment organization in treatment. *Journal of Consulting and Clinical Psychology, 62*(4), 793–800.

Dozier, M., Stovall, K. C., Albus, K. E., & Bates, B. (2001). Attachment for infants in foster care: The role of caregiver state of mind. *Child Development, 72*(5), 1467–1477.

Dozier, M., & Tyrrell, C. (1998). The role of attachment in therapeutic relationships. In J. A. Simpson & W. S. Rholes (Eds.), *Attachment theory and close relationships* (pp. 221–248). New York: Guilford Press.

Egeland, B., & Erickson, M. F. (1993). Attachment theory and findings: Implications for prevention and intervention. In S. Kramer & H. Parens (Eds.), *Prevention in mental health: Now, tomorrow, ever?* (pp. 21–50). Northvale, NJ: Aronson.

Finn, S. E., & Tonsager, M. E. (1997). Information-gathering and therapeutic models of assessment: Complementary paradigms. *Psychological Assessment, 9*(4), 374–385.

Fonagy, P., & Target, M. (1997). Attachment and reflective function: Their role in self-organization. *Development and Psychopathology, 9*(4), 679–700.

George, C., Kaplan, N., & Main, M. (1996). *Adult Attachment Interview.* Unpublished manuscript, Department of Psychology, University of California, Berkeley. (Original work developed 1985)

George, C., & West, M. (2001). The development and preliminary validation of a new measure of adult attachment: The Adult Attachment Projective. *Attachment and Human Development, 3*(1), 30–61.

Gormley, B. (2004). Application of adult attachment theory to treatment of chronically suicidal, traumatized women. *Psychotherapy: Theory, Research, Practice, Training, 41*(2), 136–143.

Hazan, C., & Shaver, P. (1987). Romantic love conceptualized as an attachment process. *Journal of Personality and Social Psychology, 52*(3), 511–524.

Hesse, E., & Main, M. (2000). Disorganized infant, child, and adult attachment: Collapse in behavioral and attentional strategies. *Journal of the American Psychoanalytic Association, 48*, 1097–1127.

Hoffman, K. T., Marvin, R. S., Cooper, G., & Powell, B. (2006). Changing toddlers' and preschoolers' attachment classifications: The Circle of Security intervention. *Journal of Consulting and Clinical Psychology, 74*(6), 1017–1026.

Horvath, A. O., & Symonds, B. D. (1991). Relation between working alliance and outcome in psychotherapy: A meta-analysis. *Journal of Counseling Psychology, 38*(2), 139–149.

Johnson, S. M. (1996). *The practice of emotionally focused marital therapy: Creating connections.* New York: Brunner/Mazel.

Johnson, S. M. (2004). Attachment theory: A guide for healing couple relationships. In W. S. Rholes & J. A. Simpson (Eds.), *Adult attachment: Theory, research, and clinical implications* (pp. 367–387). New York: Guilford Press.

Kernberg, O. F. (1975). *Borderline conditions and pathological narcissism.* New York: Aronson.

Kraemer, S., & Loader, P. (1995). "Passing through life": Alexithymia and attachment disorders. *Journal of Psychosomatic Research, 39*(8), 937–941.

Levy, K. N., Meehan, K. B., Kelly, K. M., Reynoso, J. S., Weber, M., Clarkin, J. F., et al. (2006). Change in attachment patterns and reflective function in a randomized control trial of transference-focused psychotherapy for borderline personality disorder. *Journal of Consulting and Clinical Psychology, 74*(6), 1027–1040.

Lopez, F. G., Fuendeling, J., Thomas, K., & Sagula, D. (1997). An attachment-theoretical perspective on the use of splitting defenses. *Counseling Psychology Quarterly, 10*(4), 461–472.

Main, M. (1990). Cross-cultural studies of attachment organization: Recent studies, changing methodologies, and the concept of conditional strategies. *Human Development, 33*(1), 48–61.

Main, M., & Solomon, J. (1990). Procedures for identifying infants as disorganized/disoriented during the Ainsworth Strange Situation. In M. T. Greenberg, D. Cicchetti, & E. M. Cummings (Eds.), *Attachment in the preschool years* (pp. 121–160). Chicago: University of Chicago Press.

Martin, D. J., Garske, J. P., & Davis, M. K. (2000). Relation of the therapeutic alliance with outcome and other variables: A meta-analytic review. *Journal of Consulting and Clinical Psychology, 68*(3), 438–450.

Mayseless, O. (1996). Attachment patterns and their outcomes. *Human Development, 39*, 206–223.

McBride, C., Atkinson, L., Quilty, L. C., & Bagby, R. M. (2006). Attachment as moderator of treatment outcome in major depression: A randomized control trial of interpersonal psychotherapy versus cognitive behavior therapy. *Journal of Consulting and Clinical Psychology, 74*(6), 1041–1054.

Meyer, B., & Pilkonis, P. A. (2001). Attachment style. *Psychotherapy: Theory, Research, Practice, Training, 38*(4), 466–472.

Mikulincer, M., & Shaver, P. R. (2003). The attachment behavioral system in adulthood: Activation, psychodynamics, and interpersonal processes. In M. Zenna (Ed.), *Advances in experimental social psychology* (Vol. 35, pp. 53–152). New York: Elsevier Academic Press.

Millon, T. (1996). *Disorders of personality: DSM-IV and beyond* (2nd ed.). New York: Wiley.

Murphy, B., & Bates, G. W. (1997). Adult attachment style and vulnerability to depression. *Personality and Individual Differences, 22*, 835–844.

Perry, B. D., Pollard, R. A., Blakley, T. L., Baker, W. L., & Vigilante, D. (1995). Childhood trauma, the neurobiology of adaptation, and "use dependent" development of the brain: How "states" become "traits." *Infant Mental Health Journal, 16*, 271–291.

Roth, A., & Fonagy, P. (2005). *What works for whom: A critical review of psychotherapy research* (2nd ed.). New York: Guilford Press.

Schore, A. N. (2001). The effects of early relational trauma on right brain development, affect regulation, and infant mental health. *Infant Mental Health Journal*, 22, 201–269.

Shaver, P. R., Belsky, J., & Brennan, K. A. (2000). The Adult Attachment Interview and self-reports of romantic attachment: Associations across domains and methods. *Personal Relationships*, 7(1), 25–43.

Shorey, H. S. (2006). *The interactions of hope and attachment styles in a social–cognitive–motivational model of depressive vulnerability.* Unpublished doctoral dissertation, University of Kansas, Lawrence.

Shorey, H. S., & Snyder, C. R. (2006). The role of adult attachment styles in psychopathology and psychotherapy outcomes. *Review of General Psychology*, *10*(1), 1–20.

Shorey, H. S., Snyder, C. R., Yang, X., & Lewin, M. R. (2003). The role of hope as a mediator in recollected parenting, adult attachment, and mental health. *Journal of Social and Clinical Psychology*, *22*(6), 685–715.

Siegel, D. J. (2002). Toward an interpersonal neurobiology of the developing mind: Attachment relationships, "mindsight," and neural integration. *Infant Mental Health Journal*, *22*, 67–94.

Simpson, J. A., Rholes, W. S., Oriña, M. M., & Grich, J. (2002). Working models of attachment, support giving, and support seeking in a stressful situation. *Personality and Social Psychology Bulletin*, *28*(5), 598–608.

Stovall-McClough, K. C., & Cloitre, M. (2006). Unresolved attachment, PTSD, and dissociation in women with childhood abuse histories. *Journal of Consulting and Clinical Psychology*, *74*(2), 219–228.

Toth, S. L., Rogosch, F. A., Manly, J. T., & Cicchetti, D. (2006). The efficacy of toddler–parent psychotherapy to reorganize attachment in the young offspring of mothers with major depressive disorder: A randomized preventive trial. *Journal of Consulting and Clinical Psychology*, *74*(6), 1006–1016.

Tyrell, C. L., Dozier, M., Teague G. B., & Fallot, R. D. (1999). Effective treatment relationships for persons with serious psychiatric disorders: The importance of attachment states of mind. *Journal of Consulting and Clinical Psychology*, *67*, 725–733.

Westen, D., Nakash, O., Thomas, C., & Bradley, R. (2006). Clinical assessment of attachment patterns and personality disorder in adolescents and adults. *Journal of Consulting and Clinical Psychology*, *74*(6), 1065–1085.

Whiffen, V. E., & Johnson, S. M. (1998). An attachment theory framework for the treatment of childbearing depression. *Clinical Psychology: Science and Practice*, *5*(4), 478–493.

Young, J. E. (1999). *Cognitive therapy for personality disorders: A schema-focused approach* (3rd ed.). Sarasota, FL: Professional Resource Press/Professional Resource Exchange.

# 10 Social Support

## *Basic Research and New Strategies for Intervention*

Brian Lakey

This chapter shows how basic research within the tradition of personality and social psychology informs our understanding of the links between perceived social support and psychological health and disorder and suggests new social support interventions. The social support literature is very large, dispersed across a wide range of journals, including those focusing on psychology, sociology, medicine, nursing, public health, and social work. Electronic searches conducted on January 12, 2010, found over 31,000 documents with *social support* as a keyword in FirstSearch's PsycINFO, and over 42,000 documents in ISI's Medline.

One reason for the wide interest in social support research has been the hope that it will lead to innovative interventions, possibly including strategies for preventing psychological disorder. Unfortunately, the field still lacks sufficient understanding of social support processes to create effective, new interventions. Yet, research strategies from personality and social psychology, originally developed to study person perception and person × situation interactions, have unique implications for translating social support research into new interventions. This research indicates that there is little in the way of objectively supportive people or actions; instead, perceived social support primarily reflects the unique relationships among specific support recipients and providers. Preliminary research suggests that these unique relationships can account for an important part of the link between perceived support and affect, a key component of psychological health and disorder. Thus, social support interventions might be more effective if support recipients were matched with support providers to form uniquely supportive relationships. Forecasting such relational supportive matches requires a new analytic framework that is currently under development.

## BRIEF REVIEW OF BASIC SOCIAL SUPPORT FINDINGS

Low social support is related to a wide range of psychological disorders (Barrera, 1986; Cohen & Wills, 1985; Sarason, Sarason, & Gurung, 2001). For example, low social support is linked to major depression (Lakey & Cronin, 2008), posttraumatic stress disorder (Brewin, Andrews, & Valentine, 2000), and schizophrenia (Norman et al., 2005). In addition, low social support is linked to normal variations in nonspecific psychological distress (Finch, Okun, Pool, & Ruehlman, 1999), high negative and low positive affect (Lakey & Scoboria, 2005), low self-esteem (Newcomb & Keefe, 1997), pessimism (Symister & Friend, 2003), and substance use (Wills & Cleary, 1996).

Social support is composed of three major subconstructs that are not closely interrelated (Barrera, 1986). Only one of these subconstructs is related consistently to psychological health and disorder. *Perceived support* is a support recipient's subjective judgment that friends and family would provide quality assistance during times of stress. *Enacted support* reflects the specific helping actions (e.g., advice, reassurance, tangible assistance) provided by family and friends during stressful times. *Social integration* reflects the number of different types of relationships in which recipients participate (e.g., spouse, siblings, children, friends). Although low social integration is a consistent predictor of mortality (House, Landis, & Umberson, 1988), social integration is not linked to psychological health consistently (Barrera, 1986; Finch et al., 1999). Surprisingly, receiving enacted support has been either unrelated to psychological health, or contrary to most theory, linked to worse psychological health (Barrera, 1986; Finch et al., 1999). In contrast, perceived support has been linked consistently and strongly to good psychological health and low rates of psychological disorder (Barrera, 1986; Finch et al., 1999; Sarason et al., 2001). Furthermore, the link between perceived support and psychological health does not appear to occur only in the presence of high levels of stress (Burton, Stice, & Seeley, 2004). Instead, perceived support is linked consistently to psychological health regardless of stress (Finch et al., 1999).

The consistent links between low perceived support and a wide range of disorders have raised the possibility that social support processes might be used to develop new preventive and therapeutic interventions. In fact, a sizable number of well-conducted randomized controlled trials have attempted to provide social support for a wide range of health problems (Hogan, Linden, & Najarian, 2002; Lakey & Lutz, 1996). For example, Heller, Thompson, Trueba, Hogg, and Vlachos-Weber (1991) randomly assigned low-income, rural, elderly women to a treatment condition in which participants received weekly telephone calls from a supportive staff member. Despite a well-conducted intervention, tight experimental design, and large sample, intervention participants did not display significantly greater improvements on any of the social support or psychological health measures compared to controls. Although there have been a few modest successes (Barrera, Glasgow, McKay, Boles, & Feil, 2002), the majority of these interventions have failed to provide evidence that creating large improvements in perceived support is currently possible, or that modifying perceived support leads to improvements in psychological health (Hogan et al., 2002; Lakey & Lutz, 1996). These disappointing outcomes may mean that it is not possible to modify perceived support. Another possibility is that our understanding of social support is not sufficiently developed to guide interventions.

## SOCIAL/PERSONALITY CONTRIBUTIONS TO SOCIAL SUPPORT

A number of personality and social psychologists have made important contributions to understanding social support. For example, Greg Pierce, working with the clinical psychologists Barbara and Irwin Sarason, described an attachment theory perspective of perceived support and provided evidence from several studies that perceived support operated similarly to individual difference variables (Pierce, Sarason, & Sarason, 1992; Sarason, Pierce, & Sarason, 1990). Collins and Feeney (2004) have documented how attachment styles forecast participants' reactions to social support provided by others. Feeney (2004) further developed a model of how attachment styles might influence individuals' willingness and ability to provide support to others. Gable, Gonzaga, and Strachman (2006) have documented the important role of support in response to positive events. Bolger, Zuckerman, and Kessler (2000) have shown that recipients' awareness of enacted support is linked to worsened psychological health, whereas enacted support that is not perceived is linked to improved psychological health.

Although these social/personality psychologists have contributed important insights into basic mechanisms involved in social support, the current chapter focuses on social support research derived from work on person perception and person × situation interactions. This research uses either Cronbach and colleagues' generalizability (G) theory (Cronbach, Gleser, Nanda, & Rajaratnam, 1972) or Kenny and colleagues' social relations model (SRM; Kenny, 1994; Kenny & La Voie, 1984). The G/SRM approach to social support is emphasized in this chapter because it suggests a novel approach to social support interventions. G theory is primarily a theory of reliability, although it has long been used to address other research questions as well. For example, Endler and Hunt (1969) applied G theory to isolate person × situation interactions from the main effects of persons and situations. They found that such interactions had large effects on anxiety. This research formed much of the conceptual basis of contemporary work on interactionism (Mischel & Shoda, 1995). Kenny and colleagues' SRM realized and extended Cronbach's (1955) early theoretical work on person perception by showing the importance of partitioning person perception into components that reflect (1) the dispositions of perceivers, (2) the objective features of the persons being perceived, and (3) the role of perceivers' idiosyncratic tastes in perceiving specific targets. G theory and the SRM share a fundamental similarity, in that both partition variance into components reflecting differences among research participants, differences among stimuli (e.g., other people, items, situations, or time), and the interactions between participants and stimuli.

## THE G/SRM APPROACH TO SOCIAL SUPPORT

When support recipients rate the same providers on perceived supportiveness, three important influences[1] are identified. Table 10.1 presents a schematic of a typical G study of social support. In such a design, support recipients each rate the same providers. Recipient influences (a.k.a. *perceiver components* or *perceiver effects*) reflect the extent to which recipients differ in how they perceive providers, averaged across providers ("Column means for recipi-

**TABLE 10.1. Matrix Demonstrating a Simple G Study in Which Recipients Rate the Same Providers**

| | Provider *A* | Provider *B* | Provider *C* | Column means for recipients |
|---|---|---|---|---|
| Recipient *A* | $X_{RAPA}$ | $X_{RAPB}$ | $X_{RAPC}$ | $M_{RA}$ |
| Recipient *B* | $X_{RBPA}$ | $X_{RBPB}$ | $X_{RBPC}$ | $M_{RB}$ |
| Recipient *C* | $X_{RCPA}$ | $X_{RCPB}$ | $X_{RCPC}$ | $M_{RC}$ |
| Row means for providers | $M_{PA}$ | $M_{PB}$ | $M_{PC}$ | |

*Note.* RA, recipient *A*; PB, provider *B*; etc.

ents" in Table 10.1). For example, recipient *A* may rate all providers as more supportive than does recipient *B*. Insofar as these differences are stable over time, recipient influences reflect the extent to which perceived support operates as a trait-like individual difference variable. Provider influences (a.k.a. *target components* or *target effects*) reflect the extent to which providers differ in their rated supportiveness, averaged across recipients ("Row means for providers" in Table 10.1). Phrased differently, provider influences reflect the extent to which recipients agree that some providers are more supportive than others. For example, both recipients *A* and *B* may agree that provider *B* is more supportive than provider *A*. Insofar as interrater agreement is an index of objective reality, provider components reflect the extent to which supportiveness is an objective feature of providers. Relational influences (a.k.a. *perceiver* × *target interactions*) indicate the extent to which supportiveness reflects systematic disagreement among recipients. For example, recipient *A* may see provider *A* as more supportive than provider *B*, whereas recipient *B* may see provider *B* as more supportive than provider *A*. Relational influences are reflected in the extent to which individual cell entries (e.g., "$X_{RAPA}$" in Table 10.1) differ from what would be expected given a specific recipient's tendency to see providers as supportive and a specific provider's tendency to be seen as supportive. Phrased differently, relational influences reflect the extent to which the supportiveness of providers is a matter of personal taste. In this way, perceived support is like taste in art. I like the art of Duren and Paschke, but not so much the art of Chagall, whereas the reader may have a different profile of tastes.

There are now enough G/SRM studies of perceived support to provide preliminary estimates of the relative strength of recipient, provider, and relational influences. Focusing on a range of different types of providers, studies have asked recipients to rate providers after brief conversations with strangers (Neely et al., 2006), to rate providers presented on video (Lakey, Drew, & Sirl, 1999), or to rate providers who were characters in widely viewed TV shows (Lakey, Lutz, & Scoboria, 2004). However, the most ecologically valid estimates are provided by studies in which recipients rated providers that were members of recipients' social networks. The results of five such studies are summarized in Table 10.2. These studies indicate that relational influences are overwhelmingly the most powerful determinants of perceived support, accounting for 62% of the variance in perceived support when corrected for measurement error.[2] Relatively smaller, though large in an absolute sense, are influences reflecting recipient traits, accounting for 27% of the variance. In contrast to what most social support theory emphasizes, the influence of the objective features of providers has been comparatively small, accounting for only 7%. Similar findings have been reported for communal

**TABLE 10.2. Summary of G/SRM Studies of Providers Who Are Members of Recipients' Social Networks**

| Source | Setting | Recipients and providers | Recipient influences | Provider influences | Relationship influences |
|---|---|---|---|---|---|
| Lakey et al. (1996, Study 1) | U.S. PhD program in clinical psychology | 43 graduate students rated the same four faculty members (172 dyads). | 0.11 | 0.28 | 0.61 |
| Lakey et al. (1996, Study 2) | U.S. sorority, large public university | 51 sisters rated the same 5 sisters (255 dyads). | 0.14 | 0.03 | 0.83 |
| Giblin & Lakey (in press, Study 2) | U.S. medical fellowship program | 4 groups of 6 medical fellows rated 3 clinical faculty; 1 group of 7 fellows rated three faculty (93 dyads). | 0.09 | 0.09 | 0.55 |
| Branje et al. (2002) | Dutch four-person families | Each family member rated every other family member (274 families, 3,288 dyads). | 0.34 | 0.03 | 0.59 |
| Lanz et al. (2004) | Italian four-person families | Each family member rated every other family member (108 families, 1,296 dyads). | 0.17 | 0.14 | 0.66 |
| Average weighed by number of dyads | | | 0.27 | 0.07 | 0.62 |

*Note.* Effect sizes are proportion of variance explained and are corrected for measurement error.

responsiveness, a construct very similar to perceived support, as well as enacted support (Lemay & Clark, 2008, Study 5).

One limitation of the studies described in Table 10.2 is that restricting samples to those in which recipients all know the same providers might exclude from study recipients' most important network members. For example, Lakey, McCabe, Fisicaro, and Drew (1996, Study 2) asked sorority members to rate five randomly selected sorority sisters, but these sorority sisters may not have been the most important people in any given recipient's social network. Similarly, Branje, van Aken, and van Lieshout (2002) asked members of four-person families to rate each other. Each family consisted of a mother, father, and two adolescent children. Yet, some people's most important support providers might be outside the nuclear family. To offset this potential limitation, other studies asked participants to rate their three to four most important providers (Lakey & Scoboria, 2005) or their mothers, fathers, and romantic partners (Barry, Lakey, & Orehek, 2007). Because each recipient rated different providers, providers were nested within recipients, and therefore it was not possible to separate provider from relational influences. Rather, provider and relational influences were combined into a single social influences component. Lakey and Scoboria (2005) and Barry et al. (2007) provided effect size estimates similar to the estimates provided by the studies summarized in Table 10.2, in which recipients rated the same providers. Averaged across the five samples presented in the two articles, and correcting for measurement error, recipient influences accounted for 18% of the variance in perceived support, whereas social influences (providers + relationships) accounted for 82%. It is reasonable to assume that the bulk of this 82% reflects relational influences, given the very large magnitude of relational influences compared to provider influences in the studies summarized in Table 10.2.

Thus, a number of studies have consistently found that perceived support is primarily a reflection of relational influences, but also contains a substantial portion of recipient trait influences. The objectively supportive properties of providers contribute a relatively small portion.

### Recipient, Provider, and Relationship Effects Are Statistically and Conceptually Distinct

Before reviewing the mechanisms associated with each influence and each influence's link to psychological health, it is necessary to point out that recipient, provider, and relational influences are conceptually and statistically distinct. What follows from this distinctiveness is that (1) relational influences on constructs cannot be correlated with recipient or provider influences on constructs, and (2) the same construct can have a different pattern of correlations with other constructs for each distinct influence. In the language of Cronbach and Meehl (1955), the same construct can have different nomological networks for different influences.

The conceptual distinctiveness of perceived support influences are indicated by their definitions. Recipient influences reflect recipients' tendency to perceive providers as supportive, regardless of providers' actual characteristics. Provider influences reflect the objectively supportive properties of providers. Relational influences reflect the extent to which providers' supportiveness is a matter of personal taste.

The statistical distinctness of the influences is easy to see by considering more fully the statistical meaning of each of them. Consider the matrix presented in Table 10.1 again. Recipient influences reflect mean differences among recipients, averaged across providers ("Column means for recipients"). Provider influences reflect mean differences among providers, averaged across recipients ("Row means for providers"). In contrast, relational influences are reflected in the full recipient × provider matrix. It is not possible to estimate correlations between recipient and relational influences or between provider and relational influences, because there is no way to map information represented as a row or column onto information represented as a matrix. Essentially, this limitation comes down to the preservation of information. Recipient × provider matrices contain much more information than recipient rows or provider matrices. Phrased differently, relational influences represent the residual variance, once column and row effects have been removed. As such, the relational variance is orthogonal to the column and row effects.

Each influence's nomological network can be established using multivariate generalizability (G) analyses (Brennan, 2001; Cronbach et al., 1972; Strube, 2000). Multivariate G correlations are interpreted in essentially the same way as Pearson correlations. However, multivariate G correlations estimate links between constructs for specific influences. For example, multivariate G analyses can tell investigators the extent to which perceived support is related to psychological health for each of the recipient, provider, and relational influences. Because these three influences are statistically and conceptually distinct, links between perceived support and psychological health might occur for all three, or perhaps for only one or two influences.

### Mechanisms of Recipient, Provider, and Relational Influences

Although work identifying the mechanisms underlying recipient, provider, and relational influences on perceived support has just begun, some mechanisms have already been identified.

### *Mechanisms of Recipient Influences*

Recipients may differ in their characteristic judgments of providers' supportiveness because of cognitive processes. Research in person perception indicates that perceivers do not see targets in exactly the same way, even when perceivers have identical information about targets (Kenny, 1994). One source of disagreement among perceivers is the concepts that perceivers use to think about targets (Higgins, 1996). In a given instance, one perceiver might interpret a target's actions as reflecting empathy, whereas another perceiver might interpret a target's actions as patronizing. The concepts that perceivers apply in a given instance depends upon (1) whether the concepts plausibly apply to the behavior to be considered (applicability), (2) the concepts that happen to be momentarily accessible because of recent experience (e.g., priming manipulations), and (3) the concepts that perceivers typically use in thinking about other people (chronic accessibility) (Higgins, 1996).

Recipient trait influences might emerge because recipients differ in the extent to which concepts of supportiveness are chronically accessible (Lakey & Drew, 1997). Such an explanation assumes that people with characteristically low perceived support have chronically accessible concepts that emphasize providers' typical unsupportiveness, whereas people with characteristically high perceived support have chronically accessible concepts that emphasize providers' typical supportiveness. If so, then people with low perceived support should interpret the same supportive actions and people as less supportive than people with high, perceived support. Research has consistently found evidence for such an effect (see Lakey & Drew, 1997, for a review).

For example, Lakey and colleagues presented participants with a large number of different supportive statements that providers might make in response to specific stressful situations. In Lakey and Cassady (1990, Study 2), supportive statements were written. In Lakey, Moineau, and Drew (1992) each statement was spoken by a different provider and presented via video. Recipients rated the supportiveness of each statement, and scores were averaged across all statements. Averaging ratings across all statements compounded recipient trait effects by removing effects due to the objective supportiveness of statements as well as relational influences. In both studies, recipients with characteristically low perceived support interpreted the statements as less supportive than did recipients with characteristically high perceived support, controlling for influences due to affect and social desirability. This effect is well replicated and has been observed in a range of different samples, including mildly mentally retarded adults (Lunsky & Benson, 2001), inner city, low-income children (Anan & Barnett, 1999), and community-dwelling adults (Lakey, Drew, Anan, Sirl, & Butler, 2004).

Although it is well established that recipients differ in how they characteristically interpret supportive people and actions, scholars do not yet have a description of the sequence by which this occurs. For example, support judgments might be inferred from recipients' trait-like tendencies to like other people, which might be inferred from recipients' trait-like tendencies see providers as similar to themselves in attitudes and values (Lakey, Lutz, & Scoboria, 2004; Neely et al., 2006). Alternatively, recipients might infer supportiveness on the basis of trait-like tendencies to see providers as agreeable (Branje, van Lieshout, & van Aken, 2005).

Behavioral mechanisms might also account for recipient influences on perceived support. For example, some recipients might perceive greater support across providers than do other recipients, because some recipients elicit more observable support from providers than do other recipients. So far, this mechanism has been tested in only one study. Neely et al. (2006) asked recipients to have five separate conversations with the same four providers. Both recipients and independent observers rated the supportiveness of providers. Evidence of a behavioral mechanism for recipient influences would be indicated if the recipients who characteristically perceived providers as supportive actually elicited more support from providers, as judged by independent observers. Yet, there was no evidence for such an effect. Nonetheless, Neely et al.'s (2006) sample was small, and additional studies are needed to provide more sensitive tests for behavioral mechanisms of recipient influences.

Indirect evidence also suggests that recipient influences may reflect genetic processes. For example, some research using twin studies (Kendler, 1997) has found a genetic predisposition to view others as supportive. Presumably, genetic mechanisms influence the aspect of support that is stable across time and across providers (i.e., recipient influences). However, it is unknown whether these genetic influences operate through cognitive, affective, or behavioral mechanisms.

### *Mechanisms of Provider Influences*

As described earlier, provider influences reflect interrater agreement among recipients, and therefore reflect the objective properties of providers, insofar as interrater agreement is an index of objective reality. Research on mechanisms underlying provider influences has focused on the personality characteristics of providers that lead recipients to agree that some providers are more supportive than other providers. Evidence of mechanisms involved in provider influences requires the isolation of provider influences on both provider supportiveness and provider personality characteristics. Multivariate G correlations between provider personality and supportiveness, when both reflect provider influences, offer evidence that when recipients agree about provider supportiveness, this agreement might be driven by recipients' agreement on provider personality.

Lakey et al. (1999) presented video-recorded supportive conversations to depressed inpatients and controls, and participants rated the supportiveness of providers. A separate team of observers rated providers' personality characteristics. Highly supportive providers were perceived as highly agreeable, consistent with the hypothesis that provider influences on supportiveness were driven by providers' objective agreeableness. Although this study did not use multivariate G analyses, these results reflected provider influences because scores for providers were averaged across recipients. Lakey, Lutz, and Scoboria (2004) replicated the link between supportiveness and agreeableness for provider influences using multivariate G analyses. Recipients rated well-known TV characters on likely supportiveness and personality. Again, objectively agreeable providers were perceived as objectively supportive. These two studies were limited by their artificial designs as well as by the very small number of providers sampled (four in both studies). Nonetheless, Branje et al. (2005) replicated these findings in a realistic study with a large number of providers in which family members rated each other on supportiveness and agreeableness.

Thus, although three studies have shown a link between agreeableness and supportiveness when both reflect provider influences, these correlations do not provide strong evidence that objective agreeableness causes objective supportiveness. Instead, agreeableness might be inferred from supportiveness, agreeableness and supportiveness might be the same construct when both reflect provider influences, or both might be inferred on the basis of the affect that providers elicit in recipients.

### *Mechanisms of Relational Influences*

As with recipient influences, both cognitive and behavioral mechanisms might be involved in relational influences. Relational influences occur when recipients systematically disagree about the relative supportiveness of providers. One potential cognitive mechanism for such systematic disagreement is that recipients differ in how they weigh information about providers when judging support. For example, recipient *A* might weigh provider agreeableness and conscientiousness heavily in judging support, such that agreeable and conscientious providers are perceived to be supportive. In contrast, recipient *B* might weigh provider emotional stability and openness heavily in judging support, such that emotionally stable and highly open providers are seen as supportive. If so, when recipients *A* and *B* judge the supportiveness of providers *A* and *B*, even if both recipients perceive the providers' personality characteristics in the same way, recipients *A* and *B* will arrive at different support judgments because of how recipients combine information about providers' personality characteristics.

Lutz and Lakey (2001) tested this cognitive hypothesis for relational influences in two studies by presenting participants with personality profiles of a large number of hypothetical providers and then asking participants to estimate the likely supportiveness of each provider. As in more realistic studies (e.g., Lakey et al., 2002), participants relied most heavily on provider agreeableness in judging support. In addition, however, multilevel modeling revealed significant differences in the extent to which recipients weighed each of the Big Five personality traits in judging support. Thus, although the experimental task was highly artificial, these results provide preliminary support for the hypothesis that relational influences in perceived support stem from recipients' differential weighing of provider information.

A second potential cognitive mechanism for relational influences is that recipients might base support judgments on the perceived similarity of providers to themselves. Recipients appear to use a heuristic whereby similar providers are seen as supportive providers (Lakey et al., 2002; Suitor, Pillemer, & Keeton, 1995). By definition, similarity is a relational influence, because the same features that make provider *A* similar to recipient *A*, make provider *A* dissimilar to recipient *B*. Yet, initial investigations did not use methods that distinguished among recipient, provider, and relational influences, and therefore it was impossible to know for which influence the correlation between perceived similarity and perceived support occurred (Lakey, Lutz, & Scoboria, 2004). Both Lakey, Lutz, and Scoboria (2004) and Neely et al. (2006) used methods that isolated relational influences and found strong links between recipients' perceptions of provider–recipient similarity and perceptions of provider support for relational influences specifically.

Behavioral mechanisms for relational influences are also possible. For example, recipients might systematically disagree about the supportiveness of providers because providers differ in how supportive they are to different people, as verified by independent observers. Neely et al. (2006) provide preliminary evidence of such effects. For relational influences specific to each conversation, recipients' systematic disagreement about provider supportiveness was linked to observers' ratings of providers' supportiveness. That is, on a conversation-by-conversation basis, when a given recipient found a given provider to be uniquely supportive, observers agreed that the provider acted in an especially supportive fashion. Curiously, there was no evidence of such a link when relational influences were averaged across all five conversations. Thus, additional studies are needed to confirm behavioral mechanisms of relational influences for perceived support.

In summary, some progress has been made in identifying the mechanisms underlying recipient, provider, and relational influences on perceived support. Although the findings are preliminary in some cases, relational influences appear to emerge because (1) recipients weigh information about providers differently in judging support; (2) recipients use the perceived similarity of providers to judge support, and similarity is inherently relational; and (3) on a conversation-by-conservation basis, providers behave more supportively toward some recipients than toward other recipients. Recipient influences appear to occur because recipients with high perceived support characteristically interpret specific actions of others as more supportive than do recipients with low perceived support. There is no evidence yet that high-support recipients characteristically elicit different actions from providers than do low-support recipients. Finally, provider influences appear to reflect a process whereby objectively agreeable providers are objectively supportive.

### To What Extent Are Recipient, Provider, and Relational Influences Related to Psychological Health?

If the goal is to use social support research to develop new interventions, then a key question is "To what extent is each of the recipient, provider, and relational influence linked to psychological health?" The fact that relational influences are the largest determinants of perceived support does not guarantee that relational influences are related to psychological health.[3] It might be that one of the smaller influences alone (e.g., provider influences) accounts for the correlation between perceived support and psychological health. As discussed previously, if each of the three influences can have its own nomological network, then each influence can have its own unique link to psychological health. Successfully manipulating a perceived support influence is unlikely to lead to improved psychological health if that influence itself is not related to psychological health.

Linking each of the perceived support influences to psychological health requires that psychological health itself be decomposed into recipient, provider, and relational influences. Although beyond the scope of this chapter, such a decomposition of psychological health represents a novel approach, as psychological health historically has been viewed as a property of the individual (i.e., recipient influences) rather than, for example, a result of relational influences. The exclusive focus on psychological disorder as a property of the individual probably can be traced to psychiatry's use of a disease metaphor for psychological disorder. A G/SRM approach could make a unique contribution to our understanding of psychological disorder by providing precise operational definitions and estimates of the relative magnitude of individual, provider, and relational influences on specific psychological disorders. Such an approach might be useful as psychologists consider the diagnostic categories for relational disorders (Beach & Kaslow, 2006; see also Benjamin, Chapter 19, this volume).

The first studies to examine the extent to which the different perceived support influences are related to psychological health used nested designs in which participants rated their own important network members (Barry et al., 2007; Lakey & Scoboria, 2005). As described previously, such a design combines relational and provider influences into a single social influences component. These studies have already been described with regard to their estimates of trait and social influences on perceived support. Beyond this, these studies also estimated the extent to which perceived support was linked to favorable affect for trait and social influences separately. Thus, in addition to rating the supportiveness of each provider, recipients also rated the extent to which they typically experienced positive and negative affect when with, or when thinking about, each provider. Positive and negative affects were studied as indicators of psychological health because (1) affect has been shown to be sensitive to contextual influences, (2) affect scales have valid state forms, and (3) affect is related in important ways to mood and anxiety disorders (Watson, Wiese, Vaidya, & Tellegen, 1999). In three samples Lakey and Scoboria (2005) found that perceived support was related strongly to both high positive affect and low negative affect when correlations reflected both recipient traits as well as social influences. Barry et al. (2007) replicated these results for social influences in both of their samples, but the links between perceived support and favorable affect were somewhat less consistent when correlations reflected recipient traits.

The primary advantage of the Barry et al. (2007) study as well as the Lakey and Scoboria (2005) one was that the researchers permitted recipients to rate their own important relationships; yet this feature was also the studies' primary disadvantage, because this design could not provide separate estimates for relational and provider influences. The social influence component identified by Lakey and Scoboria (2005) and Barry et al. (2007) probably reflected relational influences primarily, because as indicated on Table 10.2, nearly 90% of the combined provider + relational variance is relational. Nonetheless, studies are needed that estimate links between support and affect, isolating provider from relational influences. Such isolation requires a design in which recipients rate the same providers on perceived supportiveness and on the affect experienced when with each provider.

The Neely et al. (2006) study, described previously, permitted tests of the links between support and affect for provider and relational influences specifically, because in addition to rating supportiveness, both recipients and independent observers rated recipients' affect after each conversation with providers. There were strong and significant correlations between perceived support and positive affect when correlations reflected relational influences that generalized across conversations, as well as relational influences that were conversation specific. Moreover, correlations between positive affect and perceived support were confirmed by observer ratings when correlations reflected conversation-specific relational influences. In addition, perceived support and positive affect were strongly and significantly related when correlations reflected recipient traits. Yet, there were no significant correlations involving provider influences, indicating that the objectively supportive features of providers could not account for the link between perceived support and affect in this study.

Veenstra et al. (2010) replicated Neely et al.'s (2006) study with a sample of 40 recipients who had three separate conversations with each of three providers (a total of 360 conversations). The results for recipient ratings were remarkably consistent with Neely et al. (2006). Perceived support and positive affect were significantly and strongly related when correlations reflected relational influences that generalized across conversations, as well as relational influences that were conversation specific. In addition, perceived support was strongly and significantly related to positive affect when correlations reflected recipient traits. Again, there were no significant correlations involving provider influences.

In summary, the weight of the evidence from these seven recent studies suggests that perceived support is related to favorable affect for both recipient trait and relational influences. Studies that had participants rate their own important providers found consistent evidence that perceived support was related strongly to both positive and low negative affect when correlations reflected social influences. The results of Neely et al. (2006) and Veenstra et al. (2008) suggest that links between perceived support and favorable affect observed for social influences likely reflect relational influences. Although Lakey and Scoboria (2005) and Barry et al. (2007) found strong and consistent correlations between perceived support and low negative affect when both reflected social influences, neither Neely et al. (2006) nor Veenstra et al. (2008) observed links between low negative affect and perceived support for any influence. This inconsistency may reflect the fact that Neely et al. (2006) and Veenstra et al. (2008) studied recipients and providers who were strangers, whereas Lakey and Scoboria (2005) and Barry et al. (2007) studied providers who were important parts of recipients' social networks. Perhaps only well-established relationships can elicit a link between perceived support and low negative affect.

## Implications for Intervention

The relative magnitudes of recipient, provider, and relational influences as well as their links to affect have important implications for social support interventions intended to alleviate or prevent psychological disorder by offering new support providers to at-risk recipients. First, these findings suggest an explanation for the disappointing results of existing social support interventions. Second, the findings suggest new approaches that might be more successful.

As discussed, the results of randomized controlled trials have not yielded encouraging findings regarding the effectiveness of social support interventions in improving either perceived support or psychological health (Hogan et al., 2002; Lakey & Lutz, 1996). These interventions might have been less successful than expected because they focused on provider influences, the smallest of the three influences identified by G/SRM studies. Most social support interventions have relied on provider influences because the projects reflected an implicit assumption that most recipients would perceive intervention providers as supportive. For example, Heller et al. (1991) provided low-income, rural, elderly women with regular supportive phone calls from providers employed by the intervention. Presumably, these providers were selected because project leaders perceived the providers as supportive. Yet, the magnitude of the provider influences in G/SRM studies indicates that there is very little agreement among recipients about the supportiveness of providers (7%). Thus, one should not expect that many recipients would agree with project leaders that intervention providers were supportive. Previous randomized trials of support interventions may have been unsuccessful because recipients did not perceive providers as supportive. Thus, it is important to consider basing interventions on other social support influences.

Recipient influences might be a good focus for intervention because they account for a substantial amount of variance in perceived support (27%) and appear to be related to psychological health. Interventions targeting recipient influences might attempt to change the beliefs and perceptual biases of individuals who perceive little social support (Brand, Lakey, & Berman, 1995; Lakey & Lutz, 1996). However, recipient influences might be difficult to change because by definition, they reflect the aspect of perceived support that is stable across providers and over time. Consistent with this, Brand et al. (1995) reported statistically significant but clinically trivial changes in perceived support in a randomized trial of an intervention specifically focused on changing recipients' perceptions of social support.

Relational influences on perceived support appear to be the most promising candidates for intervention. Relational influences are overwhelmingly the strongest influences on perceived support, and there is strong preliminary evidence that relational influences on perceived support are linked to relational influences on psychological health. However, interventions focused on relational influences require a unique approach to intervention.

Interventions focused on relational influences will require matching recipients with specific providers such that uniquely supportive dyads are identified.[4] A prerequisite to such an approach is the ability to forecast which providers will be seen by which recipients as supportive. Such forecasting is parallel to psychotherapy research that attempts to match certain types of therapists with certain types of patients (e.g., ethnic matching; Sue, Fujino, Hu, Takeuchi, & Zane, 1991). Such approaches in psychotherapy research have not been especially effective, however, suggesting that developing the technology for forecasting supportive matches will be a daunting task. Fortunately, the G/SRM approach provides the analytic tools for developing this technology.

The G/SRM approach for studying how to forecast supportive matches requires a particular structure for the prediction equation. First, as described previously in this chapter, one can only forecast (i.e., correlate) relational influences on perceived support from relational influences on other constructs. Thus, studies designed to forecast supportive matches must be designed in such a way that the relational influences on any candidate predictor variable can be isolated. That is, each predictor variable must be structured so that there is a score for each provider–recipient dyad. A wide range of types of constructs could be structured in such a way. For example, it might be possible to forecast supportive matches on the basis of providers' perceived similarity to recipients, on the basis of independently determined personality similarity or complementarity, similarity in attitudes and values, or recipients' judgments of providers' supportiveness or recipients' experience of affect based on very brief interactions with providers. However, it will not be possible to use recipient or provider personality in isolation to forecast supportive matches because, as described previously, these variables are represented either as rows or columns and such configurations cannot be mapped onto the full recipient × provider matrix that defines relational influences (Table 10.1).

Two recent studies demonstrate (1) that it is possible to forecast relational supportive matches and (2) the type of design required for studying forecasting relational supportive matches.

Veenstra et al. (2010) described two studies in which relational support averaged across two later conversations were forecast from (1) recipients' judgments of providers' supportiveness based on earlier conversations, (2) recipients' perceptions of providers' supportiveness based on videotaped interviews of providers, (3) observers' ratings of early conversations between recipients and providers, and (4) recipients' experience of affect elicited by providers in earlier conversations. In Study 1, 40 recipients had three different conversations, distributed over 3 weeks, with the same three providers. In Study 2, 10 recipients had five different conversations, distributed over several months, with the same four providers. In both studies, recipients' rated the supportiveness of providers as well as their own affect after each conversation. In Study 1, recipients first viewed a 10-minute interview with each provider and rated providers' likely supportiveness. In Study 2, independent observers evaluated the supportiveness of providers during each conversation. In Study 1, the criterion was recipients' ratings of providers' supportiveness averaged across conversations 2 and 3. The criterion in Study 2 was recipients' ratings of providers' supportiveness averaged across conversations 4 and 5. In both studies, multivariate G analyses were used to isolate the relational influences of supportiveness and affect. Could recipients or observers forecast later relational support from initial conversations? Could recipients forecast later relational support from viewing a 10-minute videotaped interview?

Veenstra et al.'s (2010) results were very consistent across the two samples. Recipients could forecast later relational support with some accuracy based on an initial 10-minute (Study 1) or 20-minute (Study 2) face-to-face conversation. Forecasting was approximately equally accurate whether based on recipients' ratings of providers' supportiveness or recipients' ratings of affect during the conversation. Moreover, forecasting relational support was equally accurate when based on a 10-minute conversation (Study 1) as when based on a 20-minute conversation (Study 2), and accuracy improved minimally when based on three 20-minute conversations. Thus, preliminary evidence indicates that recipients can forecast the future supportiveness of providers based on very brief, face-to-face contact. In contrast, observers could not accurately forecast provider supportiveness from viewing conversations, and recipients could not accurately forecast providers' supportiveness from videotaped interviews of providers. Thus, Veenstra et al. (2010) demonstrated (1) that it is possible to forecast which providers will be seen by which recipients as supportive, and (2) that multivariate G analyses can be used to forecast relational supportive matches. Improving the accuracy and cost effectiveness of forecasting supportive matches should be a focus of future research.

The processes that apply to social support might also apply to psychotherapy. Hoyt (2002) presented to students videos of therapists demonstrating their approaches and asked these students to rate their expected therapeutic alliance with each therapist as well as the expertness and attractiveness of each therapist. Lakey, Cohen, and Neely (2008) presented similar videos to psychotherapy patients and students in two studies and obtained ratings of expected therapeutic alliance, as well as therapist expertness, attractiveness, and competence. In all three studies there were very strong relational influences on perceptions of therapists, suggesting that the relative importance of relational influences may extend to psychotherapy as well as to perceived support. If so, then the techniques developed for forecasting supportive matches might also be used to forecast effective client–therapist matches.

## FINAL SUMMARY

Approaches from social/personality psychology, originally developed to study person × situation interactions and person perception, suggest new approaches to interventions designed to alleviate or prevent psychological disorder by making available new support providers to recipients. Using G theory and SRM, investigators have isolated influences of perceived support that reflect the trait-like characteristics of support recipients, the objectively supportive qualities of support providers, and the unique relationships between recipients and providers. Relational influences are overwhelmingly the most powerful determinants of perceived support, and preliminary evidence indicates that relational influences on perceived support are correlated strongly with psychological health. Thus, it may be promising to focus interventions on relational influences specifically. Interventions based on relational influences require an approach that is different from interventions based on recipient or provider influences. Relational interventions require accurate forecasting of which specific providers will be seen as supportive by which specific recipients. Fortunately, multivariate G theory provides the analytic framework for studying how to forecast relational supportive matches. Recent research demonstrates that such forecasting is possible, suggesting the feasibility of new social support interventions focusing on relational influences as well as applications of these models to the assignment to clients of therapists most likely to be perceived as supportive and therefore most likely to be effective.

## NOTES

1. I use the term *influences* because univariate G/SRM studies are repeated measures of experimental designs that permit causal inferences.
2. The effect sizes presented on Table 10.2 are corrected for measurement error because those were the only results available from the Branje et al. (2002) and Lanz, Tagliabue, and Rosnati (2004) studies. Effect sizes do not sum to 1 for Branje et al. and Lanz et al. because these studies included estimates for family effects as well, which are not reported here. In addition, Branje et al. and Lanz et al. used a procedure developed by Cook (1994) for estimating variance components separately for each type of family member (mothers, fathers, older sibling, and younger sibling). In contrast, most G/SRM studies do not focus on nuclear families and thus do not draw such distinctions. To make the estimates comparable across all studies, I recalculated effect sizes for Branje et al. and Lanz et al. so that variances were pooled without regard to type of family member.
3. I am indebted to Catherine Lutz Zois for this idea.
4. It is occasionally suggested that rather than matching providers with recipients, it might be more efficient to train providers to tailor their supportive actions so that each recipient will see the actions as supportive. Yet, if providers tailored their supportive actions to the characteristics of recipients, and if providers differed in this skill, then recipients should agree that some providers (the ones who tailor their actions well) are more supportive than other providers. Such an effect would manifest itself as a provider effect rather than a relationship effect, and as we have seen, provider effects for perceived support typically are comparatively small.

## REFERENCES


Anan, R. M., & Barnett, D. (1999). Perceived social support mediates between prior attachment and subsequent adjustment: A study of urban African American children. *Developmental Psychology, 35*, 1210–1222.

Barrera, M., Jr. (1986). Distinctions between social support concepts, measures and models. *American Journal of Community Psychology, 14*, 413–445.

Barrera, M., Jr., Glasgow, R. E., McKay, H. G., Boles, S. M., & Feil, E. G. (2002). Do Internet-based support interventions change perceptions of social support? An experimental trial of approaches for supporting diabetes self-management. *American Journal of Community Psychology, 30*, 637–654.

Barry, R., Lakey, B., & Orehek, E. (2007). Links among attachment dimensions, affect and the self for broadly-generalized attachment styles and relationship-specific bonds. *Personality and Social Psychology Bulletin, 33*, 240–253.

Beach, S. R. H., & Kaslow, N. J. (2006). Relational disorders and relational processes in diagnostic practice: Introduction to the special section. *Journal of Family Psychology, 20*, 353–355.

Bolger, N., Zuckerman, A., & Kessler, R. C. (2000). Invisible support and adjustment to stress. *Journal of Personality and Social Psychology, 79*, 953–961.

Brand, E., Lakey, B., & Berman, S. (1995). A preventive, psychoeducational approach to increase perceived support. *American Journal of Community Psychology, 23*, 117–136.

Branje, S. J. T., van Aken, M. A. G., & van Lieshout, C. F. M. (2002). Relational support in families with adolescents. *Journal of Family Psychology, 16*, 351–362.

Branje, S. J. T., van Lieshout, C. F. M., & van Aken, M. A. G. (2005). Relations between agreeableness and perceived support in family relationships: Why nice people are not always supportive. *International Journal of Behavioral Development*, *29*, 120–128.

Brennan, R. L. (2001). *Generalizability theory*. New York: Springer.

Brewin, C. R., Andrews, B., & Valentine, J. D. (2000). Meta-analysis of risk factors for posttraumatic stress disorder in trauma-exposed adults. *Journal of Consulting and Clinical Psychology*, *68*, 748–766.

Burton, E., Stice, E., & Seeley, J. R. (2004). A prospective test of the stress-buffering model of depression in adolescent girls: No support once again. *Journal of Consulting and Clinical Psychology*, *72*, 689–697.

Cohen, S., & Wills, T. A. (1985). Stress, social support, and the buffering hypothesis. *Psychological Bulletin*, *98*, 310–357.

Collins, N. L., & Feeney, B. C. (2004). Working models of attachment shape perceptions of social support: Evidence from experimental and observational studies. *Journal of Personality and Social Psychology*, *87*, 363–383.

Cook, W. L. (1994). A structural equation model of dyadic relationships within the family system. *Journal of Consulting and Clinical Psychology*, *62*, 500–509.

Cronbach, L. J. (1955). Processes affecting scores on "understanding of others" and "assumed similarity." *Psychological Bulletin*, *52*, 177–193.

Cronbach, L. J., Gleser, G. C., Nanda, H., & Rajaratnam, N. (1972). *The dependability of behavioral measurements: Theory of generalizability for scores and profiles*. New York: Wiley.

Cronbach, L. J., & Meehl, P. E. (1955). Construct validity in psychological tests. *Psychological Bulletin*, *52*, 281–302.

Endler, N. S., & Hunt, J. M. (1969). Generalizability of contributions from sources of variance in the S-R inventory of anxiousness. *Journal of Personality*, *37*, 1–24.

Feeney, B. C. (2004). A secure base: Responsive support of goal strivings and exploration in adult intimate relationships. *Journal of Personality and Social Psychology*, *87*, 631–648.

Finch, J. F., Okun, M. A., Pool, G. J., & Ruehlman, L. S. (1999). A comparison of the influence of conflictual and supportive social interactions on psychological distress. *Journal of Personality*, *67*, 581–622.

Gable, S. L., Gonzaga, G. C., & Strachman, A. (2006). Will you be there for me when things go right? Supportive responses to positive event disclosures. *Journal of Personality and Social Psychology*, *91*, 904–917.

Giblin, F., & Lakey, B. (in press). Integrating mentoring and social support research within the context of stressful medical training. *Journal of Social and Clinical Psychology*.

Heller, K., Thompson, M. G., Trueba, P. E., Hogg, J. R., & Vlachos-Weber, I. (1991). Peer support telephone dyads for elderly women: Was this the wrong intervention? *American Journal of Community Psychology*, *19*, 53–74.

Higgins, E. T. (1996). Knowledge activation: Accessibility, applicability, and salience. In E. T. Higgins & A. W. Kruglanski (Eds.), *Social psychology: Handbook of basic principles* (pp. 133–168). New York: Guilford Press.

Hogan, B. E., Linden, W., & Najarian, B. (2002). Social support interventions: Do they work? *Clinical Psychology Review*, *22*, 381–440.

House, J. S., Landis, K. R., & Umberson, D. (1988). Social relationships and health. *Science*, *241*, 540–545.

Hoyt, W. T. (2002). Bias in participant ratings of psychotherapy process: An initial generalizability study. *Journal of Counseling Psychology*, *49*, 35–46.

Kendler, K. S. (1997). Social support: A genetic–epidemiologic analysis. *American Journal of Psychiatry*, *154*, 1398–1404.

Kenny, D. A. (1994). *Interpersonal perception: A social relations analysis*. New York: Guilford Press.

Kenny, D. A., & La Voie, L. (1984). The social relations model. In L. Berkowitz (Ed.), *Advances in experimental social psychology* (Vol. 18, pp. 141–182). Orlando, FL: Academic Press.

Lakey, B., Adams, K., Neely, L., Rhodes, G., Lutz, C. J., & Sielky, K. (2002). Perceived support and low emotional distress: The role of enacted support, dyad similarity, and provider personality. *Personality and Social Psychology Bulletin*, *28*, 1546–1555.

Lakey, B., & Cassady, P. B. (1990). Cognitive processes in perceived social support. *Journal of Personality and Social Psychology*, *59*, 337–343.

Lakey, B., Cohen, J. L., & Neely, L. C. (2008). Perceived support and relational influences on psychotherapy process constructs. *Journal of Counseling Psychology*, *55*, 209–220.

Lakey, B., & Cronin, A. (2008). Low social support and major depression: Research, theory, and methodological issues. In K. S. Dobson & D. Dozois (Eds.), *Risk factors for depression* (pp. 385–408). New York: Academic Press.

Lakey, B., & Drew, J. B. (1997). A social–cognitive perspective of social support. In G. R. Pierce, B. Lakey, I. G. Sarason, & B. R. Sarason (Eds.), *Sourcebook of social support and personality* (pp. 107–140). New York: Plenum Press.

Lakey, B., Drew, J. B., Anan, R., Sirl, K., & Butler, C. (2004). Negative interpretations of interpersonal situations and the relation between low perceived support and psychological distress among divorced adults. *Journal of Applied Social Psychology*, *34*, 1030–1047.

Lakey, B., Drew, J. B., & Sirl, K. (1999). Clinical depression and perceptions of supportive others: A generalizability analysis. *Cognitive Therapy and Research*, *23*, 511–533.

Lakey, B., & Lutz, C. L. (1996). Increasing social support: Preventive and therapeutic interventions. In G. R. Pierce, B. R. Sarason, & I. G. Sarason (Eds.), *Handbook of social support and the family* (pp. 435–466). New York: Plenum Press.

Lakey, B., Lutz, C. L., & Scoboria, A. (2004). The information used to judge supportiveness depends on whether the judgment reflects the personality of perceivers, the objective characteristics of targets, or their unique relationship. *Journal of Social and Clinical Psychology*, *23*, 796–814.

Lakey, B., McCabe, K., Fisicaro, S., & Drew, J. (1996). Personal and environmental determinants of social support: Three generalizability studies. *Journal of Personality and Social Psychology*, *70*, 1270–1280.

Lakey B., Moineau, S., & Drew, J. B. (1992). Perceived social support and individual differences in the interpretation and recall of supportive behavior. *Journal of Social and Clinical Psychology*, *11*, 336–348.

Lakey, B., & Scoboria, A. (2005). Trait and social influences in the links among perceived social support, affect, and self-esteem. *Journal of Personality*, *73*, 361–388.

Lanz, M., Tagliabue, S., & Rosnati, R. (2004). *Il social relations model nello studio delle relazioni familiari* [Social relations model in family relationships study]. *Testing Psicometria Metodologia*, *11*, n.p.

Lemay, E. P., Jr., & Clark, M. S. (2008). How the head liberates the heart: Projection of communal responsiveness guides relationship promotion. *Journal of Personality and Social Psychology*, *94*, 647–671.

Lunsky, Y., & Benson, B. A. (2001). Perceived social support and mental retardation: A social–cognitive approach. *Cognitive Therapy and Research*, *25*, 77–90.

Lutz, C. L., & Lakey, B. (2001). How people make support judgments: Individual differences in the traits used to infer supportiveness in others. *Journal of Personality and Social Psychology*, *81*, 1070–1079.

Mischel, W., & Shoda, Y. (1995). A cognitive–affective system theory of personality: Reconceptualizing situations, dispositions, dynamics, and invariance in personality structure. *Psychological Review*, *102*, 246–268.

Neely, L. C., Lakey, B., Cohen, J. L., Barry, R., Orehek, E., Abeare, C. A., et al. (2006). Trait and social processes in the link between social support and affect: An experimental laboratory investigation. *Journal of Personality*, *74*, 1015–1046.

Newcomb, M. D., & Keefe, K. (1997). Social support, self-esteem, social conformity, and gregariousness: Developmental patterns across 12 years. In G. R. Pierce, B. Lakey, I. G. Sarason, & B. R.

Sarason (Eds.), *Sourcebook of social support and personality* (pp. 303–333). New York: Plenum Press.

Norman, R. M. G., Malla, A. K., Manchanda, R., Harricharan, R., Takhar, J., & Northcott, S. (2005). Social support and three-year symptom and admission outcomes for first-episode psychosis. *Schizophrenia Research*, *80*, 227–234.

Pierce, G. R., Sarason, B. R., & Sarason, I. G. (1992). General and specific support expectations and stress as predictors of perceived supportiveness: An experimental study. *Journal of Personality and Social Psychology*, *63*, 297–307.

Sarason, B. R., Pierce, G. R., & Sarason, I. G. (1990). Social support: The sense of acceptance and the role of relationships. In B. R. Sarason, I. G. Sarason, & G. R. Pierce (Eds.), *Social support: An interactional view* (pp. 97–128). New York: Wiley.

Sarason, B. R., Sarason, I. G., & Gurung, R. A. R. (2001). Close personal relationships and health outcomes: A key to the role of social support. In B. R. Sarason & S. Duck (Eds.), *Personal relationships: Implications for clinical and community psychology* (pp. 15–41). New York: Wiley.

Strube, M. J. (2000). Reliability and generalizability theory. In G. G. Laurence & P. R. Yarnold (Eds.), *Reading and understanding MORE multivariate statistics* (pp. 23–66). Washington, DC: American Psychological Association.

Sue, S., Fujino, D. C., Hu, L., Takeuchi, D. T., & Zane, N. W. S. (1991). Community mental health services for ethnic minority groups: A test of the cultural responsiveness hypothesis. *Journal of Consulting and Clinical Psychology*, *59*, 533–540.

Suitor, J. J., Pillemer, K., & Keeton, S. (1995). When experience counts: The effects of experiential and structural similarity on patterns of support and interpersonal stress. *Social Forces*, *73*, 999–1014.

Symister, P., & Friend, R. (2003). The influence of social support and problematic support on optimism and depression in chronic illness: A prospective study evaluating self-esteem as a mediator. *Health Psychology*, *22*, 123–129.

Veenstra, A., Lakey, B., Cohen, J. L., Neely, L. C., Orehek, E., Barry, R., et al. (2008). *Forecasting the specific providers that recipients will perceive as uniquely supportive*. Unpublished manuscript, Grand Valley State University, Allendale, MI.

Watson, D., Wiese, D., Vaidya, J., & Tellegen, A. (1999). The two general activation systems of affect: Structural findings, evolutionary considerations, and psychobiological influence. *Journal of Personality and Social Psychology*, *76*, 820–838.

Wills, T. A., & Cleary, S. D. (1996). How are social support effects mediated? A test with parental support and adolescent substance use. *Journal of Personality and Social Psychology*, *71*, 937–952.

# 11 Social Comparison Theory

Pieternel Dijkstra
Frederick X. Gibbons
Abraham P. Buunk

Social comparison is an important, if not central, characteristic of human social life. Because of the adaptive value of adequately sizing up one's competitors, the need to compare oneself with others is phylogenetically very old, biologically very powerful, and recognizable in many species (Gilbert, Price, & Allan, 1995). Nevertheless, it was not until Festinger's (1954) classic paper that the term *social comparison* was proposed. According to Festinger, people have a fundamental desire to evaluate their opinions and abilities, and they strive for stable, accurate appraisals of themselves. Although individuals prefer to evaluate themselves using objective and nonsocial standards, they will evaluate themselves by comparison with others when such objective information is unavailable.

Since Festinger introduced it, social comparison theory has evolved considerably and has undergone numerous transitions and reformulations (e.g., Suls & Wheeler, 2000). As a result of these developments, most scholars today agree that individuals are not merely objective and unbiased self-evaluators who strive toward accurate self-perceptions. People harbor a variety of motives for comparing themselves to others, and often such motives are apt to result in biased views of the self. More specifically, in addition to self-evaluation, individuals may compare themselves with others to improve their skills or abilities (self-improvement) and to protect or enhance their self-esteem (self-enhancement; e.g., Wills, 1981; Wood, 1989). The current, broader concept of social comparison theory therefore includes "any process in which individuals relate their own characteristics to those of others" (Buunk & Gibbons, 2000, p. 491) and encompasses comparisons on many different dimensions.

## UP OR DOWN?

When comparing themselves, individuals may choose different types of comparison targets. They may compare themselves with others who are similar (lateral comparisons), with others who are better off (upward comparisons), or with others who are worse off (downward comparisons). With whom individuals choose to compare themselves depends largely on the motive for the comparison. When self-evaluation is the dominant motive, individuals typically compare themselves with others whose performance is similar to their own (the similarity hypothesis; Festinger, 1954; Suls & Wheeler, 2000), because when others' abilities are too far from one's own, either above or below, it is not possible to estimate one's own ability or opinion accurately. When self-improvement is the dominant motive, individuals typically compare themselves upwards, with others who perform better than they do (e.g., Suls & Wheeler, 2000; Wood, 1989). Observing another person who has proficiency at a task can reveal information about how to improve and may raise individuals' feelings of self-confidence and self-efficacy. Finally, when self-enhancement is the dominant motive, individuals generally prefer to compare themselves downward, with others who are worse off than themselves (e.g., Suls & Wheeler, 2000; Taylor & Lobel, 1989; Wills, 1981). Perceiving oneself as better off boosts self-esteem, reduces anxiety, and generates positive affect. In contrast, seeing someone who is better off may diminish self-esteem and produce negative affect.

## CONTRAST AND IDENTIFICATION

Buunk, Collins, Taylor, and Van Yperen (1990) and Collins (1996) have argued that the effect of social comparison information depends not only on the direction of the comparison but also on how individuals handle social comparison information. That is, individuals may contrast themselves with a comparison target (i.e., focus on the differences between themselves and the target), or they may identify with a comparison target (i.e., focus on the similarities between themselves and the comparison target). As a consequence, individuals may follow one of four strategies: upward identification, upward contrast, downward identification, and downward contrast (Buunk, Kuyper, & Van der Zee, 2005; Smith, 2000). In general, when individuals identify with a comparison target, upward comparisons (upward identification) may enhance their self-image and evoke positive feelings such as hope and admiration, whereas downward comparisons (downward identification) lower the self-image and may produce feelings of worry and fear (see also, Tesser, Miller, & Moore, 1988). Conversely, when individuals contrast with a comparison target, upward comparisons (upward contrast) may lower their self-image and evoke negative feelings, such as frustration and resentment, whereas downward comparisons (downward contrast) enhances the self-image and may produce feelings of relief and pride.

## SOCIAL COMPARISON ORIENTATION

Several researchers have theorized that people may differ in their disposition to compare themselves with others. According to Gibbons and Buunk (1999), the extent to which and the frequency with which people compare themselves with others varies from one individual to the next, an individual difference variable they call *social comparison orientation* (SCO). Relative to individuals with a low SCO, individuals with a high SCO seek out more comparisons, spend more time engaging in comparisons, experience more reactions (feelings) from comparing themselves with others, and base their personal risk perceptions (more) on comparisons with others. In summarizing the literature, Buunk and Gibbons (2006) concluded that those with high SCO are characterized by a combination of a high accessibility and awareness of the self, an interest in what others feel and think, and some degree of negative affectivity and self-uncertainty. SCO is an important individual difference variable because high-SCO individuals are not only more interested in the comparison process, but also more affected by it (Buunk & Gibbons, 2006).

This chapter discusses three clinical problems to which social comparison theory has been fruitfully applied: body image problems, depression, and occupational stress and burnout. In addition to reviewing research that has used social comparison theory as a theoretical framework, we discuss the implications of these studies for the treatment of these problems.

## BODY DISSATISFACTION

The term *body image* is used to describe the internal representation individuals have of their appearance—that is, their unique perception of their body (e.g., Thompson, Heinberg, Altabe, & Tantleff-Dunn, 2002). Body image dissatisfaction may best be conceptualized as a continuum, with levels of dissatisfaction ranging from none to extreme. Most people fall near the middle of the range, experiencing mild to moderate dissatisfaction with their bodies. Thus feelings of dissatisfaction with one's body are not necessarily problematic in nature; research suggests that it is normal to feel somewhat dissatisfied with one's appearance (e.g., Tiggeman & Slater, 2004). Low to moderate feelings of dissatisfaction may even be beneficial and lead individuals to participate in healthy behavior, such as exercising and healthy eating habits (e.g., Cash, Novy, & Grant, 1994). Nonetheless, the higher the level of body dissatisfaction, the more likely individuals are to develop clinical problems. Body dissatisfaction is one of the strongest predictors of eating disorder symptoms among women; when sufficiently severe, it may manifest itself as body dysmorphic disorder (BDD)—an excessive concern with an appearance deficit that, from an objective point of view, is small or even absent (e.g., Thompson et al., 2002).

### Social Comparison and Body Dissatisfaction

Currently, it is generally assumed that body dissatisfaction results from pervasive and unrealistic societal ideals regarding what is deemed attractive that are transmitted mostly through the mass media (e.g., Hargreaves & Tiggeman, 2004). Social comparison can be seen as an important linking process between media messages of beauty and body dissatisfaction (e.g., Tiggeman & Slater, 2004). By routinely comparing their bodies with media images of beauty, individuals become less satisfied with their bodies (for a review, see Groesz, Levine, & Murnen, 2002). In support of social comparison theory, several studies have revealed so-called contrast effects with regard to self-perceived attractiveness (e.g., Krones, Stice, Batres, & Orjada, 2005). That is, after viewing a highly attractive individual of the same sex, individuals usually experience a decrease in self-rated attractiveness and an increase in negative affect. This is especially true for women, who already perceive themselves to be unattractive (Trampe, Stapel, & Siero, 2007). The opposite is also true: Individuals who view unattractive same-sex individuals experience an increase in self-perceptions of attractiveness and a decrease in negative affect.

## Negatively Biased Social Comparisons

Although social comparison processes may lead individuals to feel both less and more satisfied with their body (depending on the comparison target), in daily life, social comparison processes more often have adverse than positive effects on individuals' body satisfaction. First, individuals often engage in evaluative and social comparison processes that are damaging to the self in the domain of weight and appearance. Specifically, individuals, especially women, frequently use a strategy of upward contrast when comparing themselves with beauty ideals (i.e., they focus on the differences between themselves and beauty ideals) and feel bad about themselves as a consequence (e.g., Engeln-Maddox, 2005; Strahan, Wilson, Cressman, & Buote, 2006). Second, the self-enhancement strategies individuals typically use to protect their self-esteem from negative social comparisons do not seem to operate when it comes to certain aspects of the body. Powell, Matacin, and Stuart (2001), for instance, found that women who rated themselves lower on a particular desirable physical trait were less inclined to rate the trait as important, except when the dimension under comparison was weight. Third, the previously mentioned contrast effect does not always occur; specifically, the positive effect of downward comparison on body satisfaction may be lost. Lin and Kulik (2002), for instance, found that, whereas exposure to a thin peer reduced body satisfaction, exposure to an oversize peer did not produce the expected increase in body satisfaction.

In sum, appearance-related comparisons make most individuals feel dissatisfied with their body. Consequently, the more often individuals compare their bodies to those of others, the less satisfied they feel with their bodies (e.g., Cattarin, Thompson, Thomas, & Williams, 2000). Once individuals compare themselves with media images of beauty, they may easily become caught in a vicious circle. Contrast comparisons with beauty ideals decrease body satisfaction, which, in turn, triggers more social comparisons in an attempt to reduce feelings of insecurity and change self-perceived shortcomings (e.g., Bessenoff, 2006). Because of the flood of media images of highly attractive individuals, these social comparisons are, however, mostly upward, and, rather than reducing feelings of insecurity, they decrease body satisfaction as a consequence.

## Moderators of Attractiveness Comparisons

Since almost everyone is exposed to societal messages of beauty, the question arises why some individuals are relatively content with their appearance, whereas others suffer from extreme appearance disparagement. Studies have revealed several variables that moderate the effect of social comparisons on body image and that may account for these individual differences. We discuss six of them.

First, the extent to which individuals have internalized society's standards of beauty seems to be a risk factor for body dissatisfaction. As individuals place greater importance on physical attractiveness, their body esteem suffers more from upward comparisons with models (e.g., for a review see Cafri, Yamamiya, Brannick, & Thompson, 2005).

Second, the negative effect of upward contrast comparisons may be moderated by the motive for the comparison. For example, in Halliwell and Ditmar's (2005) study, participants who were instructed to make self-evaluation comparisons with thin models reported higher body-focused anxiety than did participants who did not view model advertisements. Participants who were instructed to focus on self-improvement comparisons with thin models did not report higher body-focused anxiety than participants who did not view model advertisements.

Third, when individuals experience a feeling of psychological closeness to the comparison target, and thus are more likely to identify with the target, upward comparisons can lead to more positive self-appraisals of attractiveness, whereas downward comparisons can lead to more negative self-appraisals of attractiveness (Brown, Novick, Lord, & Richards, 1992).

Fourth, gender has been found to be an important moderator: Women's body image is affected more negatively by appearance-related comparisons than men's body image. In general, cultural norms for male beauty are more flexible and more realistic than those for female beauty (e.g., Hargreaves & Tiggemann, 2004). Especially the combination of a small waist and large breasts, which is characteristic of the Western female beauty ideal, is an unrealistic one. Whereas a small waist requires a relatively low amount of body fat tissue, large breasts require a relatively high amount of body fat tissue. As a consequence, contrast comparisons with the beauty ideal may be less "upward" for men than for women, resulting in a smaller reduction in body satisfaction among men than among women (e.g., Strahan et al., 2006). In addition, men simply compare their bodies across comparison targets and attributes less often than young women do (Jones, 2001), and they tend to engage in social comparison processes that are less damaging to their body image than women do. For instance, when asked to describe their appearance, men make more downward contrast than upward contrast comparisons with others, resulting in more positive than negative descriptions of their bodies, whereas women do the opposite (Strahan et al., 2006).

A fifth moderator is self-esteem. In general, high-self-esteem individuals are less likely to engage in social comparisons and are less dissatisfied with their looks than are individuals with low self-esteem (e.g., Posavac & Posavac, 2002). Individuals with high self-esteem are less sensitive to negative feedback than low-self-esteem individuals and are less likely to contrast themselves with beauty ideals (e.g., Jones & Buckingham, 2005).

Finally, a sixth moderator is individuals' level of body satisfaction: As individuals are less satisfied with their body, they are more negatively affected by social comparisons with beauty ideals. More specifically, Trampe et al. (2007) showed that body dissatisfaction increases proneness to negative social comparison effects because it increases the accessibility of self-related cognitions, which in turn increases the tendency to engage in social comparisons.

## DEPRESSION

Social comparison processes are important links between the social environment and evaluations of the self. In several ways, negative social comparison processes may give rise to and cultivate negative self-evaluations as well as feelings of inferiority and deprecatory thoughts about the self that are characteristic of depression (e.g., Santor & Yazbek, 2006; Swallow & Kuiper, 1988).

First, depressed individuals are more likely to seek upward contrasting social comparison targets that emphasize their inferiority (e.g., Buunk, Zurriaga, & Gonzalez, 2006; Heidrich & Ryff, 1993; Swallow & Kuiper, 1992). This tendency may have serious consequences. Barber (2001), for instance, found that when young men perceive that those around them are better off than are they, their inclination to commit suicide is dangerously increased.

Depressed individuals also engage relatively often in downward identification comparisons that confirm their feelings of inadequacy (Albright & Henderson, 1995; Locke, 2005). Albright and Henderson (1995), for instance, found that, relative to nondysphoric students, dysphoric students were more likely to identify with others who had less positive attributes than they had, and they were less likely to identify with others who had more positive attributes than they, causing them to engage relatively often in self-derogation and relatively seldom in self-enhancement.

In addition to seeking distressing social comparison targets, depressed individuals tend to interpret social comparison information in a less self-serving way than do nondepressed individuals. First, depressed individuals weigh upward contrast social comparison information (that emphasizes their inferiority) more than downward contrast social comparison information (that emphasizes their superiority). Ahrens (1991), for instance, found that dysphoric and nondysphoric individuals' self-evaluations did not differ when there was information about the performance of only one target. However, when they were presented with information about two targets—one performing better and one performing worse than they did—dysphoric individuals made more negative self-evaluations than did nondysphoric individuals. Depressed individuals also weigh upward contrast comparison information more than nondepressed individuals do: They show more decreased positive affect following upward contrast comparisons than nondepressed individuals (Bäzner, Brömer, Hammelstein, & Meyer, 2006).

Second, whereas nondepressed individuals have a strong tendency to see themselves as better than most others (or the "average" other) for a wide range of traits and abilities, depressed individuals do so to a lesser extent. Depressed individuals, for instance, rate themselves as less attractive, less talented, weaker, and less competent than others (e.g., Brenninkmeyer, Van Yperen, & Buunk, 2001; Cheung, Gilbert, & Irons, 2004). These negative social comparisons confirm depressed individuals' sense of inferiority and depressive state and make it hard for them to take constructive actions to solve their problems and improve their mood.

The unfavorable social comparison strategies that make individuals vulnerable to depression may be activated early in life and may reflect child-rearing (parent–child) patterns and early peer group experiences (e.g., Gilbert, 1992). For instance, childhood memories of parents behaving authoritatively and demanding submission have been found to be associated with adult depression (e.g., Gilbert, Cheung, Grandfield, & Irons, 2003). Parents who make their children believe that they are inferior to others may cause their children to seek contrasting, upward social comparisons that maintain their sense of inferiority and evoke feelings of anxiety and depression. Unfavorable social comparison strategies may then, from childhood on, dominate the internal sense of self, making it more likely that individuals, as adults, will respond with depression to negative life events (Gilbert, 1992).

## Social Comparison Frequency and Depression

According to social comparison theory, individuals who experience uncertainty are especially likely to engage in social comparisons (Festinger, 1954). Comparing oneself with others in the same situation may help reduce feelings of uncertainty and anxiety by allowing one to assess the appropriateness of one's feelings and behaviors and by providing information about the nature of the situation and one's position (e.g., Buunk & Ybema, 1997). Depressed individuals often suffer from uncertainty regarding themselves and experience low perceptions of controllability (e.g., Butzer & Kuiper, 2006; Weary, Elbin, & Hill, 1987). As a consequence, depressed individuals may be especially drawn to engage in social comparisons. Correlational studies indeed report significant, although often low, positive correlations between social comparison frequency and depression: The more depressed individuals are, the more often they compare themselves to others (e.g., Bäzner et al., 2006; Heidrich & Ryff, 1993).

Experimental studies, however, have come up with a more complex pattern of results. For example, Swallow and Kuiper (1992) found that, following bogus feedback on an intelligence test, depressed low scorers were more likely to seek social comparisons than were nondepressed low scorers. Among high scorers, the tendency to seek social comparison information was not related to depression. In contrast, Flett, Vredenburg, and Pliner (1987) found that depressed individuals, after having received a test score, were less likely to seek social comparison information in the form of other people's test scores.

A possible explanation for these discrepant findings is that depression is not always accompanied by feelings of uncertainty; some depressed individuals are certain about their negative self-concept and, consequently, do not feel the need to compare themselves constantly (Buunk & Brenninkmeyer, 2000). Evidence for this explanation was found by Butzer and Kuiper (2006), who showed that intolerance of uncertainty was a more important predictor of the frequency of social comparisons than was depression.

## Alleviating Negative Mood

Although depressed individuals relatively often seek and interpret social comparison information that confirms their inferiority, they also may use social comparisons to alleviate their negative mood. First, although depressed individuals perceive themselves as less superior than nondepressed individuals, when confronted with a reference group of other depressed individuals, depressed people do appear to show a superiority bias. Albright, Alloy, Barch, and Dykman (1993), for instance, found that, although depressed college students rated themselves less favorably on several characteristics than the "average non-depressed college student," they rated themselves more favorably on these characteristics than "the average depressed college student."

Second, depressed individuals may engage in downward comparisons, contrasting themselves to others who are worse off than they are. Downward contrast comparisons may enhance mood and self-esteem, reduce a sense of personal deviance, and help them realize that they are not the only ones with problems (Buunk & Brenninkmeyer, 2000; DeVellis, Holt, & Renner, 1990). Gibbons (1986, Study 1), for instance, found that whereas nondepressed subjects preferred information from people who were experiencing positive affect, depressed subjects preferred information from people who were experiencing negative affect, but only when they themselves were put in a relatively negative mood. In addition, whereas information indicating that another person was currently experiencing highly negative affect did not affect nondepressed individuals' mood, it improved depressed individuals' mood (Gibbons, 1986, Study 2; see also, DeVellis et al., 1990). It must be noted, however, that, as individuals are more severely depressed, they are more likely to seek upward, not downward, contrast comparisons (Butzer & Kuiper, 2006).

### Depression and Evolution

More recently, scholars (e.g., Buunk & Brenninkmeyer, 2000; Gilbert et al., 1995) have linked social comparison theory to an evolutionary psychological perspective, resulting in the *theory of involuntary subordinate strategies* (ISS). According to ISS theory, when individuals perceive a defeat or a loss in rank, social comparisons with high-status others will make them feel worthless, depressed, and anxious. In this context depression can be seen as a so-called "unconscious involuntary losing strategy" that causes the individual to accept his or her defeat or loss in rank, suppress feelings of anger toward high-status others, and accommodate to what would otherwise be an unacceptably low social rank (e.g., Sloman, Price, Gilbert, & Gardner, 1994). Support for ISS theory comes from studies among groups who have faced a loss in rank. For instance, in response to a loss of job, social comparisons have been found to be related to depressive symptoms (Sheeran, Abrams, & Orbell, 1995; Ybema, Buunk, & Heesink, 1996); the more unfavorable differences unemployed individuals perceive between themselves and significant others, the more depressed they feel and the more their self-esteem suffers.

The ISS perspective is somewhat unusual because it suggests that depression may be adaptive by helping individuals suppress their feelings of anger and accommodate themselves to an otherwise unacceptable low social rank. This would imply that individuals who do not respond to a perceived low social rank by getting depressed may be coping in a less adaptive manner. In general, however, psychologists would argue that depression is, in most cases, a maladaptive response. It becomes easier to comprehend the ISS perspective if one can see depression as part of a response pattern called *secondary control*. According to Rothbaum, Weisz, and Snyder (1982), if it is impossible to bring the environment in line with one's wishes, individuals may bring themselves into line with environmental forces in order to understand and accept their circumstances or loss of rank. They may do so by lowering their expectations and engaging in passive, withdrawn, and submissive behavior and attributions. Negative affect and depression may be seen as (but not necessarily are) part of this response pattern.

## OCCUPATIONAL STRESS AND BURNOUT

Burnout can be defined as a breakdown in adaptation to prolonged work stress and is characterized by three aspects: (1) emotional exhaustion, the core dimension of the syndrome; (2) depersonalization, that is, a negative and cynical attitude toward the recipient of one's care; and (3) a sense of reduced personal accomplishments at work (e.g., Maslach, Schaufeli, & Leiter, 2001). Nowadays social comparisons are considered one of the most important social factors involved in both the cause and maintenance of work-related stress and burnout (Buunk & Schaufeli, 1993; Michinov, 2005).

## Occupational Stress and the Need for Social Comparison Information

According to social comparison theory, individuals who experience uncertainty are especially likely to engage in social comparisons (Festinger, 1954). Because job insecurity—such as doubts about one's competence and the threat of losing one's job—plays a central role in occupational stress, individuals suffering from occupational stress and burnout should show a relatively high interest in social comparison information. This has, indeed, been found to be the case (Buunk, Schaufeli, & Ybema, 1994). However, although individuals like to know how better-performing others are doing, often individuals suffering from occupational stress and burnout are reluctant to engage in direct interactions with upward comparison targets. Sharing their experiences with another person who is doing better may be painful and may, for self-protective reasons, be avoided (Buunk et al., 1994; Buunk & Ybema, 1997). This avoidance has its advantages. Despite the potentially positive effects of contacts with others, such as social support and information exchange, social comparison that takes the form of affiliation with others may increase, rather than decrease, occupational stress and symptoms of burnout (Buunk, Janssen, & Van Yperen, 1989). Affiliation may lead to mood convergence, even in the absence of verbal communication (Buunk & Ybema, 1997), and may cause stress and burnout symptoms to be communicated from one employee to the other and to spread from one work unit to another (so-called *burnout contagion*; e.g., Bakker, Schaufeli, Sixma, & Bosveld, 2001).

The content of conversations between colleagues may play a decisive role in the effect of affiliation on burnout. When communication takes the form of burnout complaints or conversations about work-related problems, affiliation negatively affects coworkers' burnout symptoms and may lead to burnout contagion, especially among workers who are highly susceptible to the emotions of others (e.g., Bakker et al., 2001). In contrast, supportive conversations with colleagues about, for instance, how to improve one's performance and the sharing of interesting ideas about performing one's job can buffer the negative effects of upward social comparison on burnout symptoms (Halbesleben & Buckley, 2006).

## Burnout and Upward Comparisons

If individuals contrast their situation against the situation of a comparison target, upward comparison can lead to the worrying conclusion that one is worse off, which can generate negative affect. Several studies have found, for instance, that upward contrast comparisons in the form of pay or prestige inequity (i.e., feeling deprived compared to others with regard to one's income or status) result in higher levels of occupational stress and burnout (e.g., Taris, Kalimo, & Schaufeli, 2002). However, when individuals identify with the comparison target, upward comparison leads to the conclusion that it is possible and likely to become like the comparison target in the future (e.g., Van der Zee, Bakker, & Buunk, 2001).

In general, upward comparisons with coworkers have been found to evoke more positive and less negative feelings than downward comparisons (e.g., Buunk, Ybema, Gibbons, & Ipenburg, 2001; Carmona, Buunk, Peiro, Rodriguez, & Bravo, 2006). For instance, in two samples of customs and police officers, Michinov (2005) found that as officers compared themselves more often with better-off employees, their level of job satisfaction increased and they reported fewer health complaints and feelings of emotional exhaustion. Conversely, the more frequently officers compared themselves with less fortunate employees, the more dissatisfied they were and the more health problems and emotional exhaustion they reported. Individuals suffering from burnout, however, are less capable of using upward social comparison information in a self-enhancing way (Carmona et al., 2006; Van der Zee et al., 2001). They are less able to identify with, and/or to be stimulated by, better-performing others and experience more negative affect in response to upward comparisons. In a sample of Roman Catholic priests, Halbesleben and Buckley (2006), for instance, found that those with an upward social comparison pattern reported higher levels of burnout than priests with a downward social comparison pattern.

### Burnout and Downward Comparisons

Although some contradictory findings have been reported, in general, workers who are burned out seem to shift their focus from upward identifications to downward social comparisons, either downward contrast or downward identification. Burned-out individuals seem no longer to be able to identify with coworkers who are doing better; consequently, upward comparisons may become too threatening for their sense of self. In order to fulfill their need for information and certainty, then, they may shift their focus to downward comparisons. Whether this strategy is healthy or not depends on how burned-out individuals handle these downward comparisons. If they compare themselves with coworkers who are doing worse, they may come to the comforting conclusion that they are better off ("It could have been much worse"). Conversely, if they identify with coworkers who are doing worse, downward comparison is likely to lead to feelings of hopelessness and negative affect (e.g., Carmona et al., 2006; Van der Zee et al., 2001).

Evidence for both strategies—downward contrast and downward identification—has been found among burned-out individuals. In a sample of mental health workers, Buunk, Ybema, Gibbons, et al. (2001) found that individuals high in burnout with a low inclination to compare themselves with others identified more with coworkers who were doing worse and less with coworkers who were doing better. Those high in burnout who were inclined to compare themselves relatively often continued to identify with coworkers who were doing better. Furthermore, Buunk, Ybema, Van der Zee, Schaufeli, and Gibbons (2001) found that nurses who were high in burnout derived more positive affect from downward comparisons than did those with lower levels of burnout.

Social comparisons may cause and facilitate or maintain feelings of burnout. For instance, due to job uncertainty or personality characteristics, such as neuroticism, individuals may frequently compare themselves with their colleagues. Especially frequent downward identifications may lead individuals to make negative self-evaluations and experience negative affect, causing and/or contributing to feelings of burnout. Once burned out, individuals may no longer be able to make constructive social comparisons, such as upward identifications, and may rely entirely on destructive types of social comparisons that may further aggravate feelings of burnout.

## CLINICAL IMPLICATIONS

Psychological problems may arise from, and be maintained by, social comparison information. Individuals suffering from body dissatisfaction and depression tend to engage in upward contrast comparisons, focusing on the differences between themselves and others who are more beautiful/doing better, and they may feel dissatisfied and inferior as a consequence. Although individuals suffering from occupational stress and burnout do not seem to contrast themselves upward, they do seem to have lost the ability to identify with better-performing coworkers and, in the worst case, may identify with coworkers who perform worse or who are worse off.

Interventions to prevent or alleviate depression, occupational stress, and burnout may therefore encourage individuals to make more *mood-enhancing* social comparisons by promoting upward identification, which strengthens the belief that it is possible and likely for one to become like the upward comparison target, and downward contrast, which leads to the comforting conclusion that one is not so bad off after all (e.g., Buunk & Ybema, 1997; Van der Zee et al., 2001). Individuals may, for instance, be presented with oral or written information that emphasizes their similarities with others who are doing better and/or the differences with others who are doing worse. A study of Van der Zee et al. (2001), in a sample of volunteer caregivers of terminally ill patients, found such an intervention to significantly enhance positive affect among those high in emotional exhaustion.

Interventions aimed at encouraging individuals to make more mood- or self-enhancing social comparisons with others seem less effective in relieving body image problems. Physical attractiveness is a relatively uncontrollable dimension: One can only do so much to improve one's bodily attractiveness. Consequently, upward identification with beauty ideals may only provide individuals with limited, useful information to improve their appearance, whereas upward contrast may result in relatively strong feelings of self-doubt, frustration, and inadequacy. In addition, due to the ubiquitous societal ideal of beauty, downward contrast comparisons—comparing oneself to someone less attractive—which may enhance one's body satisfaction, are less likely to occur than upward comparisons. Moreover, the positive effects of downward contrasts do not always occur. Thus, the net effect of social comparisons in the domain of physical attractiveness is most likely to be negative.

Nonetheless, research on *social distancing* suggests an avenue that may help alleviate not only depression and burnout but also body image problems (e.g., Gibbons & Eggleston, 1996; Gibbons & Gerrard, 1997; Gibbons, Gerrard, Lando, & McGovern, 1991). These studies show that the mental creation of downward comparisons targets—rather than seeking external, real-life downward comparison targets—and the subsequent derogation of those targets may help people overcome their behavioral problems. Mental comparison targets influence the decision to engage or not engage in the relevant behavior via a social comparison process between oneself and the target. For example, an individual who has an unfavorable image of people who drink is less likely to drink when given the opportunity. In a similar vein, interventions to prevent or alleviate depression, burnout, and body dissatisfaction may encourage individuals to construct negative images of themselves being depressed, burned out, or dissatisfied with their body ("feared selves"; Unemori, Omoregie, & Markus, 2004), and challenge them to distance themselves from those images toward more positive images of themselves ("possible selves"; Unemori et al., 2004), such as being energetic, confident, optimistic, and/or satisfied with their body.

In addition, individuals suffering from body image problems may benefit from interventions that (1) prevent and/or interrupt appearance-related comparisons, and (2) enhance their self-esteem. First, by interrupting the social comparison process in response to media images, feelings of inferiority and body dissatisfaction may be reduced or even prevented (e.g., Posavac, Posavac, & Weigel, 2001). Second, strengthening self-esteem will help individuals feel less pressure to conform to the sociocultural ideal of beauty and become less inclined to contrast themselves with this beauty ideal (Pelletier, Dion, & Lévesque, 2004).

Cognitive-behavioral therapy contains several techniques that can be used to reach these goals (e.g., Cash & Strachan, 2002). For instance, simple thought-stopping techniques can be used to help individuals interrupt negative automatic patterns of thinking. By saying "STOP!" to oneself when noticing that one is socially comparing oneself (in a negative manner) or thinking negative thoughts (e.g., "She looks much better than I do" or "I am fat and unattractive"). In doing so, social comparisons may lose (much of) their distressing effect on body image. In addition, cognitive restructuring can help clients identify negative, appearance-related comparisons, or thoughts related to these comparisons (e.g., thoughts that increase the valence of physical appearance as a dimension of social comparison, such as "I can only be successful when I am attractive/slim/muscular" or "People dislike fat people"), and to question and refute these thoughts.

However, studies examining the effect of counterarguments against negative social comparisons in the domain of beauty have generated mixed findings. Engeln-Maddox (2005), for instance, found that comparisons with beauty ideals had negative effects on women's self-evaluations of attractiveness, despite the fact that participants were instructed to think of counterarguments, such as "Why are all these damn models toothpicks?" In contrast, Stice, Mazotti, Weibel, and Agras (2000) found that women high in internalization of the thin ideal, after having argued against the value of the thin ideal in our society, did show increases in body satisfaction and decreases in dieting behavior.

A study of Buunk and Brenninkmeijer (2001) suggests another avenue by which social comparisons may contribute specifically to recovery from depression. In their study, depressed individuals were exposed to an interview with a target individual who had overcome his or her depression either through a lot of effort ("I worked very hard at it") or without much effort ("The depression just went away"). Among depressed individuals who were inclined to compare themselves relatively often, the latter target evoked a positive mood change, whereas the target who had worked hard on overcoming his or her depression evoked a negative mood change. Providing depressed individuals with information emphasizing that, with time, they will recover by themselves may therefore elevate the mood of some depressed patients. A possible drawback of such an intervention is that depressed individuals may not seek the help they need, which in itself is a problem because only 28% of major depression sufferers seek help (Kessler et al., 1999).

The first step in helping clients, however, is to assist them in becoming aware of the social comparisons they make and the consequences these comparisons have on their self-evaluations, mood, and well-being. Therapists should explain what social comparisons are, how they influence self-evaluations, and why individuals may compare themselves to others. Helping clients to detect and observe their patterns of negative social comparisons and helping them to calmly step back from these social comparisons, rather than being absorbed by them, may enable clients not only to resolve their psychological problems but also make them more resilient to a relapse of those problems in the future.

## CONCLUSION

Social comparison—how we use others to make sense of ourselves and the world—is a vital human concern. Although originally developed as a social psychological theory, during the past decennia social comparison theory has broadened its scope to the field of clinical psychology. Research has shown that some psychological problems arise from, and can be maintained by, the use of social comparison information in a self-defeating, rather than in a self-enhancing or neutral, way. Research using social comparison theory as a theoretical framework has especially focused on the role of social comparisons in burnout, depression, and body dissatisfaction. What these three problems have in common is a negative evaluation of the self: Burnout workers experience a sense of reduced personal accomplishment at work, depressed individuals suffer from feelings of worthlessness and inferiority, and individuals who are dissatisfied with their body perceive themselves as unattractive. Because social comparisons are important links between the social environment and evaluations of the self, it is not surprising that social comparisons play such an important role in the development and maintenance of particularly these three problems. Insight into the mechanisms and patterns of social comparisons may help psychologists design interventions that exploit their positive, and minimize their negative, effects.

## REFERENCES


Ahrens, A. H. (1991). Dysphoria and social comparison: Combining information regarding others' performances. *Journal of Social and Clinical Psychology, 10*(2), 190–205.

Albright, J. S., Alloy, L. B., Barch, D., & Dykman, B. M. (1993). Social comparison by dysphoric and nondysphoric college students: The grass isn't always greener on the other side. *Cognitive Therapy and Research, 17*(6), 485–509.

Albright, J. S., & Henderson, M. C. (1995). How real is depressive realism? A question of scales and standards. *Cognitive Therapy and Research, 19*(5), 589–609.

Bakker, A. B., Schaufeli, W. B., Sixma, H. J., & Bosveld, W. (2001). Burnout contagion among general practitioners. *Journal of Social and Clinical Psychology, 20*(1), 82–98.

Barber, J. G. (2001). Relative misery and youth suicide. *Australian and New Zealand Journal of Psychiatry, 35*(1), 49–57.

Bäzner, E., Brömer, P., Hammelstein, P., & Meyer, T. D. (2006). Current and former depression and their relationship to the effects of social comparison processes. *Journal of Affective Disorders, 93*(1–3), 97–103.

Bessenoff, G. R. (2006). Can the media affect us? Social comparison, and the thin ideal. *Psychology of Women Quarterly, 30*(3), 239–251.

Brenninkmeyer, V., Van Yperen, N. W., & Buunk, B. P. (2001). Burnout and depression are not identical twins: Is decline of superiority a distinguishing feature? *Personality and Individual Differences, 30*, 873–880.

Brown, J. D., Novick, N. J., Lord, K. A., & Richards, J. M. (1992). When Gulliver travels: Social context, psychological closeness, and self-appraisals. *Journal of Personality and Social Psychology, 62*(5), 717–727.

Butzer, B., & Kuiper, N. A. (2006). Relationships between the frequency of social comparisons and self-concept clarity, intolerance of uncertainty, anxiety, and depression. *Personality and Individual Differences, 41*(1), 167–176.

Buunk, B. P., & Brenninkmeyer, V. B. (2000). Social comparison processes among depressed individuals: Evidence for the evolutionary perspective on involuntary subordinate strategies? In L. Sloman & P. Gilbert (Eds.), *Subordination and defeat: An evolutionary approach to mood disorders* (pp. 147–164). Mahwah, NJ: Erlbaum.

Buunk, B. P., & Brenninkmeyer, V. B. (2001). When individuals dislike exposure to an actively coping role model: Mood changes as related to depression and social comparison orientation. *European Journal of Social Psychology, 31*(5), 537–548.

Buunk, B. P., Collins, R. L., Taylor, S. E., & Van Yperen, N. W. (1990). The affective consequences of social comparison: Either direction has its ups and downs. *Journal of Personality and Social Psychology, 59*(6), 1238–1249.

Buunk, B. P., & Gibbons, F. X. (2000). Toward an enlightenment in social comparison theory: Moving beyond classic and Renaissance approaches. In J. Suls & L. Wheeler (Eds.), *Handbook of social comparison: Theory and research* (pp. 487–499). Dordrecht, The Netherlands: Kluwer Academic.

Buunk, B. P., & Gibbons, F. X. (2006). Social comparison orientation: A new perspective on those who do and those who don't compare with others. In S. Guimond (Ed.), *Social comparison and social psychology: Understanding cognition, intergroup relations and culture* (pp. 15–33). Cambridge, UK: Cambridge University Press.

Buunk, B. P., Janssen, P. P., & Van Yperen, N. W. (1989). Stress and affiliation reconsidered: The effects of social support in stressful and non-stressful work units. *Social Behaviour, 4*(3), 155–171.

Buunk, B. P., Kuyper, H., & Van der Zee, Y. G. (2005). Affective response to social comparison in the classroom. *Basic and Applied Social Psychology, 27*(3), 229–237.

Buunk, B. P., & Schaufeli, W. B. (1993). Burnout: A perspective from social comparison theory. In W. B. Schaufeli, C. Maslach, & T. Marek (Eds.), *Professional burnout: Recent developments in theory and research* (pp. 53–69). Philadelphia: Taylor & Francis.

Buunk, B. P., Schaufeli, W. B., & Ybema, J. F. (1994). Burnout, uncertainty, and the desire for social comparisons among nurses. *Journal of Applied Social Psychology, 24*(19), 1701–1718.

Buunk, B. P., & Ybema, J. F. (1997). Social comparisons and occupational stress: The identification contrast model. In B. P. Buunk & F. X. Gibbons (Eds.), *Health, coping, and well-being: Perspectives from social comparison theory* (pp. 359–388). Mahwah, NJ: Erlbaum.

Buunk, B. P., Ybema, J. F., Gibbons, F. X., & Ipenburg, M. (2001). The affective consequences of social comparisons as related to professional burnout and social comparison orientation. *European Journal of Social Psychology, 31*(4), 337–351.

Buunk, B. P., Ybema, J. F., Van der Zee, K. I., Schaufeli, W. B., & Gibbons, F. X. (2001). Affect generated by social comparisons among nurses high and low in burnout. *Journal of Applied Social Psychology, 31*(7), 1500–1520.

Buunk, A. P., Zurriaga, R., & Gonzalez, P. (2006). Social comparison, coping, and depression in people with spinal cord injury. *Psychology and Health, 21*(6), 791–807.

Cafri, G., Yamamiya, Y., Brannick, M., & Thompson, K. J. (2005). The influence of sociocultural factors on body image: A meta-analysis. *Clinical Psychology: Science and Practice, 12*(4), 421–433.

Carmona, C., Buunk, A. P., Peiro, J. M., Rodriguez, I., & Bravo, M. J. (2006). Do social comparison and coping styles play a role in the development of burnout? Cross-sectional and longitudinal findings. *Journal of Occupational and Organizational Psychology, 79*, 85–99.

Cash, T. F., Novy, P. L., & Grant, J. R. (1994). Why do women exercise? Factor analysis and further validation of the reasons for exercise inventory. *Perceptual and Motor Skills, 78*(2), 539–544.

Cash, T. F., & Strachan, M. D. (2002). Cognitive-behavioral approaches to changing body image. In T. F. Cash & T. Pruzinsky (Eds.), *Body image: A handbook of theory, research and clinical practice* (pp. 478–486). New York: Guilford Press.

Cattarin, J. A., Thompson, K. J., Thomas, C., & Williams, R. (2000). Body image, mood, and televised images of attractiveness: The role of social comparison. *Journal of Social and Clinical Psychology, 19*(2), 220–239.

Cheung, M. S., Gilbert, P., & Irons, C. (2004). An exploration of shame, social rank, and rumination in relation to depression. *Personality and Individual Differences, 36*(5), 1143–1153.

Collins, R. L. (1996). For better or worse: The impact of upward social comparison on self-evaluations. *Psychological Bulletin, 119*(1), 51–69.

DeVellis, R. F., Holt, K., & Renner, B. R. (1990). The relationship of social comparison to rheumatoid arthritis symptoms and affect. *Basic and Applied Social Psychology, 11*(1), 1–18.

Engeln-Maddox, R. (2005). Cognitive responses to idealized media images of women: The relationship of social comparison and critical processing to body image disturbance in college women. *Journal of Social and Clinical Psychology, 24*(8), 1114–1138.

Festinger, L. (1954). A theory of social comparison processes. *Human Relations*, *7*, 117–140.

Flett, G. L., Vredenburg, K., & Pliner, P. (1987). Depression and social comparison information-seeking. *Journal of Social Behavior and Personality*, *2*(4), 473–484.

Gibbons, F. X. (1986). Social comparison and depression: Company's effect on misery. *Journal of Personality and Social Psychology*, *51*(1), 140–148.

Gibbons, F. X., & Buunk, B. P. (1999). Individual differences in social comparison: Development of a scale of social comparison orientation. *Journal of Personality and Social Psychology*, *76*(1), 129–142.

Gibbons, F. X., & Eggleston, T. J. (1996). Smoker networks and the "typical smoker": A prospective analysis of smoking cessation. *Health Psychology*, *15*(6), 469–477.

Gibbons, F. X., & Gerrard, M. (1997). Health images and their effects on health behaviour. In B. P. Buunk & F. X. Gibbons (Eds.), *Health, coping, and well-being: Perspectives from social comparison theory* (pp. 63–94). Mahwah, NJ: Erlbaum.

Gibbons, F. X., Gerrard, M., Lando, H. A., & McGovern, P. G. (1991). Social comparison processes and smoking cessation: The role of the typical smoker. *Journal of Experimental Psychology*, *27*(3), 239–258.

Gilbert, P. (1992). *Depression: The evolution of powerlessness*. New York: Guilford Press.

Gilbert, P., Cheung, M. S., Grandfield, T., & Irons, C. (2003). Recall of threat and submissiveness in childhood: Development of a new scale and its relationship with depression, social comparison, and shame. *Clinical Psychology and Psychotherapy*, *10*(2), 108–115.

Gilbert, P., Price, J., & Allan, S. (1995). Social comparison, social attractiveness, and evolution: How might they be related? *New Ideas in Psychology*, *13*(2), 149–165.

Groesz, L. M., Levine, M. P., & Murnen, S. K. (2002). The effect of experimental presentation of thin media images on body satisfaction. *International Journal of Eating Disorders*, *31*(1), 1–16.

Halbesleben, J. R. B., & Buckley, R. M. (2006). Social comparison and burnout: The role of relative burnout and received social support. *Anxiety, Stress and Coping: An International Journal*, *19*(3), 259–278.

Halliwell, E., & Dittmar, H. (2005). The role of self-improvement and self-evaluation motives in social comparisons with idealised female bodies in the media. *Body Image*, *2*(3), 249–261.

Hargreaves, D. A., & Tiggemann, M. (2004). Idealized media images and adolescent body image: "Comparing" boys and girls. *Body Image*, *1*(4), 351–361.

Heidrich, S. M., & Ryff, C. D. (1993). The role of social comparisons processes in the psychological adaptation of elderly adults. *Journals of Gerontology*, *48*(3), 127–136.

Jones, A. M., & Buckingham, J. T. (2005). Self-esteem as a moderator of the effect of social comparison on women's body image. *Journal of Social and Clinical Psychology*, *24*(8), 1164–1187.

Jones, D. C. (2001). Social comparison and body image: Attractiveness comparisons to models and peers among adolescent girls and boys. *Sex Roles*, *45*(9–10), 645–664.

Kessler, R. C., Zhao, S., Katz, S. J., Kouzis, A. C., Frank, R. G., Edlund, M. J., et al. (1999). Past-year use of outpatient services for psychiatric problems in the National Comorbidity Survey. *American Journal of Psychiatry*, *156*, 115–123.

Krones, P. G., Stice, E., Batres, C., & Orjada, K. (2005). In vivo social comparison to a thin-ideal peer promotes body dissatisfaction: A randomized experiment. *International Journal of Eating Disorders*, *38*(2), 134–142.

Lin, L. F., & Kulik, J. A. (2002). Social comparison and women's body satisfaction. *Basic and Applied Social Psychology*, *24*(2), 115–123.

Locke, K. D. (2005). Connecting the horizontal dimensions of social comparison with self-worth and self-confidence. *Personality and Social Psychology Bulletin*, *31*(6), 795–803.

Maslach, C., Schaufeli, W. B., & Leiter, M. P. (2001). Job burnout. *Annual Review of Psychology*, *52*, 397–422.

Michinov, N. (2005). Social comparison, perceived control, and occupational burnout. *Applied Psychology: An International Review*, *54*(1), 99–118.

Pelletier, L. G., Dion, S., & Lévesque, C. (2004). Can self-determination help protect women against sociocultural influences about body image and reduce their risk of experiencing bulimic symptoms? *Journal of Social and Clinical Psychology*, *23*(1), 61–88.

Posavac, H. D., Posavac, S. S., & Weigel, R. G. (2001). Reducing the impact of media images on women at risk for body image disturbances. *Journal of Social and Clinical Psychology*, *20*(3), 324–340.

Posavac, S. S., & Posavac, H. D. (2002). Predictors of women's concern with body weight: The roles of perceived self-media ideal discrepancies. *Eating Disorders: Journal of Treatment and Prevention*, *10*(2), 153–160.

Powell, J. L., Matacin, M. L., & Stuart, A. E. (2001). Body esteem: An exception to self-enhancing illusions? *Journal of Applied Social Psychology*, *31*(9), 1951–1978.

Rothbaum, F., Weisz, J. R., & Snyder, S. S. (1982). Changing the world and changing the self: A two-process model of perceived control. *Journal of Personality and Social Psychology*, *42*(1), 5–37.

Santor, D. A., & Yazbek, A. A. (2006). Soliciting unfavourable social comparison: Effects of self-criticism. *Personality and Individual Differences*, *40*(3), 545–556.

Sheeran, P., Abrams, D., & Orbell, S. (1995). Unemployment, self-esteem, and depression: A social comparison theory approach. *Basic and Applied Social Psychology*, *17*(1–2), 65–82.

Sloman, L., Price, J., Gilbert, P., & Gardner, R. (1994). Adaptive function of depression: Psychotherapeutic implications. *American Journal of Psychotherapy*, *48*(3), 401–416.

Smith, R. H. (2000). Assimilative and contrastive emotional reactions to upward and downward social comparisons. In J. Suls & L. Wheeler (Eds.), *Handbook of social comparison: Theory and research* (pp. 173–200). Dordrecht, The Netherlands: Kluwer Academic.

Stice, E., Mazotti, L., Weibel, D., & Agras, W. S. (2000). Dissonance prevention program decreases thin-ideal internalization, body dissatisfaction, dieting, negative affect and bulimic symptoms. *International Journal of Eating Disorders*, *27*(2), 206–217.

Strahan, E. J., Wilson, A. E., Cressman, K. E., & Buote, V. M. (2006). Comparing to perfection: How cultural norms for appearance affect social comparisons and self-image. *Body Image*, *3*(3), 211–227.

Suls, J., & Wheeler, L. (2000). A selective history of classic and neo-social comparison theory. In J. Suls & L. Wheeler (Eds.), *Handbook of social comparison: Theory and research* (pp. 1–23). Dordrecht, The Netherlands: Kluwer Academic.

Swallow, S. R., & Kuiper, N. A. (1988). Social comparison and negative self-evaluations: An application to depression. *Clinical Psychology Review*, *8*(1), 55–76.

Swallow, S. R., & Kuiper, N. A. (1992). Mild depression and frequency of social comparison behaviour. *Journal of Social and Clinical Psychology*, *11*(2), 167–180.

Taris, S. E., Kalimo, R., & Schaufeli, W. B. (2002). Inequity at work: Its measurement and associations with worker health. *Work and Stress*, *16*(4), 287–301.

Taylor, S. E., & Lobel, M. (1989). Social comparison activity under threat: Downward evaluation and upward contacts. *Psychological Review*, *96*(4), 569–575.

Tesser, A., Miller, M., & Moore, J. (1988). Some affective consequences of social comparison and reflection processes. *Journal of Personality and Social Psychology*, *54*(1), 49–61.

Thompson, K. J., Heinberg, L. J., Altabe, M., & Tantleff-Dunn, S. (2002). *Exacting beauty: Theory, assessment, and treatment of body image disturbances*. Washington, DC: American Psychological Association.

Tiggemann, M., & Slater, A. (2004). Thin ideals in music television: A source of social comparison and body dissatisfaction. *International Journal of Eating Disorders*, *35*(1), 48–58.

Trampe, D., Stapel, D. A., & Siero, F. W. (2007). On models and vases: Body dissatisfaction and proneness to social comparison effects. *Journal of Personality and Social Psychology*, *92*(1), 106–118.

Unemori, P., Omoregie, H., & Markus, H. R. (2004). Self-portraits: Possible selves in European-American, Chilean, Japanese, and Japanese-American cultural contexts. *Self and Identity*, *3*(4), 321–328.

Van der Zee, K. I., Bakker, A. B., & Buunk, B. P. (2001). Burnout and reactions to social comparison information among volunteer caregivers. *Anxiety, Stress, and Coping: An International Journal*, *14*(4), 391–430.

Weary, G., Elbin, S., & Hill, M. G. (1987). Attributional and social comparison processes in depression. *Journal of Personality and Social Psychology, 52*(3), 605–610.

Wills, T. A. (1981). Downward comparison principles in social psychology. *Psychological Bulletin, 90*(2), 245–271.

Wood, J. V. (1989). Theory and research concerning social comparisons of personal attributes. *Psychological Bulletin, 106*(2), 231–248.

Ybema, J. F., Buunk, B. P., & Heesink, J. A. M. (1996). Affect and identification in social comparison after loss of work. *Basic and Applied Social Psychology, 18*(2), 151–169.

# 12 Self-Disclosure and Psychological Well-Being

Denise M. Sloan

Humans have a natural tendency to share their thoughts and feelings with others, and this tendency is even stronger when they experience a very unpleasant or pleasant life event. Disclosing our deepest thoughts and feelings to people around us serves an evolutionary function of strengthening our interpersonal relationships. In addition to facilitating social bonds, self-disclosure also produces a wide variety of health benefits, and self-disclosure in psychotherapy is thought to play a critical role in successful treatment outcome. This chapter reviews the health benefits associated with self-disclosure, including that which occurs in psychotherapy, highlights factors that appear to be important for maximizing the benefits of self-disclosure, reviews theories proposed to account for why self-disclosure results in health benefits, discusses the clinical implications of the empirical findings on self-disclosure, and offer suggestions for future research.

## DEFINING SELF-DISCLOSURE

*Self-disclosure* refers to the communication of personally relevant information, thoughts, and feelings to another. Self-disclosure can vary along a dimension of depth (Derlega, Metts, Petronio, & Margulis, 1993). An example of minimal-depth self-disclosure might be a person disclosing that he or she encountered a lot of traffic on the way into work. An example of self-disclosure of greater depth would be a person disclosing that he or she spent several hours crying the previous night after receiving bad news. The first example involves self-disclosure of factual information, whereas the second involves emotional information about the self. Emotional disclosures reveal one's private feelings, opinions, and judgments (Derlega et al., 1993; Reis & Patrick, 1996). Although both types of disclosures involve revealing information about oneself, only disclosures involving emotions and feelings appear to promote physical and psychological health (e.g., Collins & Miller, 1994; Laurenceau, Barrett, & Pietromonaco, 1998; Sloan, Marx, Epstein, & Lexington, 2007).

## SELF-DISCLOSURE AND WELL-BEING

A wealth of research indicates that self-disclosure results in a variety of health benefits, including psychological well-being. Self-disclosure of physical health conditions has been found to be important to overall health and disease progression. For instance, studies with both adults and children have found that disclosure of HIV status is associated with greater psychological well-being, improved quality of social support, and increases in CD4 T-lymphocyte percentage (e.g., Sherman, Bonanno, Wiener, & Battles, 2000; Zea, Reisen, Poppen, Bianchi, & Echeverry, 2005). Similarly, failure to disclose concerns regarding a recent cancer diagnosis is related to poorer psychological well-being and social support (e.g., Figueiredo, Fries, & Ingram, 2004).

One of the more systematic lines of work investigating the benefits of self-disclosure involves written emotional disclosure. The focus of this work is been a procedure originally used by Pennebaker and Beall (1986), which involves writing about a stressful or traumatic experience with as much emotion and feeling as possible over several occasions, for at least 20 minutes each session. Since Pennebaker and Beall's (1986) original report demonstrating the beneficial effects on overall physical health and a reduction in the number of illness visits to a medical clinic resulting from written disclosure, many studies have examined the benefits of written disclosure with a wide range of populations and outcome measures. In general, these studies have found that individuals assigned to write, with as much emotion as possible, for several occasions about stressful or traumatic experiences show improvements in psychological health (e.g., decrease in depression, anxiety, anger, and distress; increase in subjective well-being), physical health (e.g., decreases in physical health symptom complaints, ratings of pain, and in disability ratings), decrease in health care utilization, improved immune functioning, and improvement in academic performance, compared with individuals randomly assigned to a nondisclosure control condition (see Sloan & Marx, 2004b, for a review). These wide-ranging health benefits associated with written disclosure have been obtained for a variety of populations, including college students, individuals with chronic health conditions (e.g., chronic pain, asthma, arthritis, cancer), prison inmates, and trauma survivors. The use of a randomized experimental design in these studies allows for a cause–effect interpretation of the findings.

In addition to the wide range of benefits and the variety of individuals who appear to benefit from written disclosure, the brevity of the intervention is also remarkable. Most evidence-based treatment protocols suggest the use of at least eight sessions in order for improvement in functioning to be observed. Yet, the written disclosure procedure typically includes only three sessions, with each session consisting of approximately 20 minutes. Although written disclosure has not been uniformly successful in symptom amelioration (e.g., Batten, Follette, Rasmussen Hall, & Palm, 2002; Gidron, Peri, Connolly, & Shalev, 1996; Stroebe, Stroebe, Schut, Zech, & van den Bout, 2002), several meta-analyses have found that, overall, written disclosure is associated with psychological and physical health benefits (Frattaroli, 2006; Frisina, Borod, & Lepore, 2004; Smyth, True, & Souto, 2001).

For example, a recent meta-analysis of 146 randomized disclosure studies indicated a positive and significant average effect size ($r$ = .075; Frattaroli, 2006). Importantly, this meta-analysis used a random effects approach, from which the results are more generalizable than a fixed meta-analysis approach. That is, with a random effects approach one can generalize the effects to similar studies not included in the analysis and to future studies.

Given the wealth of data demonstrating the benefits derived from self-disclosure, investigators have begun to turn their attention to understanding factors that affect self-disclosure outcome. The most comprehensive examination of moderators of self-disclosure outcome is a meta-analysis conducted by Frattaroli (2006), who examined 22 possible moderators in 146 self-disclosure studies. Her findings indicated that a greater number of self-disclosure sessions (at least three sessions), longer disclosure sessions (at least 15 minutes), and more detailed disclosure instructions (i.e., the person is instructed to disclose regarding a specific negative life event, rather than allowing the person to select the disclosure topic) are associated with stronger effects. In addition, self-disclosure studies in which individuals self-disclose within their homes had greater effect sizes compared with self-disclosure studies that are conducted in a controlled setting, such as a clinic or laboratory. This finding is somewhat unexpected, as investigators generally believe that providing a controlled setting is essential for ensuring that individuals comply with the disclosure instructions (e.g., disclose for the specified time period) and for minimizing distractions. The larger effect size for disclosures at home reported by Frattaroli may reflect that individuals are more relaxed and better able to engage in the disclosure task when the session is conducted within their homes. Frattaroli also found that the effects of disclosure are greater for individuals reporting high stress and for individuals whose self-disclosure focuses on a more recent trauma or stressful life event.

Lastly, Frattaroli (2006) found that time to follow-up assessment moderated the effects of disclosure, with shorter follow-up assessment intervals (e.g., less than 1 month) being associated with stronger effects than longer intervals (e.g., more than 1 month). This finding suggests that psychosocial interventions that are brief and that focus only on or emphasize self-disclosure may not yield long-lasting symptom or behavior changes. However, this meta-analysis examined studies in which disclosure took place only on a handful of occasions. It seems likely that self-disclosure that takes place over a longer period of time (on repeated occasions), such as is typical of psychotherapy, would be associated with longer-lasting benefits.

Also noteworthy are factors that do *not* appear to moderate the beneficial impact of self-disclosure. The meta-analysis conducted by Frattaroli (2006) indicated that several factors did not moderate, including demographic characteristics (e.g., age, gender, racial background), time between the disclosure sessions (e.g., disclosure once a week, disclosure on consecutive days), and mode of disclosure (e.g., talking, handwriting, typing). Frattaroli's findings provide potentially important information regarding for whom self-disclosure works best and under what conditions, but these findings should be regarded as a starting point for further exploration. The reason for caution is that Frattaroli indirectly examined moderator effects. That is, most studies included in the meta-analysis did not directly examine whether the variables affected outcome. As a result, Frattaroli compared studies that varied in methodological procedures, such as setting of disclosure and mode of disclosure. This approach to examining moderator variables can result in a third variable accounting for the moderator findings. For instance, the finding that disclosure at home has a higher overall effect size relative to disclosure that takes place in a controlled setting could be attributable to the setting of disclosure (home vs. clinic); however, the finding might also be attributable to some other variable in which the studies differed (e.g., the participant sample, time to follow-up assessment, number of writing sessions). Therefore, Frattaroli's findings are not definitive, but they do provide us with directions for future research.

A handful of studies of the written disclosure procedure have directly examined variables that moderate outcome. Radcliffe, Lumley, Kendall, Stevenson, and Beltran (2007) examined the importance of an audience for self-disclosure. Radcliffe et al. (2007) randomly assigned participants to one of four conditions. Participants were assigned to a disclosure condition in which they shared their written disclosure narratives (i.e., submitted to an experimenter), a disclosure condition in which they did not share their written disclosure narratives (i.e., not submitted), or to one of two nondisclosure control groups. Participants assigned to one of the disclosure conditions were informed prior to the writing sessions whether or not they would be required to submit their disclosure narratives. Although both disclosure groups showed greater improvements in cognitive intrusion and avoidance symptoms than did the control groups, individuals who shared their disclosure narrative displayed a broader range of psychological and physical health benefits than did the individuals who did not share their disclosure narrative. The findings by Radcliffe and colleagues suggest that people do benefit from disclosure whether or not there is an audience. However, those who share their disclosures with someone else, even if it is a relative stranger, enjoy the greater benefits.

Consistent with Frattaroli's moderator findings, several studies have found that written disclosure is equally beneficial for males and females (Epstein, Sloan, & Marx, 2005; Sheese, Brown, & Graziano, 2004). However, women are more likely to self-disclose than men (see Dindia & Allen, 1992, for a review) and consequently may derive more benefits from self-disclosure. Nevertheless, when men do self-disclose, they experience benefits that are comparable to those experienced by women.

Social relationships also moderate outcomes associated with written disclosure. Sheese and colleagues (2004) found that the more extraverted participants were and the more social supports they had, the more likely they were to derive benefits from written disclosure. This finding may support Pennebaker's speculation that the benefits associated with written disclosure are maintained through increases in social bonding. That is, Pennebaker (1997) proposed that writing about traumatic or upsetting experiences may prompt individuals to disclose these events to individuals in a social support capacity, resulting in increased social bonds. The social bonding hypothesis seems feasible given the long line of research demonstrating the positive effects of self-disclosure on social relationships. However, it is unknown whether individuals subsequently disclose more in their real life following participation in these studies. This would be an important area to further investigate. Nonetheless, there is clear evidence that self-disclosure substantially impacts social relationships, as is reviewed next.

## SELF-DISCLOSURE AND SOCIAL RELATIONSHIPS

Self-disclosure plays a critical role in the development and maintenance of social relationships. For example, intimacy is formed when a person discloses personal information, thoughts, and feelings to a partner, the partner responds, and the person then interprets his or her partner's responses as accepting and caring (Reis & Shaver, 1988). In this manner, intimacy is a dynamic process that begins with self-disclosure. The type of self-disclosure is central in predicting whether intimacy develops. Specifically, a study by Laurenceau and colleagues (1998) indicates that emotional self-disclosures are a more important predictor of the development of intimacy than are self-disclosures of facts or information. Self-disclosures also increase the degree to which the discloser is liked (see Collins & Miller, 1994). The more intimate disclosures a person makes, the more the person is liked, although this relationship appears to be stronger in ongoing relationships relative to initial encounters (Collins & Miller, 1994). Self-disclosure also increases the likelihood that other people will disclose in return (Collins & Miller, 1994). Thus, the positive effects of self-disclosure on social relationships are derived from a dynamic process in which self-disclosure facilitates intimacy and reciprocity in sharing.

## SELF-DISCLOSURE OF POSITIVE LIFE EXPERIENCES

The majority of self-disclosure research has focused on the effect of disclosing negative life experiences, such as traumatic events and diagnosis of chronic health conditions. However, benefits also occur from self-disclosure of positive events. Replicating findings from Langston (1994), Gable and colleagues (2004) found that communicating personal positive experiences is related to increases in daily positive affect and well-being, beyond the impact of the positive event itself. Further, when others are perceived to respond positively (not passively or negatively), the benefits of positive self-disclosure are further enhanced. In two additional studies Gable, Reis, Impett, and Asher (2004) found that greater relationship satisfaction occurs when one's close partner responds positively to positive self-disclosures. These researchers also found that positive events that are disclosed to others are more likely to be recalled by the discloser than are positive events that are not disclosed. This is an important finding, given that remembering positive life experiences is associated with greater overall well-being (Taylor & Stanton, 2007). In contrast, negative events that are disclosed to others are not more likely to be recalled than are negative events that are not disclosed.

Taken together, self-disclosure of positive events is related to increases in psychological well-being and strengthens social bonds via a dynamic process that is similar to the process involved in self-disclosure of negative experiences. The findings of Gable and colleagues (2004) also indicate that positive life events become more accessible in memory when a person tells others of his or her positive experiences.

## WHEN SELF-DISCLOSURE IS NOT BENEFICIAL

Although a wealth of research demonstrates the various benefits resulting from self-disclosure of both positive and negative life events and feelings, there are circumstances in which self-disclosure can be detrimental. Within social relationships, several factors determine whether or not self-disclosure will yield desired changes in psychological and physical health, including to whom we disclose, the degree to which we disclose, and the context of the self-disclosure. For example, depressed individuals display the tendency to self-disclose too much personal negative information ("I spent hours crying alone in my bedroom last night"), and such inappropriate self-disclosures partially account for why depressed individuals are socially isolated

(Segrin, 2000; Segrin & Abramson, 1994). As noted previously, to whom one discloses is also important. Self-disclosures to individuals with whom we have an ongoing relationship can result in increases in psychological well-being and can strengthen our relationships with them (Reis & Shaver, 1988). However, self-disclosures to a relative stranger can be viewed as odd or inappropriate and, as a result, the stranger may be unlikely to respond in a positive manner, ultimately leaving the self-discloser feeling unsupported (Reis & Shaver, 1988).

Research also indicates that in some situations it is best to suppress or inhibit self-disclosures. In a longitudinal investigation of adjustment to the death of a spouse, Bonanno and colleagues (2002) found that greater disclosure of distress was related to greater reports of grief several months later. Paradoxically, bereaved adults who displayed initial suppression of emotional disclosures (in terms of their feelings of grief surrounding the death of their spouse) showed minimal grief several months later and improved self-reported physical health. These findings suggest that suppression of self-disclosure can be adaptive. An important methodological aspect of the Bonnano et al. study is that the disclosure of grief was made to a relative stranger (i.e., an experimenter). As noted earlier, disclosure to a relative stranger may differ from disclosure to someone with whom one has an ongoing relationship. It is unclear whether different results would have obtained by Bonnano et al. if the bereaved adults had disclosed their feelings of grief and sadness to individuals with whom they had an ongoing relationship. Nonetheless, Pennebaker and colleagues (Cohn, Mehl, & Pennebaker, 2004; Pennebaker, Mayne, & Francis, 1997) have noted the adaptive value of fluctuating between positive and negative self-disclosure in order for the disclosure to lead to beneficial outcomes. That is, physical and psychological health benefits are greatest when individuals disclose both positive and negative information rather than solely focusing on just negative information or only positive information. In general, it appears that people derive the most benefits from self-disclosure when they can balance their disclosures in terms of positive and negative information and emotion.

## SELF-DISCLOSURE IN PSYCHOTHERAPY

Of particular interest to psychotherapists is how self-disclosure affects the psychotherapy process. Although we generally think about client self-disclosure, the topic of therapist self-disclosure has drawn considerable attention and debate. Important issues include the content of therapist self-disclosure, under what conditions should such self-disclosures occur, and the effect of therapist self-disclosures on treatment outcome and the therapist–client relationship. In general, therapists engage in self-disclosures infrequently, and their self-disclosures are typically about factual information (e.g., training background) rather than personal and intimate topics (e.g., Hill & Knox, 2002). Therapists who adhere to a humanistic/experiential therapy approach engage in self-disclosure more frequently than do psychoanalytic therapists (e.g., Edwards & Murdock, 1994; Geller & Farber, 1997). There are no differences in the frequency of therapist self-disclosures between male and female therapists and between therapists of different racial backgrounds (Edwards & Murdock, 1994).

Therapist self-disclosures can have positive or negative effects on the psychotherapy process. In general, therapist self-disclosure reduces severity of psychological symptoms displayed by the client and results in the client liking the therapist more (e.g., Barrett & Berman, 2001; Farber, Berano, & Capobianco, 2004; Hill & Knox, 2002). These findings are consistent with the overall positive outcome associated with self-disclosure in the general population, including the effects found for strengthening social relationships (Collins & Miller, 1994). However, therapist self-disclosures are not always useful or helpful. As with self-disclosures that occur outside of psychotherapy, the content and timing of the disclosure are important (Hill & Knox, 2002). Therapist self-disclosures that serve the purpose of immediate goals for therapy appear to be the most beneficial in terms of treatment outcome and of strengthening the therapist–client relationship. Examples of such disclosures are those that serve the purpose of normalizing a client's experiences and those that model appropriate behavior (e.g., Knox, Hess, Petersen, & Hill, 1997). In contrast, self-disclosures that shift the focus of attention from the client to the therapist, and those that are made to satisfy the needs of the therapist can result in burdening the client and blurring the therapist–client boundary (Hill & Knox, 2002). Consequently, these types of therapist self-disclosures are likely to impede treatment progress and damage the therapist–client relationship.

Studies on therapist self-disclosure provide useful information about the conditions under which therapists might use disclosure to facilitate successful treatment outcome, although some caution must be taken when interpreting these data. The research on therapist disclosures has been sparse and is fraught with methodological limitations. Studies widely vary in their definition of self-disclosure, making it difficult to compare results from different studies. Some studies have relied on analog designs in which college student participants were asked, if they were a client, how they would feel in response to various hypothetical therapist self-disclosures, whereas other studies have examined actual therapy sessions. Studies also have emphasized examining the frequency of therapist self-disclosures rather than examining more critical aspects of disclosures, such as timing, content, and quality.

Despite the obvious importance of client self-disclosures, strikingly little research has been conducted in this area. Not surprisingly, clients disclose far more frequently in psychotherapy than they do in other settings, such as in medical interviews and cross-examinations (Stiles, 1995). Many therapists believe that self-disclosure is an essential factor in successful psychotherapy outcome, although psychotherapy research has not supported this contention (Farber, 2006; Stiles, 1995). Specifically, psychological distress is related to client disclosure, with greater distress related to greater frequency of disclosure (e.g., Burchill & Stiles, 1988; Weintraub, 1981). The relation between disclosure and distress has also been observed outside of the psychotherapy setting, with individuals displaying greater severity of depression and anxiety symptoms showing a greater frequency of self-disclosures, particularly when describing their depression and anxiety symptoms (e.g., Stiles, Shuster, & Harrigan, 1992). Although client disclosure increases with increased levels of distress, several studies have shown that the degree of client disclosure in psychotherapy is unrelated to treatment outcome (e.g., Orlinsky, Grawe, & Parks, 1994; Stiles & Shapiro, 1994).

In summary, studies have shown that therapist self-disclosures that are made to achieve immediate therapy goals are generally beneficial both in terms of successful treatment outcome and of strengthening the therapist–client relationship. Clients display a high frequency of self-disclosures in psychotherapy, with greater distress related to greater disclosure. Nonetheless, in contrast to the wealth of data demonstrating the benefits of self-disclosure to psychological well-being, a similar relationship has not been found for psychotherapy clients. The factors likely to be most important, such as content and timing of client self-disclosure, have not been investigated. Self-disclosure in psychotherapy is clearly an understudied topic.

Overall, research has indicated that self-disclosure does indeed result in improved psychological well-being, as well as improvements in a variety of other areas of functioning. In addition, a number of factors affecting whether or not benefits are derived has been identified. What is less clear is why self-disclosure is beneficial. A number of theories has been proposed to account for the beneficial outcomes associated with self-disclosure, although empirical attention to this issue has been scant.

## THEORIES OF WHY SELF-DISCLOSURE ENHANCES PSYCHOLOGICAL WELL-BEING

### Emotional Inhibition

Freud's theory of emotional inhibition is perhaps the first theory that emphasized the importance of self-disclosure to psychological well-being. Freud (see Breuer & Freud, 1895/1957) suggested that inhibition of emotions leads to psychological distress and that the way to treat psychological problems is by allowing a person to talk freely about whatever comes to his or her mind. Freud's contention that emotional inhibition leads to psychological problems has received empirical support. For instance, individuals who inhibit their emotions are more likely to suffer serious health conditions such as hypertension and coronary heart disease (e.g., Smith, 1992; Steptoe, 1993).

Based on the emotional inhibition theory, Pennebaker (1989) proposed that disclosure of previously inhibited thoughts and feelings surrounding negative life experiences leads to a reduction in stress, which, in turn, produces greater psychological and physical well-being. Although psychologists have long assumed that the mere self-disclosure of previously inhibited thoughts and feelings results in beneficial outcome, this notion has received limited empirical support. Although disclosure (or expression) of emotions does appear to have beneficial effects, disclosure in and of itself does not appear to account for the observed benefits in psychological well-being. Specifically, disclosure of negative life events that have been previously disclosed is as likely to result in beneficial outcomes as is disclosure of negative life events that have not been previously disclosed (Greenberg & Stone, 1992; Pennebaker, 1989). Thus, emotional inhibition does not appear to solely account for the observed benefits associated with disclosure.

### Social Support

As described previously, there is some speculation that the benefits associated with self-disclosure are the result of increases in social bonding. That is, when a person discloses personal and intimate aspects of his or her life to another person, the social bond between the two individuals is strengthened. The person to whom one discloses is apt to feel emotionally closer to the discloser, and, in return, is more likely to self-disclose. Consequently, the benefits of self-disclosure are the indirect result of improvement in one's social support system. The contention that self-disclosure is beneficial through the improvement of social relationships does not yet have empirical support (Sloan & Marx, 2004b). However, one must first have close relationships in order for social relationships to be further strengthened by self-disclosure. If a person is socially isolated or has a limited social support system, then that person is not likely to derive as broad of an array of benefits from self-disclosure (Radcliffe et al., 2007; Sheese et al., 2004). Specifically, as noted previously, Sheese and colleagues (2004) found that people who have greater social supports are more likely to benefit from self-disclosure than are people with limited social support. It should be noted that the findings of Sheese et al. does not directly address whether social support serves as an underlying mechanism of self-disclosure outcome. It is also the case that people with fewer social supports still derive some benefits from disclosure, though the benefits may not be as great as among those with more social supports. Despite the work that needs to be conducted in this area, there does appear to be a clear connection between self-disclosure and positive social relationships. However, the exact nature of the relation, and how one affects the other, still needs to be determined.

### Cognitive Adaptation

Cognitive adaptation theory and related theories such as cognitive assimilation theory and cognitive restructuring theory share the premise that coming to terms with a negative life event requires an integration of, or change in, one's current worldview or schema. According to Janoff-Bulman (1992), humans hold several core beliefs that are challenged when a traumatic life event occurs. These core beliefs include the notion that we are invulnerable, the world is meaningful and comprehensible, and we are good people. Within this set of beliefs are additional assumptions, such as the world is a safe place and other people are basically good. When a serious life event occurs, our core beliefs are challenged and may even be shattered. Thus, according to this theory, coping with a traumatic life event requires us to reformulate our core beliefs in order to make sense of the negative experience that has occurred. Until the person is able to integrate the negative life event into his or her core beliefs, he or she will experience distress and likely some disruption to daily life. Once the event has been integrated into the person's worldview, however, the psychological distress diminishes.

Using the premise of cognitive adaptation, several researchers have proposed that self-disclosure leads to psychological well-being because the disclosure allows a person to provide organization, structure, and cohesion to a stressful life experience that did not take place when the experience initially occurred (e.g., Pennebaker, 1997; Smyth et al., 2001). The opportunity to organize and synthesize a negative life experience, in turn, allows one to integrate the experience into one's core set of beliefs about the world. Cognitive adaptation is also a central premise of evidence-based therapy approaches for trauma, such as cognitive processing therapy (e.g., Resick & Schnicke, 1996). However, the research examining cognitive adaptation as an underlying mechanism for beneficial outcome associated with self-disclosure in the general population is not as convincing as the research conducted with trauma populations. The lack of support for the cognitive adaptation model is mainly due to the manner in which this model has been tested. Usually, the research design is correlational rather than mediational. The research also suffers from problems with the assessment of changes in cognition. Although cognitive adaptation is an internal process, investigators have had to rely on external methods to examine this process, such as coding disclosure narratives for linguistic variables. The sensitivity of such procedures to capture the cognitive adaptation process is questionable.

### Exposure

Principles of learning have been used to explain the development of pathological fear-based disorders, such as posttraumatic stress disorder (e.g., Foa & Kozak, 1986; Keane, Zimering,

& Caddell, 1985). Specifically, when an aversive unconditioned stimulus (UCS), which elicits an unconditioned response (UCR; e.g., fear), is paired (usually repeatedly) with nonthreatening, neutral stimuli, these neutral stimuli (conditioned stimulus; CS) may come to elicit a conditioned response (CR) that is similar to the UCR (fear). Further, avoidance of the CS is thought to maintain the CR. Based on these assumptions, behavioral scientists and therapists have developed a treatment model in which an individual is repeatedly exposed to the CS in the absence of the UCS, so that the CS and UCS become unpaired and the CR extinguishes (Rachman, 1980).

Some investigators have proposed that self-disclosure results in psychological well-being as a result of exposure to the CS in the absence of the UCS (Bootzin, 1997; Sloan & Marx, 2004a). For instance, if a person is instructed to disclose thoughts and feelings surrounding the traumatic memory that he or she had previously been avoiding, then the opportunity for unpairing of the CS and the UCS is presented. As a result of such exposure and decoupling of the CS and UCS, the person would no longer display the heightened fear response when faced with the CS.

There are a wealth of data supporting the development of pathological fear-based disorders and data indicating that exposure therapies are effective treatments for anxiety (e.g., Rothbaum, Meadows, Resick, & Foy, 2000). In addition, among individuals displaying posttraumatic stress symptoms, self-disclosure of traumatic life experiences often leads to improvement in psychological health (Sloan & Marx, 2004a; Sloan, Marx, & Epstein, 2005). However, the exposure model is based on the premise that pathological fear has developed. Using an exposure model to account for psychological health benefits resulting from self-disclosure among individuals who do not display pathological fear is inconsistent with the exposure theory. Thus, exposure may be an underlying mechanism of self-disclosure for individuals who experience pathological fear, but the exposure model would not make sense in the absence of pathological fear.

In sum, the scant available evidence for the theories proposed to account for beneficial effects of self-disclosure is unconvincing. To be fair, the research that has been conducted examining underlying mechanisms of psychological well-being resulting from self-disclosure has been sparse. Thus, primary underlying mechanisms that have been suggested, such as cognitive assimilation and emotional inhibition, need to be further investigated. In future work, it will be important to examine multiple possible underlying mechanisms as well as to examine whether these mechanisms vary with time and with different populations.

## CLINICAL IMPLICATIONS

Self-disclosure by a client is generally regarded as a critical factor in predicting psychotherapy outcome (Farber, 2006). Despite this widely held belief, there is no empirical evidence that greater self-disclosure in psychotherapy results in greater improvement. However, this important topic has received surprisingly little research attention; thus, the null findings obtained may have more to do with the sparse attention this area has received rather than whether the relationship between client self-disclosure and treatment outcome exists. Perhaps a more informative research area to consider is the general literature on the effect of self-disclosure on psychological and physical health. This literature has shown a robust effect in which self-disclosure results in improved psychological health, physical health, and social relationships.

There is also evidence that the conditions under which self-disclosure occurs and the quality of the disclosure are more critical factors in determining outcome than whether or not self-disclosure occurs.

The literature on the benefits obtained from self-disclosure has revealed a number of other important findings as well. Disclosing factual information is not as beneficial as disclosing information about personal emotions and feelings. Findings from studies of imaginal-based exposure therapies also highlight the importance of client disclosures of emotional reactions to a traumatic event, in addition to disclosing factual information (e.g., Meadows & Foa, 1999). These findings underscore the importance of therapists' attending to the content of a client's disclosure, with specific attention to disclosures regarding emotions. Research also indicates that disclosure of both pleasant and unpleasant experiences leads to beneficial outcome. Therefore, client disclosures of pleasant experiences may be as important as their disclosures of unpleasant life experiences. Disclosures of positive life events are likely to facilitate the development of the therapist–client relationship (Lyubomirsky & Dickerhoof, Chapter 13, this volume), which would increase the likelihood that clients would later disclose negative life experiences.

It is important for therapists to be aware of the fact that people disclose more when they are experiencing greater distress but that greater disclosure does not necessarily lead to greater benefits. Level of distress may moderate the ultimate effects of disclosure. For example, disclosure that occurs when one is experiencing moderate distress may be more beneficial than disclosure that takes place in low and high levels of distress (Farber, 2006; Stiles, 1995).

Research has also shown that some inhibition of disclosure can lead to the most successful outcomes. Consequently, a client's tendency to refrain from disclosing at various points in the psychotherapy process should not be viewed negatively. The findings of Frattaroli (2006) and Sheese et al. (2004) suggest that it is important that the client believes she or he has control over when and what he or she discloses. Accordingly, therapists should carefully consider when they want to allow clients to choose the timing of their disclosures in session and when they believe it is important to press the client for additional details that are not spontaneously offered. Timing of disclosures is also important in determining whether or not psychological benefits are achieved.

Recent research indicates that the greatest benefits are derived from written self-disclosure when a person shares his or her disclosure with someone else (Radcliffe et al., 2007). Thus, although clients would likely benefit from writing about their negative life experiences, they would gain additional psychological benefits if they subsequently share their written stories. Some therapy protocols require that clients engage in written disclosure (e.g., trauma narratives) outside of session, to be subsequently read together by therapist and client (Resick & Schnicke, 1996). Given the findings on self-disclosure, the approach of requesting that clients bring in their written disclosure to be read in session may be helpful only once a trusting therapy relationship has been established. Another clinically relevant research finding from the self-disclosure literature is that benefits from self-disclosure are more apt to occur when the disclosure is responded to in an accepting and nonjudgmental manner.

One area of self-disclosure in psychotherapy that has received considerable attention is the use of therapist self-disclosure. Although the research regarding therapist self-disclosures has methodological limitations, what can be gleaned from the findings is that therapists should use caution when self-disclosing to clients and should be mindful about when they are self-disclosing and why.

## FUTURE DIRECTIONS

Although a number of aspects related to self-disclosure have been examined, there are several topics that have received little or no scientific study. We know very little about how culture impacts self-disclosure, an area of considerable importance for psychotherapy. It is also unclear how the increasing use of electronic mail and internet blogs, which are shared online diaries that can be viewed by anyone online, may be changing society's comfort level with self-disclosure. The increased use of electronic means to self-disclose, mainly to strangers, will likely affect people's general comfort level and willingness to disclose. There is evidence that too much self-disclosure can have deleterious effects, and we will need to carefully evaluate the impact of electronic self-disclosure on psychological well-being, and whether the use of electronic self-disclosure decreases the degree to which people self-disclose within ongoing relationships.

## REFERENCES


Barrett, M. S., & Berman, J. S. (2001). Is psychotherapy more effective when therapists disclose information about themselves? *Journal of Consulting and Clinical Psychology*, *69*, 597–603.

Batten, S. V., Follette, V. M., Rasmussen Hall, M. L., & Palm, K. M. (2002). Physical and psychological effects of written disclosure among sexual abuse survivors. *Behavior Therapy*, *33*, 107–122.

Bonanno, G. A., Wortman, C. B., Lehman, D. R., Tweed, R. G., Haring, M., Sonnega, J., et al. (2002). Resilience to loss and chronic grief: A prospective study from pre-loss to 18 months post-loss. *Journal of Personality and Social Psychology*, *83*, 1150–1164.

Bootzin, R. R. (1997). Examining the theory and clinical utility of writing about emotional experiences. *Psychological Science*, *8*, 167–169.

Breuer, J., & Freud, S. (1957). *Studies on hysteria* (J. Strachey, Trans.). New York: Basic Books. (Original work published 1895)

Burchill, S. A. L., & Stiles, W. B. (1988). Interactions of depressed college students with their roommates: Not necessarily negative. *Journal of Personality and Social Psychology*, *55*, 410–419.

Cohn, M. A., Mehl, M. R., & Pennebaker, J. W. (2004). Linguistic markers of psychological change surrounding September 11, 2001. *Psychological Science*, *15*, 687–693.

Collins, N. L., & Miller, L. C. (1994). Self-disclosure and liking: A meta-analytic review. *Psychological Bulletin*, *116*, 457–475.

Derlega, V. J., Metts, S., Petronio, S., & Margulis, S. T. (1993). *Self-disclosure*. Newbury Park, CA: Sage.

Dindia, K., & Allen, M. (1992). Sex differences in self-disclosure. A meta-analysis. *Psychological Bulletin*, *112*, 106–124.

Edwards, C. E., & Murdock, N. L. (1994). Characteristics of therapist self-disclosure in the counseling process. *Journal of Counseling and Development*, *72*, 384–389.

Epstein, E. M., Sloan, D. M., & Marx, B. P. (2005). Getting to the heart of the matter: Written disclosure, gender, and heart rate. *Psychosomatic Medicine*, *67*, 413–419.

Farber, B. A. (2006). *Self-disclosure in psychotherapy*. New York: Guilford Press.

Farber, B. A., Berano, K. C., & Capobianco, J. A. (2004). Clients' perceptions of the process and consequences of self-disclosure in psychotherapy. *Journal of Counseling Psychology*, *51*, 340–346.

Figueiredo, M. I., Fries, E., & Ingram, K. M. (2004). The role of disclosure patterns and unsupportive social interactions in the well-being of breast cancer patients. *Psycho-Oncology*, *13*, 96–105.

Foa, E. B., & Kozak, M. (1986). Emotional processing of fear: Exposure to corrective information. *Psychological Bulletin*, *99*, 20–35.

Frattaroli, J. (2006). Experimental disclosures and its moderators: A meta-analysis. *Psychological Bulletin, 132*, 823–865.

Frisina, P. G., Borod, J. C., & Lepore, S. J. (2004). A meta-analysis of the effects of written emotional disclosure on the health outcomes in clinical populations. *Journal of Nervous and Mental Disease, 192*, 629–634.

Gable, S. L., Reis, H. T., Impett, E. A., & Asher, E. R. (2004). What do you do when things go right? The intrapersonal and interpersonal benefits of sharing positive events *Journal of Personality and Social Psychology, 87*, 228–245.

Geller, J. D., & Farber, B. A. (1997, August). *Why therapists do and don't disclose.* Paper presented at the annual meeting of the American Psychological Association, Chicago.

Gidron, Y., Peri, T., Connolly, J. F., & Shalev, A. Y. (1996). Written emotional disclosure in posttraumatic stress disorder: Is it beneficial for the patient? *Journal of Nervous and Mental Disease, 184*, 505–507.

Greenberg, M. A., & Stone, A. A. (1992). Emotional disclosure about traumas and its relation to health: Effects of previous disclosure and trauma severity. *Journal of Personality and Social Psychology, 63*, 75–84.

Hill, C. E., & Knox, S. (2002) Self-disclosure. In J. C. Norcross (Ed.), *Psychotherapy relationships that work* (pp. 249–259). New York: Oxford University Press.

Janoff-Bulman, R. (1992). *Shattered assumptions: Towards a new psychology of trauma.* New York: Free Press.

Keane, T. M., Zimering, R. T., & Caddell, J. M. (1985). A behavioral formulation of posttraumatic stress disorder in Vietnam veterans. *Behavior Therapist, 8*, 9–12.

Knox, S., Hess, S., Peterson, D., & Hill, C. E. (1997). A qualitative analysis of client perceptions of the effects of helpful therapist self-disclosure in long-term therapy. *Journal of Counseling Psychology, 44*, 274–283.

Langston, C. A. (1994). Capitalizing on and coping with daily-life events: Expressive responses to positive events. *Journal of Personality and Social Psychology, 67*, 1112–1125.

Laurenceau, J. P., Barrett, L. F., & Pietromonaco, P. R. (1998). Intimacy as an interpersonal process: The importance of self-disclosure, partner disclosure, and perceived partner responsiveness in interpersonal exchanges. *Journal of Personality and Social Psychology, 74*, 1238–1251.

Meadows, E. A., & Foa, E. B. (1999). Cognitive-behavioral treatment of traumatized adults. In P. A. Saigh & D. J. Bremner (Eds.), *Posttraumatic stress disorder: A comprehensive text* (pp. 376–390). Needham Heights, MA: Allyn & Bacon.

Orlinsky, D. E., Grawe, K., & Parks, B. K. (1994). Process and outcome in counseling: *Noch einmal.* In A. E. Bergin & S. L. Garfield (Eds.), *Handbook of psychotherapy and behavior change* (4th ed., pp. 270–376). New York: Wiley.

Pennebaker, J. W. (1989). Cognition, inhibition, and disease. In L. Berkowitz (Ed.), *Advances in experimental social psychology* (Vol. 22, pp. 211–244). New York: Academic Press.

Pennebaker, J. W. (1997). Writing about emotional experiences as a therapeutic process. *Psychological Science, 8*, 162–166.

Pennebaker, J. W., & Beall, S. K. (1986). Confronting a traumatic event: Toward an understanding of inhibition and disease. *Journal of Abnormal Psychology, 95*, 274–281.

Pennebaker, J. W., Mayne, T. J., & Francis, M. E. (1997). Linguistic predictors of adaptive bereavement. *Journal of Personality and Social Psychology*, 72, 863–871.

Rachman, S. (1980). Emotional processing. *Behaviour Research and Therapy, 18*, 51–60.

Radcliffe, A. M., Lumley, M. A., Kendall, J., Stevenson, J. K., & Beltran, J. (2007). Written emotional disclosure: Testing whether social disclosure matters. *Journal of Social and Clinical Psychology, 26*, 362–384.

Reis, H. T., & Patrick, B. C. (1996). Attachment and intimacy: Component processes. In E. T. Higgins & A. W. Kruglanski (Eds.), *Social psychology: Handbook of basic principles* (pp. 523–563). New York: Guilford Press.

Reis, H. T., & Shaver, P. (1988). Intimacy as an interpersonal process. In S. Duck (Ed.), *Handbook of personal relationships* (pp. 367–389). Chichester, UK: Wiley.

Resick, P. A., & Schnicke, M. K. (1996). *Cognitive processing therapy for rape victims: A treatment manual.* Newbury Park, CA: Sage.

Rothbaum, B. O., Meadows, E. A., Resick, P., & Foy, D. W. (2000). Cognitive-behavioral therapy. In E. B. Foa, T. M. Keane, & M. J. Friedman (Eds.), *Effective treatments for PTSD* (pp. 60–83). New York: Guilford Press.

Segrin, C. (2000). Social skills deficits associated with depression. *Clinical Psychology Review, 20,* 379–403.

Segrin, C., & Abramson, L. Y. (1994). Negative reactions to depressive behaviors: A communication theories analysis. *Journal of Abnormal Psychology, 103,* 655–668.

Sheese, B. E., Brown, E. L., & Graziano, W. G. (2004). Emotional expression in cyberspace: Searching for moderators of the Pennebaker disclosure effect via e-mail. *Health Psychology, 23,* 457–464.

Sherman, B. F., Bonanno, G. A., Wiener, L. S., & Battles, H. B. (2000). When children tell their friends they have AIDS: Possible consequences for psychological well-being and disease progression. *Psychosomatic Medicine, 62,* 238–247.

Sloan, D. M., & Marx, B. P. (2004a). A closer examination of the structured written disclosure procedure. *Journal of Consulting and Clinical Psychology, 72,* 165–175.

Sloan, D. M., & Marx, B. P. (2004b). Taking pen to hand: Evaluating theories underlying the written disclosure paradigm. *Clinical Psychology: Science and Practice, 11,* 121–137.

Sloan, D. M., Marx, B. P., & Epstein, E. M. (2005). Further examination of the exposure model underlying the efficacy of written emotional disclosure. *Journal of Consulting and Clinical Psychology, 73,* 549–554.

Sloan, D. M., Marx, B. P., Epstein, E. M., & Lexington, J. M. (2007). Does altering the instructional set affect written disclosure outcome? *Behavior Therapy, 38,* 155–168

Smith, T. W. (1992). Hostility and health: Current status of a psychosomatic hypothesis. *Health Psychology, 11,* 139–150.

Smyth, J. M., True, N., & Souto, J. (2001). Effects of writing about traumatic experiences: The necessity for narrative structuring. *Journal of Social and Clinical Psychology, 20,* 161–172.

Steptoe, A. (1993). Stress and the cardiovascular system: A psychosocial perspective. In S. C. Stanford & P. Salmon (Eds.), *Stress: From synapse to syndrome* (pp. 119–141). San Diego, CA: Academic Press.

Stiles, W. B. (1995). Disclosure as a speech act: Is it psychotherapeutic to disclose? In J. W. Pennebaker (Ed.), *Emotion, disclosure, and health* (pp. 71–91). Washington, DC: American Psychological Association.

Stiles, W. B., & Shapiro, D. A. (1994). Disabuse of the drug metaphor: Psychotherapy process–outcome correlations. *Journal of Consulting and Clinical Psychology, 62,* 942–948.

Stiles, W. B., Shuster, P. L., & Harrigan, J. A. (1992). Disclosure and anxiety: A test of the fever model. *Journal of Personality and Social Psychology, 63,* 980–988.

Stroebe, M., Stroebe, W., Schut, H., Zech, E., & van den Bout, J. (2002). Does disclosure of emotions facilitate recovery from bereavement? Evidence from two prospective studies. *Journal of Consulting and Clinical Psychology, 70,* 169–178.

Taylor, S. E., & Stanton, A. L. (2007). Stress, coping, and mental health. *Annual Review of Clinical Psychology, 3,* 377–401.

Weintraub, W. (1981). *Verbal behavior: Adaptation and psychopathology.* New York: Springer-Verlag.

Zea, M. C., Reisen, C. A., Poppen, P. J., Bianchi, F. T., & Echeverry, J. J. (2005). Disclosure of HIV status and psychological well-being among Latino gay and bisexual men. *AIDS and Behavior, 9,* 15–26.

# Social Cognition and Emotion

# 13 A Construal Approach to Increasing Happiness

Sonja Lyubomirsky
Rene Dickerhoof

Seeking ever-greater happiness—or what researchers refer to as "subjective well-being" (SWB; Diener, 1984; Diener, Suh, Lucas, & Smith, 1999)—is an important goal for people in almost every nation (Diener, 2000). Indeed, ever since the pursuit of happiness was immortalized in the Declaration of Independence as an inalienable right for all citizens, it has become ingrained in U.S. culture. Yet, many appear unsuccessful in this pursuit. Although everyone undoubtedly knows friends, colleagues, neighbors, and acquaintances who are consistently positive and upbeat, it is not difficult to identify other individuals who are chronically down-and-out and dissatisfied with life. What accounts for these two affective predispositions? That is, why are some people happier than others, and is it possible to shift from being a generally unhappy person to a happier one?

To address these questions, we begin by discussing two contrasting theories of the determinants of happiness—*bottom-up* and *top-down*—and then introduce a new framework that incorporates both of these perspectives. Next, we describe several potential happiness-increasing practices and provide empirical evidence from our laboratory that supports their use to improve well-being in healthy individuals. Finally, weaving social and clinical psychology together, we consider how particular interventions to bolster happiness can inform interventions to alleviate clinical problems such as major depressive disorder and generalized anxiety disorder. Future directions for research on the pursuit of happiness and its applications to the clinical arena are then discussed.

## DETERMINANTS OF HAPPINESS

The fast-growing area of positive psychology has focused on investigating positive human emotions (e.g., awe), positive behaviors (e.g., acts of kindness), and positive cognitions (e.g., optimistic thinking). To be sure, one of its central aims has been to elucidate the causes of well-being. Efforts to understand what drives happiness have come to be guided by two major theoretical perspectives (Diener, 1984). The first, referred to as the *bottom-up* theory, postulates that happiness is rooted in an individual's life circumstances—for example, in day-to-day uplifts and hassles, as well as factors such as socioeconomic status, educational attainment, physical health, and demographic variables such as age, gender, and race. According to the bottom-up perspective, happy people are the privileged and fortunate. They are simply those individuals who encounter relatively more positive and satisfying life events and those who have accrued the greatest advantages in life. Complicating matters, the causal pathway between happiness and advantages in life is bidirectional, as happy people have been documented to be more likely to attain success in work, social relationships, and health (Lyubomirsky, King, & Diener, 2005). All in all, although the bottom-up theory is fairly intuitive, it has not received much support in the literature (Myers & Diener, 1995). Rather, studies have consistently shown that the average person's objective circumstances are less predictive than one might expect of how happy he or she is likely to be (for classic reviews, see Andrews & Withey, 1976; Campbell, Converse, & Rodgers, 1976).

In contrast, the *top-down* theory argues that happiness is not caused by external variables (such as people's objective life circumstances), but, rather, is the product of biological or temperamental factors that direct behaviors and cognitions (Diener, 1984). These top-down forces are thought to act on individuals' personalities and ultimately to color their everyday perceptions of the world.

Not surprisingly, support for the top-down theory of happiness comes from research investigating the biological, or temperamental, underpinnings of well-being. For example, in an oft-cited study from the field of behavioral genetics, Lykken and Tellegen (1996) showed that identical twins reared apart are substantially more similar in well-being than are fraternal twins reared either together or apart, suggesting that genes may have a powerful effect on happiness. Remarkably, as these researchers reported, the well-being of one's identical twin, either today or 10 years earlier, is a better predictor of one's happiness than one's current educational attainment, income, or status. Thus, there appears to be a strong innate biological component to happiness that is likely to have a global "trickle-down" effect on how people think about, behave, and experience the world around them.

The top-down theory of happiness is further supported by the study of personality. Several personality traits, which are by definition stable across time and consistent across situations (Allport, 1955), have been shown to be related to two aspects of well-being: positive affect (PA) and negative affect (NA). Numerous studies have demonstrated that people who are extraverted have high levels of PA, and people who are neurotic have high levels of NA (Costa & McCrae, 1980; Emmons & Diener, 1985). Furthermore, these associations are so strong that whether or not a particular individual is extraverted or neurotic predicts how happy he or she will be 10 years down the line (Costa, McCrae, & Zonderman, 1987). Hence, evidence connecting personality traits to well-being also points to the possibility that happiness may be largely driven by top-down temperamental forces.[1]

In their seminal review, Diener and colleagues (1999) summed up the current state of research on theories of well-being as following a trend from a focus on bottom-up perspectives to top-down perspectives. Of course, much like the dichotomy between nature and nurture, the distinction between top-down and bottom-up theories is likely overstated and not necessarily constructive. Indeed, the integration of these two theories is essential to providing the most comprehensive portrayal of happiness (Brief, Butcher, George, & Link, 1993; Diener, Larsen, & Emmons, 1984; Emmons, Diener, & Larsen, 1986; Headey & Wearing, 1989; Lyubomirsky, 2001). Our *construal model of happiness* is essentially a top-down model that incorporates the importance of bottom-up factors.

## THE CONSTRUAL MODEL OF HAPPINESS

The construal model of happiness holds that objective life circumstances indeed play a critical role in well-being but are poor predictors of happiness because their effect on happiness depends largely on how they are construed, perceived, or compared to others (i.e., on top-down processes; Lyubomirsky, 2001). For example, being married or an accountant or a city dweller will make a person happy only if he or she actively judges these circumstances to be positive, satisfying, and meaningful. Similarly, having an annual income of $100K might be construed as satisfying if one's peers are making $50K but dissatisfying if one's peers are making $250K (e.g., Solnick & Hemenway, 1998). In these instances, the *interpretation* of one's circumstances plays an integral role in determining well-being.

Accordingly, both bottom-up and top-down forces influence how happy or unhappy people are—that is, both circumstances (e.g., being married or wealthy) and temperaments (e.g., possessing a generally positive perspective or an extraverted disposition) affect well-being. Their joint effect is a property of the interaction between people's objective social worlds and the way that they subjectively interpret them.

According to the construal model, people are happier when they interpret their life circumstances in an optimistic "glass-is-half-full" fashion (e.g., "I am an excellent candidate for the job"), and this is true regardless of how "ideal" their circumstances may actually be (i.e., whether or not they are truly qualified and competitive for the job). Indeed, a wealth of research suggests that the way people construe their circumstances can have an impact on their well-being (for reviews, see Diener et al., 1999; Lyubomirsky, 2001). As just one example, a strong positive relationship exists between how satisfied people are with their life circumstances averaged across various domains (e.g., finances, health, friendships, family relations, education, etc.) and how happy overall they report themselves to be (Argyle, 1987; Campbell, 1981; Dickerhoof & Lyubomirsky, 2008; Diener et al., 1999). That is, although abundant data show that objective life circumstances (e.g., socioeconomic status, educational attainment) are not strongly related to well-being, *subjective* appraisals (i.e., how people feel about these circumstances) *are* correlated with well-being. Furthermore, the effect of life circumstances on happiness depends on whether people have an optimistic outlook on life (a top-down factor)—particularly when life circumstances are seen to be relatively poor (a bottom-up factor; see Figure 13.1[2]). That is, having an optimistic disposition seems to buffer relatively less fortunate individuals from their less-than-ideal lives and prevents them from being unhappy (Dickerhoof & Lyubomirsky, 2008).

In sum, how people construe and think about (using top-down processes) objective events and situations in their lives plays an important role in determining how happy they

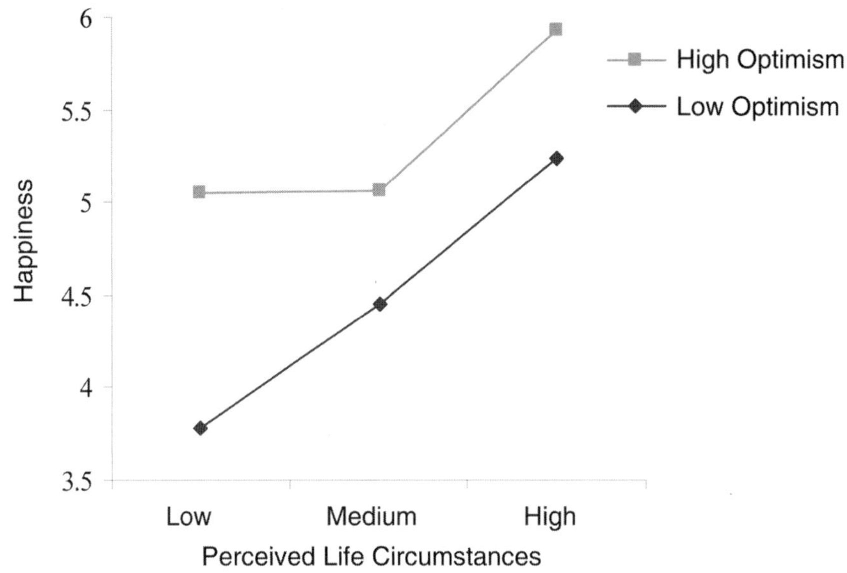


**FIGURE 13.1.** The effect of perceived life circumstances on happiness in individuals with high versus low optimism.

are. A valuable practical question to ask concerns what unhappy people can learn from their happier peers about more adaptive ways to interpret and experience their social realities. Happy and unhappy individuals respond differently (in a top-down fashion) to their social environments, and these responses appear to reinforce happiness in happy individuals and maintain or even bolster unhappiness in unhappy ones (Lyubomirsky, 2001). For example, happy people report higher self-esteem and greater optimism (e.g., Lucas, Diener, & Suh, 1996; Lyubomirsky & Lepper, 1999; Lyubomirsky, Tkach, & DiMatteo, 2006; Tarlow & Haaga, 1996), are better able to derive positive meaning from negative events (Folkman, 1997; Lyubomirsky & Tucker, 1998), and feel a stronger sense of mastery or control over their own lives (Bandura, 1997; Grob, Stetsenko, Sabatier, Botcheva, & Macek, 1999; Lyubomirsky et al., 2006). Furthermore, happy people have more confidence about their abilities and skills (Totterdell, 2000), are more assertive (Schimmack, Oishi, Furr, & Funder, 2004), and use more humor (e.g., Martin & Lefcourt, 1983; Nezu, Nezu, & Blissett, 1988), spirituality, and faith when coping with life stressors than do their unhappy counterparts (e.g., McCrae & Costa, 1986; McIntosh, Silver, & Wortman, 1993; Myers, 2000). Finally, happy people are less likely to be characterized by two tendencies that have a negative impact on well-being: namely, dwelling excessively on themselves and their problems (Lyubomirsky, Boehm, Kasri, & Zehm, 2010; Lyubomirsky, Caldwell, & Nolen-Hoeksema, 1998; Lyubomirsky, Tucker, Caldwell, & Berg, 1999) and regularly comparing themselves to others (Lyubomirsky & Ross, 1997; Lyubomirsky, Tucker, & Kasri, 2001).

The correlational research described thus far does not establish the causal direction between happiness and positive and adaptive behaviors and cognitions. Alternative methods are necessary to determine whether happiness causes positive thinking and constructive coping or, alternatively, whether optimistic interpretations of the environment make people happy. Thus, the question remains whether employing strategies that promote adaptive interpretations (e.g., positive thinking) and that inhibit maladaptive construals (e.g., pessimistic rumination) can inform interventions to improve well-being. This possibility, and the small but growing number of experimental studies supporting it, is addressed next.

## CAN LESS HAPPY PEOPLE BECOME LASTINGLY HAPPIER?

Using adaptive strategies to cope with daily experiences and to interpret circumstances in relatively positive ways—for example, thinking optimistically or avoiding upward social comparisons—appears to come naturally to happy people. Those who are predisposed to be unhappy, however, appear to be characterized by relatively more maladaptive and negatively biased cognitions and behaviors, suggesting that a top-down, hardwired, genetically determined, and stable "setpoint" or happiness baseline contributes to how people interpret their realities. If this is true, then increasing happiness may be a very difficult, if not futile, endeavor (Lykken & Tellegen, 1996). Indeed, unlike many clinically diagnosed disorders, which are generally treatable to varying degrees, a person's level of happiness has not always been viewed as a state that he or she can elevate with a little effort and hard work.

Challenging this pessimistic perspective, we argue that a predisposition for unhappiness is a condition that can be effectively "treated" using a number of behavioral and cognitive therapies. (For a classic meta-analysis on the effectiveness of such therapies, see Smith, Glass, & Miller, 1980). That is, happiness too can be changed for the better (Lyubomirsky, Sheldon, & Schkade, 2005). Indeed, some positive psychologists argue that helping people become lastingly happier should be the field's ultimate goal (e.g., Seligman, Steen, Park, & Peterson, 2005).

Yet, our scientific understanding of how to actively pursue and attain happiness is still in its infancy. That is, although a plethora of research is devoted to the alleviation of maladaptive conditions such as anxiety or depression, only a handful of studies at present has empirically addressed the possibility of increasing people's happiness (e.g., see Fordyce, 1977, 1983; Lyubomirsky, Dickerhoof, Boehm, & Sheldon, 2009; Seligman et al., 2005; Sheldon & Lyubomirsky, 2006; Tkach, 2005).

Lyubomirsky, Sheldon, and Schade (2005) recently developed the sustainable happiness model, which argues that the most promising route to increasing happiness is through the intentional and committed practice of cognitive, behavioral, and goal-based activities associated with enhanced well-being. Evidence is mounting to support this model. For example, work by Lyubomirsky and colleagues has shown that well-being can be improved over both short-term periods (such as 4 weeks) and longer durations (up to 9 months) when people are motivated to engage in adaptive or positive behaviors and cognitions (see Lyubomirsky et al., 2009; Lyubomirsky, Sheldon, et al., 2005; Sheldon & Lyubomirsky, 2006; Tkach, 2005). The sustainable happiness model further has predictions about the variables that moderate and mediate the effectiveness of any particular happiness-enhancing activity. In other words, the ways in which the activities are ultimately carried out should affect their efficacy. Specifically, the timing, variety, and frequency with which these activities are practiced—as well as the degree of authentic motivation that one has to engage in them—are hypothesized to have an impact on their ability to be effective. These issues are addressed next.

For example, supporting the role of timing in the efficacy of happiness-enhancing strategies, Lyubomirsky, Sheldon, et al. (2005) showed that practicing five acts of kindness in 1 day (e.g., opening the door for a stranger, doing a roommate's dishes, or taking out a neighbor's trash) increased well-being over a 6-week period relative to a no-treatment control group. This effect was not found, however, for those asked to carry out five kind acts sporadically over a 7-day period, suggesting that optimal timing may affect a person's ability to benefit from this behavioral happiness-enhancing strategy.

A subsequent relatively more intensive 10-week intervention examined the benefits of engaging in acts of kindness toward others (Tkach, 2005). In this experiment, regularly and faithfully engaging in generous acts also improved well-being; however, varying the types of acts committed (i.e., consistently bestowing different kindnesses) was more happiness-promoting than engaging in the same activities week to week. This study thus highlights the importance of taking advantage of *variety* when practicing acts of kindness toward others.

Another 6-week intervention was designed to test the effects of practicing the cognitive happiness-increasing strategy of grateful thinking (Emmons & McCullough, 2003; Lyubomirsky, Sheldon, et al., 2005). In this study, participants were asked simply to focus on things for which they were grateful (e.g., "a healthy body," "parents," "friends"). This strategy improved well-being (relative to controls) when practiced once a week but not when overpracticed (i.e., when performed three times a week). Thus, *frequency* may play a critical role in the effect of expressing gratitude on well-being; specifically, excessive engagement in this cognitive strategy (or, potentially, any other known happiness-enhancing activity) could actually be unhelpful or even detrimental (however, see Emmons & McCullough, 2003, for somewhat divergent results, although their dependent variables involved transient feelings of well-being immediately after participants counted their blessings as opposed to pre- vs. postintervention).

A 4-week experimental study examined the short-term effects of expressing gratitude and yet another cognitive strategy—practicing optimistic thinking—on positive and negative affect (Sheldon & Lyubomirsky, 2006). In this study, people who practiced gratitude and optimism (relative to controls) experienced greater self-concordance (i.e., identification with and interest in continuing these exercises; Sheldon & Elliot, 1999), which, in turn, was associated with more frequent practice of these activities. Finally, and most important, the more frequently participants practiced these exercises, the greater gains in positive affect they obtained. Thus, intrinsic drive and interest in a given happiness strategy, as well as the effort invested in it, appear to contribute to its effectiveness.

To build on our findings with respect to self-concordance (or "intrinsic interest"), we sought to examine the effect of motivation to become happier on the extent to which a person is likely to benefit from practicing a happiness-enhancing activity. To this end, we asked students to choose between two posted studies: one purported to be a "happiness intervention" and the other advertised to be a "cognitive exercises" experiment. (In reality, these were both the same study; Lyubomirsky et al., 2009.) The purpose of providing two study options was to divide our participants into two groups: those who were intrinsically motivated to become happier (i.e., those who chose the happiness intervention) and those who were relatively less motivated or interested in becoming happier (i.e., those who chose the study about cognitive exercises). To ensure that students who signed up for the "happiness intervention" would not report greater gains in happiness simply due to expectancy effects, at an initial lab meeting, all participants—regardless of the "study" in which they chose to participate—were told that the experiment should make them happier. At this point, students were randomly assigned to participate in one of three experimental conditions for 15 minutes a week over an 8-week period—to express gratitude, to practice optimism, or to engage in a comparison control activity (i.e., keeping a list of what happened over the past 7 days). The results of this experiment revealed that people who were more motivated to become happier began the study with the same baseline levels of happiness but were generally more likely to benefit from the happiness activities than were those who were relatively less motivated. Indeed, our "motivated" participants who practiced either optimism or gratitude continued to report gains in well-being up to 9 months after completing this experiment, relative to both "nonmotivated" participants and controls. This pattern of results suggests that intrinsic desire to be happier may be crucial to accomplishing this goal.

Growing evidence thus supports the notion that people can indeed become happier by intentionally and willfully practicing positive behavioral and cognitive strategies (e.g., focusing on strengths rather than weaknesses, working to think more positively, demonstrating gratitude, or doing things for others; for details about happiness-enhancing activities performed in other laboratories, see Fordyce, 1977, 1983; Seligman et al., 2005; Seligman, Rashid, & Parks, 2006). Furthermore, the research evidence speaks to the importance of considering variables such as timing, variety, frequency, self-concordance, and motivation when practicing happiness-increasing strategies. That is, there appear to be optimal ways to carry out any given strategy (e.g., not to overpractice gratitude), and knowing what is optimal can help people magnify the benefits obtained from engaging in these activities. Additionally, elucidating precisely *how* these activities lead to increases in well-being has potentially important ramifications. That is, why does practicing positive behaviors and cognitions make people happier (or less unhappy)? What underlying mechanisms are brought about by engaging in these activities that ultimately cause gains in well-being?

Although this question has not been well studied to date, a few investigations are beginning to examine potential mediators of the effects of practicing happiness-enhancing strategies on well-being. For example, in his kindness intervention, Tkach (2005) demonstrated that one potential mechanism (or mediator) of the effects of practicing acts of kindness on gains in happiness is the perception of gratitude from the target of the kindness. That is, participants who dispensed kindnesses in this experiment recognized that the recipients were grateful and appreciative of their help, and this perceived appreciation led them to experience greater boosts in happiness. Likewise, in Lyubomirsky et al.'s (2009) intervention examining the importance of motivation, expressing optimism or gratitude on a weekly basis led people to report feeling happier, and this effect was mediated by increases in positive perceptions of their lives (see Figure 13.2). In other words, the participants became happier after expressing gratitude or optimism precisely because these activities prompted them to interpret their lives in a more positive manner. Indeed, by the end of the experiment, participants reported that they were more satisfied with their life experiences than they had been at the beginning of the study, even though independent raters judged that their circumstances were not objectively improving.[3] Thus, both these studies suggest that one potential explanation for why happiness strategies increase well-being is that intentional happiness-enhancing activities change (for the better) how people construe their situations.

Consistent with these findings, Lichter, Hayes, and Kammann (1980) attempted to increase happiness by using two cognitive activities to "retrain" participants' mindsets to think more positively. The first retraining activity had participants engage in eight 2-hour discussion sessions (conducted over a 4-week period) focused on how to combat irrational beliefs about the self. As predicted, participating in these discussion groups led to improvements in

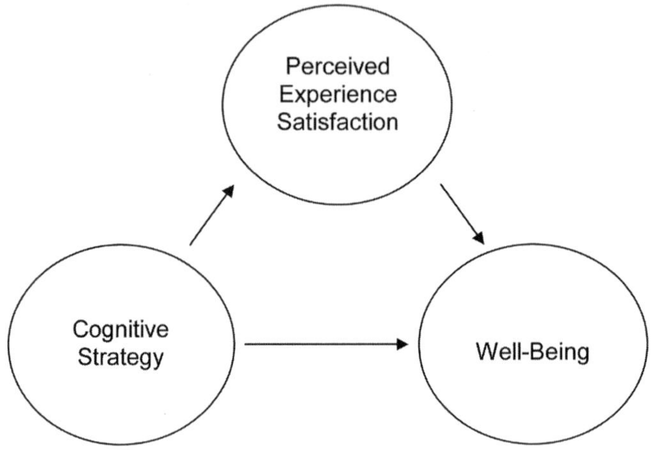


**FIGURE 13.2.** Perceived experience satisfaction mediates the relation between practicing a happiness-increasing cognitive strategy and gains in well-being.

happiness relative to a control group, both immediately after completing the intervention and 6 weeks later. In the second retraining activity, participants were asked to rehearse positive statements about the self over a 2-week period. Not surprisingly, people who "retrained" their thinking in this manner reported gains in well-being, as well as reductions in depressive symptoms, relative to control participants. Although a number of alternative explanations may account for the effectiveness of these activities (e.g., placebo effects, demand characteristics, group support effects), it is reasonable to assume that the "retraining" activities did change participants' construals, which ultimately made them happier.

Thus, in line with a construal approach to happiness, practicing positive intentional activities may directly combat the effects of negative construals (which characterize generally unhappy people), while simultaneously promoting the effects of positive construals (which tend to characterize generally happy people). In turn, such newly acquired positive perceptions of their circumstances may ultimately make people feel happier in much the same way that cognitive-behavioral therapy (CBT) alleviates depression (Beck, 1967; Beck, Rush, Shaw, & Emery, 1979).

## CLINICAL IMPLICATIONS

Converging research shows that happiness can be increased—even over relatively long periods of time—when people engage in a variety of adaptive behavioral and cognitive activities. A question for clinical and counseling psychologists is whether these findings are relevant only to efforts to improve well-being in healthy individuals or whether they may also be useful to apply to interventions designed to alleviate clinical disorders such as generalized anxiety or major depression. That is, does understanding how to improve well-being help us better understand how to treat ill-being?

To be sure, some researchers have proposed that an important root of depression—as well as social anxiety—is a deficit in positive affect (Brown, Chorpita, & Barlow, 1998; Chorpita, Plummer, & Moffitt, 2000; Davidson, 1993; Kashdan, 2002; Watson, Clark, & Carey, 1988). That is, evidence suggests that depressed people with the greatest positive affect deficits are the least likely to recover from their debilitating condition (Rottenberg, Kasch, Gross, & Gotlib, 2002). Accordingly, because positive practices like expressing gratitude, practicing optimism, and being generous can enhance positive emotions (Lyubomirsky et al., 2009; Sheldon & Lyubomirsky, 2006; Tkach, 2005), they may also be able to effectively alleviate depression and other problems (e.g., generalized anxiety or social anxiety). However, little is currently known regarding which goal—enhancing positive emotions versus decreasing negative ones—is more important.

Studies testing Fredrickson's (2001) broaden-and-build model of positive emotions have demonstrated that positive emotions can "undo" the detrimental effects of negative emotions (Fredrickson & Levenson, 1998; Fredrickson, Mancuso, Branigan, & Tugade, 2000). Furthermore, daily positive emotion can mediate a person's ability to recover from stressful experiences (Ong, Bergeman, Bisconti, & Wallace, 2006). Thus, the positive affect produced by practicing intentional happiness-enhancing activities may mitigate the negative effects of depressive symptoms.

Furthermore, research in our laboratory (Lyubomirsky et al., 2009) shows that expressing gratitude and optimism not only increases happiness, but also reduces depressive symptomatology, as measured by the Center for Epidemiological Studies Depression Scale (Radloff, 1977). Specifically, practicing either gratitude or optimism over an 8-week period led to increases in positive affect 3 months after the intervention, which ultimately led to reductions in depressive symptoms at an even later date (6 months postintervention; see Figure 13.3). These findings indicate that one potential mechanism by which cognitive strategies alleviate depressive symptoms is the ability of the strategies to increase positive emotions.

Given this knowledge, we believe that targeting *positive* behaviors can contribute to progress in developing effective strategies for reducing negative or maladaptive thoughts, behaviors, and emotions. Indeed, Parloff, Kelman, and Frank (1954) noted a half century

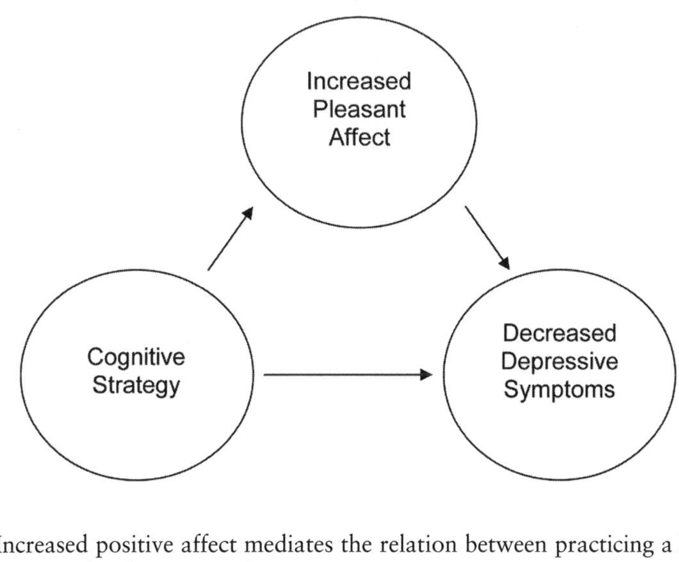


**FIGURE 13.3.** Increased positive affect mediates the relation between practicing a happiness-increasing cognitive strategy and reductions in depressive symptoms.

ago that therapy should not simply be about the reduction of illness, but also about increasing personal effectiveness and comfort. Others point out that the road to recovering from adversity lies not just in repairing the negative, but also in engendering the positive (Ryff & Singer, 1996). Moreover, these researchers warn that the absence of positive well-being may actually make people more vulnerable to the presence of ill-being.

Fortunately, clinicians have already acknowledged the importance of focusing on and nurturing positive behaviors and emotions in clinical populations, ranging from individuals suffering from schizophrenia (Ahmed & Boisvert, 2006) to incarcerated sex offenders (Ward & Stewart, 2003; for an overview of this burgeoning paradigm focused on positive practices, see Tedeschi & Kilmer, 2005). As one example of this growing literature, Fava and his colleagues (Fava, Rafanelli, Cazzaro, Conti, & Grandi, 1998; Fava et al., 2005) used a positive psychological approach, referred to as well-being therapy (WBT), to treat clients who are in the residual (i.e., recovery) phase of a number of affective disorders. This research suggests that a focus on positive experiences and adaptive functioning during a period when clients may begin to experience residual symptoms of their disorder may be valuable in helping to reduce relapse rates.

The primary purpose of WBT is to help clients maintain—and possibly even improve on—the psychological benefits obtained from standard therapy such as CBT. To this end, Fava and his colleagues (1998) randomly assigned clients experiencing residual symptoms of affective disorders to receive either WBT or standard CBT. Both therapies consisted of eight 40-minute sessions once every other week; however, in the first and second week of WBT (in contrast to CBT), clients were asked to identify only positive life experiences, no matter how short-lived, and to record those experiences in a diary. During the next three sessions (i.e., sessions 3–5), clients were asked to identify negative feelings and beliefs that interrupt thoughts about these initial positive experiences. Finally, in the last three sessions (i.e., sessions 6–8), clients were assessed on six dimensions of positive psychological functioning—autonomy, environmental mastery, personal growth, purpose in life, self-acceptance, and positive relations with others (Ryff, 1989)—and impairment in each domain was discussed. The results of this experiment showed that WBT was at least as effective as CBT during the residual phase, and some evidence suggested that it was even more effective.

In another study examining the effects of WBT relative to CBT (Fava et al., 2005), clients who suffered from generalized anxiety disorder reported greater improvement in their illness immediately after treatment and 1 year later if they had received a combination of four CBT treatments followed by four WBT treatments (vs. having received eight CBT treatments only). These results suggest that not only do positive psychotherapies work, but that using these types of therapies in conjunction with standard pathology-alleviating therapies (e.g., CBT) to alleviate mental illness may be more effective than focusing on alleviating pathology alone.

Another group of researchers has also begun to test the promise of practicing positive psychological strategies not only to increase well-being but to combat psychological disorders (Seligman et al., 2006). In the first of two studies to test this possibility, mildly to moderately depressed individuals engaged in a 6-week group intervention, 2 hours-per-week, that required them to practice a novel positive strategy each week. These activities were (1) using personal strengths (e.g., empathy, courage, creativity) during daily life, (2) thinking of three good things that happened recently (as well as their causes), (3) writing a hypothetical positive obituary of themselves, (4) making a "gratitude visit" (i.e., personally telling someone how grateful they are to them), (5) using "active-constructive" responding (i.e., reacting in a visibly positive and enthusiastic way to someone else's good news), and (6) practicing savoring (i.e., taking time to truly enjoy something that they normally take for granted).

The results of this experiment provided clear-cut evidence that practicing positive psychological activities can not only increase life satisfaction but can also alleviate symptoms of depression. Indeed, mildly depressed people who participated in this intervention were no longer depressed (and more satisfied with their lives) as long as 1 year after completing this study, whereas control participants continued to report mild to moderate depression levels.

In the second intervention to alleviate depressive symptoms, Seligman and his colleagues (2006) focused on individuals who met criteria for major depressive disorder. In the first two conditions of this experiment, participants were randomly assigned to receive so-called *positive psychotherapy* (PPT) or *treatment as usual* (TAU)—that is, any nonspecific traditional strategy that the therapist found appropriate. Additionally, a third nonrandomized condition, *treatment as usual plus medication* (TAUMED),[4] was included to compare receiving the combination of traditional therapy and drug therapy with the PPT group and the TAU group, respectively.

Unlike the first study, which used a group approach to therapy, participants in this study met individually with a therapist in 14 sessions that took place over 12 weeks or less. Although the therapy sessions were tailored to each client's specific issues and needs, for clients who received PPT the therapist followed a protocol written and designed by Rashid and Seligman (in press). Generally speaking, the key distinction between PPT and TAU (or TAUMED) was a focus on positive, rather than negative, circumstances, behaviors, and emotions (for further details, see Seligman et al., 2006).

Again, the results of this study provided support for the use of positive psychological techniques in efforts to lift symptoms of mental disorders. Not only did PPT work to decrease symptoms of depression (as well as to increase happiness), it actually proved to be more effective than traditional therapy (the TAU group) and than traditional therapy used in conjunction with drug therapy (the TAUMED group). Furthermore, PPT led to higher remission rates relative to both TAU and TAUMED conditions.

Thus, initial evidence supports the contention that positive psychological practices can effectively combat mental disorders such as depression, in addition to boosting levels of happiness in clinical populations (for additional examples of positive psychological therapies, see Compton, 2004; Frisch, 2005; Lopez et al., 2004; Wong, 2006). We propose that the same mechanism that triggers increases in happiness in nonclinical samples also operates to decrease maladaptive symptoms, such as anxiety and depression, in clinical samples. That is, one potential explanation for these findings is that positive practices have the ability to change (for the better) how people perceive their social worlds. This thesis—that positive construals have an impact on happiness—is, of course, entirely consistent with theories of depression that suggest that negative interpretations of life circumstances contribute to depressed mood (Abramson, Metalsky, & Alloy, 1989; Beck, 1967, 1991).

Indeed, the construal model of happiness converges well with clinical interventions that have alleviated ill-being by focusing on positive human attributes and behaviors. The success of such interventions points to the importance of jump-starting positive thoughts and experiences in order to shift ingrained negative cognitions and enhance well-being (Fredrickson, 2001). For example, Fava and colleagues (1998, 2005) attempt to reframe clients' negative cognitions about positive circumstances and experiences (e.g., "He only asked me out because he wanted to meet my friend" or "She offered me the promotion because no one else wanted it"), whereas Seligman and colleagues (2006) ask participants to practice positive strategies (e.g., using active-constructive logic and thinking about good things) that should combat negative thinking. Both activities draw on changing perceptions, interpretations, and construals.

Happiness-elevating activities such as practicing optimism, expressing gratitude, or committing acts of kindness can also be used alone or in conjunction with psychotherapies or pharmacological therapies to alleviate affective disorders. By promoting adaptive construals that may lead to gains in well-being (e.g., "I've been a very fortunate person" or "My future goals are more attainable than I had thought"), such activities offer a valuable approach to tackling maladaptive construals that fuel depressed mood. As described above, several studies have already employed positive psychological strategies to alleviate problematic thoughts and behaviors symptomatic of clinical and subclinical depression and anxiety (in addition to successfully increasing happiness). Although it is not yet clear precisely how these activities "work," changes in construals are likely to play a critical role (Lyubomirsky et al., 2009).

## CONCLUSIONS AND FUTURE QUESTIONS

Although research is beginning to reveal the applications of happiness interventions in both nonclinical and clinical settings, we are still a long way from fully understanding *when* positive psychological practices should be implemented to optimize their effects and *how* these activities actually work to increase happiness and mitigate disorders such as major depression. For example, Fava and colleagues (1998, 2005) have noted that practicing positive strategies can be most effective in the residual phase of affective disorders; however, other researchers have demonstrated that positive psychotherapies may be used as the primary form of treatment (Seligman et al., 2006). Furthermore, much more work is needed to directly test the critical mediators underlying the effectiveness of happiness-enhancing activities in alleviating depression—namely, variables such as positive construals (Lyubomirsky, 2001) and increases in positive emotions (cf. Lyubomirsky, Dickerhoof, et al., 2007). Finally, the value of applying happiness interventions to other mental disorders with an affective component, such as addictions, eating disorders, and personality disorders, remains an open question for future research.

Future research in this area should focus on understanding the precise mechanisms through which positive psychological strategies produce gains in happiness and reduce symptoms of affective disorders. It is not enough to know which practices improve happiness and alleviate distress and pathology; rather, we need to understand the specific processes that account for such effects. To the extent that this aim is realized, researchers will be able to optimize positive psychological practices to make people happier and to help those suffering from affective disorders to achieve a higher and lasting level of well-being.

## NOTES

1. Notably, although personality and well-being are related to one another and both are fairly stable, research suggests that these two constructs are empirically distinct and that personality traits appear to be stabler than PA and NA (Vaidya, Gray, Haig, & Watson, 2002).

2. Because the quality of life circumstances (low, medium, and high) were judged by the participants themselves (as opposed to independent observers), this bottom-up factor presumably has an added subjective component here.
3. Our preliminary research findings suggest that adaptive cognitive strategies (e.g., expressing gratitude and optimism) improve the way in which people construe their environments, which ultimately leads to gains in well-being. However, it is also plausible that such cognitive activities may create an influx of positive experiences or encounters (e.g., practicing optimism may help people achieve goals, or expressing gratitude may improve social relationships), which may also act to increase well-being. Future interventions to increase happiness need to explore and distinguish these two potential mediators—positive change in thoughts (i.e., subjective change in circumstances) and positive change in experiences (i.e., objective change in circumstances).
4. Random assignment was not used in the TAUMED group due to ethical concerns about administering medication without acknowledging clients' preferences for drug treatment.

## REFERENCES


Abramson, L. Y., Metalsky, G. I., & Alloy, L. B. (1989). Hopelessness depression: A theory-based subtype of depression. *Psychological Review, 96*, 358–372.

Ahmed, M., & Boisvert, C. M. (2006). Using positive psychology with special mental health populations. *American Psychologist, 61*, 333–335.

Allport, G. W. (1955). *Becoming: Basic considerations for a psychology of personality.* New Haven, CT: Yale University Press.

Andrews, F. M., & Withey, S. B. (1976). *Social indicators of well-being: America's perception of life quality.* New York: Plenum Press.

Argyle, M. (1987). *The psychology of happiness.* London: Methuen.

Bandura, A. (1997). *Self-efficacy: The exercise of control.* New York: Freeman.

Beck, A. T. (1967). *Depression: Clinical, experimental, and theoretical aspects.* New York: Harper & Row.

Beck, A. T. (1991). Cognitive therapy: A 30-year retrospective. *American Psychologist, 46*, 368–375.

Beck, A. T., Rush, A. J., Shaw, B. F., & Emery, G. (1979). *Cognitive therapy of depression: A treatment manual.* New York: Guilford Press.

Brief, A. P., Butcher, A. H., George, J. M., & Link, K. E. (1993). Integrating bottom-up and top-down theories of subjective well-being: The case of health. *Journal of Personality and Social Psychology, 64*, 646–653.

Brown, T. A., Chorpita, B. F., & Barlow, D. H. (1998). Structural relationships among dimensions of the DSM-IV anxiety and mood disorders and dimensions of negative affect, positive affect, and autonomic arousal. *Journal of Abnormal Psychology, 107*, 179–192.

Campbell, A. (1981). *The sense of well-being in America.* New York: McGraw-Hill.

Campbell, A., Converse, P. E., & Rodgers, W. L. (1976). The quality of American life: Perceptions, evaluations, and satisfactions. New York: Sage.

Chorpita, B. F., Plummer, C. P., & Moffitt, C. (2000). Relations of tripartite dimensions of emotion to childhood anxiety and mood disorders. *Journal of Abnormal Child Psychology, 28*, 299–310.

Compton, W. C. (2004). *An introduction to positive psychology.* Belmont, CA: Wadsworth.

Costa, P. T., Jr., & McCrae, R. R. (1980). Influence of extraversion and neuroticism on subjective well-being: Happy and unhappy people. *Journal of Personality and Social Psychology, 38*, 668–678.

Costa, P. T., Jr., McCrae, R. R., & Zonderman, A. B. (1987). Environmental and dispositional influences on well-being: Longitudinal follow-up of an American national sample. *British Journal of Psychology, 78*, 299–306.

Davidson, R. J. (1993). The neuropsychology of emotion and affective style. In M. Lewis & J. M. Haviland (Eds.), *Handbook of emotion* (pp. 143–154). New York: Guilford Press.

Dickerhoof, R., & Lyubomirsky, S. (2008). [*Mediators of the effect of expressing optimism and gratitude on well-being and depressive symptoms*]. Unpublished raw data.

Diener, E. (1984). Subjective well-being. *Psychological Bulletin, 95*, 542–575.

Diener, E. (2000). Subjective well-being: The science of happiness and a proposal for a national index. *American Psychologist, 55*, 34–43.

Diener, E., Larsen, R. J., & Emmons, R. A. (1984). Person × situation interactions: Choice of situations and congruence response models. *Journal of Personality and Social Psychology, 47*, 580–592.

Diener, E., Suh, E. M., Lucas, R. E., & Smith, H. L. (1999). Subjective well-being: Three decades of progress. *Psychological Bulletin, 125*, 276–302.

Emmons, R. A., & Diener, E. (1985). Personality correlates of subjective well-being. *Personality and Social Psychology Bulletin, 11*, 89–97.

Emmons, R. A., Diener, E., & Larsen, R. J. (1986). Choice and avoidance of everyday situations and affect congruence: Two models of reciprocal interactionism. *Journal of Personality and Social Psychology, 51*, 815–826.

Emmons, R. A., & McCullough, M. E. (2003). Counting blessings versus burdens: An experimental investigation of gratitude and subjective well-being in daily life. *Journal of Personality and Social Psychology, 84*, 377–389.

Fava, G. A., Rafanelli, C., Cazzaro, M., Conti, S., & Grandi, S. (1998). Well-being therapy: A novel psychotherapeutic approach for residual symptoms of affective disorders. *Psychological Medicine, 28*, 475–480.

Fava, G. A., Ruini, C., Rafanelli, C., Finos, L., Salmaso, L., Mangelli, L., et al. (2005). Well-being therapy of generalized anxiety disorder. *Psychotherapy and Psychosomatics, 74*, 26–30.

Folkman, S. (1997). Positive psychological states and coping with severe stress. *Social Science and Medicine, 45*, 1207–1221.

Fordyce, M. W. (1977). Development of a program to increase happiness. *Journal of Counseling Psychology, 24*, 511–521.

Fordyce, M. W. (1983). A program to increase happiness: Further studies. *Journal of Counseling Psychology, 30*, 483–498.

Fredrickson, B. L. (2001). The role of positive emotions in positive psychology: The broaden-and-build theory of positive emotions. *American Psychologist, 56*, 218–226.

Fredrickson, B. L., & Levenson, R. W. (1998). Positive emotions speed recovery from the cardiovascular sequelae of negative emotions. *Cognition and Emotion, 12*, 191–220.

Fredrickson, B. L., Mancuso, R. A., Branigan, C., & Tugade, M. M. (2000). The undoing effect of positive emotions. *Motivation and Emotion, 24*, 237–258.

Frisch, M. B. (2005). *Quality of life therapy: Applying a life satisfaction approach to positive psychology and cognitive therapy*. New York: Wiley.

Grob, A., Stetsenko, A., Sabatier, C., Botcheva, L., & Macek, P. (1999). A cross-national model of subjective well-being in adolescence. In F. D. Alsaker, A. Flammer, & N. Bodmer (Eds.), *The adolescent experience: European and American adolescents in the 1990s* (pp. 115–130). New York: Erlbaum.

Headey, B., & Wearing, A. (1989). Personality, life events, and subjective well-being: Toward a dynamic equilibrium model. *Journal of Personality and Social Psychology, 57*, 731–739.

Kashdan, T. B. (2002). The neglected relationship between social interaction anxiety and hedonic deficits: Differentiation from depressive symptoms. *Journal of Anxiety Disorders, 18*, 719–730.

Lichter, S., Hayes, K., & Kammann, R. (1980). Increasing happiness through cognitive retraining. *New Zealand Psychologist, 9*, 57–64.

Lopez, S. J., Snyder, C. R., Magyar-Moe, J. L., Edwards, L. M., Pedrotti, J. T., Janowski, K., et al. (2004). Strategies for accentuating hope. In P. A. Linley & S. Joseph (Eds.), *Positive psychology in practice* (pp. 388–404). Hoboken, NJ: Wiley.

Lucas, R. E., Diener, E., & Suh, E. M. (1996). Discriminant validity of well-being measures. *Journal of Personality and Social Psychology, 71*, 616–628.

Lykken, D., & Tellegen, A. (1996). Happiness is a stochastic phenomenon. *Psychological Science, 7,* 186–189.

Lyubomirsky, S. (2001). Why are some people happier than others? The role of cognitive and motivational processes in well-being. *American Psychologist, 56,* 239–249.

Lyubomirsky, S., Boehm, J. K., Kasri, F., & Zehm, K. (2010). *The cognitive and hedonic costs of dwelling on achievement-related negative experiences.* Manuscript submitted for publication.

Lyubomirsky, S., Caldwell, N. D., & Nolen-Hoeksema, S. (1998). Effects of ruminative and distracting responses to depressed mood on retrieval of autobiographical memories. *Journal of Personality and Social Psychology, 75,* 166–177.

Lyubomirsky, S., Dickerhoof, R., Boehm, J. K., & Sheldon, K. M. (2009). *Becoming happier takes both a will and a proper way: An experimental longitudinal intervention to boost well-being.* Manuscript submitted for publication.

Lyubomirsky, S., King, L., & Diener, E. (2005). The benefits of frequent positive affect: Does happiness lead to success? *Psychological Bulletin, 131,* 803–855.

Lyubomirsky, S., & Lepper, H. S. (1999). A measure of subjective happiness: Preliminary reliability and construct validation. *Social Indicators Research, 46,* 137–155.

Lyubomirsky, S., & Ross, L. (1997). Hedonic consequences of social comparison: A contrast of happy and unhappy people. *Journal of Personality and Social Psychology, 73,* 1141–1157.

Lyubomirsky, S., Sheldon, K. M., & Schkade, D. (2005). Pursuing happiness: The architecture of sustainable change. *Review of General Psychology, 9,* 111–131.

Lyubomirsky, S., Tkach, C., & DiMatteo, R. M. (2006). What are the differences between happiness and self-esteem? *Social Indicators Research, 78,* 363–404.

Lyubomirsky, S., & Tucker, K. L. (1998). Implications of individual differences in subjective happiness for perceiving, interpreting, and thinking about life events. *Motivation and Emotion, 22,* 155–186.

Lyubomirsky, S., Tucker, K. L., Caldwell, N. D., & Berg, K. (1999). Why ruminators are poor problem solvers: Clues from the phenomenology of dysphoric rumination. *Journal of Personality and Social Psychology, 77,* 1041–1060.

Lyubomirsky, S., Tucker, K. L., & Kasri, F. (2001). Responses to hedonically-conflicting social comparisons: Comparing happy and unhappy people. *European Journal of Social Psychology, 31,* 1–25.

Martin, R. A., & Lefcourt, H. M. (1983). Sense of humor as a moderator of the relation between stressors and moods. *Journal of Personality and Social Psychology, 45,* 1313–1324.

McCrae, R. R., & Costa, P. T., Jr. (1986). Personality, coping, and coping effectiveness in an adult sample. *Journal of Personality, 54,* 385–405.

McIntosh, D. N., Silver, R. C., & Wortman, C. B. (1993). Religion's role in adjustment to a negative life event: Coping with the loss of a child. *Journal of Personality and Social Psychology, 65,* 812–821.

Myers, D. G. (2000). The funds, friends, and faith of happy people. *American Psychologist, 55,* 56–67.

Myers, D. G., & Diener, E. (1995). Who is happy? *Psychological Science, 6,* 10–19.

Nezu, A. M., Nezu, C. M., & Blissett, S. E. (1988). Sense of humor as a moderator of the relation between stressful events and psychological distress: A prospective analysis. *Journal of Personality and Social Psychology, 54,* 520–525.

Ong, A. D., Bergeman, C. S., Bisconti, T. L., & Wallace, K. A. (2006). Psychological resilience, positive emotions, and successful adaptation to stress in later life. *Journal of Personality and Social Psychology, 91,* 730–749.

Parloff, M. B., Kelman, H. C., & Frank, J. D. (1954). Comfort, effectiveness, and self-awareness as criteria of improvement in psychotherapy. *American Journal of Psychiatry, 111,* 343–352.

Radloff, L. S. (1977). The CES-D Scale: A self-report depression scale for research in the general population. *Applied Psychological Measurement, 1,* 385–401.

Rashid, T., & Seligman, M. E. P. (in press). *Positive psychotherapy: A treatment manual.* New York: Oxford University Press.

Rottenberg, J., Kasch, K. L., Gross, J. J., & Gotlib, I. H. (2002). Sadness and amusement reactivity differentially predict concurrent and prospective functioning in major depressive disorder. *Emotion, 2,* 135–146.

Ryff, C. D. (1989). Happiness is everything, or is it? Explorations on the meaning of psychological well-being. *Journal of Personality and Social Psychology, 57,* 1069–1081.

Ryff, C. D., & Singer, B. (1996). Psychological well-being: Meaning, measurement, and implications for psychotherapy research. *Psychotherapy and Psychosomatics, 65,* 14–23.

Schimmack, U., Oishi, S., Furr, M. R., & Funder, D. C. (2004). Personality and life satisfaction: A facet-level analysis. *Personality and Social Psychological Bulletin, 30,* 1062–1075.

Seligman, M. E. P., Rashid, T., & Parks, A. C. (2006). Positive psychotherapy. *American Psychology, 61,* 774–788.

Seligman, M. E. P., Steen, T. A., Park, N., & Peterson, C. (2005). Positive psychology progress: Empirical validation of interventions. *American Psychologist, 60,* 410–421.

Sheldon, K. M., & Elliot, A. J. (1999). Goal striving, need satisfaction, and longitudinal well-being: The self-concordance model. *Journal of Personality and Social Psychology, 76,* 482–497.

Sheldon, K. M., & Lyubomirsky, S. (2006). How to increase and sustain positive emotion: The effects of expressing gratitude and visualizing best possible selves. *Journal of Positive Psychology, 1,* 73–82.

Smith, M. L., Glass, G. V., & Miller, T. I. (1980). *The benefits of psychotherapy.* Baltimore, MD: Johns Hopkins University Press.

Solnick, S., & Hemenway, D. (1998). Is more always better? A survey on positional concerns. *Journal of Economic Behaviour and Organisation, 37,* 373–383.

Tarlow, E. M., & Haaga, D. A. F. (1996). Negative self-concept: Specificity to depressive symptoms and relation to positive and negative affectivity. *Journal of Research in Personality, 30,* 120–127.

Tedeschi, R. G., & Kilmer, R. P. (2005). Assessing strengths, resilience, and growth to guide clinical interventions. *Professional Psychology: Research and Practice, 36,* 230–237.

Tkach, C. (2005). *Unlocking the treasury of human kindness: Enduring improvements in mood, happiness, and self-evaluations.* Unpublished doctoral dissertation, University of California, Riverside.

Totterdell, P. (2000). Catching moods and hitting runs: Mood linkage and subjective performance in professional sport teams. *Journal of Applied Psychology, 85,* 848–859.

Vaidya, J. G., Gray, E. K., Haig, J., & Watson, D. (2002). On the temporal stability of personality: Evidence for differential stability and the role of life experiences. *Journal of Personality and Social Psychology, 83,* 1469–1484.

Ward, T., & Stewart, C. A. (2003). The treatment of sex offenders: Risk management and good lives. *Professional Psychology: Research and Practice, 34,* 353–360.

Watson, D., Clark, L. A., & Carey, G. (1988). Positive and negative affectivity and their relations to anxiety and depressive disorders. *Journal of Abnormal Psychology, 97,* 346–353.

Wong, Y. J. (2006). Strength-centered therapy: A social constructionist, virtues-based psychotherapy. *Psychotherapy: Theory, Research, Practice, Training, 43,* 133–146.

# 14 Emotions of the Imperiled Ego

## *Shame, Guilt, Jealousy, and Envy*

June Price Tangney
Peter Salovey

In recent years investigators working at the interface of social and clinical psychology have delved into a range of clinically relevant emotions. This chapter focuses on developments in the scientific study of four negatively valenced emotions—two "self-conscious" emotions (shame and guilt) and two "social-comparative" emotions (jealousy and envy), with a special emphasis on the clinical implications of this work. To be sure, social psychologists have conducted vital work on other clinically relevant emotions—most notably anger, fear, joy, and sadness are the emotions most commonly induced in laboratory experiments investigating the influence of feeling states on other psychological processes.

However, we have selected shame, guilt, jealousy, and envy as the focus of this chapter for three reasons. First, these emotions are often encountered in clinical settings. Not infrequently, clients enter therapy seeking relief from troubling excesses of shame, guilt, jealousy, and/or envy. Second, until recently these emotions have received relatively little empirical attention from researchers in the field of emotion research. Much of the initial research on emotion focused on so called "basic" emotions that emerge early in life and that are readily identified by unique facial expressions (thus circumventing the need to rely solely on self-report of internal phenomena). Third, shame, guilt, jealousy, and envy are of special interest to both social and clinical psychologists because they are, above all, "self-" or "ego-relevant" emotions. At issue, in each case, is some threat to the self.

## ARE SHAME, GUILT, JEALOUSY, AND ENVY "PROBLEMATIC" EMOTIONS?

Some years ago we wrote a similar chapter entitled "Shame, Guilt, Jealousy, and Envy: Problematic Emotions" (Tangney & Salovey, 1999). In retrospect, we think we may have overstated the point. All emotions are potentially problematic when experienced too intensely, too often, or in inappropriate and unhelpful contexts. This is most obviously the case for negative emotions. A similar, though perhaps less immediately obvious, case can be made for positive emotions. Positive emotions of joy and pride may be welcomed in the moment, but too much joy or pride experienced out of proportion with the realities of the individual's circumstance or situation (as, e.g., among some individuals diagnosed with bipolar disorder or narcissistic personality disorder) can set the stage for serious problems for the person and his or her functioning in the interpersonal realm. Consider, as well, the social impact of subclinical but obnoxious expressions of hubris, or "pride in self" (Tracy & Robins, 2007).

In our view, such clinical manifestations represent instances of normal human emotions gone awry. In the normal realm, the rich palate of human emotions serves important adaptive functions. All human emotions—both pleasant and unpleasant—provide critical salient "fast track" (near-immediate) information about environmental events important to the person experiencing them. In turn, these human emotions—both pleasant and unpleasant—form the basis of human motivation (Frijda, 2006). Emotions also serve useful social signaling functions—most obviously in the case of emotions that are paired with universally recognized facial expressions (e.g., anger, disgust, fear, joy), but also in the case of emotions marked by easily decoded postural features, such as pride and shame (Darwin, 1872). Thus, although this chapter focuses on clinically relevant aspects of shame, guilt, jealousy, and envy, we wish to emphasize that these are normal human emotions that nearly everyone experiences in the course of daily life.

In this chapter we examine adaptive and maladaptive aspects of these ego-relevant emotions, drawing on current psychological theory and recent empirical work. We consider the implications of these emotions for both individual adjustment and interpersonal behavior in the normal realm. We then examine the special challenges that arise among troubled and distressed individuals—for example, clients who seek therapy—when the utility of these emotions breaks down, and offer some tentative suggestions on how therapists, counselors, friends, or distressed individuals themselves might consider "realigning" problematic experiences of shame, guilt, jealousy, and/or envy into their right and useful place vis-à-vis our relationship with our "self" and others.

## SHAME VERSUS GUILT AND JEALOUSY VERSUS ENVY: WHAT ARE THE SIMILARITIES AND DIFFERENCES?

A significant advance in the scientific study of emotion has been the clarification of emotion terms often used loosely—both in everyday conversation and in psychological writings. Our lexicon for negative emotions is richer than for positive emotions. Nonetheless, people—psychologists and nonspecialists alike—are often imprecise in their use of emotion terms. It is not uncommon to see the terms *jealousy* and *envy* used interchangeably or the term *jealousy* used generically even in situations where jealousy and envy can be differentiated. Similarly, the distinction between *shame* and *guilt* is often unclear in everyday conversation and in the writings of many investigators. But a growing body of emotions theory and research has underscored crucial differences between these often-confused emotional dyads.

## Similarities between Shame and Guilt

Shame and guilt are members of a family of emotions termed "self-conscious emotions" (Tangney & Fischer, 1995). In contrast to the basic emotions (e.g., anger, fear, joy) that emerge very early in life and are characterized in part by unique, universally recognizable facial expressions, as well as evidenced in nonhuman animals, the self-conscious emotions have been described as "secondary," "derived," or "complex" emotions because they emerge later in development, require several key cognitive abilities, and may be uniquely human (Fischer & Tangney, 1995; Lewis, 1992; Lewis, Sullivan, Stanger, & Weiss, 1989).

First, self-conscious emotions require the development of a sense of self—a recognition of oneself as separate and distinct from others. In fact, most emotion theorists believe that a recognized self is a *prerequisite* for emotions such as embarrassment, shame, guilt, and pride (Lewis, 1992; Stipek, 1995; Stipek, Recchia, & McClintic, 1992; Tracy & Robins, 2004; Wallbott & Scherer, 1995; see Barrett, 1995, however, for an opposing view). For this reason, very young children (e.g., prior to age 15 months) do not have the cognitive capacity to experience self-conscious emotions because there is not yet a developed conscious sense of self.

Second, self-conscious emotions require the development of a set of standards against which the self is evaluated, because self-conscious emotions involve not only *consciousness* (awareness) of the self but also *evaluation* of the self vis-à-vis standards. Such standards need not be fully internalized (i.e., owned by the self as intrinsic values and standards); they may rely heavily on significant others in the social environment. But a sense of what constitutes "good" and "bad," "acceptable" and "unacceptable," "desirable" and "inappropriate" is a precondition for experiences of shame and guilt.

Third, shame and guilt are evoked by failures or transgressions in some significant domain. That is, both shame and guilt are *negatively valenced* self-conscious emotions that arise when people recognize that they have violated a standard of consequence. For this reason, shame and guilt are sometimes referred to as "moral emotions" because they presumably inhibit hurtful, socially undesirable behaviors (e.g., Damon, 1988; Eisenberg, 1986; Harris, 1989).

## Distinguishing between Shame and Guilt

Most people do not clearly differentiate between shame and guilt (Tangney & Dearing, 2002). In Western contexts, people are inclined to use *guilt* as a nonspecific term to refer to aspects of both emotions. Alternatively, people refer to "shame and guilt" in one breath, as an inseparable pair of emotion terms.

When people do make a distinction between shame and guilt, they often refer to differences in the content or structure of *events* that elicit shame versus guilt. The notion is that certain *kinds of situations* lead to shame, whereas other *kinds of situations* lead to guilt. There are two types of "situation-based" accounts of the difference between shame and guilt.

First, and most notably, shame has been conceptualized as the more "public" emotion, arising from public exposure and disapproval, whereas guilt has been conceptualized as a more "private" experience arising from self-generated pangs of conscience (Ausubel, 1955; Benedict, 1946). From this perspective, a person would feel guilt about lashing out at a romantic partner at home in private, but that person would feel shame for doing so at a party with family or friends.

As it turns out, research does not support this public–private distinction. In a study of people's autobiographical accounts of personal shame and guilt experiences, there was no difference in the frequency with which shame and guilt experiences occurred when people were alone versus *not* in the presence of others (Tangney, Marschall, Rosenberg, Barlow, & Wagner, 1994). Among both children and adults, shame and guilt were *both* most often experienced in the presence of others, and there were no differences in the degree to which others were *aware* of shame- and guilt-inducing transgressions and failures. In fact, in a study of adults' narrative accounts of personal shame, guilt, and embarrassment experiences, shame was somewhat *more* likely (18.2%) than guilt (10.4%) to occur outside of the presence of an observing audience (Tangney, Miller, Flicker, & Barlow, 1996).

Shame and guilt do not differ substantially in the *types* of the transgressions or failures that elicit them, either. Analyses of personal shame and guilt experiences described by both children and adults revealed very few, if any, "classic" shame-inducing or guilt-inducing situations (Tangney, 1992; Tangney et al., 1994). Most types of events (e.g., lying, cheating, stealing, hurting someone) are cited by some people in connection with feelings of shame and by other people in connection with guilt. Nonmoral failures and shortcomings (e.g., socially inappropriate behavior or dress) are somewhat more likely to elicit shame. Nonetheless, failures in work, school, or sport settings and violations of social conventions are cited by a significant number of children and adults in connection with guilt.

So how *do* shame and guilt differ? The weight of empirical evidence supports Helen Block Lewis's (1971) distinction between these two closely related emotions. From Lewis's perspective, what matters is not so much what was done (or not done) but rather whether people focus on themselves (their character) or their behavior. When people feel shame, their focus is on the self ("*I* did that horrible thing"), whereas when people feel guilt, their focus is on a behavior ("I *did* that horrible *thing*"). According to Lewis, this differential focus on self versus behavior gives rise to quite distinct emotional experiences.

Feelings of shame are apt to be especially painful and overwhelming because the focus is broadly on oneself, as a person—the sense that *I* am unworthy, incompetent, or just plain bad. People in the midst of a shame experience often report a sense of shrinking or of "being small." They feel worthless and powerless. There's also a sense of being "exposed." Although shame does not necessarily involve an actual observing audience present to witness one's shortcomings, people are inclined to imagine how their defective self would appear to others. As in guilt, feelings of shame arise from a specific behavior or transgression, but the implications of that behavior extend to something broader and more enduring. The "bad behavior" is seen as a reflection, more generally, of a defective, objectionable self.

Feelings of guilt involve a negative evaluation of some specific behavior (or failure to act). The failure or transgression is self-relevant, in the sense that the person feels responsible, but it does not carry with it an indictment of the self. With this focus on a specific behavior comes a sense of tension, remorse, and regret. People in the midst of a guilt experience often report a nagging focus or preoccupation with the specific transgression—thinking of it over and over, wishing they had behaved differently or could somehow undo the bad deed that was done.

From Lewis's perspective, the distinction between shame and guilt lies not in the nature of the emotion-eliciting event (type of event, public vs. private), but rather in the way the event is construed. As reviewed by Tangney and Dearing (2002), this "self versus behavior" distinction between shame and guilt has received impressive empirical support from research using a range of methods—including qualitative case study analyses (Lewis, 1971; Lindsay-Hartz, 1984; Lindsay-Hartz, De Rivera, & Mascolo, 1995), content analyses of shame and guilt narratives (Ferguson, Stegge, & Damhuis, 1990; Tangney, 1992; Tangney et al., 1994), quantitative ratings of autobiographical accounts of shame and guilt experiences (e.g., Ferguson, Stegge, & Damhuis, 1991; Tangney, 1993; Tangney, Miller, et al., 1996; Wallbott & Scherer, 1995; Wicker, Payne, & Morgan, 1983), and analyses of participants' counterfactual thinking (Niedenthal, Tangney, & Gavanski, 1994). Most recently, Tracy and Robins (2006) used both experimental and correlational methods to demonstrate that internal, stable, uncontrollable self attributions of failure (i.e., depressogenic attributions) are associated with shame, whereas internal, unstable, controllable (i.e., behavioral) attributions are associated with guilt. Together, these studies underscore that shame and guilt are distinct emotional experiences, differing substantially along cognitive, affective, and motivational dimensions.

## Similarities between Jealousy and Envy

One reason why the words *jealousy* and *envy* are sometimes used interchangeably is that social comparison processes are often implicated in both. In envy-producing situations, a person observes the possessions, attributes, or relationships of another and wishes he or she possessed the object (and that the other person did not). The possession could be, in fact, a material object such as a house, car, or money, but it could also be a human attribute such as an extraverted personality or even a friendship or romance with another person. We feel envy when someone has something we would like for ourselves, and we would like the other person not to have it. Sometimes we wonder, "what is it about this other person that I don't have that allows him or her to have the desired attribute, possession, or relationship?"

Jealousy often has a similar underlying dynamic, though the nature of who possesses what is different. In jealousy-provoking situations, the person actually possesses the desired attribute, tangible object, or relationship, and is concerned that another person will take it from him or her. Once again social comparison is implicated as the person tries to imagine what it is about the other person that would allow him or her to be successful in "stealing away" what is desirable. Often what is "possessed" is a relationship with another person, and the person experiencing jealousy wonders, "What is it about the other person that could lead to his or her success in replacing me in this relationship?"

So, jealousy and envy are similar in that both involve a reflection on one's personal qualities and a comparison with those of another person. In fact, many situations that produce jealousy also have a component of envy in them, as one feels that he or she is not measuring up to another person. Not surprisingly, feelings of anger and sorrow are common in both envy and jealousy, though fear is probably more common in jealousy (Salovey & Rodin, 1986).

## Distinguishing between Jealousy and Envy

There are important distinctions between jealousy and envy, nonetheless. Envy is derived from the Latin, *invidere*, to look upon another person with malice. Envy represents a discontent with and desire for the possessions of another (Salovey & Rodin, 1986, 1989). The word *jealous* is derived from the same Greek root as that for *zealous*, a fervent devotion to the promotion of some person or object. Jealousy refers to the belief or suspicion that what one has is in danger of being lost. When we perceive that a rival threatens the stability of a close relationship and subsequently feel some combination of anger, fear, and sorrow as a result, we usually say that we are jealous. Mere displeasure at the advantages of another *and* the desire to have those advantages for oneself result in envy (DeSteno & Salovey, 1995; Salovey, 1991).

Situations that provoke envy or jealousy are of a specific nature. We do not envy just anyone's random attributes that we have not attained ourselves. Nor are we invariably jealous when our lovers threaten to leave us for just any other person. Rather, envy is most likely experienced when comparisons are made in domains that are especially important and relevant to how we define ourselves (Salovey & Rodin, 1984), an observation first made in psychology by William James (1890). Likewise, jealousy is most likely experienced when an important relationship is threatened by a rival, and we worry that we don't measure up in domains that are especially important to us (DeSteno & Salovey, 1996; Salovey & Rodin, 1991).

Following Heider (1958), we find it useful to conceptualize differences between jealousy and envy using the familiar triad involving persons *P* and *O* and an object or person *X* (Bryson, 1977; Salovey & Rodin, 1989). The crucial factor discriminating between jealousy and envy is whether there is a previously established sentimental relationship between two elements in the triad. Person *P* is said to feel jealousy when he or she believes that his or her previously established unique relationship with *X* is threatened by real (or imagined) attempts between O and *X* to form an equivalent relationship. Person *P* is said to feel envy when person O has a previously established relationship with *X*, and *P* attempts to supplant O in that relationship or tries to denigrate O, *X*, or the relationship between *X* and O.

The terms *jealousy* and *envy* are often used synonymously but asymmetrically; people are apt to use *jealousy* when they mean *envy*, but rarely use *envy* to mean *jealousy*. One reason the term *jealousy*, but not *envy*, is used generically in both romantic and social comparison situations is that there is generally a part–whole relationship between the two. When one compares oneself to another and does not measure up, one experiences envy. But, when one's relationship with another person is threatened by a rival, one experiences jealousy as one imagines the loss of that relationship *and* envy when one reflects on the relatively superior attributes of the rival that have allowed him or her to threaten the relationship. Jealousy is thus used generically because jealousy often includes envy with the addition of other distressing elements as well. Jealousy is the whole, and envy is a part. Jealousy's power lies in the simultaneous threat to a valued relationship and threat to self-evaluation via negative social comparison (Spinoza, 1675/1949).

## SHAME, GUILT, JEALOUSY, AND ENVY: SOME COMMON THEMES

We've grouped together shame, guilt, jealousy, and envy because they share certain psychological features. First, each emotion arises from a comparison with some standard—a comparison in which the individual comes up short. The nature of the comparison varies across these four emotions, but in each case, some aspect of the individual or his or her behavior is found wanting. Second, shame, guilt, jealousy, and envy are each fundamentally *interpersonal* emotions. For example, Tangney et al. (1994) and Tangney, Miller, et al. (1996) observed that the vast majority of shame and guilt experiences reported by both children and adults occurred in social contexts. And by their very nature, experiences of jealousy and envy arise in relation to others. Moreover, shame, guilt, jealousy, and envy all have significant implications for subsequent interpersonal behavior.

Although considerable research has examined interpersonal aspects of these four emotions, the *emphasis* of studies on jealousy and envy differs considerably from the emphasis of studies on shame and guilt. In the case of jealousy and envy, theory and research have focused on interpersonal factors *contributing to* the experience of these emotions. To what degree does the likelihood and intensity of jealous and envious feelings hinge on aspects of the interpersonal situation and the type of comparison being made? In the case of shame and guilt, theory and research have focused instead on the interpersonal *outcomes* of these emotions. What kinds of interpersonal behaviors are motivated by these two "moral" emotions? And how do individual differences in proneness to shame versus proneness to guilt relate to various aspects of social adjustment? We next summarize work conducted in these two important areas.

### The Interpersonal Context of Jealousy and Envy

#### *A Self-Evaluation Maintenance Perspective*

In empirical work on jealousy and envy (e.g., DeSteno & Salovey, 1996; Salovey & Rodin, 1984, 1991), we have found self-evaluation maintenance theory (SEM; Tesser, 1986, 1988) a most useful conceptual starting point. A major premise of SEM theory is that individuals are motivated to maintain or raise their positive self-evaluation. When faced with a situation in which another has possessions that one desires or performs well on some task, two opposing processes are possible. In the first, *comparison*, another's superior performance or possessions lowers one's self-evaluation. In the second process, called *reflection*, the good performance or possessions of another raise one's self-evaluation. That is, we bask in reflected glory (cf. Cialdini et al., 1976).

According to SEM theory, the *relevance* of the other's performance to one's self-definition determines whether comparison or reflection results. If the domain of the other person's performance is self-definitionally relevant, comparison is likely. Reflection follows when the domain is irrelevant. Because, according to SEM theory, we are motivated to maintain (or raise) our self-evaluation, we are apt to bask in reflected glory at our friends' nonthreatening successes in domains not centrally relevant to the self. When self-relevance is high, however, we feel a press to maintain self-esteem by engaging in any of a number of coping strategies, such as negatively reevaluating the quality of the other's performance, disengaging from the relationship with the comparison other, changing our self-definition to reduce the relevance of the other's performance, or actually maliciously preventing the other's good performance (e.g., Salovey & Rodin, 1988; Tesser, Millar, & Moore, 1988; Tesser, Pilkington, & McIntosh, 1989).

We have generated data supporting an SEM view of jealousy and envy in both survey and experimental research. For example, in a magazine survey some years ago (Salovey & Rodin, 1991), we asked respondents questions concerning what attributes were particularly important to them, how they would ideally like to be on these attributes, and how they actually perceived themselves. We measured self-esteem using a standard instrument and then obtained respondents' reports of their likelihood of engaging in a variety of jealous and envious behaviors as well as indications of the situations in which they would experience the most jealousy or envy. Envy and jealousy and the behaviors associated with them were predicted by the importance of a domain to self-definition and by large discrepancies between actual and ideal self-descriptions on the relevant attribute—wealth, fame, being well-liked, or physical attractiveness. Domain importance and real–ideal discrepancies in each domain predicted jealousy and envy in that domain, even accounting for global self-esteem. Real–ideal self-discrepancies were most closely associated with envy and jealousy in those domains rated as most important. A person with a large real–ideal discrepancy about personal wealth, for example, tended to report great jealousy if his or her spouse showed an interest in someone very wealthy, especially if that domain was rated as important. This pattern was particularly robust when the self-definitional area was physical attractiveness.

As another way of testing an SEM model of jealousy, DeSteno and Salovey (1996) conducted two experiments exploring how the characteristics of the rival in a jealousy situation determine the amount of jealousy experienced. To the extent that a romantic rival excels on dimensions identified as especially self-relevant to an individual, that individual should experience greater jealousy, as such an individual would represent an especially great threat to self-evaluation. We presented participants with hypothetical rivals excelling in three domains: athleticism, intelligence, or popularity. Participants were asked to imagine a situation in which they and their boyfriend or girlfriend were at a party and the rival and beloved flirted with each other. The question: Which rivals elicit the most jealousy? According to the SEM model of jealousy, a match between participants' self-relevant domains and the domain of achievement of the rival would maximize jealousy.

In a first study (DeSteno & Salovey, 1996, Experiment 1), participants were most jealous when the rival was successful in the domain that the participant rated as most important to his or her own sense of self. This effect was especially strong when the domain was athleticism or popularity. Now this is not merely a social comparison effect; it is not simply that being compared with a relevant rival makes people feel bad. In fact, when we asked participants how much they liked the rivals, putting the flirtation incident aside, they actually liked matching rivals the most! So, it's not that they are put off merely because someone else excels in a domain that is important to the self ... at least not until that person threatens the stability of a valued relationship.

A limitation of this experiment, however, is that we provided participants with descriptions of individuals that we felt were excellent in the specified domains. However, there was no way of knowing whether the participants conceived of them in the same way. Therefore we conducted a second experiment that used a new set of scenarios, and participants indicated whom they believed to be the most intelligent, athletic, and popular (DeSteno &

Salovey, 1996, Experiment 2). In the second study, not enough of the participants indicated that popularity was the most important domain to them, so we only included participants for whom either intelligence or athleticism was their self-defining domain. Once again, romantic rivals who excelled on a matching dimension elicited more jealousy. Athletic students were jealous when an athlete honed in on a date. The ones who valued intelligence were threatened by smart rivals. And the matching relationship seems "dose dependent." The more important a domain, the greater the jealousy in the presence of a matching rival.

Taken together, results from these studies are consistent with an SEM perspective for understanding envy and jealousy. People appear to be especially vulnerable to experiences of envy and jealousy when the domain of comparison is important to their self-definition, and when there are substantial real–ideal discrepancies in that domain. In other words, our worst rival excels in highly valued areas—particularly those in which we feel ourselves to be inadequate or less adequate.

### *Contrasting Motivations and Concerns*

The situations that give rise to shame and guilt are objectively quite similar in terms of the types of failures and transgressions involved and the degree to which others are aware of the event (Tangney et al., 1994). Nonetheless, people's *interpersonal concerns* differ, depending on whether they are experiencing shame (about the self) or guilt (about a specific behavior). For example, in a study of children's and adults' autobiographical accounts of personal shame and guilt experiences (Tangney et al., 1994), there were systematic differences in people's interpersonal focus as they described past failures, misdeeds, and transgressions, depending on whether they were describing shame or guilt events. Among adults, especially, shame experiences were more likely to involve a concern with others' evaluations of the self, whereas guilt experiences were more likely to involve a concern with the effect of one's behavior on others. This difference in "egocentric" versus "other-oriented" interpersonal concerns likely derives from shame's self-focus versus guilt's more specific behavioral focus. A shamed person who is focusing on negative *self*-evaluations would naturally be concerned with others' evaluations of the self, as well. In contrast, a person experiencing guilt is already less self-absorbed (focusing on a negative *behavior* somewhat apart from the self) and thus is more likely to recognize (and become concerned with) the effects of that behavior on others.

Along similar lines, when people describe guilt-inducing events, they convey more other-oriented empathy than when describing shame-inducing events (Leith & Baumeister, 1998; Tangney et al., 1994). In contrast, people induced to feel shame exhibit less empathy (Marschall, 1996). The acute self-focus of shame may interfere with an other-oriented empathic connection, whereas the processes involved in guilt are more congruent with perspective taking and empathic concern.

The differential relationship of shame and guilt to empathy is evident not only when considering *situation-specific* episodes, but also when considering more general affective traits or *dispositions*. Across numerous studies of children, adolescents, college students, and adults from many walks of life, proneness to guilt has been positively associated with a dispositional capacity for empathy. That is, guilt-prone individuals are generally empathic individuals. In contrast, shame proneness is unrelated or negatively related to other-oriented empathy and positively associated with problematic "self-oriented" personal distress responses (Leith

& Baumeister, 1998; Tangney, 1991, 1995; for a review, see Tangney, Stuewig, & Mashek, 2007).

Not only do shame and guilt differ in the type of interpersonal concerns aroused and in the degree to which other-oriented empathy is facilitated. There is a good deal of evidence that they also give rise to very different motivations or "action tendencies" for subsequent interpersonal behavior (Ketelaar & Au, 2003; Lewis, 1971; Lindsay-Hartz, 1984; Tangney, 1993; Tangney, Miller, et al., 1996; Wallbott & Scherer, 1995; Wicker et al., 1983; for a review, see Tangney et al., 2007). On one hand, shame has been consistently linked with motivations to deny, hide, or escape the shame-inducing situation. In fact, recent physiological research has linked the shame experience with elevated levels of pro-inflammatory cytokine and cortisol (Dickerson, Gruenewald, & Kemeny, 2004), which can trigger postural signs of deference and self-concealment. Guilt, on the other hand, is consistently linked with the motivation to take reparative action (e.g., confessing, apologizing, undoing the harmful consequences of the bad behavior). In short, guilt promotes constructive, proactive pursuits, whereas shame promotes defensiveness and an inclination to sever interpersonal contact. Barrett and colleagues (Barrett, 1995; Barrett, Zahn-Waxler, & Cole, 1993) use avoidant versus reparative patterns of behavior as early markers of shame-prone versus guilt-prone styles among toddlers, behavior patterns that significantly relate to independent parental reports of children's displays of shame and guilt in the home.

## IN WHAT WAYS ARE SHAME, GUILT, JEALOUSY, AND ENVY USEFUL?

### Adaptive Functions of Shame and Guilt

As fundamentally social beings, we spend much of our lives involved in relationships of significance, interacting with people who matter to us. Given such ongoing social interaction, mistakes and transgressions—tactless remarks, unintended slights, flashes of anger, betrayals large and small—are inevitable. Feelings of shame and guilt can serve as immediate, painful feedback that we have "done wrong" and that some kind of action is necessary.

The adaptive functions of guilt are most obvious. As described above, guilt directs people's attention toward their effect on others (vs. the more self-focused concerns associated with shame), thus facilitating an other-oriented empathic connection, which in turn motivates reparative action—confessing, apologizing, in some way undoing the harm that was done. In other words, guilt orients us in a constructive, proactive, future-oriented direction, encouraging us to repair relationships and make changes for the better in the wake of inevitable rifts and transgressions in social life.

Baumeister, Stillwell, and Heatherton (1994) identified several other "relationship-enhancing functions" of guilt. First, Baumeister et al. (1994) observed that, in feeling guilty, people "affirm their social bonds," signaling to one another that the relationship and each other's welfare are important. We feel guilty because we care—an important message of reassurance for those whom we've hurt or offended. Second, feelings of guilt can serve to restore equity in a relationship. Baumeister et al. observe that it is usually the less powerful person in a relationship or situation who behaves in a manner to induce guilt in a relationship partner; concessions or reallocations often follow, thereby moving the dyad closer to a state of equality. Third, guilt may serve to "redistribute" emotional distress. In instances of interpersonal harm, the victim is initially the distressed party. (And in many instances, the perpetrator may experience significant benefits from the transgression.) Guilt can level the emotional playing field. When perpetrators subsequently experience negative emotions of guilt (spontaneously or in response to guilt-inducing behaviors of the victim), and especially when perpetrators express guilt, victims feel *better*. In effect, negative affect is redistributed, so that the affective experiences of victim and perpetrator are closer in valence. As Baumeister et al. point out, similarity breeds empathy and attraction. Thus, the relationship in the moment is strengthened.

The adaptive functions of shame are less readily apparent. Much theory and research has emphasized the dark side of shame (Harder & Lewis, 1987; Lewis, 1971; Tangney, Burggraf, & Wagner, 1995; Tangney & Dearing, 2002; Tangney et al., 2007), underscoring the negative consequences of shame both for psychological adjustment and interpersonal behavior. Why do we have the capacity to experience this emotion? What adaptive purpose might it serve?

One possible function of shame may be in aiding self-regulation via disengagement. Tomkins (1963) saw shame as a means of regulating excessive interest and excitement in early infant–caregiver interactions, the notion being that some mechanism is needed to "put the brakes on" interest and excitement in social interactions when one is rebuffed or ignored, especially at early stages of development (see also, Nathanson, 1987; Schore, 1991). More recently, Dickerson, Kemeny, Aziz, Kim, & Fahey (2004) suggested the utility of shame in fostering self-regulation beyond the social domain—in performance domains as well. Shame may serve adaptive functions by encouraging people to disengage appropriately from goals that require skills or resources they do not possess, or in situations that are uncontrollable (see also, Tracy & Robins, 2006). That is, feelings of shame, and the attendant sense of inferiority, lead people to make the adaptive choice to abandon efforts that are pointless or ineffectual.

A second view, based in evolutionary psychology, regards shame as a relatively primitive emotion that served adaptive "appeasement" functions in the distant past, among ancestors whose cognitive processes were less sophisticated and in the context of much simpler societies (Tangney, 2003). This sociobiological approach taken by Gilbert (1997) and others (de Waal, 1996; Fessler, 2007; Keltner, 1995; Leary, Britt, Cutlip, & Templeton, 1992; Leary, Landel, & Patton, 1996) emphasizes the appeasement functions of shame, humiliation, or embarrassment displays, observed among human and nonhuman primates. In brief, displays of shame and embarrassment communicate subordinates' submission and recognition of offense (deviations from expected patterns of behavior). Such communications reaffirm the relative rank in a dominance hierarchy and minimize harmful intragroup aggression. That is, shame-like submissive displays have been shown to diffuse anger and aggressive retaliation from dominant peers (de Waal, 1996). Furthermore, the motivation to withdraw—so often a component of the shame experience—may be a useful response, interrupting potentially threatening social interactions, further allowing shamed subordinates to escape imminent threats of attack, and permitting parties to later regroup once the conflict has deescalated. In short, from this perspective, shame evolved as an important "damage limitation strategy" in contexts where the likelihood of aggression was high and the consequences were often life-threatening.

Humankind, however, has evolved not only in terms of physical characteristics but also in terms of emotional, cognitive, and social complexity. With increasingly complex perspective-taking and attributional abilities, modern human beings have the capacity to distinguish between self and behavior, to take another person's perspective, and to empathize with others' distress. Whereas early moral goals centered on reducing potentially lethal aggression, clarifying social rank, and enhancing conformity to social norms, modern morality centers on the ability to acknowledge one's wrongdoing, accept responsibility, and take reparative action. In this sense, guilt may be the moral emotion of the new millennium (Tangney, 2003).

Fessler (2007) recently proposed a third potentially adaptive function of shame, this one also arising from an evolutionary perspective. Fessler observed that as human society has evolved, dominance hierarchies have been replaced by "prestige hierarchies." Whereas in dominance hierarchies, an elevated social position is acquired by threat or force, in prestige hierarchies, individuals are selected to elevated positions *by* observers (the lower rank and file): "In short, a dominant position is taken from others, but a prestigious position is given by others" (p. 176). Fessler points out that the "appeasement" functions of shame thus became less relevant as a means of avoiding bodily injury, since prestige competitions generally do not involve physical aggression. Nonetheless, such signs of appeasement may play an important role in modern society by signaling that one is a trustworthy partner who takes seriously social norms. Modern prestige hierarchies rely heavily on cooperative ventures, in which participants risk significant cost by investing time, energy, and/or resources, and by passing up other opportunities, in order to behave in a fashion that will benefit all involved. Thus, the potential for exploitation is high. For this reason, one's reputation as a trustworthy partner is extremely important. Individuals who transgress, but then express clear signs of shame, protect their reputation as a trustworthy potential partner who is still "on the same page" as others. In contrast, the reputations of apparently shameless transgressors (e.g., Bernie Madoff) are severely tarnished. They are no longer attractive as trustworthy cooperative partners. Our sense is that expressions of guilt (especially when accompanied by apologies and efforts to make reparation) can serve the same important reputation-repairing function. The degree to which expressions of shame or guilt are more effective in this regard remains to be examined empirically.

A fourth view is that because shame is such a painful emotion, fear of shame helps people avoid "doing wrong" (Barrett, 1995; Ferguson & Stegge, 1995; Zahn-Waxler & Robinson, 1995), decreasing the likelihood of transgression and impropriety. There is, however, surprisingly little direct evidence of this inhibitory function of shame. Research indicates that guilt, but not shame, is effective in serving a moral, self-regulatory function (for reviews, see Stuewig & Tangney, 2007; Tangney et al., 2007). For example, among felony offenders, an impaired capacity to experience guilt predicts reoffense during the first year postrelease; shame proneness is unrelated to subsequent recidivism (Tangney et al., 2007). Similarly, college students' self-reported moral behavior was substantially positively correlated with proneness to guilt but unrelated to shame proneness (Tangney & Dearing, 2002).

Although shame may not be as effective as guilt in motivating moral behavior across most situations, shame may be useful in some circumstances. No doubt, there *are* instances when individuals are faced with fundamental shortcomings of the self (moral or otherwise) that require substantial and meaningful change. The acute pain of shame and corresponding self-focus may, in some cases, motivate productive soul-searching. The challenge is to remain engaged in introspection and self-repair without becoming sidetracked by the defensive reactions so often engendered by shame. Such adaptive experiences of shame seem most likely to arise from private, self-generated experiences of shame as opposed to public, other-imposed shame episodes, and among high "ego-strength" individuals with a solid sense of self.

Ferguson, Brugman, White, and Eyre (2007) have suggested that the combination of shame and guilt might be especially effective in this regard. She theorizes that "*joint* tendencies to offer repair and apologies (as opposed to *primarily* ruminating about one's guilt or shame) and genuine acceptance of one's guilt combined with meditations about ourselves and how we could improve one's self or behavior (as opposed to externalizing, minimizing, or rationalizing) serves individuals most adaptively in the realm of morality *and* honest self-assessment" (p. 339). In one study, Ferguson found that "the *dual* presence of guilt and shame in the narratives was associated with the most beneficial consequences (and fewest detrimental consequences) than either experience in isolation" (p. 340). (Notably, the beneficial effect of co-occurring shame and guilt was primarily evident when another person purposely made respondents feel shamed and guilty.) In contrast, analyses of dispositional tendencies to experience shame and/or guilt indicate that it is the propensity to feel guilt, absent experiences of shame, that is most adaptive. The propensity to experience *both* shame and guilt is similarly related to less adaptive outcomes as is the propensity to experience shame (Tangney, Youman, & Stuewig, 2009).

## Adaptive Functions of Jealousy and Envy

Regarding envy and jealousy, several intriguing adaptive functions have been suggested. A sociological perspective views envy as having adaptive significance in promoting economic development in (usually developed) societies (Schoeck, 1969). Envy is thought to motivate individuals to better their lot, improve their talents and abilities, and be more productive (Rorty, 1971). Although envy is an acknowledged motivator, admitting to it is still highly stigmatized and so most societies conceive of envy as a necessary evil. This conception of envy emphasizes what Foster (1972) terms the "competitive axis" of envy. Competitive envy underscores wants and desires for the self rather than those things one wants to take from others. Envy expressed in this manner is expected to motivate self-improvement. The denigration of others and their possessions that embodies the dark side of envy is not featured in this formulation. Schoeck (1969) argues that developed societies promote envy specifically to motivate their citizens to improve themselves, and advertising is an excellent window from which to view how societies attempt to motivate individuals to differentiate themselves from those around them.

We can consider this argument at the individual level as well. When of moderate intensity and limited duration, envy can be a motivator. One way individuals can become motivated to accomplish new goals is to harness their envy to energize goal-directed behavior. The social comparisons involved in envy can highlight areas in need of development. Perhaps at first, Salieri's envy of Mozart's obvious talents and productivity motivated his attempts to compose.

A second adaptive function of envy is its potential role in the formation and clarification of one's identity. Most individuals recognize that some situations are more likely to induce envy than others. This emotional feedback informs one about dimensions of self that are especially crucial to one's unique identity. What does one learn when one's envy of a Nobel Prize-winning colleague involves rumination about how one would spend the prize money, but little attention to her new-found fame? It would seem that a core part of one's identity includes a desire for material wealth but not necessarily for the admiration of others.

Jealousy, too, can have adaptive significance; perhaps that is why Freud (1922/1955, p. 32) noted that it is "one of those affective states, like grief, that may be described as normal." For one, it is an early warning sign in relationships, signaling that attention needs to be paid to threats to the stability of that relationship and/or to the self-esteem of a relationship partner. Only in the fantasy world of the Harlequin romance novels is jealousy actually a sign of love itself. Nonetheless, jealousy is a signal that someone about whom we care very much is in danger of being lost. If we never experienced jealousy, we must either be very sure that losing a loved one to another is impossible, or we must not care very much about this partner in the first place.

## WHEN DO SHAME, GUILT, JEALOUSY, AND ENVY BECOME PROBLEMATIC?

Although shame, guilt, jealousy, and envy are emotions that can serve quite a range of adaptive functions for both individuals and groups, there are obviously darker sides to these emotions. When do these emotions become problematic? Intensity of affective reaction may seem the most obvious dimension of importance here. However, although brief flareups of intense jealousy, envy, shame, or guilt can represent unpleasantness for oneself and significant others, these experiences may be short-lived and of relatively little consequence to ongoing relationships and to the mental stability of the individual. Duration and pervasiveness, on the other hand, strike us as more significant warning signs of these emotions gone awry. It is not the intensity of one's guilt that drives one to seek therapy, but rather the number of situations in which one finds oneself feeling guilt, and the persistence with which these guilt experiences eat away at one's peace of mind. By the same token, a brief albeit intense flash of jealousy may simply reveal the depths of one's passion, but chronic obsessive jealousy can become all-consuming psychologically and can even land one in jail.

A closely related issue here concerns the appropriateness of the context eliciting these feelings. A person who is prone to pervasive feelings of shame across a multitude of situations is no doubt experiencing shame in situations that do not warrant such reactions. Daily reactions signaling fundamental flaws in the self are, by definition, overgeneralizations and overreactions to failures and transgressions. Thus, in assessing clinically relevant problems with these four emotions, one must attend more to their *appropriateness*, *pervasiveness*, and *duration* than the short-term intensity of these experiences, per se.

A second set of issues concern people's ability to cope constructively with these feelings and resolve them satisfactorily. A person may experience guilt in an appropriate context, and the intensity of these feelings might be commensurate with the transgression. But that same person may lack the coping skills to express these feelings adaptively and/or to resolve them. For example, college students' reports of "useful" short-lived experiences of guilt were much more likely to involve active reparation of the harm done or a heart-felt resolution to change one's behavior for the better in the future (Tangney, 1996). In contrast, nagging chronic experiences of guilt were not typically accompanied by constructive changes in one's behavior. It seems that some people are more adept at identifying avenues of reparation or change, whereas others obsess unproductively ad infinitum. This may be a useful point of intervention with clients troubled by chronic feelings of guilt. Therapy may include helping distressed clients develop problem-solving skills aimed specifically at identifying proactive solutions or other constructive means of atoning for their transgressions.

Similarly, an effective method of coping with envy is to reframe the domain in which envy is elicited as not as important to one's sense of self. Alternatively, one can develop a multidimensional sense of self so that one can reflect on successes in one domain when another is threatened. The individual chronically smitten with envy is the person for whom all life domains are defined as equally significant in determining one's self-worth. Perhaps it is for these reasons that therapists dealing with envious clients may ask them to fantasize about trading their life for that of the envied other. Salieri may have envied Mozart's profound musical talents. But would he really have wanted to be Mozart, where being Mozart entailed psychological immaturity, physical infirmities, and abject poverty, along with his obvious musical gifts? Salieri might have benefited from this reframing, but, alas, we do not have the opportunity to ask his therapist! One can envy the specific attributes of another, but this envy may resolve when one entertains the possibility of *being* that other person.

## Links to Psychopathology

What kinds of psychological symptoms and disorders are likely to arise when tendencies to experience shame, guilt, envy, or jealousy take a turn for the worse? Research consistently demonstrates a relationship between proneness to shame and a whole host of psychological symptoms, including depression, anxiety, obsessive thought, paranoid ideation, eating disorder symptoms, and low self-esteem (Allan, Gilbert, & Goss, 1994; Cook, 1991; Gramzow & Tangney, 1992; Harder, 1995; Harder, Cutler, & Rockart, 1992; Harder & Lewis, 1987; Hoblitzelle, 1987; Sanftner, Barlow, Marschall, & Tangney, 1995; Tangney, 1993; Tangney et al., 1995; Tangney, Wagner, & Gramzow, 1992). These findings are robust across a range of measurement methods and across diverse age groups and populations.

The research is more mixed regarding the relationship of guilt to psychopathology. In fact, two very different views of guilt are represented in the theoretical literature, and two types of measures are employed in empirical studies. The traditional view, rooted in the psychoanalytic tradition (e.g., Freud, 1909/1955, 1924/1961), is that guilt contributes significantly to symptoms of psychopathology (Blatt, D'Afflitti, & Quinlin, 1976; Harder, 1995; Harder & Lewis, 1987; Rodin, Silberstein, & Striegel-Moore, 1985; Weiss, 1993; Zahn-Waxler, Kochanska, Krupnick, & McKnew, 1990). On the other hand, recent theory and research have emphasized the adaptive functions of guilt, particularly for interpersonal behavior (Baumeister et al., 1994; Hoffman, 1982; Tangney, 1991, 1994, 1995). Tangney and colleagues (Tangney, Wagner, & Gramzow, 1992; Tangney et al., 1995) have argued that once one makes the critical distinction between shame and guilt, there is no compelling theoretical reason to expect tendencies to experience guilt over specific behaviors to be associated with poor psychological adjustment (unless such experiences of guilt become chronic and intractable).

And, in fact, when measures are used that are sensitive to Lewis's (1971) self versus behavior distinction (e.g., scenario-based methods assessing shame and guilt with respect to specific situations), the tendency to experience "shame-free" guilt is essentially unrelated to psychological symptoms (Gramzow & Tangney, 1992; Tangney, 1994; Tangney et al., 1995; Tangney, Wagner, & Gramzow, 1992). Studies employing adjective checklist-type (and other globally worded) measures of shame and guilt find both shame-prone and guilt-prone styles associated with psychological symptoms (Harder, 1995; Harder et al., 1992; Harder & Lewis, 1987; Kugler & Jones, 1992; Meehan et al., 1996).

Jealousy and envy have also been linked to various psychological symptoms. Currently, the only disorder listed in the *Diagnostic and Statistical Manual of Mental Disorders, Fourth Edition* (DSM-IV) in which jealousy or envy is the primary symptom is delusional disorder, jealous type, what was once called "pathological jealousy" (American Psychiatric Association, 1994). In this disorder, the individual is convinced, even in the absence of supporting data, that his or her spouse is unfaithful or likely to be unfaithful. Often, trivial incidents—a partner's slip of the tongue, a piece of paper with a name written on it—are exaggerated and presented as evidence for the supposed infidelity. The delusionally jealous individual often confronts the partner with such evidence and may, in fact, take dramatic actions, such as to telephone presumed rivals, attempt to injure the partner, throw the partner out of the home, or even file for divorce. Such individuals may resort to stalking the partner, or a presumed rival, and attempt to curtail the freedom of the partner to associate with others or to even leave the house.

Although delusional jealousy is the only mental disorder in which jealousy or envy is the primary symptom, these emotions may feature in other psychological difficulties. For example, in paranoid personality disorder, the individual may ceaselessly question, without justification, the fidelity of a spouse or other sexual partner or may be focused excessively and resentfully on the attainments of others. Alternatively, the hypersensitivity to others' evaluation that characterizes individuals with narcissistic personality disorder can sometimes involve extremes of envy. Such individuals generally feel that successful others do not deserve their success, despite chronically envying these successes, and may fantasize about injuring their rivals or in other ways interfering with their rivals' accomplishments. Because such people rarely experience the pleasurable accomplishment of their ambitions, envy of others is often chronic and unremitting. The DSM-IV, in fact, lists explicitly preoccupation with feelings of envy as one of the possible diagnostic symptoms of narcissistic personality disorder (American Psychiatric Association, 1994).

Several empirical studies have examined psychosocial correlates of the propensity to experience envy. Together, these studies confirm that the tendency to feel envy frequently is not a happy or healthy trait. In studies of undergraduates, Smith, Parrott, Diener, Hoyle, and Kim (1999) found that their Dispositional Envy Scale (which includes elements of inferiority and ill will) was positively correlated with depression, neuroticism, hostility, and resentment, and negatively correlated with self-esteem, life satisfaction, and happiness. In a study of 167 employed master's degree students, Vecchio (2000) found that frequency of envy in the workplace was associated with low self-esteem and Machiavellianism (the tendency to be cunning, scheming, and unscrupulous, as assessed by the MACH-IV). In Boone's (2005) study of 154 employed adults, the propensity to experience workplace envy was positively related to depression, paranoid ideation, self-oriented personal distress reactions, and negatively correlated with self-esteem and perspective taking. (There was no correlation between job satisfaction and envy.)

Several investigators have examined adaptive and/or maladaptive efforts to cope with envy. In their larger study of jealousy and envy among undergraduates, Salovey and Rodin (1988) examined positive strategies for coping with envy in the domain of work/school. They identified three clusters. *Self-reliance* includes efforts at emotional control, perseverance, and tenacity in the face of hardship. *Self-bolstering* includes thinking positively about the self compared to others and doing something nice for oneself. *Selective ignoring* refers to minimizing the importance of the envy-inducing event. Results suggested that focusing on one's own motivation (self-reliance) to achieve a goal may be the most effective method of coping, whereas attempting to build up the self (self-bolstering) appeared least effective.

Whereas Salovey and Rodin (1988) focused exclusively on constructive strategies for coping with envy, Vecchio (1995, 1997) attempted to capture the full range of envy coping strategies—the good, the bad, and the ugly. Elaborating on White and Mullen's (1989) research on coping with romantic jealousy, Vecchio identified 12 strategies for coping with envy in the workplace. Multidimensional scaling indicated two coping dimensions: constructive–destructive and engaging others–disengaging from others (Vecchio, 1997). For example, the response "Try to make myself more valuable to my employer" is both constructive and engaging; "Seek social support of a colleague, friend or family member in order to discharge my emotions" is constructive but disengaged from the work environment. "Criticize the successful person to others" is engaging but destructive; "Take mood altering drugs (i.e., alcohol) to cope with the stress of the situation" is destructive to the individual and disengaging from the work context.

Finally, Boone (2005) extended this work, developing the scenario-based Coping with Occupational and Professional Envy (COPE), which assesses (1) the domain relevance of occupational scenarios, (2) the propensity to experience occupational envy, and (3) characteristic ways of coping with envy. In Boone's (2005) study of 154 employed adults, constructive coping styles (both engaging and disengaging responses) to deal with workplace envy were positively related to job satisfaction, self-esteem, other-oriented empathy, and perspective taking. Destructive engaging responses were associated with anxiety, paranoid ideation, hostility, depression, low empathic concern, and difficulties taking another person's perspective. Destructive disengaging coping methods were associated with job dissatisfaction, low self-esteem, anxiety, depression, somatic concerns, and paranoid ideation. Overall, these finding suggest that envy is not necessarily destructive. Depending on one's style of coping, envy can be adaptive, consistent with a functionalist perspective of emotion, or pose serious problems for the individual and his or her social relationships.

## Links to Aggression

Research has shown that three of these emotions—shame, jealousy, and envy—can motivate aggressive behavior. (If anything, guilt appears to be inversely associated with aggression.) In fact, the situations in which these emotions are most likely to come to the attention of clinicians are precisely those that involve aggression or threats of aggression.

Many legal scholars have argued that unbridled envy and jealousy are at the root of much criminal activity. Unfortunately, this issue has received little systematic attention by social scientists. Consideration of crimes of passion is fraught with political overtones. Many commentators (e.g., Jordan, 1985) have noted that the classic crime of passion, the murder of a lover and rival upon discovering them in the midst of a sexual indiscretion, is a myth. Rather, such so-called crimes of passion are preceded by years of psychological abuse and physical battering, and, in fact, very little passion at all.

Nonetheless, homicide committed in the alleged heat of passion is considered manslaughter rather than murder in many states (Dressler, 1982). The American Law Institute's Model

Penal Code still lists manslaughter as any intentional killing committed under the influence of extreme mental or emotional disturbance for which there is a reasonable explanation or excuse. Yet confusion characterizes the courts' interpretation of the law in what are called "sight of adultery" cases. For example, a married person who kills upon "sight of adultery" can be convicted of manslaughter, but an unmarried person who kills under similar circumstances has committed murder (Dressler, 1982). There is no real evidence that "sight of adultery" by a married person arouses any more intense and putatively cognitively disrupting "passion" than that in the unmarried. As Dressler noted, "This rule is really a judgment by courts that adultery is a form of injustice perpetrated upon the killer which merits a violent response, whereas 'mere' sexual unfaithfulness out of wedlock does not" (p. 438).

The psychiatric literature is the source of many case studies of jealous murderers, despite the legal confusion over the proper use and disposition of a "heat-of-passion" defense. Typically, murderers experience intense jealousy immediately preceding the killing (Cuthbert, 1970; Lehrman, 1939). Psarska's (1970) analysis of homicide cases found that in nearly one-fourth, nondelusional jealousy was a causal factor. Among these 38 cases, 16 involved actual unfaithfulness and the remaining 22 cases comprised situations where longstanding marital conflicts developed into jealousy. Moreover, delusional jealousy has been reported one of the leading motives of murderers judged insane (Mowat, 1966). Only a few social scientists have addressed these disturbing trends. Most place the blame on several interrelated factors: (1) societal sanctioning of aggression and battering (mostly by men) in the context of marital relationships, (2) an emphasis on exclusivity rather than permanence in what couples value in their marital relationships, (3) a lack of resolution of how couples should deal rationally with the availability of extramarital sexuality, and (4) unrealistic visions of what can be expected in a normal marital relationship (Whitehurst, 1971).

There is essentially no social scientific literature on envy as the motive for aggression against persons or property, but one imagines such possibilities. Indeed, some have argued that "hate crimes" against ethnic or other minority group members are, at times, motivated by (often false) perceptions of the growing power of such individuals vis-à-vis the majority group and an envy of this power (or, perhaps, a jealous guarding of one's own power).

There also appears to be a special link between shame and anger. Helen Block Lewis (1971) first noted the link between shame and anger (or humiliated fury) in her clinical case studies, and empirical studies of children, adolescents, and adults have confirmed that individuals prone to the ugly feeling of shame are also prone to feelings of outwardly directed anger and hostility (Tangney, 1995; Tangney, Wagner, Barlow, Marschall, & Gramzow, 1996; Tangney, Wagner, Fletcher, & Gramzow, 1992). (In contrast, proneness to "shame-free" guilt is negatively or negligibly correlated with anger and hostility.)

Not only are shame-prone individuals more prone to anger, in general, than their non-shame-prone peers. Once angered, they are also more likely to manage their anger in an unconstructive fashion. In a cross-sectional developmental study of children, adolescents, college students, and adults (Tangney, Wagner, et al., 1996), shame was clearly related to maladaptive and nonconstructive responses to anger, across individuals of all ages. Consistent with Scheff's (1987, 1995) and Retzinger's (1987) descriptions of the "shame–rage spiral," shame proneness was related to malevolent intentions; direct, indirect, and displaced aggression; self-directed hostility; and projected negative long-term consequences of everyday episodes of anger. (In contrast, guilt was generally associated with constructive means of handling anger.) Similar findings have been observed at the situational level, too. For example, Wicker et al. (1983) found that college students reported a greater desire to punish others involved in personal shame versus guilt experiences. And in a study of specific real-life episodes of anger among romantically involved couples, shamed partners were significantly angrier, more likely to engage in aggressive behavior, and less likely to elicit conciliatory behavior from their significant other (Tangney & Dearing, 2002).

What accounts for this counterintuitive link between shame and anger? Shame is a painful, ugly feeling that involves a global negative evaluation of the entire self. When people feel shame, they feel devalued. Their sense of self—and self-efficacy—is impaired. And their awareness of others' negative evaluations (real or imagined) is highlighted. This is an extremely distressing experience that motivates people to suppress or eliminate the pain associated with shame. There are at least two routes open for shamed individuals to manage their feelings of shame. The more passive route involves withdrawal—hiding from the shame-eliciting situation. The more active route involves other-directed blame and anger. When feeling shame, people initially direct hostility inward ("*I'm* such a bad person"). But this hostility can easily be redirected outward in a defensive attempt to protect the self (Tangney, 1995; Tangney, Wagner, Fletcher, et al., 1992).

In contrast, feelings of guilt are less likely to invoke a defensive retaliation and anger. Because guilt involves a negative evaluation of a specific behavior, somewhat apart from the global self, guilt is less threatening to the self. And because the experience of guilt is less likely to interfere with feelings of empathy for others, guilty individuals are more apt to take the other person's perspective, thus further reducing the likelihood of aggression.

## CLINICAL IMPLICATIONS

### Shame and Guilt

Because feelings of shame are inevitable in clinical settings, the ability to identify and resolve shameful feelings constructively can be an invaluable clinical skill. Clinicians may find it useful to consider shame-related issues on several levels.

First, given the vast empirical research linking shame proneness to a range of psychological problems (Harder & Lewis, 1987; Tangney, Wagner, & Gramzow, 1992), it stands to reason that clients entering therapy are likely to be prone to shame from the start. Moreover, the context of psychotherapy is, by its nature, shame inducing. People who seek psychological help have essentially identified themselves as deficient, defective, or in some way in need of repair. The process of psychotherapy, especially insight-oriented therapy, then further encourages an acute focus on self—especially the feared, problematic aspects of self. Clients are encouraged to reveal their most painful secrets and flaws. To make matters worse, these painful, shame-inducing revelations are made in front of a therapist who is assumed to be the paragon of mental health. Not only is the *reality* of the therapeutic context likely to induce feelings of shame. Clients' experiences in therapy are often complicated by the process of "transference," typically associated with painful relationships from their past. In their quest for help, clients are apt to import more shame into this already shame-laden situation, and some of this shame may arise from envying the positive qualities (e.g., emotional stability) of the therapist.

Second, client experiences of shame are apt to impact the process and course of therapy in significant ways. The wish to hide, escape, or externalize blame so often associated with shame may be seen in episodes of "resistance" or in negative "transference reactions" (Tangney & Dearing, 2002). Thus, when the flow of therapeutic interaction grinds to a halt, when the client responds to the therapist with seemingly irrational anger, or when the client suddenly and inexplicably misses sessions or decides to discontinue treatment, the possibility of an underlying sense of shame might be considered. Although shame is a common emotion (especially in the therapy room), people rarely announce that they are feeling shame (Lewis, 1971). In fact, shame is one of the most frequently overlooked emotions—by the person experiencing shame, as well as by others in the immediate social context. In treating clients, it is helpful to listen with a "third ear" for shame-based experiences. Clients often provide subtle cues that signal the possibility of shame. There may be an abrupt interruption in the client's account of previous events; the client may have difficulty articulating his or her experience of the moment. There may be signs of discomfort or agitation, nervous laughter, and/or downcast eyes. Other potential markers of unexpressed shame include gaze aversion, face touching, lip manipulation, and a slumped posture (Keltner, 1995; Keltner & Buswell, 1996; Lewis, 1992). Or there may be expressions of disproportionate anger, especially vis-à-vis the therapist.

Third, clinicians can take a variety of steps to help clients cope with shame. Gentle, empathic encouragement to simply verbalize shame-inducing events and associated experiences can help reduce the pain of unacknowledged shame. As clients translate into words their preverbal, global shame reaction, they bring to bear a more logical, differentiated thought process that may prompt them to spontaneously reevaluate their global negative self-attributions associated with the experience. The therapist can further assist the client in making such cognitive reevaluations using key cognitive-behavioral interventions, for example, as described by Beck, Epstein, and Harris (1983) and Ellis (1962), challenging internal, stable, and global attributions (irrational beliefs) that are associated with shame (Tracy & Robins, 2006). It's a fact that most flaws, setbacks, and transgressions really *don't* warrant global feelings of worthlessness or shame.

Another potentially powerful intervention is to explicitly educate clients about the difference between shame and guilt. We have been surprised to find in our clinical work that many clients haven't considered the difference between condemning a behavior versus condemning the self. They hadn't considered the possibility that there might be "good ways" and "bad ways" to feel bad in response to failures and transgressions. Given an explicit choice, many spontaneously shift to more adaptive (and less aversive) behavior-focused feelings of guilt.

In addition, we cannot overemphasize the importance of therapists' empathy, acceptance, and positive regard, especially as clients experience and share significant episodes of shame. By providing warmth and acceptance of the client as a *person*, while acknowledging the client's need and desire for behavioral change (Linehan, 1993), therapists can provide a shame-reducing atmosphere that simultaneously readies the person for change. By responding to the client with compassion and respect, the therapist can encourage new experiences of self-compassion and self-respect—a powerful antidote to crippling experiences of shame that leaves open the possibility of more adaptive feelings of guilt, leading to constructive, proactive, future-oriented change.

Finally, it's worth noting that shame can be a two-way street in the emotionally charged therapy room. Therapists, too, are vulnerable to shame. Most therapists' identities center on being empathic, wise, and effective helping professionals. On a bad day, a therapist may confront multiple shaming experiences—from one client after another. Shamed clients may lash out at therapists in ways that can be shame inducing—for example, questioning their skills or credentials, blaming the therapist for lack of progress, reproaching the therapist for "not really understanding," or leaving therapy altogether. As human beings, therapists may feel shame and/or anger in response to such affronts, and owing to their professional role, may feel further shame for reacting with such negative feelings. Therapists' effectiveness may be enhanced to the extent that they can recognize such negative "countertransference" reactions and work through associated feelings of shame.

### Envy and Jealousy

In addition to problematic experiences of envy and jealousy that may bring clients into therapy, feelings of envy and jealousy may arise in the course of psychotherapy—within the psychotherapeutic relationship itself. Therapists' awareness of dynamics involving clients' experiences of envy and jealousy in the therapeutic relationship can greatly enhance their effectiveness. Clients, for example, may envy the qualities of their therapists that allow them to appear emotionally stabler or healthier than they feel. This may lead to an idealization of the therapist that is not constructive for the course of therapy. The therapist as a model of how best to think about and cope with difficult situations may be an appropriate component of more directive therapies, but only if the client believes he or she could also acquire and master these skills. Clients may want to learn to think and behave in a manner similar to their therapists, but they should not hope to *be* their therapists.

Jealousy in the therapeutic relationship—for example, a client feeling jealous that a therapist sees other clients or is involved in successful personal relationships—likely needs to be dealt with explicitly. Such a reaction suggests problems with interpersonal boundaries on the part of the client and, in extreme cases, may be a symptom of psychopathology, such as in borderline personality disorder. It may reflect a problematic transferential relationship such that the client has fantasies of being in some kind of other relationship with the therapist. Depending on the nature of the therapy being conducted, this transference may need to be addressed systematically.

There is little literature on feelings of envy (or jealousy, for that matter) by therapists toward their clients. It would seem natural that certain attributes of clients—wealth, fame, relationships—might be desired by their therapists. These countertransferential feelings may be meaningful and relevant to the manner in which the client behaves in interpersonal settings more generally (e.g., does the client actively try to provoke the envy of others?) or may be more specific to the private fantasies of the therapist him- or herself. Either way, therapists can enhance their effectiveness by acknowledging and considering feelings of envy and jealousy as they arise by both participants in the therapeutic context.

## COMMENTARY

In this chapter we've described some of the antecedents and consequences of feelings of jealousy, envy, shame, and guilt. These four emotions can result from similar stimuli and can produce intertwined affective reactions. However, investigators and clinicians who specialize in these emotions typically do not consider all four emotions in the same package. Shame and guilt experts do not typically collaborate with jealousy and envy experts along theoretical, empirical, or clinical lines, and vice versa. This chapter emphasizes how a richer understanding of the adaptive and maladaptive aspects of envy, jealousy, shame, and guilt can inform basic theory and research on emotions. Similarly, clinical interventions that draw on an integrated consideration of these "emotions of the imperiled ego" may be especially effective.

## REFERENCES

Allan, S., Gilbert, P., & Goss, K. (1994). An exploration of shame measures II: Psychopathology. *Personality and Individual Differences*, *17*, 719–722.

American Psychiatric Association. (1994). *Diagnostic and statistical manual of mental disorders* (4th ed.). Washington, DC: Author.

Ausubel, D. P. (1955). Relationships between shame and guilt in the socializing process. *Psychological Review*, *62*, 378–390.

Barrett, K. C. (1995). A functionalist approach to shame and guilt. In J. P. Tangney & K. W. Fischer (Eds.), *Self-conscious emotions: The psychology of shame, guilt, embarrassment, and pride* (pp. 25–63). New York: Guilford Press.

Barrett, K. C., Zahn-Waxler, C., & Cole, P. M. (1993). Avoiders versus amenders: Implications for the investigation of shame and guilt during toddlerhood? *Cognition and Emotion*, *7*, 481–505.

Baumeister, R. F., Stillwell, A. M., & Heatherton, T. F. (1994). Guilt: An interpersonal approach. *Psychological Bulletin*, *115*, 243–267.

Beck, A. T., Epstein, N., & Harrison, R. (1983). Cognitions, attitudes and personality dimensions in depression. *British Journal of Cognitive Psychotherapy*, *1*(1), 1–16.

Benedict, R. (1946). *The chrysanthemum and the sword*. Boston: Houghton Mifflin.

Blatt, S. J., D'Afflitti, J. P., & Quinlin, D. M. (1976). Experiences of depression in normal young adults. *Journal of Abnormal Psychology*, *86*, 203–223.

Boone, A. L. (2005). *The green-eyed monster at work: An investigation of how envy relates to behavior in the workplace*. Unpublished doctoral dissertation, George Mason University, Fairfax, VA.

Bryson, J. B. (1977, September). *Situational determinants of the expression of jealousy*. Paper presented at the meeting of the American Psychological Association, San Francisco.

Cialdini, R. B., Borden, R. J., Thorne, A., Walker, M. R., Freeman, S., & Sloan, L. R. (1976). Basking in reflected glory: Three (football) field studies. *Journal of Personality and Social Psychology*, *34*, 366–375.

Cook, D. R. (1991). Shame, attachment, and addictions: Implications for family therapists. *Contemporary Family Therapy*, *13*, 405–419.

Cuthbert, T. M. (1970). A portfolio of murders. *British Journal of Psychiatry*, *116*, 1–10.

Damon, W. (1988). *The moral child: Nurturing children's natural moral growth*. New York: Free Press.

Darwin, C. (1872). *The expression of the emotions in man and animals*. London: John Murray.

DeSteno, D. A., & Salovey, P. (1995). Jealousy and envy. In A. S. R. Manstead & M. Hewstone (Eds.), *The Blackwell encyclopedia of social psychology* (pp. 342–343). Oxford, UK: Basil Blackwell.

DeSteno, D. A., & Salovey, P. (1996). Jealousy and the characteristics of one's rival: A self-evaluation maintenance perspective. *Personality and Social Psychology Bulletin*, *22*, 920–932.

de Waal, F. B. M. (1996). *Good natured: The origins of right and wrong in humans and other animals*. Cambridge, MA: Harvard University Press.

Dickerson, S. S., Gruenewald, T. L., & Kemeny, M. E. (2004). When the social self is threatened: Shame, physiology, and health. *Journal of Personality*, *72*(6), 1191–1216.

Dickerson, S. S., Kemeny, M. E., Aziz, N., Kim, K. H., & Fahey, J. L. (2004). Immunological effects of induced shame and guilt. *Psychosomatic Medicine*, *66*(1), 124–131.

Dressler, J. (1982). Rethinking the heat of passion: A defense in search of a rationale. *Journal of Criminal Law and Criminology*, *73*, 421–470.

Eisenberg, N. (1986). *Altruistic cognition, emotion, and behavior.* Hillsdale, NJ: Erlbaum.

Ellis, A. (1962). *Reason and emotion in psychotherapy.* Oxford, UK: Lyle Stuart.

Ferguson, T. J., Brugman, D., White, J., & Eyre, H.L. (2007). Shame and guilt as morally warranted experiences. In J. L. Tracy, R. W. Robins, & J. P. Tangney (Eds.), *The self-conscious emotions: Theory and research* (pp. 330–348). New York: Guilford Press.

Ferguson, T. J., & Stegge, H. (1995). Emotional states and traits in children: The case of guilt and shame. In J. P. Tangney & K. W. Fischer (Eds.), *Self-conscious emotions: The psychology of shame, guilt, embarrassment, and pride* (pp. 174–197). New York: Guilford Press.

Ferguson, T. J., Stegge, H., & Damhuis, I. (1990). Guilt and shame experiences in elementary school-age children. In R. J. Takens (Ed.), *European perspectives in psychology* (Vol. 1, pp. 195–218). New York: Wiley.

Ferguson, T. J., Stegge, H., & Damhuis, I. (1991). Children's understanding of guilt and shame. *Child Development, 62,* 827–839.

Fessler, D. M. T. (2007). From appeasement to conformity: Evolutionary and cultural perspectives on shame, competition, and cooperation. In J. L. Tracy, R. W. Robins, & J. P. Tangney (Eds.), *The self-conscious emotions: Theory and research* (pp. 174–193). New York: Guilford Press.

Fischer, K. W., & Tangney, J. P. (1995). Self-conscious emotions and the affect revolution: Framework and overview. In J. P. Tangney & K. W. Fischer (Eds.), *Self-conscious emotions: The psychology of shame, guilt, embarrassment, and pride* (pp. 3–22). New York: Guilford Press.

Foster, G. (1972). The anatomy of envy: A study in symbolic behavior. *Current Anthropology, 13,* 165–202.

Freud, S. (1955). Notes upon a case of obsessional neurosis. In J. Strachey (Ed. & Trans.), *The standard edition of the complete psychological works of Sigmund Freud* (Vol. 10, pp. 155–318). London: Hogarth Press. (Original work published 1909)

Freud, S. (1955). Some neurotic mechanisms in jealousy, paranoia, and homosexuality. In J. Strachey (Ed. & Trans.), *The standard edition of the complete psychological works of Sigmund Freud* (Vol. 18, pp. 221–232). London: Hogarth Press. (Original work published 1922)

Freud, S. (1961). The dissolution of the Oedipus complex. In J. Strachey (Ed. & Trans.), *The standard edition of the complete psychological works of Sigmund Freud* (Vol. 19, pp. 173–182). London: Hogarth Press. (Original work published 1924)

Frijda, N. (2006). *The laws of emotion.* Hillsdale, NJ: Erlbaum.

Gilbert, P. (1997). The evolution of social attractiveness and its role in shame, humiliation, guilt, and therapy. *British Journal of Medical Psychology, 70,* 113–147.

Gramzow, R., & Tangney, J. P. (1992). Proneness to shame and the narcissistic personality. *Personality and Social Psychology Bulletin, 18,* 369–376.

Harder, D. W. (1995). Shame and guilt assessment and relationships of shame and guilt proneness to psychopathology. In J. P. Tangney & K. W. Fischer (Eds.), *Self-conscious emotions: The psychology of shame, guilt, embarrassment, and pride* (pp. 368–392). New York: Guilford Press.

Harder, D. W., Cutler, L., & Rockart, L. (1992). Assessment of shame and guilt and their relationship to psychopathology. *Journal of Personality Assessment, 59,* 584–604.

Harder, D. W., & Lewis, S. J. (1987). The assessment of shame and guilt. In J. N. Butcher & C. D. Spielberger (Eds.), *Advances in personality assessment* (Vol. 6, pp. 89–114). Hillsdale, NJ: Erlbaum.

Harris, P. L. (1989). *Children and emotion: The development of psychological understanding.* New York: Basil Blackwell.

Heider, F. (1958). *The psychology of interpersonal relations.* New York: Wiley.

Hoblitzelle, W. (1987). Attempts to measure and differentiate shame and guilt: The relation between shame and depression. In H. B. Lewis (Ed.), *The role of shame in symptom formation* (pp. 207–235). Hillsdale, NJ: Erlbaum.

Hoffman, M. L. (1982). Development of prosocial motivation: Empathy and guilt. In N. Eisenberg-Berg (Ed.), *Development of prosocial behavior* (pp. 281–313). New York: Academic Press.

James, W. (1890). *The principles of psychology.* New York: Holt.

Jordan, N. (1985). Till murder do us part. *Psychology Today, 19*(7), 7.

Keltner, D. (1995). Signs of appeasement: Evidence for the distinct displays of embarrassment, amusement, and shame. *Journal of Personality and Social Psychology, 68*, 441–454.

Keltner, D., & Buswell, B. N. (1996). Evidence for the distinctness of embarrassment, shame, and guilt: A study of recalled antecedents and facial expressions of emotion. *Cognition and Emotion, 10*(2), 155–171.

Ketelaar, T., & Au, W. T. (2003). The effects of feelings of guilt on the behavior of uncooperative individuals in repeated social bargaining games: An affect-as-information interpretation of the role of emotion in social interaction. *Cognition and Emotion, 17*(3), 429–453.

Kugler, K., & Jones, W. H. (1992). On conceptualizing and assessing guilt. *Journal of Personality and Social Psychology, 62*, 318–327.

Leary, M. R., Britt, T. W., Cutlip, W. D., II., & Templeton, J. L. (1992). Social blushing. *Psychological Bulletin, 112*, 446–460.

Leary, M. R., Landel, J. L., & Patton, K. M. (1996). The motivated expression of embarrassment following a self-presentational predicament. *Journal of Personality, 64*, 619–637.

Lehrman, P. R. (1939). Some unconscious determinants in homicide. *Psychiatric Quarterly, 13*, 605–621.

Leith, K. P., & Baumeister, R. F. (1998). Empathy, shame, guilt, and narratives of interpersonal conflicts: Guilt-prone people are better at perspective taking. *Journal of Personality, 66*, 1–37.

Lewis, H. B. (1971). *Shame and guilt in neurosis.* New York: International Universities Press.

Lewis, M. (1992). *Shame: The exposed self.* New York: Free Press.

Lewis, M., Sullivan, M. W., Stanger, C., & Weiss, M. (1989). Self-development and self-conscious emotions. *Child Development, 60*, 146–156.

Lindsay-Hartz, J. (1984). Contrasting experiences of shame and guilt. *American Behavioral Scientist, 27*, 689–704.

Lindsay-Hartz, J., de Rivera, J., & Mascolo, M. (1995). Differentiating shame and guilt and their effects on motivation. In J. P. Tangney & K. W. Fischer (Eds.), *Self-conscious emotions: The psychology of shame, guilt, embarrassment, and pride* (pp. 274–300). New York: Guilford Press.

Linehan, M. M. (1993). *Cognitive-behavioral treatment of borderline personality disorder.* New York: Guilford Press.

Marschall, D. E. (1996). *Effects of induced shame on subsequent empathy and altruistic behavior.* Unpublished master's thesis, George Mason University, Fairfax, VA.

Meehan, M. A., O'Connor, L. E., Berry, J. W., Weiss, J., Morrison, A., & Acampora, A. (1996). Guilt, shame, and depression in clients in recovery from addiction. *Journal of Psychoactive Drugs, 28*, 125–134.

Mowat, R. R. (1966). *Morbid jealousy and murder: A psychiatric study of morbidly jealous murderers at Broadmoor.* London: Tavistock.

Nathanson, D. L. (1987). A timetable for shame. In D. L. Nathanson (Ed.), *The many faces of shame* (pp. 1–63). New York: Guilford Press.

Niedenthal, P. M., Tangney, J. P., & Gavanski, I. (1994). "If only I weren't" versus "If only I hadn't": Distinguishing shame and guilt in counterfactual thinking. *Journal of Personality and Social Psychology, 67*, 585–595.

Psarska, A. D. (1970). Jealousy factor in homicide in forensic psychiatric material. *Polish Medical Journal, 6*, 1504–1510.

Retzinger, S. R. (1987). Resentment and laughter: Video studies of the shame–rage spiral. In H. B. Lewis (Ed.), *The role of shame in symptom formation* (pp. 151–181). Hillsdale, NJ: Erlbaum.

Rodin, J., Silberstein, L., & Striegel-Moore, R. (1985). Women and weight: A normative discontent. In T. B. Sondregger (Ed.), *Psychology and gender: Nebraska symposium on motivation, 1984.* Lincoln: University of Nebraska Press.

Rorty, A. O. (1971). Some social uses of the forbidden. *Psychoanalytic Review, 58*, 497–510.

Salovey, P. (1991). Social comparison processes in envy and jealousy. In J. Suls & T. A. Wills (Eds.), *Social comparison theory: Contemporary theory and research* (pp. 261–285). Hillsdale, NJ: Erlbaum.

Salovey, P., & Rodin, J. (1984). Some antecedents and consequences of social-comparison jealousy. *Journal of Personality and Social Psychology*, *47*, 780–792.

Salovey, P., & Rodin, J. (1986). The differentiation of romantic jealousy and social-comparison jealousy. *Journal of Personality and Social Psychology*, *50*, 1100–1112.

Salovey, P., & Rodin, J. (1988). Coping with envy and jealousy. *Journal of Social and Clinical Psychology*, *7*, 15–33.

Salovey, P., & Rodin, J. (1989). Envy and jealousy in close relationships. *Review of Personality and Social Psychology*, *10*, 221–246.

Salovey, P., & Rodin, J. (1991). Provoking jealousy and envy: Domain relevance and self-esteem threat. *Journal of Social and Clinical Psychology*, *10*, 395–413.

Sanftner, J. L., Barlow, D. H., Marschall, D. E., & Tangney, J. P. (1995). The relation of shame and guilt to eating disorders symptomatology. *Journal of Social and Clinical Psychology*, *14*, 315–324.

Scheff, T. J. (1987). The shame–rage spiral: A case study of an interminable quarrel. In H. B. Lewis (Ed.), *The role of shame in symptom formation* (pp. 109–149). Hillsdale, NJ: Erlbaum.

Scheff, T. J. (1995). Conflict in family systems: The role of shame. In J. P. Tangney & K. W. Fischer (Eds.), *Self-conscious emotions: The psychology of shame, guilt, embarrassment, and pride* (pp. 393–412). New York: Guilford Press.

Schoeck, H. (1969). *Envy: A theory of social behavior*. New York: Harcourt, Brace & World.

Schore, A. N. (1991). Early superego development: The emergence of shame and narcissistic affect regulation in the practicing period. *Psychoanalysis and Contemporary Thought*, *14*, 187–250.

Smith, R. H., Parrott, W. G., Diener, E. F., Hoyle, R. H., & Kim, S. H. (1999). Dispositional envy. *Journal of Personality and Social Psychology*, *25*(8), 1007–1020.

Spinoza, B. (1949). *Ethics* (J. Gutmann, Ed. & Trans.). New York: Hafner. (Original work published 1675)

Stipek, D. (1995). The development of pride and shame in toddlers. In J. P. Tangney & K. W. Fischer (Eds.), *Self-conscious emotions: The psychology of shame, guilt, embarrassment, and pride* (pp. 274–300). New York: Guilford Press.

Stipek, D., Recchia, S., & McClintic, S. (1992). Self-evaluation in young children. *Monographs of the Society for Research in Child Development*, *57*(1), 100.

Stuewig, J., & Tangney, J.P. (2007). Shame and guilt in antisocial and risky behaviors. In J. L. Tracy, R. W. Robins, & J. P. Tangney (Eds.), *The self-conscious emotions: Theory and research* (pp. 371–388). New York: Guilford Press.

Tangney, J. P. (1990). Assessing individual differences in proneness to shame and guilt: Development of the self-conscious affect and attribution inventory. *Journal of Personality and Social Psychology*, *59*, 102–111.

Tangney, J. P. (1991). Moral affect: The good, the bad, and the ugly. *Journal of Personality and Social Psychology*, *61*, 598–607.

Tangney, J. P. (1992). Situational determinants of shame and guilt in young adulthood. *Personality and Social Psychology Bulletin*, *18*, 199–206.

Tangney, J. P. (1993). Shame and guilt. In C. G. Costello (Ed.), *Symptoms of depression* (pp. 161–180). New York: Wiley.

Tangney, J. P. (1994). The mixed legacy of the super-ego: Adaptive and maladaptive aspects of shame and guilt. In J. M. Masling & R. F. Bornstein (Eds.), *Empirical perspectives on object relations theory* (pp. 1–28). Washington, DC: American Psychological Association.

Tangney, J. P. (1995). Shame and guilt in interpersonal relationships. In J. P. Tangney & K. W. Fischer (Eds.), *Self-conscious emotions: The psychology of shame, guilt, embarrassment, and pride* (pp. 114–139). New York: Guilford Press.

Tangney, J. P. (1996, August). *Functional and dysfunctional guilt*. In J. Bybee & J. P. Tangney (Chairs), *Is guilt adaptive? Functions in interpersonal relationships and mental health*. Symposium presented at the American Psychological Association meetings, Toronto.

Tangney, J. P. (2003). Self-relevant emotions. In M. R. Leary & J. P. Tangney (Eds.), *Handbook of self and identity* (pp. 384–400). New York: Guilford Press.

Tangney, J. P., Burggraf, S. A., & Wagner, P. E. (1995). Shame-proneness, guilt-proneness, and psychological symptoms. In J. P. Tangney & K. W. Fischer (Eds.), *Self-conscious emotions: The psychology of shame, guilt, embarrassment, and pride* (pp. 343–367). New York: Guilford Press.

Tangney, J. P., & Dearing, R. L. (2002). *Shame and guilt.* New York: Guilford Press.

Tangney, J. P., & Fisher, K. W. (Eds.). (1995). *Self-conscious emotions: The psychology of shame, guilt, embarrassment, and pride.* New York: Guilford Press.

Tangney, J. P., Marschall, D. E., Rosenberg, K., Barlow, D. H., & Wagner, P. E. (1994). *Children's and adults' autobiographical accounts of shame, guilt, and pride experiences: An analysis of situational determinants and interpersonal concerns.* Unpublished manuscript.

Tangney, J. P., Miller, R. S., Flicker, L., & Barlow, D. H. (1996). Are shame, guilt and embarrassment distinct emotions? *Journal of Personality and Social Psychology, 70,* 1256–1269.

Tangney, J. P., & Salovey, P. (1999). Problematic social emotions: Shame, guilt, jealousy, and envy. In R. M. Kowalski & M. R. Leary (Eds.), *The social psychology of emotional and behavioral problems: Interfaces of social and clinical psychology* (pp. 167–195). Washington, DC: American Psychological Association.

Tangney, J. P., Stuewig, J., & Mashek, D. J. (2007). Moral emotions and moral behavior. *Annual Review of Psychology, 58,* 345–372.

Tangney, J. P., Wagner, P. E., Barlow, D. H., Marschall, D. E., & Gramzow, R. (1996). The relation of shame and guilt to constructive vs. destructive responses to anger across the lifespan. *Journal of Personality and Social Psychology, 70,* 797–809.

Tangney, J. P., Wagner, P. E., Fletcher, C., & Gramzow, R. (1992). Shamed into anger? The relation of shame and guilt to anger and self-reported aggression. *Journal of Personality and Social Psychology, 62,* 669–675.

Tangney, J. P., Wagner, P. E., & Gramzow, R. (1992). Proneness to shame, proneness to guilt, and psychopathology. *Journal of Abnormal Psychology, 103,* 469–478.

Tangney, J. P., Youman, K., & Stuewig, J. (2009). Proneness to shame and proneness to guilt. In M. R. Leary & R. H. Hoyle (Eds.), *Handbook of individual differences in social behavior* (pp. 192–209). New York: Guilford Press.

Tesser, A. (1986). Some effects of self-evaluation maintenance on cognition and action. In R. M. Sorrentino & E. T. Higgins (Eds.), *Handbook of motivation and cognition: Foundations of social behavior* (Vol. 1, pp. 435–464). New York: Guilford Press.

Tesser, A. (1988). Toward a self-evaluation maintenance model of social behavior. In L. Berkowitz (Ed.), *Advances in experimental social psychology* (Vol. 21, pp. 181–227). New York: Academic Press.

Tesser, A., Millar, M., & Moore, J. (1988). Some affective consequences of social comparison and reflection processes: The pain and pleasure of being close. *Journal of Personality and Social Psychology, 54,* 49–61.

Tesser, A., Pilkington, C. J., & McIntosh, W. D. (1989). Self-evaluation maintenance and the mediational role of emotion: The perception of friends and strangers. *Journal of Personality and Social Psychology, 57,* 442–456.

Tomkins, S. (1963). *Affect, imagery, consciousness: Vol. 2. The negative affects.* New York: Springer.

Tracy, J. L., & Robins, R. W. (2004). Putting the self into self-conscious emotions: A theoretical model. *Psychological Inquiry, 15*(2), 103–125.

Tracy, J. L., & Robins, R. W. (2006). Appraisal antecedents of shame and guilt: Support for a theoretical model. *Personality and Social Psychology Bulletin, 32,* 1339–1351.

Tracy, J. L., & Robins, R. W. (2007). The psychological structure of pride: A tale of two facets. *Journal of Personality and Social Psychology, 92,* 506–525.

Vecchio, R. P. (1995). It's not easy being green: Jealousy and envy in the workplace. In R. P. Vecchio (Ed.), *Leadership: Understanding the dynamics of power and influence in organizations* (pp. 542–562). Notre Dame, IN: University of Notre Dame Press.

Vecchio, R. P. (1997). Categorizing coping responses for envy: A multidimensional analysis of workplace perceptions. *Psychological Reports, 81*, 137–138.

Vecchio, R. P. (2000). Negative emotion in the workplace: Employee jealousy and envy. *International Journal of Stress Management*, 7(3), 161–179.

Wallbott, H. G., & Scherer, K. R. (1995). Cultural determinants in experiencing shame and guilt. In J. P. Tangney & K. W. Fischer (Eds.), *Self-conscious emotions: The psychology of shame, guilt, embarrassment, and pride* (pp. 465–487). New York: Guilford Press.

Weiss, J. (1993). *How psychotherapy works.* New York: Guilford Press.

White, G. L., & Mullen, P. E. (1989). *Jealousy: Theory, research, and clinical strategies.* New York: Guilford Press

Whitehurst, R. N. (1971). Violence potential in extramarital sexual responses. *Journal of Marriage and the Family, 33*, 683–691.

Wicker, F. W., Payne, G. C., & Morgan, R. D. (1983). Participant descriptions of guilt and shame. *Motivation and Emotion, 7*, 25–39.

Zahn-Waxler, C., Kochanska, G., Krupnick, J., & McKnew, D. (1990). Patterns of guilt in children of depressed and well mothers. *Developmental Psychology, 26*, 51–59.

Zahn-Waxler, C., & Robinson, J. (1995). Empathy and guilt: Early origins of feelings of responsibility. In J. P. Tangney & K. W. Fischer (Eds.), *Self-conscious emotions: The psychology of shame, guilt, embarrassment, and pride* (pp. 143–173). New York: Guilford Press.

# 15 Social Cognitive Vulnerability to Depression and Anxiety

John H. Riskind
Lauren B. Alloy
Brian M. Iacoviello

Why do some people repeatedly get depressed or anxious? Many people who become depressed become anxious as well. Others develop just one or the other. Do social cognitive factors play a role in vulnerability to these emotional problems? Are there both nonspecific as well as specific risk factors? Answers to these questions, which are some of the most important faced by clinical researchers and practitioners, have been proposed by current social cognitive theories of vulnerability to emotional disorders. The present chapter reviews issues, concepts, and research concerning social cognitive vulnerability to emotional problems and disorders. These factors, and their interactions with stressful life events, can set the stage for the onset, escalation, and maintenance of these emotional problems. We begin by briefly describing some of the basic suppositions of social cognitive appraisal models in understanding individuals' emotions and reactions to stressful events. We next consider the roles of vulnerability–stress interactions, cognitive activation of vulnerabilities, and specificity, as well as behavioral coping patterns that contribute to vulnerability to depression and anxiety. We then conclude with examples of social cognitive vulnerability variables that have been examined in contemporary research.

## BASIC SUPPOSITIONS OF SOCIAL COGNITIVE MODELS OF VULNERABILITY

Social psychological and cognitive emotions theories suggest that cognitive phenomena such as appraisals and information processing play an important intermediary role that comes between situation and response (e.g., Fridja, 1987; Lazarus, 1991; Ortony, Clore, & Collins, 1988; Roseman, Spindel, & Jose, 1990). Such social cognitive models have direct clinical applications that have been elaborated by cognitive clinical models (e.g., Abramson, Metalsky, & Alloy, 1989; Beck, 1967; Beck & Clark, 1997). For example, an individual who attributes unusual body sensations to heart conditions or a stroke will react differently than an individual who does not, or an individual who ascribes social rejection to inherent personal defects is likely to respond differently (e.g., experience more depression) than an individual who does not. Social cognitive models assume that ordinary emotions and pathological states such as severe depression or anxiety are rooted in the same psychological mechanisms. For example, Beck (e.g., 1967, 1976) suggested that the same cognition–emotion links appear to play a role in clinically severe anxiety and depression, and the extremes of emotion are simply "exaggerations of normal adaptive processes" (Beck, 1991, p. 370).

Abramson et al. (1989) distinguished between distal and proximal factors that influence the onset and course of emotional problems. *Distal factors* typically refer to more trait-like dispositional characteristics (e.g., dysfunctional attitudes or depressive thinking styles) to respond to stressful situations in maladaptive ways; such factors might also include habitual dysfunctional ways of coping or responding to others. Distal features of vulnerability set the stage for anxiety or depression at points in the future when the specific stressful events that trigger problems are encountered. Thus, they are seen as a risk factor in the development of future anxiety and depression. In contrast, *proximal* factors refer to more immediate or situation-based thought processes or behaviors that occur very close to, or even during, episodes of pathological emotional states (e.g., an increase in attention to possible signs of rejection). Such proximal factors emerge after distal factors become triggered by stressful events.

## VULNERABILITY–STRESS INTERACTIONS IN DEPRESSION AND ANXIETY

Anxiety and depression often arise from combinations of internal and external factors. For example, some individuals develop high levels of these syndromes after the occurrence of stressful life events, whereas other people develop no significant emotional problems at all. Most contemporary researchers adopt a *vulnerability–stress* paradigm in which the ways that different individuals respond to stressful events depends on their underlying cognitive or interpersonal vulnerabilities. In other words, stressful events (e.g., social rejection, failure, physical illness) can precipitate, escalate, or maintain states of depression or anxiety for some individuals (e.g., see Alloy & Abramson, 1999), but the degree and even direction of response can differ enormously from person to person, depending on their distal predispositions. In conjunction with that, most individuals who are exposed to precipitating stressful events do not develop disorders. Further, when disorders or problems emerge, the specific outcomes differ for different individuals and are not dictated by the precipitating stress alone. For some individuals, stressful events may trigger depression (Brown & Harris, 1978; Paykel, 1982), whereas for others the events may trigger bipolar disorder (Johnson & Roberts, 1995), anxiety disorders (Last, Barlow, & O'Brien, 1984; Roy-Byrne, Geraci, & Uhde, 1986), or even schizophrenia (Zuckerman, 1999).

Thus, vulnerability models are proposed to help explain why most people don't develop emotional problems or other problems after stress, and why those who do develop affliction may differ so much in the particular problems they develop (e.g., depression vs. eating disorder, etc.; Riskind & Alloy, 2006). In some cases, cognitive styles or vulnerabilities may be specific to depression or anxiety, whereas in others, there may be nonspecific, common vulnerability factors that cut across both disorders.

Social cognitive researchers prefer to use the term *vulnerability* rather than *diathesis* because vulnerability can reflect cognitive and interpersonal patterns, whereas diathesis often refers to genetic or biological traits (e.g., Just, Abramson, & Alloy, 2001). Vulnerabilities can be developed before emotional problems and can be seen as premorbid risk factors. Beck (1967, 1976) proposed one of the first examples of a nonbiological vulnerability factor: An individual's cognitive vulnerability to later stressful difficulties is due to maladaptive schemas comprised of distorted or dysfunctional core beliefs, attitudes, and concepts developed from earlier experiences. Although some schemas might contain cognitive content that promotes social adjustment, other schemas are distorted and/or dysfunctional and have a highly adverse influence on the individual's perceptions, interpretations, and subsequent responses to events.

## SOCIAL COGNITIVE FACTORS: A UNIFIED PERSPECTIVE

The etiology of emotional disorders can involve complex interactions between many different factors. Because any list of possible cognitive or social factors is beyond the scope of this chapter, we focus on cognitive factors that have been conceptualized as vulnerabilities and on intermediary proximal processes that may reflect activation of such vulnerabilities, such as biased information processing as well as problematic coping and interpersonal behavior (see also, Riskind & Alloy, 2006). Also considered are developmental factors (e.g., early peer victimization) that have been proposed as antecedents of enduring maladaptive cognitive predispositions or interpersonal behaviors and coping patterns (e.g., dysfunctional beliefs or attitudes) (e.g., Alloy et al., 2004; Alloy, Abramson, Safford, & Gibb, 2006; Gibb et al., 2001, 2006).

Some cognitive vulnerabilities to emotional problems may be evident to outside observers without much effort, whereas others may be latent and detectable only after exposure to stressful events (e.g., Ingram, Miranda, & Segal, 1998; Riskind & Rholes, 1984). Once activated, such cognitive vulnerabilities are thought to influence proximal cognitive processes such as how persons interpret events, make inferences from the events, or remember and plan from the events. Moreover, a cognitive vulnerability can influence depression and anxiety in a broad, nonspecific sense or in a specific sense that is distinct to each syndrome. Thus, any distal vulnerability factors and their interaction with stressful events can potentially differ and manifest themselves differently in important ways for different emotional problems. For example, theorists have suggested that depression is associated with cognitive content and negative styles involving a blanket sense of hopelessness and/or worthlessness (Abramson et al., 1989; Abramson et al., 2002; Beck, 1967, 1987), whereas anxiety is presumed to be associated with content and negative styles related to a sense of vulnerability to threatening or dangerous situations where harm or a noxious outcome is as yet not realized (Beck, 1976; Riskind, 1997).

In terms of proximal information processing that occurs close to, or even during, episodes of emotional problems, some researchers have suggested that depression and anxiety differ in attention and memory biases (Mathews & Macleod, 2005). That is, it has been proposed that depressed individuals show a stronger bias in later selective memory for negative information concerned, for instance, with past failure or loss, whereas anxious individuals show a stronger attentional bias for threat cues ("hypervigilance") at an early stage of processing these cues (e.g., Williams, Watts, MacLeod, & Mathews, 1997). Other recent studies, however, suggest a more complicated story (Bar-Haim et al., 2007; Cisler, Bacon, & Williams, 2009). Indeed, attentional biases have been observed in connection with depression. For example, although anxious individuals may be initially drawn to threatening stimuli, they may then shift their attention away, unlike depressed individuals who have difficulty disengaging attention from such stimuli (Koster, De Raedt, Goeleven, Frank, & Crombez, 2005; Mathews & MacLeod, 2005). As another example, depressed and formerly depressed persons show a bias to attend to sad faces, whereas nondepressed controls show a bias to orient toward happy ones (e.g., Joorman & Gotlib, 2007).

Cognitive vulnerability models suggest that maladaptive cognitive structures such as schemas and styles influence attentional bias. However, several intriguing studies suggest that attentional biases can be directly trained and can alter mood states. For example, individuals can be trained to attend to nonthreatening stimuli rather than threatening ones, and this attentional training can affect subsequent mood changes a short time later (e.g., MacLeod, Rutherford, Campbell, Ebsworthy, & Holker, 2002; Mathews & MacLeod, 2002). It would appear somewhat unlikely that retraining attentional bias alone will have long-term protective capacity for preventing future emotion disorders, but this remains to be determined. Our present central focus is on negative cognitive styles that are conceptualized as shaping information processing that occurs in attention or memory processes for example.

In addition to differences in negative cognitive styles, interpersonal behavior (e.g., withdrawal, confrontation) may also influence the escalation of symptoms (e.g., Joiner, 2000). Recent research, to be considered shortly, suggests that cognitive vulnerabilities may well play an active role in instigating social behaviors and interactions with others that are themselves stressful (Joiner, 2000).

## COMMON AND DISTINCT SOCIAL COGNITIVE FACTORS

Depression and anxiety may have common features that reflect the high degree of co-occurrence or comorbidity of the syndromes. The typically high correlations between depression and anxiety may indicate that they are subsumed by a common or nonspecific negative affectivity factor (e.g., Brown, Chorpita, & Barlow, 1998; Mineka, Watson, & Clark, 1998). However, "common factor" researchers also propose that anxiety and depression are not equivalent. In addition to the common features, such researchers recognize that there are features that distinguish them. For example, hyperarousal may be more characteristic of anxiety, whereas lack of positive affectivity may characterize depression.

Some researchers have proposed that the common or nonspecific features of anxiety, depression, or other syndromes may reflect "transdiagnostic" cognitive features—that is, features that cut across boundaries (Harvey, Watkins, Mansell, & Shafran, 2004). For example, depression and anxiety both typically involve repetitive, often irresistible, negative thinking. Greater knowledge of such transdiagnostic aspects of anxiety and depression may facilitate advances in the prevention and treatment of important features of both emotional conditions

(Harvey et al., 2004). Nevertheless, the majority of contemporary researchers and clinical practitioners continue to believe that it is important to distinguish depression and anxiety and to seek better understanding of their specific as well as common features. Therefore, achieving greater strides in understanding specific cognitive and interpersonal factors may help to elucidate what is relatively *unique* about each of these emotional conditions, as well as help in designing specific interventions that are tailored for each of the conditions.

Many of the cognitive factors have been studied in relation to anxiety and depression seem to be nonspecific, held in common, and perhaps function as proximal factors as well. The belief that one is lacking in control over outcomes may be a nonspecific factor that is characteristic of both conditions (Riskind & Alloy, 2006). Like lack of control, low self-efficacy is related to both depression and anxiety (Muris, 2002), perhaps because it arises from early experiences in which control over the environment was lacking. Similarly, perfectionism has been found to be a common feature of depression and anxiety (Hewitt, Caelian, & Flett, 2002; Kawamura, Hunt, & Frost, 2002). Nonetheless, some evidence suggests that specific dimensions of self-efficacy or perfectionism may provide some discrimination. Muris (2002) found that depression and anxiety were both related to low self-efficacy with respect to managing negative thoughts and emotional states, whereas low self-efficacy over academic performance was mainly related to depression. Kawamura et al. (2002) found evidence of an aspect of perfectionism that is related to anxiety independent of depression, and a separate aspect of perfectionism that is related to depression, independent of anxiety.

Muris, Schmidt, Lanbrichs, and Meesters (2001) found some evidence from structural equation modeling that depressive cognitive vulnerability styles were the primary source of depressive symptoms in adolescents. Self-efficacy was a more proximal mediator of the effects of such depressive styles. Some research indicates that perfectionism may serve as a vulnerability factor for depression (e.g., Enns, Cox, & Clara, 2005). However, this work is in its early stages, and Enns et al. found that perfectionism did not contribute to prediction of depression beyond the effects of neuroticism. Several other extant bodies of research represent programmatic studies of factors that have been explicitly proposed as vulnerability factors for depression and anxiety.

## DEPRESSION

Major contemporary cognitive theories of depression maintain that negative cognitive styles—the ways in which people typically construe their lives—have major influences on their vulnerability to depression. In particular, theories of hopelessness (Abramson et al., 1989) and depression (Beck, 1967) contain a "cognitive vulnerability hypothesis" in which individuals who exhibit particular maladaptive thinking patterns are at increased risk for depression when they experience negative life events.

According to the hopelessness theory (Abramson et al., 1989), people who exhibit characteristic styles of inferring stable and global causes, negative consequences, and negative self-characteristics in response to a negative life event are more likely to develop depression—particularly, "hopelessness depression"—than people who don't exhibit these negative inferential styles. People who exhibit these hypothesized depressogenic inferential styles should be more likely to make negative inferences about the causes, consequences, and self-implications of any particular negative life event they experience, thereby increasing the likelihood that they will develop hopelessness, the proximal cause of the symptoms of depression, particularly hopelessness depression. For example, individuals who are prone to depression tend to attribute failures or rejections to causal factors that are stable or enduring (as opposed to unstable or temporary) and global or all-pervasive (as opposed to highly specific). Moreover, they then infer that these negative events have enduring and pervasive impact on their own lives and mean that they are unworthy or flawed in some way. This negative cognitive style tends to make them much more vulnerable to hopelessness when undesirable events occur.

Beck's (1967) cognitive theory hypothesizes that negative self-schemas revolving around themes of failure, loss, inadequacy, and worthlessness establish a cognitive vulnerability to depression. Such negative self-schemas are often represented as a set of dysfunctional attitudes, such as that one's worth depends on being perfect or on others' approval. When they confront negative life events that impinge on these beliefs, individuals who possess dysfunctional attitudes are hypothesized to develop negatively biased construals of the self, world, and future (hopelessness) and, in turn, depression. Thus, both theories hypothesize that people with negative cognitive styles are at greater risk for depression onset than people with positive cognitive styles because of the former group's tendency to appraise life events negatively.

A large body of research has examined whether negative cognitive styles actually contribute vulnerability to clinically significant depression. Many of the initial studies showed convincing and robust associations between depression symptoms or clinical depression and negative cognitive styles, and some studies showed that the negative cognitive styles predicted depressive symptoms over time (for reviews, see Abramson et al., 2002; Alloy, Abramson, Safford, et al., 2006). Subsequent studies showed that currently non-depressed individuals with a history of past depressive disorders had elevated negative cognitive styles (for a review, see Just et al., 2001). Although supportive of the cognitive vulnerability hypothesis of cognitive theories, these different correlational and retrospective findings do not adequately address the question of whether negative cognitive styles serve as a vulnerability to develop depression, because they are also consistent with the alternate hypothesis that negative cognitive styles are a consequence of past depression.

## The Temple–Wisconsin Cognitive Vulnerability to Depression Project

Importantly, the most definitive evidence for the prospective development of depression has been provided by the Temple–Wisconsin Cognitive Vulnerability to Depression (CVD) project (Alloy & Abramson, 1999). This two-site study has examined the cognitive vulnerability hypotheses of hopelessness (Abramson et al., 1989) and Beck's (1967) theories of depression. Using a sample of college freshmen, this study selected two groups: those at high or low cognitive risk for developing depression, based on the presence or absence of negative inferential styles and dysfunctional attitudes. The groups were compared in terms of the rates of past and prospective depression (Alloy et al., 2000; Alloy, Abramson, Whitehouse, et al., 2006). Alloy, Abramson, Safford, et al. (2006) followed prospectively 347 college freshmen with no initial psychiatric disorders, at high risk versus low risk for depression, based on their cognitive styles, for 2.5 years. Controlling for initial depression symptoms, they found that the high-risk participants had odds of major, minor, and hopelessness depression that were 3.5–6.8 times higher than low-risk individuals during the follow-up. Negative cognitive styles were similarly predictive of first onsets and recurrences of major depression and hopelessness depression, but predicted first onsets of minor depression more strongly than recurrences. The results, then, suggested that the depressive cognitive styles were particularly important vulnerability factors for predicting prospective rates for the *first* time that previously "never depressed" individuals developed clinically significant major depression, and also predicted rates of *subsequent recurrences* of major depressive episodes in individuals with such episodes in the past. Interestingly, although the depressive cognitive styles also predicted first-time occurrence of minor depression, they did not predict recurrences as well. A further interesting finding of this study is that it suggested that the specific cognitive risk factors in depression are different than those in anxiety. Thus, the risk groups did not differ in incidence of anxiety disorders not comorbid with depression or in incidence of other disorders, although high-risk participants were more likely to have an onset of anxiety comorbid with depression.

Thus, both retrospective and prospective data from the CVD project highlight the role of negative cognitive styles as a vulnerability to depression, supporting the cognitive vulnerability hypothesis of depression. Other data from this CVD project have suggested a number of other factors that seem to represent a cognitive vulnerability to depression.

Beck has proposed a refined vulnerability model in which the predisposing beliefs can be differentiated by whether they are primarily "autonomous" or "sociotropic." *Autonomy* refers to an investment in protecting one's independence and control, whereas *sociotropy* refers to an investment in maintaining positive interactions with other people. Beck (1987) hypothesized that sociotropic and autonomous attitudes confer specific vulnerability to developing depression in response to different kinds of precipitating events that threaten these beliefs (e.g., interpersonal stressors for sociotropy and achievement stressors for autonomy). This specific vulnerability hypothesis has received some empirical support, although the evidence for the sociotropy × interpersonal stressors combination leading to depression is more consistent than for the autonomy × achievement stressors combination (for a review, see Zuroff, Mongrain, & Santor, 2004).

## The Role of Rumination in Cognitive Vulnerability to Depression

Nolen-Hoeksema's (1991) response styles theory of depression hypothesizes that individuals who tend to ruminate in response to dysphoria, as opposed to those who distract themselves from the dysphoria, will experience longer and severer depressions. In this theory, rumination refers to "behaviors and thoughts that focus one's attention on one's depressive symptoms and on the implications of these symptoms" (Nolen-Hoeksema, 1991, p. 569). *Distraction*, on the other hand, refers to actively ignoring depressive symptoms by focusing on other, neutral or positive, activities. In support of this theory, several studies have demonstrated that rumination was associated with increased likelihood of major depression and longer and severer episodes of depression (e.g., Just & Alloy, 1997; Nolen-Hoeksema, 2000; Spasojevic & Alloy, 2001).

In describing the expected relation between the cognitive vulnerabilities featured in their and Beck's theories of depression and rumination, Abramson and colleagues (2002) hypothesized that rumination would mediate the effect of cognitive vulnerability on the development of depressive episodes. Indeed, Spasojevic and Alloy (2001) determined that a ruminative response style, as measured at time 1 of the CVD project, mediated the effect of cognitive risk status in predicting prospective episodes of major depression. Moreover, rumination also mediated the effects of other risk factors (past history of depression, self-criticism, maladaptive dependency) in predicting major depression. Further, expanding upon the response styles theory, Robinson and Alloy (2003) proposed that individuals who have a negative inferential style and who also tend to ruminate about these negative cognitions in response to the occurrence of negative life events (i.e., stress-reactive rumination) might be more likely to develop episodes of depression in the first place. Essentially, a negative cognitive style would provide the negative content, but one would be more likely to become depressed when this negative content is "on one's mind" than when it is not. Thus, Robinson and Alloy hypothesized that stress-reactive rumination would exacerbate the effect of negative cognitive styles, predicting the onset of depression. Using CVD project data, they demonstrated that stress-reactive rumination, when assessed at time 1, interacted with cognitive risk to predict prospective onsets of major depression and hopelessness depression episodes. Among high-risk participants, those who were also high in stress-reactive rumination experienced a higher incidence of major and hopelessness depression episodes than high-risk participants who did not tend to ruminate in response to stressors. Among the low-risk participants, there were no such differences.

### Does Cognitive Vulnerability to Depression Onset Also Impact the Course of the Disorder?

As important as understanding factors that contribute to the onset or recurrence of depression is an understanding of factors that influence the course of the disorder. That is, what factors maintain or worsen the disorder, once onset or a recurrence has occurred? Some research suggests that the factors that maintain depression may be different from those that initiate it (Daley, Hammen, & Rao, 2000; Lewinsohn, Allen, Seeley, & Gotlib, 1999). Iacoviello, Alloy, Abramson, Whitehouse, Hogan, et al. (2006) hypothesized that cognitive vulnerability to depression onset would predict a worse course of depression, including a greater number, longer duration, and greater severity of depressive episodes experienced, as well as greater chronicity of the depression overall. Indeed, using prospective data from the CVD project, Iacoviello et al. found that high-risk individuals with negative cognitive styles experienced a greater number of episodes, severer episodes, and more chronic depressions during the study than did low-risk individuals who exhibit positive cognitive styles. This evidence strongly indicates that the same cognitive factors shown to confer risk for the development of depression also predict aspects of its course.

In summary, findings from the CVD project provide strong support for the cognitive vulnerability hypothesis of hopelessness and Beck's theories of depression. In particular, results from the CVD project indicate that cognitive factors, namely, a negative cognitive style and dysfunctional attitudes, can predict the eventual onset and recurrence of depression as well as indicators of its course. Additionally, it was demonstrated that rumination mediates the effect of cognitive risk, predicting prospective onset of depression, and stress-reactive rumination interacts with cognitive risk to predict depression onset as well. Other research has emphasized Beck's distinction between autonomy and sociotropy as cognitive predisposition, but evidence from prospective studies is still scanty.

## ANXIETY

### Cognitive Vulnerability to Anxiety

Cognitive models of anxiety propose that anxiety is related to distorted cognitive appraisals and beliefs that reflect overestimation of threat as well as underestimation of resources for coping with threat. According to Beck's cognitive model, distorted beliefs and appraisals, embedded or derived in distorted danger schemas, lead to the overestimation of the dangerousness in environmental (e.g., rejection or failure) or internal bodily stimuli (e.g., physical cues of a heart attack) (e.g., Beck & Clark, 1997). In addition, Beck argued that each form of disorder (e.g., loss in depression, threat in anxiety) as well as each specific or distinct form of anxiety is related to its own "*disorder-specific cognitive profile.*" For example, social anxiety is related to the overestimation of the threat of public humiliation (e.g., "looking like a fool"); panic is concerned with the perception of imminent catastrophe (e.g., a heart attack or stroke); generalized anxiety is related to widespread overestimation of danger; whereas specific phobias are associated with overestimations of danger with regard to very specific phobic stimuli (e.g., "All dogs are dangerous"). Although the appraisals and beliefs in anxiety may be verbal thoughts, they can also be accessed through memories and imagery (Beck, 1976).

A substantial body of literature has shown that anxious persons and patients report threat-related thoughts and distorted mental images that reflect systematic biases in the ways in which they process and attend to threat-related information (Beck & Clark, 1997; Mathews & MacLeod, 2002). Moreover, as in the case of depression, cognitive therapy outcome trials provide evidence that restructuring maladaptive cognitions produces symptomatic relief from anxiety (e.g., Hofmann & Smits, 2008). Notwithstanding the extensive evidence for Beck's model, most of the evidence for cognitive vulnerability to anxiety is largely based on cross-sectional data (see Riskind & Williams, 2006), and there is more evidence, though scanty, available from prospective longitudinal studies such as those of the Temple–Wisconsin CVD project.

Furthermore, the ability to distinguish anxious individuals from depressed ones with self-report measures of cognition is mixed. For example, Beck and Perkins, (2001) conducted a meta-analysis on both clinical and nonclinical studies and found that depression-related cognitions discriminated depression from anxiety, but anxiety-related (threat) cognitions, as well as worry, did not distinguish anxiety from depression. Therefore, the demonstration of cognitive vulnerability factors for anxiety, as well as anxiety-specific cognitive content that distinguishes it from depression, has lagged the advances in equivalent work on cognition in depression. Indeed, research on explicit cognitive vulnerability to anxiety rather than depression has only recently begin to blossom.

### The Role of Anxiety Sensitivity in Anxiety Disorders

The construct of *anxiety sensitivity* has been explicitly proposed as a cognitive vulnerability factor for anxiety and panic (Reiss & McNally, 1985; Schmidt & Woolaway-Bickel, 2006; Taylor, 1999). This construct, which has received substantial attention in recent years, refers to a person's perception that physiological symptoms may produce adverse or harmful consequences. For example, individuals with high anxiety sensitivity may perceive anxiety-related sensations as signs of imminent physical catastrophe, such as a heart attack or stroke, a catastrophic paralysis of cognitive control, or negative evaluation, whereas those with low anxiety sensitivity experience these sensations as unpleasant but nonthreatening. Anxiety sensitivity is distinguished from most other cognitive conceptualizations of anxiety because it has been proposed to be a stable trait-like premorbid characteristic that may precede the development of panic attacks or clinical anxiety.

Anxiety sensitivity has been found to be associated with several information-processing biases, including interpretive biases for ambiguous body-relevant information and memory biases (Teachman, 2005). For example, false feedback studies have shown that emotional responding occurs to the mere perception of increased heart rate or other physical sensations in the absence of any actual bodily changes (Barsky, Cleary, Sarnie, & Ruskin, 1994; Ehlers, Margraf, Roth, Taylor, & Birbaumer, 1988; Story & Craske, 2008). However, evidence for attentional biases has been mixed (Teachman, 2005).

Prospective studies have shown that anxiety sensitivity is a predictor of future spontaneous panic attacks over time in individuals with a minimal (Schmidt, Lerew, & Jackon, 1997, 1999) or no history of panic (Ehlers, 1995). A number of studies show that individuals with anxiety sensitivity are sensitive to experimental provocations, such as exposure to $CO_2$ (Telch, Silverman, & Schmidt, 1996). In addition, a study by Schmidt, Zvolensky, and Maner (2006) has reported that anxiety sensitivity predicted the later onset or development of anxiety disorders in college students over a 2-year follow-up period.

Although anxiety sensitivity was initially proposed to be specific to panic disorder, it has been found to be elevated in depression (Schmidt et al., 1997; Taylor, Koch, Woody, & McLean, 1996) as well as other anxiety disorders (Deacon & Abramowitz, 2006; Kearney, Albano, Eisen, Allan, & Barlow, 1997; Keogh, Ayers, & Francis, 2002; Taylor, 2003). In addition, anxiety sensitivity or some aspect of it may be a risk factor for depression (Schmidt et al., 1997). In this regard, recent research reveals that anxiety sensitivity can be broken down into several factors (for a review, see Zinbarg, Mohlman, & Hong, 1999). Of these, depression may be related to a fear of loss of cognitive control (Blais et al., 2001; Taylor et al., 1996; Zinbarg, Barlow, & Brown, 1997), whereas panic disorder is related to elevated fears on a somatic sensations factor (Taylor et al., 1996; Zinbarg, Brown, Barlow, & Rapee, 2001), and social anxiety is most strongly related to the fear of negative evaluation (McWilliams, Stewart, & MacPherson, 2000; Zinbarg et al., 1997).

## Looming Cognitive Style

A growing body of evidence also supports another construct, the "looming cognitive style," as a potential cognitive vulnerability to anxiety. *Looming vulnerability* refers to a psychological phenomenon involving anxiety marked by dynamic perceptions of a threatening stimulus as moving rapidly toward oneself in time or space. An anxious person imagines threatening stimuli as an escalating process that is rising in risk (Riskind, 1997; Riskind, Tzur, Williams, Mann, & Shahar, 2007; Riskind & Williams, 2006; Riskind, Williams, Gessner, Chrosniak, & Cortina, 2000). According to the looming vulnerability model, people who are at risk for anxiety can develop anxiety-oriented looming cognitive styles that lead them to habitually form perceptions and generate mental scenarios of possible threats as rapidly becoming more threatening by the moment. For example, people who have social anxiety may have this anxiety partly because they play out dynamic scenes in which social humiliation or rejection is rapidly developing and approaching. Dynamic perceptions and simulations of threat have a behavioral urgency and activate worry and other defensive behavior. Thus, people who exhibit characteristic styles (or looming cognitive styles) of forming perceptions or internal simulations of stimuli as becoming more threatening by the moment (even when they aren't) are more likely to develop anxiety and worry than people who don't exhibit these negative styles. According to this model, looming vulnerability is less specifically related to depression states, which are more concerned with helplessness/hopelessness and passive disengagement and/or accommodation to inescapable aversive circumstances (Riskind et al., 2000; Riskind, Williams, & Joiner, 2006).

Remarkably consistent evidence has been found that the looming cognitive style is related specially to anxiety, even when controlling for depression, but the reverse is not true (Adler & Strunk, 2010; Riskind & Williams, 2006; Riskind et al., 2000). Moreover, consistent with the proposal that the looming cognitive style functions as a danger schema and a vulnerability factor, college students with this style were shown to exhibit a variety of information-processing biases, even when anxiety is controlled. For example, students with the looming cognitive style showed a schematic interpretive bias when providing spellings of tape-recorded homophones, including high-threat words, when more than one spelling was possible (e.g., *die* rather than *dye*), and a variety of memory biases (e.g., pictorial images) for threat information (Riskind et al., 2000). Moreover, the looming cognitive style is a common theme across a spectrum of anxiety syndromes, including social anxiety, obsessive–compulsive disorder (OCD), generalized anxiety, and posttraumatic stress disorder (PTSD) (Reardon & Williams, 2007; Riskind et al., 2007; Williams, Shahar, Riskind, & Joiner, 2005), and is reported across the spectrum of classic anxiety syndromes in clinical patients (Riskind & Rector, 2010; Riskind & Williams, 2005).

The looming cognitive style predicts future anxiety symptom changes over short periods of a week (Adler & Strunk, 2010; Riskind et al., 2007) and longer periods of up to 7 months (Black, Balaban, & Riskind, 2002), and prospectively predicts short-term increases in anxiety (Adler & Strunk, 2010; Riskind et al., 2007) and worry and OCD symptoms in college undergraduates (Riskind et al., 2007). The looming cognitive style also heightens the risk of increased anxiety after the occurrence of stressful life events. Adler & Strunk (2010) found that stressful life events prospectively predicted increases in anxiety for individuals who had the looming cognitive style but not for individuals who did not have the style. But the stress-vulnerability interaction did not predict increases in depression. The looming style is related to previous lifetime history of anxiety disorders, controlling for present symptoms of anxiety and depression, as well as the presence of current anxiety disorders (Black, Riskind, & Kleiman, in press). However, it is not related to previous lifetime history of depression disorders.

In relation to cognitive specificity, maladaptive looming styles can also be seen in relation to specific fears in different anxiety disorders or subtypes. For instance, there are looming styles of fears for spiders, (Riskind & Maddux, 1994; Riskind, Moore, & Bowley, 1995), cancer (Levin, Li, & Riskind, 2007), contamination (Dorfin & Woody, 2006; Riskind, Abreu, Strauss, & Holt, 1997; Riskind & Rector, 2007; Riskind, Wheeler & Picerno, 1997; Tolin, Worhunsky, & Maltby, 2004), and social anxiety (Brown & Stopa, 2008). People with spider phobias appear to spontaneously generate mental scenarios and images of spiders moving toward them. Individuals may experience looming vulnerability in connection with the dangers that they typically fear, but not in relation to other dangers (Riskind, Kelly, Harman, Moore, & Gaines, 1992).

According to the looming vulnerability model, the perceived or imagined movement of phobic stimuli can impede habituation (Riskind, 1997). Consistent with this prediction, Dorfin and Woody (2006) demonstrated that individuals who received instructions regarding moving imagery (i.e., to visualize urine as moving and spreading) after drops of sterilized urine were placed on their arms steadily increased in emotional distress ratings over time. This was in contrast to individuals who received instructions regarding static imagery (i.e., to visualize urine as unmoving from its site of contamination), or safety imagery (i.e., the urine contains no harmful germs), who exhibited habituation and decreased ratings of emotional distress. Tolin et al. (2004) also found evidence that looming vulnerability impedes habituation. They used a different methodology in which patients with OCD touched a clean pencil to a contaminated object (e.g., a toilet) and then touched that pencil with secondary contamination to another clean pencil. OCD patients, as compared to panic disorder patients or normal controls, apparently believed in an endless transfer or chain of contagion from initially contaminated stimulus to other stimuli. Perceptions of looming vulnerability, or the imagined movement of contaminants, fully mediated this effect.

The looming cognitive style and anxiety sensitivity are negative appraisal styles that are considered to be cognitive vulnerabilities for the broader classic spectrum of anxiety syndromes (e.g., generalized anxiety, OCD) and not just limited to any single form of anxiety. Although support for these putative vulnerability factors comes from a growing body of evidence, the work on vulnerability to anxiety is much less advanced than the Temple–Wisconsin depression research project.

Another approach developed by Wells (e.g., Wells, 2000; Wells & Matthews, 1996) contains some elements of self-monitoring and interpretation of internal processes reminiscent of anxiety sensitivity but with a much broader and elaborate focus. Wells maintains that metacognitive processes and beliefs, self-attentional processes, and worry/rumination strategies are central to the development and maintenance of anxiety disorders. *Metacognition* refers to higher-level cognitive functions that are involved in the ability to monitor, control, or interpret one's own thinking. Wells argues that dysfunctional beliefs about one's own cognitive activities can detrimentally guide these activities in psychological disorders. For example, "worry about worry" (i.e., the belief that worry itself is harmful) can lead to a self-focus and intensification of worry and rumination that then traps people in cycles and contributes to an escalation of symptoms in anxiety disorders such as generalized anxiety disorder. Research has supported that particular metacognitions are associated with pathological worry (Wells & Papageorgiou, 1998) and several anxiety disorders, including generalized anxiety disorder and OCD (Wells & Carter, 2001), but also with other disorders, including depression (Papageorgiou & Wells, 2003). Further research is needed to investigate the vulnerability role of metacognitive beliefs.

## Beyond Appraisal Theories

Beyond cognitive appraisal theories of vulnerabilities, another productive line of recent investigation in anxiety research has begun to attend to the self-protective processes involved in the anxiety experience (e.g., cognitive avoidance, avoidance of negative affect). Several groups of investigators have focused on the central idea that the exposure to threatening stimuli causes active patterns of avoidance to arise for negative emotions and internal experience. Borkovec has argued that worry serves as a method of avoiding emotional fear imagery of perceived danger and aversive body sensations (Borkovec, Ray, & Stoeber, 1998;

Sibrava & Borkovec, 2006). He asserts that worry is associated with verbal thoughts rather than imagery, and that it reduces, at least in the short term, cardiovascular arousal associated with emotionally laden fearful images of perceived dangers. A series of experimental and self-report studies provides support for aspects of Borkovec's model. For example, research indicates that verbal thoughts elicit little cardiovascular arousal, whereas images of emotional stimuli elicit a significantly greater response (Borkovec & Inz, 1990; Vrana, Cuthbert, & Lang, 1986).

Other researchers have begun to extend the avoidance function of worry to consider more generally the construct that people engage in experiential avoidance of negative internal experiences in other forms of dysfunctional emotion regulation (e.g., regarding anger or sadness, not just fear). Several researchers maintain that maladaptive attempts to control or suppress aversive emotional experience play a significant role in emotional disorders (e.g., Amstadter, 2008; Mennin, Heimberg, & Turk, 2002; Roemer, Salters, Raffa, & Orsillo, 2005). Such researchers have suggested that "experiential avoidance" of internal experience may be an important causal factor in maintaining and/or escalating generalized anxiety and other forms of anxiety states.

## INTERPERSONAL PROCESSES AND POTENTIAL FEEDBACK LOOPS IN DEPRESSION AND ANXIETY

Any person's vulnerability to depression or anxiety is not just influenced by cognitive processes but also by dysfunctional patterns of behavior and coping. In many instances, the manifestation of such maladaptive interpersonal behaviors ebbs and wanes in a state-dependent manner with symptoms (e.g., some individuals withdraw from others when depressed). However, there may be important individual differences, and some people may engage in faulty avoidance coping or other dysfunctional behavior that increases susceptibility to emotional disorders. For example, avoidance coping (i.e., wanting situations to "go away") has been found to be a predictor of higher rates of future stressful life events as well as depression (Holahan, Moos, Holahan, Brennan, & Schutte, 2005).

Research has shown that depressed or anxious individuals often behave in dysfunctional ways, such as withdrawing from others (Joiner, 2000) or avoiding eye contact, that may be perceived as aloofness or oddness and elicit negative reactions from other people. Joiner (2000) has described how self-propagating interpersonal processes influence episode duration, relapse, and recurrence of depression. Such self-propagatory processes entail active behaviors that exacerbate existing symptoms or that instigate recurrence of depression, including (1) stress-generating behaviors whereby individuals actively produce stress for themselves; (2) negative feedback-seeking behaviors wherein individuals actually seek negative feedback to verify their low self-concept; (3) excessive reassurance-seeking behaviors whereby individuals repeatedly seek assurance, inducing frustration and irritation in others; (4) interpersonal conflict avoidance wherein individuals avoid addressing situations and thus lose social support; and (5) blame maintenance behaviors wherein individuals are continually viewed by others in a negative way due to symptoms of depression despite positive changes.

Having special relevance in this connection, recent studies suggest that depressive cognitive styles, and not just depressive symptoms, actively influence the stress-generation process.

Safford, Alloy, Abramson, & Crossfield (2007) found that negative cognitive styles predicted greater stress generation, controlling for past, current, and future depression. Thus negative cognitive styles can contribute to stress propagation and interpersonal problems, which, in turn, might actually reinforce the cognitive biases and result in the maintenance or recurrence of psychopathology.

A recent study of anxiety vulnerability reports the interesting finding that stress generation may not be limited to cognitive vulnerability to depression. Indeed, a study by Riskind, Black, and Shahar (2010) found that the looming cognitive style and anxiety sensitivity augmented each other's effects in predicting stress generation, after adjusting for earlier levels of such events. Similar to Safford et al.'s (2007) finding, this stress-generation effect seemed to be predicted by the negative cognitive styles, not by anxiety. Like cognitive vulnerability to depression, the findings of this interesting study imply that anxiety-related cognitive styles are vulnerabilities that help to generate interpersonal and other problems, which, in turn, might help to propagate these vulnerabilities, leaving the person at risk of future depression and anxiety.

## ORIGINS OF COGNITIVE VULNERABILITY TO DEPRESSION AND ANXIETY

There has been increasing attention to the possible origins of cognitive vulnerabilities. Several studies emanating from the Temple–Wisconsin CVD project have shown that a history of childhood maltreatment, parental inferential feedback, and parenting styles have a potential role in the development of negative cognitive vulnerability styles. Negative cognitive styles may be, at least in part, the internal representations of actual maltreatment experienced rather than cognitive distortions. For example, a cognitively vulnerable freshman who infers that negative consequences will follow a low grade may be a person who was abused as a child after getting low grades. Rose and Abramson (1992) hypothesized that emotional maltreatment may be even more likely than physical or sexual abuse to contribute to the development of negative cognitive styles because with emotional maltreatment, negative cognitions are directly supplied to the child by the abuser (e.g., "You're so stupid—you'll never amount to anything").

In line with such predictions, recent reviews of studies examining the relation between childhood maltreatment and cognitive vulnerability to depression showed that a history of both sexual and emotional maltreatment, but not physical abuse, was associated with negative cognitive styles (Alloy, Abramson, Smith, Gibb, & Neeren, 2006; Gibb, 2002). In addition, the presence versus absence of a negative cognitive style seemed to fully, or at least partially, explain the relationship between reported levels of emotional maltreatment and prospective onsets of major depression and hopelessness depression episodes (Gibb et al., 2001). Moreover, a reported history of childhood emotional abuse and, for women, of childhood sexual abuse was related to a ruminative response style (Spasojevic & Alloy, 2002).

Alloy and colleagues (2001) found that according to individuals' and parents' reports, both mothers and fathers of high-risk individuals provided more negative (stable, global) attributional feedback regarding negative events in their child's life than did mothers and fathers of individuals without negative cognitive styles, and this predicted the likelihood of their child developing an episode of a depressive disorder over a 2.5-year prospective follow-up period. Thus, evidence is accumulating that points to the role of parents in contributing to the development of negative cognitive styles and vulnerability to depression by providing negative inferential feedback to their child regarding negative events in the child's life (for a review, see Alloy et al., 2004).

Cognitive vulnerability to depression could also arise as the result of other negative parenting practices. In particular, a parenting style that lacks emotional warmth or incorporates negative psychological control (criticism, intrusiveness, and guilt-induction), a pattern referred to as "affectionless control" by Parker (1983), has been implicated as a risk factor for depression (for reviews, see Alloy et al., 2001; Alloy, Abramson, Safford, et al., 2006; Garber & Flynn, 1988). Consistent with the lack of emotional warmth component of the affectionless control pattern, Alloy et al. (2001) found that less warmth and acceptance from fathers predicted negative cognitive styles in their offspring, but there was no effect like this for mothers' parenting. In addition, low warmth or acceptance from fathers predicted prospective onsets of depression disorders in their offspring during a 2.5-year follow-up, and negative psychological control from either parent was associated with a ruminative response style among CVD project participants (Spasojevic & Alloy, 2002). Rumination mediated the relationship between overcontrolling parenting and prospective onsets of major depression. Thus, both lack of emotional warmth and overcontrolling parenting were related to offspring's cognitive vulnerability to depression, via negative cognitive styles and rumination, respectively.

Work on the origins of cognitive vulnerability to anxiety is less developed, but several studies have given it attention. Williams and Riskind (2004) examined the pattern of relationships between adult romantic attachment patterns, the looming cognitive style, anxiety symptoms, and both general and specific relationship outcomes. Insecure adult attachment styles (preoccupied and/or fearful), reflecting a negative view of self in romantic relationships, were associated with higher levels of the looming cognitive style and anxiety symptoms. Moreover, the results suggested that the effect of romantic attachment patterns on anxiety depended partially on their relationships with the looming cognitive style (e.g., partial mediation). Riskind et al. (2004) reported two additional studies on the links between parenting, attachment variables, and cognitive vulnerability. They found that low levels of maternal overprotection and high levels of paternal overprotection predicted significant variance in looming cognitive style, beyond the effects of current anxious and depressive symptoms. Moreover, retrospective reports of maternal attachment insecurity were associated with significantly higher looming cognitive style scores as well as anxious and depressive symptoms. In addition, attachment insecurity and cognitive styles were related to adult romantic attachment insecurity and potentially high-risk relationship behaviors.

Most studies on the origins of cognitive vulnerability so far are retrospective, and accordingly, these developmental findings should be viewed as tentative (but see Gibb et al., 2006, for prospective evidence that emotional maltreatment contributes to development of a negative inferential style). However, these preliminary results support the necessity for further prospective tests of the role that maltreatment, maladaptive inferential feedback, and negative parenting practices may play in the development of negative cognitive styles and ruminative response styles, and ultimately, vulnerability to depression and anxiety.

## CLINICAL IMPLICATIONS: CAN COGNITIVE VULNERABILITY BE TREATED AND/OR PREVENTED?

To understand how depression or anxiety can be adequately treated, it may be crucial to address these underlying cognitive vulnerabilities. Clinical interventions designed to ameliorate cognitive vulnerabilities should decrease the emotional conditions. Likewise, preventive interventions designed to thwart the development of such vulnerabilities in the first place could reduce the likelihood of developing depression or anxiety in the face of negative life events. Cognitive-behavioral therapy (CBT) has been shown to be an effective treatment for depression, with recent findings suggesting that it may also reduce risk for relapse and recurrence in adults (Hollon, Thase, & Markowitz, 2002; Hollon et al., 2005). In addition, research suggests that CBT for depression is an effective treatment insofar as it can reduce the negativity of individuals' attributional styles (DeRubeis & Hollon, 1995; Hollon & Beck, 1994). This finding suggests that the effectiveness of CBT in reducing the risk for relapses or recurrences of depression (presumably anxiety) may stem from its ability to ameliorate negative cognitive styles, decrease cognitive vulnerability for these states, and thwart subsequent episodes of disorder. This research lends support to the notion that interventions could be implemented to prevent the development of cognitive vulnerabilities. Moreover, preventive efforts might ideally be directed at children, before they reach early adolescence and puberty, to prevent the formation and consolidation of cognitive vulnerability to depression and anxiety. Some evidence has been found that early prevention interventions reduce the risk of future depression in adolescents (Gillham, Reivich, Jaycox, & Seligman, 1995; Jaycox, Reivich, Gillham, & Selligman, 1994; Yu & Seligman, 2002).

The construct of social cognitive vulnerability, therefore, has a central role in understanding and treating these emotional disorders as well as preventing their relapse. Unless the underlying cognitive vulnerabilities (e.g., negative cognitive styles or attitudes) are adequately treated or prevented, the factors that cause these psychological problems to develop or persist will remain. This chapter has presented an overarching framework for synthesizing available knowledge and has pointed to additional research that is needed.

## REFERENCES

Abramson, L. Y., Alloy, L. B., Hankin, B. L., Haeffel, G. J., MacCoon, D. G., & Gibb, B. E. (2002). Cognitive vulnerability–stress models of depression in a self-regulatory and psychobiological context. In I. H. Gotlib & C. L. Hammen (Eds.), *Handbook of depression* (3rd ed., pp. 268–294). New York: Guilford Press.

Abramson, L. Y., Metalsky, G., & Alloy, L. B. (1989). Hopelessness depression: A theory based subtype of depression. *Psychological Review*, *96*, 358–372.

Adler, A. D., & Strunk, D. R. (2010). Looming maladaptive style as a moderator of risk factors for anxiety. *Cognitive Therapy and Research*, *34*, 59–68.

Alloy, L. B., & Abramson, L. Y. (1999). The Temple–Wisconsin Cognitive Vulnerability to Depression (CVD) project: Conceptual background, design, and methods. *Journal of Cognitive Psychotherapy: An International Quarterly*, *13*, 227–262.

Alloy, L. B., Abramson, L. Y., Gibb, B. E., Crossfield, A. G., Pieracci, A. M., & Spasojevic, J., et al. (2004). Developmental antecedents of cognitive vulnerability to depression: Review of findings from the Cognitive Vulnerability to Depression Project. *Journal of Cognitive Psychotherapy: An International Quarterly*, *18*, 115–133.

Alloy, L. B., Abramson, L. Y., Hogan, M. E., Whitehouse, W. G., Rose, D., Robinson, M., et al. (2000). The Temple–Wisconsin Vulnerability to Depression project: Lifetime history of Axis I psychopathology in individuals at high and low cognitive risk for depression. *Journal of Abnormal Psychology, 109*, 403–418.

Alloy, L. B., Abramson, L. Y., Safford, S. M., & Gibb, B. E. (2006). The Cognitive Vulnerability to Depression (CVD) project: Current findings and future directions. In L. B. Alloy & J. H. Riskind (Eds.), *Cognitive vulnerability to emotional disorders* (pp. 33–61). Mahwah, NJ: Erlbaum.

Alloy, L. B., Abramson, L. Y., Smith, J. B., Gibb, B. E., & Neeren, A. M. (2006). Role of parenting and maltreatment histories in unipolar and bipolar mood disorders: Mediation by cognitive vulnerability to depression. *Clinical Child and Family Psychology Review, 9*, 23–64.

Alloy, L. B., Abramson, L. Y., Tashman, N., Berrebbi, D. S., Hogan, M. E., Whitehouse, W. G., et al. (2001). Developmental origins of cognitive vulnerability to depression: Parenting, cognitive, and inferential feedback styles of the parents of individuals at high and low cognitive risk for depression. *Cognitive Therapy and Research, 25*, 397–423.

Alloy, L. B., Abramson, L. Y., Whitehouse, W. G., Hogan, M. E., Panzarella, C., & Rose, D. (2006). Prospective incidence of first onsets and recurrences of depression in individuals at high and low cognitive risk for depression. *Journal of Abnormal Psychology, 115*, 145–156.

Amstadter, A. (2008). Emotion regulation and anxiety disorders. *Journal of Anxiety Disorders, 22*, 211–221.

Bar-Haim, Y., Lamy, D., Pergamin, L., Bakermans-Kranenburg, M. H., & van IJzendoorn, M. H. (2007). Threat-related attentional bias in anxious and non-anxious individuals: A meta-analytic study. *Psychological Bulletin, 133*, 1–24.

Barsky, A. J., Cleary, P. D., Sarnie, M. K., & Ruskin, J. N. (1994). Panic disorder, palpitations, and the awareness of cardiac activity. *Journal of Nervous and Mental Disorders, 182*, 63–67.

Beck, A. T. (1967). *Depression: Clinical, experimental, and theoretical aspects.* New York: Harper & Row.

Beck, A. T. (1976). *Cognitive therapy and the emotional disorders.* New York: International Universities Press.

Beck, A. T. (1987). Cognitive models of depression. *Journal of Cognitive Psychotherapy: An International Quarterly, 1*, 5–37.

Beck, A. T. (1991). Cognitive therapy: A 30-year retrospective. *American Psychologist, 46*, 368–375.

Beck, A. T., & Clark, D. A. (1997). An information processing model of anxiety: Automatic and strategic processes. *Behaviour Research and Therapy, 35*, 49–58.

Beck, R., & Perkins, T. S. (2001). Cognitive content-specificity for anxiety and depression: A meta-analysis. *Cognitive Therapy and Research, 25*, 651–663.

Black, D. O., Balaban, M. S., & Riskind, J. H. (2002, November). *Vulnerability to anxiety and life events: A nine-month prospective study.* Poster presentation at the annual meeting of the Association for Advancement of Behavior Therapy, New Orleans.

Black, D., Riskind, J. H., & Kleiman, E. M. (in press). Lifetime history of anxiety and mood disorders predicted by cognitive vulnerability to anxiety. *International Journal of Cognitive Therapy.*

Blais, M. A., Otto, M. W., Zucker, B. G., McNally, R. M., Schmidt, N. B., Fava, M., et al. (2001). The anxiety sensitivity index: Item analysis and suggestions for refinement. *Journal of Personality Assessment, 77*, 272–294.

Borkovec, T. D., & Inz, J. (1990). The nature of worry in generalized anxiety disorder: A predominance of thought activity. *Behaviour Research and Therapy, 28*, 153–158.

Borkovec, T. D., Ray, W. J., & Stoeber, J. (1998). Worry: A cognitive phenomenon intimately linked to affective, physiological, and interpersonal behavioral processes. *Cognitive Therapy and Research, 22*, 561–576.

Brown, G. W., & Harris, T. O. (1978). *Social origins of depression.* London, UK: Tavistock.

Brown, M. A., & Stopa, L. (2008). The looming maladaptive style in social anxiety. *Behavior Therapy*, *39*, 57–64.

Brown, T. A., Chorpita, B. F., & Barlow, D. H. (1998). Structural relationships among dimensions of the DSM-IV anxiety and mood disorders and dimensions of negative affect, positive affect, and autonomic arousal. *Journal of Abnormal Psychology*, *107*, 179–192.

Cisler, J. M., Bacon, A. K., & Williams, N. L. (2009). Phenomenological characteristics of attentional biases towards threat: A critical review. *Cognitive Therapy and Research*, *33*, 221–234.

Daley, S. E., Hammen, C., & Rao, U. (2000). Predictors of first onset and recurrence of major depression in young women during the 5 years following high school graduation. *Journal of Abnormal Psychology*, *109*, 525–533.

Deacon, B., & Abramowitz, J. (2006). Anxiety sensitivity and its dimensions across the anxiety disorders. *Journal of Anxiety Disorders*, *20*, 837–857.

DeRubeis, R. J., & Hollon, S. D. (1995). Explanatory style in the treatment of depression. In G. M. Buchanan & M. E. P. Seligman (Eds.), *Explanatory style* (pp. 99–111). Hillsdale, NJ: Erlbaum.

Dorfin, N. M., & Woody, S. R. (2006). Does threatening imagery sensitize distress during contaminant exposure? *Behaviour Research and Therapy*, *44*, 395–413.

Ehlers, A. (1995). A 1-year prospective study of panic attacks: Clinical course and factors associated with maintenance. *Journal of Abnormal Psychology*, *104*, 164–172.

Ehlers, A., Margraf, J., Roth, W. T., Taylor, C. B., & Birbaumer, N. (1988). Anxiety induced by false heart rate feedback in patients with panic disorder. *Behaviour Research and Therapy*, *26*, 1–11.

Enns, M. W., Cox, B. J., & Clara, I. P (2005). Perfectionism and neuroticism: A longitudinal study of specific vulnerability and diathesis–stress models. *Cognitive Therapy and Research*, *29*, 463–478.

Fridja, N. (1987). *The emotions*. New York: Cambridge University Press.

Garber, J., & Flynn, C. (1988). Origins of the depressive cognitive style. In D. Routh & R. J. DeRubeis (Eds.), *The science of clinical psychology: Evidence of a century's progress* (pp. 53–93). Washington, DC: American Psychological Association

Gibb, B. E. (2002). Childhood maltreatment and negative cognitive styles: A quantitative and qualitative review. *Clinical Psychology Review*, *22*, 223–246.

Gibb, B. E., Alloy, L. B., Abramson, L. Y., Rose, D. T., Whitehouse, W. G., Donovan, P., et al. (2001). History of childhood maltreatment, negative cognitive styles, and episodes of depression in adulthood. *Cognitive Therapy and Research*, *25*, 425–446.

Gibb, B. E., Alloy, L. B., Walshaw, P. D., Comer, J. S., Shen, G. H. C., & Villari, A. G. (2006). Predictors of attributional style change in children. *Journal of Abnormal Child Psychology*, *34*, 425–439.

Gillham, J. E., Reivich, K. J., Jaycox, L. H., & Seligman, M. E. P. (1995). Prevention of depressive symptoms in schoolchildren: Two-year follow-up. *Psychological Science*, *6*, 343–351.

Harvey, A., Watkins, E., Mansell, W., & Shafran, R. (2004). *Cognitive behavioural processes across psychological disorders: A transdiagnostic approach to research and treatment*. Oxford, UK: Oxford University Press.

Hewitt, P. L., Caelian, C. F., & Flett, G. L. (2002). Perfectionism in children: Associations with depression, anxiety, and anger. *Personality and Individual Differences*, *32*, 1049–1061.

Hofmann, S. G., & Smits, J. A. (2008). Cognitive-behavioral therapy for adult anxiety disorders: A meta-analaysis of randomized placebo-controlled trials. *Journal of Clinical Psychiatry*, *69*, 621–632.

Holahan, C. J., Moos, R. H., Holahan, C. K., Brennan, P. L., & Schutte, K. K. (2005). Stress generation, avoidance coping, and depressive symptoms: A 10-year model. *Journal of Consulting and Clinical Psychology*, *73*, 658–666.

Hollon, S. D., & Beck, A. T. (1994). Cognitive and cognitive-behavioral therapies. In A. E. Bergin & S. L. Garfield (Eds.), *Handbook of psychotherapy and behavior change* (4th ed., pp. 428–466). New York: Wiley.

Hollon, S. D., DeRubeis, R. J., Shelton, R. C., Amsterdam, J. D., Salomon, R. M., O'Reardon, J. P., et al. (2005). Prevention of relapse following cognitive therapy vs. medications in moderate to severe depression. *Archives of General Psychiatry*, *62*, 417–422.

Hollon, S. D., Thase, M. E., & Markowitz, J. C. (2002). Treatment and prevention of depression. *Psychological Science and Public Interest*, *3*, 39–77.

Iacoviello, B. M., Alloy, L. B., Abramson, L. Y., Whitehouse, W. G., & Hogan, M. E. (2006). The course of depression in individuals at high and low cognitive risk for depression: A prospective study. *Journal of Affective Disorders*, *93*, 61–69.

Ingram, R. E., Miranda, J., & Segal, Z. (1998). *Cognitive vulnerability to depression.* New York: Guilford Press.

Jaycox, L. H., Reivich, K. J., Gillham, J., & Seligman, M. E. P. (1994). Prevention of depressive symptoms in school children. *Behavior Research and Therapy*, *32*, 801–816.

Johnson, S. L., & Roberts, J. E. (1995). Life events and bipolar disorder: Implications from biological theories. *Psychological Bulletin*, *117*, 434–449.

Joiner, T. E., Jr. (2000). Depression's vicious scree: Self-propagating and erosive processes in depression chronicity. *Clinical Psychology: Science and Practice*, *7*, 203–218.

Joorman, J., & Gotlib, I. H. (2007). Selective attention to emotional faces following recovery from depression. *Journal of Abnormal Psychology*, *116*, 80–85.

Just, N., Abramson, L. Y., & Alloy, L. B. (2001). Remitted depression studies as tests of the cognitive vulnerability hypotheses of depression onset: A critique and conceptual analysis. *Clinical Psychology Review*, *21*, 63–83.

Just, N., & Alloy, L. B. (1997). The response styles theory of depression: Tests and an extension of the theory. *Journal of Abnormal Psychology*, *106*, 221–229.

Kawamura, K. Y., Hunt, S. L., & Frost, R. O. (2002). Perfectionism, anxiety, and depression: Are the relationships independent? *Cognitive Therapy and Research*, *25*, 291–301.

Kearney, C. A., Albano, A. M., Eisen, A. R., Allan, W. D., & Barlow D. H. (1997). The phenomenology of panic disorder in youngsters: An empirical study of a clinical sample. *Journal of Anxiety Disorders*, *11*, 49–62.

Keogh, E., Ayers, S., & Francis, H. (2002). Does anxiety sensitivity predict posttraumatic stress symptoms following childbirth? A preliminary report. *Cognitive Behaviour Therapy*, *31*, 145–155.

Koster, E., De Raedt, R., Goeleven, E., Franck, E., & Crombez, G. (2005). Mood-congruent attentional bias in dysphoria: Maintained attention to and impaired disengagement from negative information. *Emotion*, *5*, 446–455.

Last, C. G., Barlow, D. H., & O'Brien, G. T. (1984). Precipitants of agoraphobia: Role of stressful life events. *Psychological Reports*, *54*, 567–570.

Lazarus, R. (1991). *Emotion and adaptation.* New York: Oxford University Press.

Levin, T., Li, Y., & Riskind, J. H. (2007) Looming threat-processing style in a cancer cohort. *General Hospital Psychiatry*, *29*, 32–38.

Lewinsohn, P. M., Allen, N. B., Seeley, J. R., & Gotlib, I. H. (1999). First onset versus recurrence of depression: Differential processes of psychosocial risk. *Journal of Abnormal Psychology*, *108*, 483–489.

MacLeod, C., Rutherford, E., Campbell, L., Ebsworthy, G., & Holker, L. (2002). Selective attention and emotional vulnerability: Assessing the causal basis of their association through the experimental manipulation of attentional bias. *Journal of Abnormal Psychology*, *111*, 107–123.

Mathews, A., & MacLeod, C. (2002). Induced processing biases have causal effects on anxiety. *Cognition and Emotion*, *16*, 331–354.

Mathews, A., & MacLeod, C. (2005). Cognitive vulnerability to emotional disorders. *Annual Review of Clinical Psychology*, *1*, 167–195.

McWilliams, L. A., Stewart, S. H., & MacPherson, P. S. R. (2000). Does the social concerns component of the Anxiety Sensitivity Index belong to the domain of anxiety sensitivity or negative evaluation sensitivity? *Behaviour Research and Therapy*, *38*, 985–992.

Mennin, D. S., Heimberg, R. G., & Turk, C. L. (2002). Applying an emotion regulation framework to integrative approaches to generalized anxiety disorder. *Clinical Psychology: Science and Practice*, *9*, 85–90.

Mineka, S., Watson, D., & Clark, L. A. (1998). Comorbidity of anxiety and unipolar mood disorders. *Annual Review of Psychology*, *49*, 377–412.

Muris, P. (2002). Relationships between self-efficacy and symptoms of anxiety disorders and depression in a normal adolescent sample. *Personality and Individual Differences*, *32*, 337–348.

Muris, P., Schmidt, H., Lanbrichs, R., & Meesters, C. (2001). Protective and vulnerability factors of depression in normal adolescents. *Behaviour Research and Therapy*, *39*, 555–565.

Nolen-Hoeksema, S. (1991). Responses to depression and their effects on the duration of the depressive episode. *Journal of Abnormal Psychology*, *100*, 20–28.

Nolen-Hoeksema, S. (2000). Ruminative responses predict depressive disorders. *Journal of Abnormal Psychology*, *109*, 504–511.

Ortony, A., Clore, G. L., & Collins, A. (1988). *The cognitive structure of emotions*. New York: Cambridge University Press.

Papageorgiou, C., & Wells, A. (2003). An empirical test of a clinical metacognitive model for rumination and depression. *Cognitive Therapy and Research*, *27*, 261–273.

Parker, G. (1983). Parental "affectionless control" as an antecedent to adult depression. *Archives of General Psychiatry*, *34*, 138–147.

Paykel, E. S. (Ed.). (1982). *Handbook of affective disorders*. New York: Guilford Press.

Reardon, J. M., & Williams, N. L. (2007). The specificity of cognitive vulnerabilities to emotional disorders: Anxiety sensitivity, looming vulnerability, and explanatory style. *Journal of Anxiety Disorders*, *21*, 625–643.

Reiss, S., & McNally, R. J. (1985). Expectancy model of fear. In S. Reis & R. R. Bootzin (Eds.), *Theoretical issues in behavior therapy* (pp. 107–121). San Diego, CA: Academic Press.

Riskind, J. H. (1997). Looming vulnerability to threat: A cognitive paradigm for anxiety. *Behaviour Research and Therapy*, *35*, 386–404.

Riskind, J. H., Abreu, K., Strauss, M., & Holt, R. (1997). Looming vulnerability to spreading contamination in subclinical OCD. *Behaviour Research and Therapy*, *35*, 405–414.

Riskind, J. H., & Alloy, L. B. (2006). Cognitive vulnerability to emotional disorders: Theory, design, and methods. In L. B. Alloy & J. H. Riskind (Eds.), *Cognitive vulnerability to emotional disorders* (pp. 1–29). Mahwah, NJ: Erlbaum.

Riskind, J. H., Black, D., & Shahar, G. (2010). Cognitive vulnerability to anxiety in the stress generation process: Interaction between the looming cognitive style and anxiety sensitivity. *Journal of Anxiety Disorders*, *24*, 124–128.

Riskind, J., Kelly, K., Harman, W., Moore, R., & Gaines, H. (1992). The loomingness of danger: Does it discriminate focal fear and general anxiety from depression? *Cognitive Therapy and Research*, *16*, 603–622.

Riskind, J. H., & Maddux, J. E. (1994). The loomingness of danger and the fear of AIDS: Perceptions of motion and menace. *Journal of Applied Social Psychology, 24*, 432–442.

Riskind, J. H., Moore, R., & Bowley, L. (1995). The looming of spiders: The fearful perceptual distortion of movement and menace. *Behavior Research and Therapy*, *33*, 171–178.

Riskind, J. H., & Rector, N. A. (2007). Beyond belief: Incremental prediction of OCD by looming vulnerability illusions. *Journal of Cognitive Psychotherapy*, *21*, 243–256.

Riskind, J. H., & Rector, N. A. (2010). *Looming vulnerability to threat across the anxiety disorders.* Manuscript in preparation.

Riskind, J. H., & Rholes, W. S. (1984). Cognitive accessibility and the capacity of cognitions to predict future depression: A theoretical note. *Cognitive Therapy and Research*, *8*, 1–12.

Riskind, J. H., Tzur, D., Williams, N., Mann, B., & Shahar, G. (2007). Short-term predictive effects of the looming cognitive style on anxiety disorder symptoms under restrictive methodological conditions. *Behaviour Research and Therapy*, *45*, 1765–1777.

Riskind, J. H., Wheeler, D. J., & Picerno, M. R. (1997). Using mental imagery with subclinical OCD to "freeze" contamination in its place: Evidence for looming vulnerability theory. *Behaviour Research and Therapy*, *35*, 757–768.

Riskind, J. H., & Williams, N. L. (2005). The looming maladaptive style in generalized anxiety disorder: Distinctive danger schema and phenomenology. *Cognitive Therapy and Research*, *29*, 7–27.

Riskind, J. H., & Williams, N. L. (2006). A unique vulnerability common to all anxiety disorders: The looming maladaptive style. In L. B. Alloy & J. H. Riskind (Eds.), *Cognitive vulnerability to emotional disorders* (pp. 175–206). Mahwah, NJ: Erlbaum.

Riskind, J. H., Williams, N. L., Altman, M. D., Black, D. O., Balaban, M. S., & Gessner, T. L. (2004). Developmental antecedents of the looming maladaptive style: Parental bonding and parental attachment insecurity. *Journal of Cognitive Psychotherapy: An International Quarterly*, *18*, 43–52.

Riskind, J. H., Williams, N. L., Gessner, T., Chrosniak, L. D., & Cortina, J. (2000). The looming maladaptive style: Anxiety, danger, and schematic processing. *Journal of Personality and Social Psychology*, *79*, 837–852.

Riskind, J. H., Williams, N. L., & Joiner, T. E. (2006). A unique overarching vulnerability for the anxiety disorders: The looming maladaptive style. *Journal of Social and Clinical Psychology*, *25*, 779–801.

Robinson, M. S., & Alloy, L. B. (2003). Negative cognitive styles and stress-reactive rumination interact to predict depression: A prospective study. *Cognitive Therapy and Research*, *27*, 275–291.

Roemer, L., Salters, K., Raffa, S. D., & Orsillo, S. M. (2005). Fear and avoidance of internal experiences in GAD: Tests of a conceptual model. *Cognitive Therapy and Research*, *29*, 71–88.

Rose, D. T., & Abramson, L. Y. (1992). Developmental predictors of depressive cognitive style: Research and theory. In D. Cicchetti & S. L. Toth (Eds.), *Rochester symposium on developmental psychopathology* (Vol. IV, pp. 323–349). Hillsdale, NJ: Erlbaum.

Roseman, I. J., Spindel, M. S., & Jose, P. E. (1990). Appraisals of emotion-soliciting events: Testing a theory of discrete emotions. *Journal of Personality and Social Psychology*, *59*, 899–915.

Roy-Byrne, P. B., Geraci, M., & Uhde, T. W. (1986). Life events and the onset of panic disorder. *American Journal of Psychiatry*, *143*, 1424–1427.

Safford, S. M., Alloy, L. B., Abramson, L. Y., & Crossfield, A. G. (2007). Negative cognitive style as a predictor of negative life events in depression-prone individuals: A test of the stress generation hypothesis. *Journal of Affective Disorders*, *99*, 147–154.

Schmidt, N. B., Lerew, D. R., & Jackson, R. J. (1997). The role of anxiety sensitivity in the pathogenesis of panic: Prospective evaluation of spontaneous panic attacks during acute stress. *Journal of Abnormal Psychology*, *106*, 355–364.

Schmidt, N., Lerew, D., & Jackson, R. (1999). Prospective evaluation of anxiety sensitivity in the pathogenesis of panic: Replication and extension. *Journal of Abnormal Psychology*, *108*, 532–537.

Schmidt, N. B., & Woolaway-Bickel, K. (2006). Cognitive vulnerability to panic disorder. In L. B. Alloy & J. H. Riskind (Eds.), *Cognitive vulnerability to emotional disorders* (pp. 207–234). Mahwah, NJ: Erlbaum.

Schmidt, N. B., Zvolensky, M. J., & Maner, J. K. (2006). Anxiety sensitivity: Prospective prediction of panic attacks and Axis I pathology. *Journal of Psychiatric Research*, *40*, 691–699.

Sibrava, N. J., & Borkovec, T. D. (2006). The cognitive avoidance theory of worry. In G. Davey & A. Wells (Eds.), *Worry and its psychological disorders: Theory, assessment and treatment* (pp. 239–256). Hoboken, NJ: Wiley.

Spasojevic, J., & Alloy, L. B. (2001). Rumination as a common mechanism relating depressive risk factors to depression. *Emotion*, *1*, 25–37.

Spasojevic, J., & Alloy, L. B. (2002). Who becomes a depressive ruminator? Developmental antecedents of ruminative response style. *Journal of Cognitive Psychotherapy: An International Quarterly*, *16*, 405–419.

Story, T. J., & Craske, M. (2008). Responses to false physiological feedback in individuals with panic attacks and elevated anxiety sensitivity. *Behaviour Research and Therapy*, *46*, 1001–1008.

Taylor, S. (Ed.). (1999). *Anxiety sensitivity: Theory, research, and treatment of the fear of anxiety.* Mahwah, NJ: Erlbaum.

Taylor, S. (2003). Anxiety sensitivity and its implications for understanding and treating PTSD. *Journal of Cognitive Psychotherapy, 17,* 179–186.

Taylor, S., Koch, W. J., Woody, S., & McLean, P. (1996). Anxiety sensitivity and depression: How are they related? *Journal of Abnormal Psychology, 105,* 474–479.

Teachman, B. A. (2005). Information processing and anxiety sensitivity: Cognitive vulnerability to panic reflected in interpretation and memory biases. *Cognitive Therapy and Research, 29,* 479–499.

Telch, M. J., Silverman, A., & Schmidt, N. B. (1996). The relationship between anxiety sensitivity and perceived control in a caffeine challenge. *Journal of Anxiety Disorders, 10,* 21–35.

Tolin, D. F., Worhunsky, P., & Maltby, N. (2004). Sympathetic magic in contamination-related OCD. *Journal of Behavior Therapy and Experimental Psychiatry, 35,* 193–205.

Vrana, S. R., Cuthbert, B. N., & Lang, P. J. (1986). Fear imagery and text processing. *Psychophysiology, 23,* 247–253.

Wells, A. (2000). *Emotional disorders and metacognition: Innovative cognitive therapy.* New York: Wiley.

Wells, A., & Carter, K. (2001). Further tests of a cognitive model of generalized anxiety disorder: Metacognitions and worry in GAD, panic disorder, social phobia, depression, and nonpatients. *Behavior Therapy, 32,* 85–102.

Wells, A., & Matthews, G. (1996). Modelling cognition in emotional disorder: The S-REF model. *Behaviour Research and Therapy, 32,* 867–870.

Wells, A., & Papageorgiou, C. (1998). Relationship between worry and obsessive–compulsive symptoms and meta-cognitive beliefs. *Behaviour Research and Therapy, 36,* 899–913.

Williams, J. M. G., Watts, F. N., MacLeod, C., & Mathews, A. (1997). *Cognitive psychology and emotional disorders* (2nd ed.). Chichester, UK: Wiley.

Williams, N. L., & Riskind, J. H. (2004). Cognitive vulnerability and attachment. *Journal of Cognitive Psychotherapy: An International Quarterly, 18,* 3–6.

Williams, N. L., Shahar, G., Riskind, J. H., & Joiner, T. E. (2005). The looming maladaptive style predicts shared variance in anxiety disorder symptoms: Further support for a cognitive model of vulnerability to anxiety. *Journal of Anxiety Disorders, 19,* 157–175.

Yu, D. L., & Seligman, M. E. P. (2002). Preventing depression symptoms in Chinese children. *Prevention and Treatment, 5,* Article 9. Available at *journals.apa.org/prevention/volume5/pre0050009a.html.*

Zinbarg, R. E., Barlow, D. H., & Brown, T. A. (1997). Hierarchical structure and general factor saturation of the anxiety sensitivity index: Evidence and implications. *Psychological Assessment, 9,* 277–284.

Zinbarg, R. E., Brown, T. A., Barlow, D. H., & Rapee, R. M. (2001). Anxiety sensitivity, panic, and depressed mood: A reanalysis teasing apart the contributions of the two levels in the hierarchical structure of the Anxiety Sensitivity Index. *Journal of Abnormal Psychology, 110,* 372–377.

Zinbarg, R. E., Mohlman, J., & Hong, N. N. (1999). Dimensions of anxiety sensitivity. In S. Taylor (Ed.), *Anxiety sensitivity: Theory, research, and treatment of the fear of anxiety* (pp. 83–114). Mahwah, NJ: Erlbaum.

Zuckerman, M. (1999). *Vulnerability to psychopathology: A biosocial model.* Washington, DC: American Psychological Association.

Zuroff, D. C., Mongrain, M., & Santor, D. (2004). Conceptualizing and measuring personality vulnerability to depression: Comment on Coyne and Whiffen (1995). *Psychological Bulletin, 130,* 489–511.

# PART III

# SOCIAL PSYCHOLOGY OF PSYCHOLOGICAL ASSESSMENT AND DIAGNOSIS

# 16 The Social Psychology of Clinical Judgment

Howard N. Garb

In his bestselling book *Blink: The Power of Thinking without Thinking*, Malcolm Gladwell (2005, p. 15) stated that the "important task of this book is to convince you that our snap judgments and first impressions can be educated and controlled.... Just as we can teach ourselves to think logically and deliberately, we can also teach ourselves to make better snap judgments."

Should mental health professionals make snap judgments? To answer this and other questions, we can turn to research on social psychology and clinical psychology. Findings from social psychology describe how individuals in everyday life make judgments. Many studies on how mental health professionals make judgments in clinical settings are based on ideas and methods from social psychology.

Two general topics are addressed in this chapter. The first area of inquiry relates to how mental health professionals make judgments. For example, the fact that cognitive processes lie largely outside the realm of awareness poses challenges for improving clinical judgment and for understanding and explaining clients' emotions, motivations, and behaviors. The second area of inquiry relates to the influence of social factors. For example, one can ask if mental health professionals sometimes make less valid judgments for black clients than for white clients. And, as another example, one can wonder if the type of treatment provided by mental health professionals depends on the context in which the decisions are made.

## COGNITIVE PROCESSES AND BIASES

The study of how mental health professionals make judgments has been strongly influenced by research on social psychology, social cognition, and cognitive psychology. Results are described for (1) the primacy effect, (2) awareness of cognitive processes, (3) cognitive heuristics, (4) confirmatory hypothesis testing, (5) causal reasoning, and (6) biases and errors.

### The Primacy Effect

As already mentioned, Gladwell (2005) encouraged people to make snap judgments. Interestingly, people already do this; in everyday life, people often make judgments about other people very quickly. This phenomenon is called the *primacy effect*, and it is also true of clinical judgment. In one review of studies on social and clinical judgment (Ambady & Rosenthal, 1992), predictions based on observations under 30 seconds did not differ significantly from predictions based on 4- and 5-minute observations. As described by Kendell (1973, p. 444), "Accurate diagnoses can often be reached very early in an interview, even within the first two minutes, and after five or ten minutes further expenditure of time is subject to a law of rapidly diminishing returns."

Making judgments quickly is efficient, in that it saves time and energy. And those judgments may frequently be correct. But if someone quickly forms a negative impression of us, we might complain that the person did not get to know us. And when a client seeks help, he or she might object to learn that the mental health professional very quickly formed impressions that were unlikely to change.

### Awareness of Cognitive Processes

Judgments, feelings, and motives occur largely outside the realm of cognitive awareness (Wilson, 2002). For this reason, it can be difficult for mental health professionals to know exactly how they make clinical judgments and decisions. In a classic study (Einhorn, Kleinmuntz, & Kleinmuntz, 1979), an expert psychologist was instructed to examine the Minnesota Multiphasic Personality Inventory (MMPI) protocols to rate level of adjustment. The psychologist was asked to think aloud into a tape recorder as he made judgments regarding the profiles. The experimenter listened to the clinician's statements and constructed a list of decision rules to reflect how the clinician said he made his judgments. When these decision rules were used to predict his judgments, the correlation between the predictions and the clinician's judgments was low. Presumably this happened because much of cognitive processing occurs outside of conscious awareness. That is, although the psychologist described his thoughts while examining the MMPI protocols and making ratings of level of adjustment, his statements did not accurately reflect how his judgments were made. As observed by Wilson (2002), "The mind operates most efficiently by relegating a good deal of high-level, sophisticated thinking to the unconscious" (p. 6). Unfortunately, we do not have direct access to these nonconscious processes.

If clinicians are often unaware of how they make judgments, this can make it difficult for them to correct errors in judgment. For example, clinicians who prescribe medication differently for minority clients may not be aware of their bias, and this lack of awareness will make it difficult for them to improve their decisions.

Clinicians face a second handicap. Not only is it difficult for mental health professionals to know exactly how they make judgments and decisions, but they face the difficult task of helping their clients better understand their feelings and motives—even though feelings and motives occur largely outside the realm of cognitive awareness (Bem, 1972; Gazzaniga &

LeDoux, 1978; Wilson, 2002). This makes it more difficult for both clients and therapists to explain clients' behaviors. In addition, uncertainty can make anyone anxious, and people are most comfortable when they can explain things. The temptation to accept case formulations and explanations of a client's behavior is strong, even though research suggests that this is the most difficult task facing clinicians (Garb, 1998, 2005).

## Cognitive Heuristics

Cognitive heuristics are simple rules for making judgments and decisions. Although they allow us to efficiently process vast amounts of information, they can also cause us to make characteristic types of mistakes. Cognitive heuristics include the affect, representativeness, and availability heuristics.

The *affect heuristic* refers to the fact that people often make judgments and decisions based, in part, on their feelings. *Affect* refers to a feeling, such as fear or pleasure, which occurs rapidly and is short in duration. The effect of the affect heuristic may be especially pronounced when someone bases a judgment on his or her "gut instinct" or intuition. Early theoretical and empirical work on cognitive heuristics (e.g., Tversky & Kahneman, 1974) led to a Nobel prize for Daniel Kahneman, but did not include descriptions of the affect heuristic. Kahneman (2003, p. 703) subsequently wrote that the formulation of the affect heuristic is "probably the most important development in the study of judgment heuristics in the past few decades."

The affect heuristic has grown in importance to our understanding of social judgments made in everyday life, but its role in the cognitive processes of mental health professionals has been studied only indirectly (Slovic, Monahan, & MacGregor, 2000). One reason it has been difficult to learn about the effect of feelings on judgments is because their influence can lie outside of our awareness.

Gladwell (2005) has argued that one way people can make better snap judgments is by trusting their emotions. For example, in his book *Blink: The Power of Thinking without Thinking* (2005), he described how several experts in the world of art had a strong negative emotional response upon seeing a statue that had been bought by the Getty Museum (a response that Gladwell labeled "intuitive repulsion"). It later became clear that the emotional response of these experts was correct: The statue was a forgery.

Can mental health professionals be trained to make better judgments by relying on their emotions? Everyone, including mental health professionals, already makes judgments and decisions that are based, in part, on their feelings. A training intervention to help mental health professionals make better judgments by changing the way they rely on their emotions has not yet been described and evaluated in the research literature.

Interestingly, research on clinical judgment supports strategies that can run counter to relying on one's emotions to guide judgments. Studies indicate that clinicians too often become overconfident and satisfied with their judgments. To counter their overconfidence, rather than being told to attend to their feelings, they are typically advised to (1) consider more alternatives, (2) ask more questions, and (3) attend more closely to criteria when making diagnoses (e.g., Arkes, 1981; Garb, 1998, 2005). Similarly, a large body of research exists on statistical prediction (Grove, Zald, Lebow, Snitz, & Nelson, 2000; Meehl, 1954). For example, statistically based instruments incorporating objective and clinically derived measures are available for the prediction of violent behavior (Harris,

Rice, & Quinsey, 1993) and sexual reoffense (Hanson, 1998). When predictions based on statistical rules are compared to clinicians' predictions, the statistical predictions are typically more accurate than, or as accurate as, the clinicians' predictions. Of course, statistical prediction rules are not "attending to their feelings" when making judgments. The implications of these results are not that clinicians should focus more on their feelings, but that clinicians should be more willing to incorporate statistical prediction rules into their assessment practice.

The *representativeness heuristic* (Kahneman, Slovic, & Tversky, 1982) is said to be descriptive of cognitive processes when a judgment is made by deciding if a person is representative of a category. For example, when considering whether someone is a good friend, one could compare the person to a stereotype or prototype for the category of friends (e.g., a hypothetical or actual person with all or many of the positive qualities associated with being a good friend). The representativeness heuristic is oftentimes descriptive of how judgments are made in everyday life (e.g., Gilovich, Griffin, & Kahneman, 2002).

Although mental health professionals are supposed to attend to criteria when making diagnoses, the representativeness heuristic is sometimes more descriptive of what they actually do. In one study (Garb, 1996), psychologists and psychology interns read case histories and then made similarity ratings and diagnostic ratings. Similarity ratings could range from 0 to 10, with 0 indicating that the client is not at all similar to the typical person with the disorder and a rating of 10 indicating that the client exemplifies the disorder. Diagnostic ratings could range from 0 to 10, with 0 indicating that the client definitely does not have the disorder, a rating of 5 indicating that the client has a "50/50" chance of having the disorder, and a rating of 10 indicating that the client definitely has the disorder. Similarity ratings and diagnostic ratings were highly correlated ($r = .92$), indicating that the representativeness heuristic is descriptive of how many clinicians make diagnoses. Because clinicians' mental representations of the typical person with a particular mental disorder often diverge from the relevant DSM criteria, only 25% of the clinicians in this study made diagnoses that one would expect them to make if they had adhered to the DSM criteria.

According to the *availability heuristic*, information that can be more easily remembered will have a greater influence on judgment. The ease with which information is remembered can be related to the vividness of the information. For example, when clinicians try to determine if a particular test result is a strong indicator of a personality trait or diagnosis, they typically remember instances when a client with the test result had, or did not have, the trait or diagnosis (true positives and false positives). They are less likely to remember instances when a client did not have the test result (true negatives and false negatives.)

The ease with which information is remembered can also be related to the strength of verbal associative connections between events. For the interpretation of projective drawings, many suggested signs and interpretations have strong verbal associative connections. For example, for house–tree–person drawings, Hammer (1964) argued that a "Tree with an open base [no line drawn under the tree] suggests inadequate reality contact" (p. 14) and "the neck of the Person overemphasized reflects conflict between intellectual control and expression of bodily drives" (p. 11). The sign approach for interpreting projective drawings has not been supported by research (e.g., Lilienfeld, Wood, & Garb, 2000). The availability heuristic may be, in part, responsible for the generation of these interpretations.

### Confirmatory Hypothesis Testing

*Confirmatory hypothesis testing* refers to a tendency to seek, use, and remember information that can confirm, but not refute, an initial hypothesis. In a well-designed study (Haverkamp, 1993), clinical and counseling psychology graduate students watched a videotape of an initial counseling session. They listed their (1) hypotheses (specifically, they were asked to list the major theme or problem they would address in counseling this client), (2) questions they would like to ask the client, and (3) reasons for wanting to ask these questions. The nature of each question was coded as confirmatory, neutral, or disconfirmatory by an independent panel of psychologists. Confirmatory questions could confirm that their initial hypothesis did describe the client's main problem (e.g., asking about sleep problems to help confirm suspected depression); disconfirmatory questions addressed whether a different problem could best be thought of as being a client's main problem (e.g., asking about anxiety in social situations, given initial impressions of depression). The graduate students' style of hypothesis testing was confirmatory 64% of the time, neutral 21% of the time, and disconfirmatory 15% of the time. The results suggest that clinicians may zero in on a single hypothesis before exploring a range of alternatives.

### Causal Reasoning

Causal reasoning—that is, judgments about cause and effect relations—underlies much of clinical judgment. For example, when clinicians make diagnoses, they are influenced not only by diagnostic criteria but also by their implicit causal theories (e.g., Kim & Ahn, 2002; Pottick, Kirk, Hsieh, & Tian, 2007). For example, Kim and Ahn (2002) had clinicians describe their causal theories for different mental disorders. They then had clinicians make diagnoses for a group of clients. They found that clinicians weighed diagnostic criteria more heavily when the criteria described symptoms and behaviors that were part of their implicit causal model for a disorder. This is not supposed to occur: Clinicians making DSM diagnoses are supposed to weigh each criterion equally. Kim and Ahn also found that clinicians' implicit theories of causation influenced their memories of a client's mental status. The clinicians recalled causally central symptoms more often than symptoms that are diagnostic but were not part of their implicit theories of causation. In addition, when clinicians falsely remembered a client as having symptoms the client did not really have, the symptoms they were most likely to falsely remember were those that were causally central to their theories of different disorders.

Causal reasoning is also important in making predictions. In particular, there is evidence that clinicians make fairly sophisticated use of information about the client and the context. In one study (Mulvey & Lidz, 1998), staff members at a mental health emergency room estimated the probability that patients would become violent within the next 6 months. Near-verbatim transcripts were recorded of the interactions among clinicians, patients, and families. The assessment interviews were then coded and analyzed both qualitatively and quantitatively. Mulvey and Lidz observed:

> Clinicians did not appear to be making simple "yes" or "no" judgments of dangerousness. Rather, they seemed to be making contextualized judgments regarding future violence. Instead of stating whether they thought someone was highly likely or unlikely to be involved in violence, the clinicians gave what we called "conditional judgments" regarding future

> violence. ... In other words, they saw the violence as dependent upon certain conditions in the person's life. (p. S108)

Thus, when making predictions, clinicians may often attend to the *person* and *situation*, rather than only to the *person*.

When clinicians cannot construct a compelling case formulation to help them make predictions, they may simply rely on the *past behavior heuristic* (Garb, 1996). That is, they may simply decide that the best predictor of future behavior is past behavior. The assumption underlying this approach is that for any particular client, only unimportant changes have occurred over time on both person and situation factors.

Just as clinicians often make causal judgments when making diagnoses and predictions, causal judgments also underlie treatment decisions. For example, Witteman and Koele (1999) had 56 psychotherapists formulate treatment plans for a group of depressed clients. Treatment plans were highly variable. Specific symptoms and seriousness of depression were largely unrelated to treatment plan. Similarly, theoretical background of the psychotherapist was a weak predictor of treatment plan. For example, for one of the cases, some of the client-centered therapists proposed that client-centered therapy be used, but others recommended that the client be offered family therapy or psychoanalytic treatment. In contrast, the best predictor of treatment plan was related to the implicit theories of the psychotherapists. As observed by Witteman and Koele, "The best explanations of the treatment proposals seemed to be the therapist's theory-inspired interpretations of the patient complaints" (p. 100).

In summary, clinicians often make causal judgments when determining diagnoses, predictions, and treatment decisions. This is ironic because clinicians are not very good at making causal judgments (Garb 1998, 2005). In fact, making causal judgments is the most difficult task for clinicians. One reason statistical prediction rules are often more accurate than clinicians is because statistical prediction typically relies on an actuarial approach (observing patterns of events for a prior sample) rather than on a causal theory.

### Biases and Errors

Biases and errors that are associated with clinical judgment include confirmatory bias, covariation misestimation (or illusory correlation), the anchoring and adjustment effect, the halo effect, hindsight bias, and the conjunction effect. All of these biases and errors occur in social judgment as well as clinical judgment.

*Confirmatory bias* occurs when confirmatory hypothesis testing leads to mistakes in judgment. Research describing the occurrence of confirmatory hypothesis testing was described earlier. Hypothesis testing underlies all clinical judgment, and it is likely that confirmatory bias has occurred in many instances when clinicians have made errors in judgment. For example, it is likely that racial bias is due, in part, to a failure to collect information that would lead clinicians to consider additional hypotheses about their clients. The occurrence of racial bias is described later in this chapter.

The terms *covariation misestimation* and *illusory correlation* refer to the same phenomenon. They are said to occur when an individual believes that two classes of events are correlated when, in reality, they are (1) not correlated, (2) correlated to a lesser extent than believed, or (3) correlated in the reverse direction from that which is reported. Arkes (1981) described the following example:

> Assume that you suspect that a certain MMPI profile is diagnostic of an impending psychotic break. To check this suspicion, you keep track of how many people with this profile do or do not have a subsequent psychotic episode. Would you also consider keeping track of those without that profile in order to test the hypothesis? Since the hypothesis deals only with people having a certain profile, disregarding those without it appears sensible. Yet those instances need to be recorded to test the hypothesis adequately. (p. 324)

In many instances, clinicians will continue to use a set of invalid test scores, incorrectly believing the test scores are correlated with important patient characteristics because they fail to notice instances when the patient characteristics occur in the absence of presumably diagnostic test scores (Chapman & Chapman, 1967, 1969).

The *anchoring and adjustment effect* can occur in two ways. First, a clinician can be influenced by whether an item of information is collected early or late in the course of psychotherapy. For example, after reading the summaries of five therapy sessions, therapists rated clients as more maladjusted and having a worse prognosis when information about suicide ideation or anorexia was presented in the summary of the first session rather than in the summary of the fourth session (Friedlander & Phillips, 1984). Second, clinicians can be influenced by the range of clients with whom they work. In Rich, Paul, and Mariotto (1988), when two patients on different psychiatric units had a similar level of adjustment (as meticulously determined by research staff), the ratings of adjustment made by clinical staff varied as a function of the level of adjustment of other patients on the unit. (Higher ratings of adjustment were given to patients who were on units with patients who were functioning relatively poorly.)

The *halo effect* occurs when a salient characteristic of a patient inappropriately influences judgments about a patient's other characteristics. For example, the observation of depressed nonverbal behavior should not lead clinicians to make severe ratings for symptoms of depression that are not reflected by nonverbal behavior. Yet Mumma (2002) reported that when psychologists watched videotapes of interviews with patients who showed clear-cut depressed nonverbal behavior, their ratings became more severe for symptoms such as appetite/weight change and suicidal ideation.

Judgments made in everyday life and in clinical practice sometimes violate axioms of probability theory. For example, *hindsight bias* occurs when individuals overestimate the likelihood that they would have predicted an outcome after they have become aware of the outcome (Arkes, Faust, Guilmette, & Hart, 1988; Fischhoff, 1975). Thus, if a client kills someone and an investigation is conducted, the investigators may conclude that the homicide could have been predicted—but they may reach this conclusion in part because of hindsight bias.

The *conjunction effect* (Tversky & Kahneman, 1983) occurs when individuals rate the likelihood of events $A$ and $B$ both occurring as greater than the likelihood of event $A$ occurring or the likelihood of event $B$ occurring. According to probability theory, the probability of events $A$ and $B$, $P(A \cap B)$, cannot be greater than the probability of event $A$, $P(A)$, or the probability of event $B$, $P(B)$. For example, the likelihood of a client having posttraumatic stress disorder and a chronic pain disorder cannot be greater than the likelihood of the client having posttraumatic stress disorder or the likelihood of the client having a chronic pain disorder. (Every time a client has both posttraumatic stress disorder and a chronic pain disorder, the client must necessarily have posttraumatic stress disorder.) In a recent clinical judgment study (Garb, 2006), when the judgment task was to rate the likelihood of different combinations of test results being obtained, violations of the conjunction rule were relatively large in magnitude and occurred for 58% of the clinicians. These results are not entirely surprising because we know that clinicians do not make ratings in a manner that emulates a strictly empirically based approach such as actuarial prediction. Instead, cognitive heuristics, confirmatory hypothesis testing, and causal reasoning shape how judgments are made.

## SOCIAL FACTORS

Some of the most famous studies that have ever been conducted on clinical judgment have described how social factors affect clinical judgment. Social factors include client characteristics (e.g., the race of the client) and context effects (e.g., whether the treatment a client receives depends on clinic setting).

### Client Characteristics

Judgments and decisions made by mental health professionals are said to be biased when their *accuracy* varies as a function of the group membership of a client. For example, if diagnoses of schizophrenia and bipolar disorder are more accurate for white clients than for black clients, then racial bias is said to be present. Notice that bias is not necessarily present when a diagnosis is given more often to members of one group than another. If a *disorder* is more prevalent for one group than another (e.g., depression among females), then the diagnosis for that disorder should be made more frequently for that group.

#### *Gender Bias*

Early research suggested that mental health professionals viewed female clients as less psychologically healthy than male clients. In the most highly cited study on gender bias (cited more than 500 times), Broverman, Broverman, Clarkson, Rosenkrantz, and Vogel (1970) had clinicians rate the social desirability of different traits. Clinicians rated which qualities would be desirable for a female, which would be desirable for a male, and which would be desirable for an adult without gender specified. Broverman et al. (1970) concluded that clinicians are significantly less likely to attribute traits that characterize "normal adults" to women than to men.

Subsequent research indicates that clinicians are *not* biased to view female clients as being less psychologically healthy than male clients (Kelley & Blashfield, 2009). Widiger and Settle (1987) repeated the Broverman et al. (1970) study, except they used a questionnaire that contained more items that describe socially desirable female stereotype traits than items that describe socially desirable male stereotype traits. Using this questionnaire, ratings of healthy females were similar to ratings for the healthy adult with gender unspecified, and ratings of healthy males were dissimilar to the ratings for the healthy adult with gender unspecified. Despite the importance of these findings, the study by Widiger and Settle has been cited fewer than 25 times.

Evidence of gender bias has generally been absent for ratings of level of adjustment and for differential diagnoses, with the exception of diagnosing histrionic personality disorder and antisocial personality disorder (Garb, 1997). In all of the studies, different groups of mental health professionals were given identical case vignettes except for the identification of gender. For rating *level of adjustment*, judgments were not significantly different for female and male clients in 12 studies; they were better for female clients than male clients in four studies; and mixed results were obtained in two studies (Garb, 1997, p. 110). With regard to *diagnosis*, male clients were more likely to be diagnosed as having an antisocial personality disorder and female clients were more likely to be diagnosed as having a histrionic personality disorder, even when the clients were described by the same information, except for the designation of gender (e.g., Ford & Widiger, 1989). Gender bias has typically not been reported for Axis I or Axis II disorders other than antisocial and histrionic personality disorders.

Gender bias may occur for the differential diagnosis of antisocial personality disorder and histrionic personality disorder because gender is closely tied to the stereotypes for these two disorders. Thus, if male gender forms part of a clinician's stereotype for antisocial personality disorder and female gender forms part of a clinician's stereotype for histrionic personality disorder, then gender bias is likely to occur when the representativeness heuristic is descriptive of how the diagnoses are made.

### *Social Class Bias*

Psychological problems occur most frequently, and with greatest severity, among the poor. Stressors associated with poverty can contribute to psychological disorders, and the occurrence of psychological disorders can contribute to a downward spiral in socioeconomic status. Hollingshead and Redlich (1958) proposed another possible explanation for why psychological disorders occur most frequently among the poor: They suggested that diagnoses and ratings of level of adjustment may be biased.

Fifty years of research indicates that social class bias does not occur when clinicians describe clients or make diagnoses (e.g., Garb, 1997). Nor does it occur when mental health professionals make decisions about whether a client should be hospitalized (e.g., Rabinowitz, Massad, & Fennig, 1995). However, social class does influence decisions made by clinicians regarding psychotherapy (Garb, 1997; Smith, 2005). Historically, lower socioeconomic clients are less likely to be referred for psychotherapy, perhaps because middle-class therapists experience greater success (or believe they will experience greater success) with middle-class clients than lower-class clients. When referred, lower-class clients are more likely to be seen for supportive therapy than for insight-oriented therapy.

This is not to mean that other forms of discrimination based on socioeconomic status (SES) do not occur. Social class bias is not evident when clinicians describe clients or make diagnoses, but the rich have more resources than the poor. Certainly the wealthier receive better health care than the poor (owing to better health coverage, not necessarily because of the biases of individual clinicians). But the popular saying "When you're rich you're called eccentric, when you're poor you're called crazy" does not seem true. Instead, when you're rich, you will sometimes be appropriately diagnosed and treated because you will have good health coverage, whereas when you're poor, available health care resources are likely to be considerably less.

### *Racial Bias*

Research on clinical judgment suggests that racial bias is more pervasive than gender bias and social class bias. For this reason, it is not surprising that recent research on bias in clinical judgment has focused on this topic. It is an especially important area of research in psychiatry, particularly with regard to the use of psychotropic medication. The methodology of the research has been strong, and it is notable that racial bias has been found when investigators have examined judgments made in real-life settings.

Racial bias most frequently occurs with the diagnosis and treatment of psychotic patients. In half a dozen studies, white patients with a psychotic mood disorder were more likely to be correctly diagnosed than black and Hispanic patients with a psychotic mood disorder (e.g., Pavkov, Lewis, & Lyons, 1989). Subsequent research has focused on the effect of race on the use of psychotropic medication. For example, the Schizophrenia Patient Outcome Research Team, using a stratified random sample of 719 persons diagnosed with schizophrenia, showed that black were less likely than white patients to receive treatment in accordance with recommended practices (Lehman & Steinwachs, 1998). Similarly, black patients with bipolar disorder were less likely than white patients with bipolar disorder to receive lithium and selective serotonin reuptake inhibitors (SSRIs; Kilbourne & Pincus, 2006), and black patients with schizophrenia were less likely than white patients with schizophrenia to receive second-generation antipsychotics (e.g., Mallinger, Fisher, Brown, & Lamberti, 2006). More generally, black patients are at greater risk for excessive antipsychotic dosing compared to white patients (e.g., Walkup et al., 2000).

In conclusion, it does appear that black patients sometimes receive lower-quality medical care than other patients. It is difficult to disentangle all of the reasons why this occurs, but results from one study (Segal, Bola, & Watson, 1996) are illuminating. In this study, black patients, compared to white, Hispanic, and Asian patients, received a significantly larger number of psychotropic medications, a significantly larger number of injections of antipsychotic medication, and a significantly larger number of doses of antipsychotic medicine. These differences in treatment were obtained even though the investigators controlled for (1) level of functioning, (2) presence of a psychotic disorder, (3) danger to self or others or gravely disabled, (4) history of mental disorder, and (5) whether physical restraints were used. Clinicians spent significantly less time with the black patients than the other patients. When they spent more time evaluating the black patients, the dosage of antipsychotic medication decreased.

### Context Effects

The best known clinical judgment study ever conducted was on the effect of context on psychodiagnosis and treatment. In this study (Rosenhan, 1973), research confederates with no known psychopathology went to the emergency rooms of different psychiatric hospitals. They were all hospitalized after complaining of hearing voices. None were committed to the hospital: All entered voluntarily. Each confederate initially complained of hearing a voice that said "empty," "hollow," and "thud." Once they were hospitalized, they no longer reported hearing the voice, and they consistently reported that they were feeling fine. The confederates answered all questions in a truthful manner except when asked why they had come to the hospital, whether they had heard voices, and their name, vocation, and place of employment. Remarkably, 11 of the 12 confederates were diagnosed at admission as having schizophrenia, and length of hospitalization ranged from 7 to 52 days with an average stay of 19 days. Rosenhan (1973) argued that behavior that would seem normal in the community was seen as being consistent with schizophrenia when viewed in the context of a psychiatric hospital. He concluded that "we cannot distinguish the sane from the insane in psychiatric hospitals" (1973, p. 257) and that a psychiatric diagnosis reveals "little about the patient but much about the environment in which an observer finds him" (1973, p. 251).

Rosenhan's assertions strike at the heart of mental health practice. If the effect of context is so overpowering that clinicians cannot adequately evaluate a client, then the value of their interventions will be undermined. However, while the results from Rosenhan's study have had an important impact on mental health practice, his conclusions from the data are widely viewed by mental health professionals as being overstated (see the special section that appeared in the *Journal of Abnormal Psychology* in 1975; see also, Davis, 1976; Spitzer, 1975).

The results from Rosenhan's classic study are important because they were one factor that led to the development of explicit and specific criteria for making diagnoses. Explicit and specific criteria became widely available only with the publication of the American Psychiatric Association's (1980) *Diagnostic and Statistical Manual of Mental Disorders*, third edition (commonly referred to as DSM-III). If a person's sole presenting symptom is hearing voices, clinicians will not assign a diagnosis of schizophrenia if they adhere to current diagnostic criteria. Put another way, the harmful effects of context on diagnoses described by Rosenhan are minimized when clinicians adhere to explicit diagnostic criteria. Although Rosenhan (1975, p. 467) argued that "my own preference runs to omitting diagnoses entirely," it is more credible to argue that clinicians should adhere to criteria when making diagnoses. At the same time, there is a growing realization that clinicians should not adhere to DSM criteria in a rote manner, and that it is important to consider the context of a client's life when using the DSM criteria (Horwitz & Wakefield, 2007). Finally, it can be pointed out that hospitalization for these pseudo-patients was not inappropriate. If someone complains of hearing voices and the reason for the complaint is unknown, then a complete evaluation needs to be performed. But it is difficult to rationalize the length of stay. Undoubtedly, context was exerting an impact on clinicians.

As empirical data have been collected, we have learned more about when context effects are, and are not, important for understanding clinical judgment. For example, recent work reveals that clinicians do not simply attend to symptoms when making diagnoses, they also rely on case formulations and context (Kim & Ahn, 2002; Pottick et al., 2007). For example, Pottick et al. (2007) found that diagnoses of conduct disorder decreased by 80% when contextual information suggested that a youth's problematic behaviors disappeared when he was not in a dangerous environment filled with gang violence.

To a surprising extent, type of treatment provided depends just as much on the particular clinic where a client is seen as it does on empirical evidence about what type of treatment works best for what type of patient. For example, in a study of 338 patients with major depressive disorder (Keller et al., 1986), large differences in the amount and type of treatment (medicine, electroconvulsive therapy, psychotherapy) were found across five medical centers. The best predictor of the type and amount of treatment received was not the severity of depression but the hospital setting where the patient went for treatment.

Even whether someone is committed to a hospital against his or her will depends, in part, on context. In one study (Lidz, Coontz, & Mulvey, 2000), 96 clinicians made 432 different emergency room assessments. Investigators recorded a range of data, including whether the individual (1) was able to care for self, (2) had made a recent suicide attempt, (3) had recently been violent, or (4) had been self-referred or was accompanied to the emergency room by police, medics, or family members. The strongest predictor of both admission and involuntary commitment was whether the individual was self-referred or accompanied. Individuals were almost always committed when the police were involved or when the first steps of the commitment had already been taken. In contrast, when individuals arrived on their own volition, they were referred for outpatient treatment more than half of the time. Individuals who were accompanied by family or a friend fell between the two groups, often being referred for outpatient treatment but also being voluntarily or involuntarily hospitalized. As noted by the authors, "The presence of violence against others or suicide appears to have considerable influence, but even these do not appear as strong as who accompanies the patient" (p. 50). These results illustrate the role social factors play in psychiatric hospitalization decisions.

## IMPLICATIONS FOR CLINICAL PRACTICE

Can we teach ourselves to make better snap judgments, as urged by Gladwell (2005)? In the review of the literature conducted for this chapter, no evidence was found on how this can be done. Gladwell implied that one can become better at making snap judgments by attending to one's emotions (which clinicians already do) and by gaining a variety of experiences. For example, he recounted how an expert recognized that a statue was a forgery because the statue did not resemble long-buried statuary that the expert had unearthed. However, one of the most interesting findings on clinical judgment is that it can be very difficult to learn from clinical experience. This is true for medical doctors (Choudhry, Fletcher, & Soumerai, 2005), mental health professionals (Garb, 1989), and neuropsychologists (Garb & Schramke, 1996). It is difficult to learn from experience, in part, because clinicians often do not receive accurate feedback on whether their judgments are right or wrong, but also because clinicians are not always aware of how social factors affect their judgments, and because cognitive processes are imperfect.

Research on the social psychology of clinical judgment suggests that clinicians should be very careful about making snap judgments. Racial bias decreased when clinicians spent more time, not less time, with patients (Segal et al., 1996). Cognitive heuristics are related to making snap judgments because they all involve using a simple rule to make judgments. But while reliance on cognitive heuristics is efficient in terms of time and cognitive resources, their use can lead to the systematic occurrence of certain types of errors. For example, mental health professionals can make diagnoses very quickly by relying on the representativeness heuristic, but this can lead to their drifting from the DSM criteria, which in turn can lead to low interrater reliability. Finally, cognitive biases may occur more frequently when clinicians make snap judgments. For example, confirmatory bias occurs when clinicians make judgments and decisions relatively quickly. When they take the time to collect comprehensive information and consider alternative hypotheses, they are less likely to stick with their initial impression.

Forming sudden impressions and being influenced by one's feelings are an ingrained part of the process of how we make judgments. This is unlikely to change. Nor should it. But after quickly forming an impression of a client, clinicians should collect additional information and consider alternative hypotheses. Valuable information can be collected in a range of ways, such as by using statistical prediction rules (Grove et al., 2000), systematically monitoring the progress (or lack of progress) of clients receiving mental health treatment (e.g.,

Lambert, Harmon, Slade, Whipple, & Hawkins, 2005), and using computers to administer structured interviews (Garb, 2007). By using these and other information-gathering tools, we will be performing a service for our clients.

## AUTHOR NOTE

The views expressed in this chapter are those of the author and are not the official policy of the Department of Defense or the United States Air Force.

## REFERENCES

Ambady, N., & Rosenthal, R. (1992). Thin slices of expressive behavior as predictors of interpersonal consequences: A meta-analysis. *Psychological Bulletin, 111*, 256–274.

American Psychiatric Association. (1980). *Diagnostic and statistical manual of mental disorders* (3rd ed.). Washington, DC: Author.

Arkes, H. R. (1981). Impediments to accurate clinical judgment and possible ways to minimize their impact. *Journal of Consulting and Clinical Psychology, 49*, 323–330.

Arkes, H. R., Faust, D., Guilmette, T. J., & Hart, K. (1988). Eliminating the hindsight bias. *Journal of Applied Psychology, 73*, 305–307.

Bem, D. J. (1972). Self-perception theory. In L. Berkowitz (Ed.), *Advances in experimental social psychology* (Vol. 6, pp. 1–62). New York: Academic Press.

Broverman, I., Broverman, D., Clarkson, F., Rosenkrantz, P., & Vogel, S. (1970). Sex-role stereotypes and clinical judgments of mental health. *Journal of Consulting and Clinical Psychology, 34*, 1–7.

Chapman, L. J., & Chapman, J. P. (1967). Genesis of popular but erroneous psychodiagnostic observations. *Journal of Abnormal Psychology, 72*, 193–204.

Chapman, L. J., & Chapman, J. P. (1969). Illusory correlation as an obstacle to the use of valid psychodiagnostic signs. *Journal of Abnormal Psychology, 74*, 271–280.

Choudhry, N. K., Fletcher, R. H., & Soumerai, S. B. (2005). Systematic review: The relationship between clinical experience and quality of health care. *Annals of Internal Medicine, 142*, 260–273.

Davis, D. A. (1976). On being detectably sane in insane places: Base rates and psychodiagnosis. *Journal of Abnormal Psychology, 85*, 416–422.

Einhorn, H. J., Kleinmuntz, D. N., & Kleinmuntz, B. (1979). Linear regression and process-tracing models of judgment. *Psychological Review, 86*, 465–485.

Fischhoff, B. (1975). Hindsight/foresight: The effect of outcome knowledge on judgment under uncertainty. *Journal of Experimental Psychology: Human Perception and Performance, 1*, 288–299.

Ford, M. R., & Widiger, T. A. (1989). Sex bias in the diagnosis of histrionic and antisocial personality disorders. *Journal of Consulting and Clinical Psychology, 57*, 301–305.

Friedlander, M. L., & Phillips, S. D. (1984). Preventing anchoring errors in clinical judgment. *Journal of Consulting and Clinical Psychology, 52*, 366–371.

Garb, H. N. (1989). Clinical judgment, clinical training, and professional experience. *Psychological Bulletin, 105*, 387–396.

Garb, H. N. (1996). The representativeness and past-behavior heuristics in clinical judgment. *Professional Psychology, 27*, 272–277.

Garb, H. N. (1997). Race bias, social class bias, and gender bias in clinical judgment. *Clinical Psychology: Science and Practice, 4*, 99–120.

Garb, H. N. (1998). *Studying the clinician: Judgment research and psychological assessment*. Washington, DC: American Psychological Association.

Garb, H. N. (2005). Clinical judgment and decision making. *Annual Review of Clinical Psychology, 1*, 67–89.

Garb, H. N. (2006). The conjunction effect and clinical judgment. *Journal of Social and Clinical Psychology*, *25*, 1048–1056.

Garb, H. N. (2007). Computer-administered interviews and rating scales. *Psychological Assessment*, *19*, 4–13.

Garb, H. N., & Schramke, C. J. (1996). Judgment research and neuropsychological assessment: A narrative review and meta-analyses. *Psychological Bulletin*, *120*, 140–153.

Gazzaniga, M. S., & LeDoux, J. E. (1978). *The integrated mind*. New York: Plenum Press.

Gilovich, T., Griffin, D., & Kahneman, D. (Eds.). (2002). *Heuristics and biases*. New York: Cambridge University Press.

Gladwell, M. (2005). *Blink: The power of thinking without thinking*. New York: Little, Brown.

Grove, W. M., Zald, D. H., Lebow, B. S., Snitz, B. E., & Nelson, C. (2000). Clinical versus mechanical prediction: A meta-analysis. *Psychological Assessment*, *12*, 19–30.

Hammer, E. F. (1964). *The House–Tree–Person clinical research manual*. Los Angeles: Western Psychological Services.

Hanson, R. K. (1998). What do we know about offender risk assessment? *Psychology, Public Policy, and Law*, *4*, 50–72

Harris, G. T., Rice, M. E., & Quinsey, V. L. (1993). Violent recidivism of mentally disordered offenders: The development of a statistical prediction instrument. *Criminal Justice and Behavior*, *20*, 315–335.

Haverkamp, B. E. (1993). Confirmatory bias in hypothesis testing for client-identified and counselor self-generated hypotheses. *Journal of Counseling Psychology*, *40*, 303–315.

Hollingshead, A. B., & Redlich, F. C. (1958). *Social class and mental illness: A community study*. New York: Wiley.

Horwitz, A. V., & Wakefield, J. C. (2007). *The loss of sadness: How psychiatry transformed normal sorrow into depressive disorder*. New York: Oxford University Press.

Kahneman, D. (2003). A perspective on judgment and choice: Mapping bounded rationality. *American Psychologist, 58*, 697–720.

Kahneman, D., Slovic, P., & Tversky, A. (Eds.). (1982). *Judgment under uncertainty: Heuristics and biases*. New York: Cambridge University Press.

Keller, M. B., Lavori, P. W., Klerman, G. L., Andreasen, N. C., Endicott, J., Coryell, W., et al. (1986). Low levels and lack of predictors of somatotherapy and psychotherapy received by depressed patients. *Archives of General Psychiatry*, *43*, 458–466.

Kelley, L. P., & Blashfield, R. K. (2009). An example of psychological science's failure to self-correct. *Review of General Psychology*, *13*, 122–129.

Kendell, R. E. (1973). Psychiatric diagnoses: A study of how they are made. *British Journal of Psychiatry*, *122*, 437–445.

Kilbourne, A. M., & Pincus, H. A. (2006). Patterns of psychotropic medication use by race among veterans with bipolar disorder. *Psychiatric Services*, *57*, 123–126.

Kim, N. S., & Ahn, W. (2002). Clinical psychologists' theory-based representations of mental disorders predict their diagnostic reasoning and memory. *Journal of Experimental Psychology: General*, *131*, 451–476.

Lambert, M. J., Harmon, C., Slade, K., Whipple, J. L., & Hawkins, E. J. (2005). Providing feedback to psychotherapists on their patients' progress: Clinical results and suggestions. *Journal of Clinical Psychology/In Session*, *61*, 165–174.

Lehman, A. F., & Steinwachs, D. M. (1998). Patterns of usual care for schizophrenia: Initial results from the Schizophrenia Patient Outcomes Research Team (PORT) client survey. *Schizophrenia Bulletin*, *24*, 11–20.

Lidz, C. W., Coontz, P. D., & Mulvey, E. P. (2000). The "pass-through" model of psychiatric emergency room assessment. *International Journal of Law and Psychiatry*, *23*, 43–51.

Lilienfeld, S. O., Wood, J. M., & Garb, H. N. (2000). The scientific status of projective techniques. *Psychological Science in the Public Interest*, *1*, 27–66.

Mallinger, J. B., Fisher, S. G., Brown, T., & Lamberti, J. S. (2006). Racial disparities in the use of second-generation antipsychotics for the treatment of schizophrenia. *Psychiatric Services*, *57*, 133–136.

Meehl, P. E. (1954). *Clinical vs. statistical prediction*. Minneapolis: University of Minnesota Press.

Mulvey, E. P., & Lidz, C. W. (1998). Clinical prediction of violence as a conditional judgment. *Social Psychiatry and Psychiatric Epidemiology*, *33*, S107–S113.

Mumma, G. H. (2002). Effects of three types of potentially biasing information on symptom severity judgments for major depressive episode. *Journal of Clinical Psychology*, *58*, 1327–1345.

Pavkov, T. W., Lewis, D. A., & Lyons, J. S. (1989). Psychiatric diagnoses and racial bias: An empirical investigation. *Professional Psychology*, *20*, 364–368.

Pottick, K. J., Kirk, S. A., Hsieh, D. K., & Tian, X. (2007). Judging mental disorder in youths: Effects of client, clinician, and contextual differences. *Journal of Consulting and Clinical Psychology*, *75*, 1–8.

Rabinowitz, J., Massad, A., & Fennig, S. (1995). Factors influencing disposition decisions for patients seen in a psychiatric emergency service. *Psychiatric Services*, *46*, 712–718.

Rich, B. E., Paul, G. L., & Mariotto, M. J. (1988). Judgmental relativism as a validity threat to standardized psychiatric rating scales. *Journal of Psychopathology and Behavioral Assessment*, *10*, 241–257.

Rosenhan, D. L. (1973). On being sane in insane places. *Science*, *179*, 250–258.

Rosenhan, D. L. (1975). The contextual nature of psychiatric diagnosis. *Journal of Abnormal Psychology*, *84*, 462–474.

Segal, S. P., Bola, J. R., & Watson, M. A. (1996). Race, quality of care, and antipsychotic prescribing practices in psychiatric emergency services. *Psychiatric Services*, *47*, 282–286.

Slovic, P., Monahan, J., & MacGregor, D. G. (2000). Violence risk assessment and risk communication: The effects of using actual cases, providing instruction, and employing probability versus frequency formats. *Law and Human Behavior*, *24*, 271–296.

Smith, L. (2005). Psychotherapy, classism, and the poor: Conspicuous by their absence. *American Psychologist*, *60*, 687–696.

Spitzer, R. L. (1975). On pseudoscience in science, logic in remission, and psychiatric diagnosis: A critique of Rosenhan's "On Being Sane in Insane Places." *Journal of Abnormal Psychology*, *84*, 442–452.

Tversky, A., & Kahneman, D. (1974). Judgments under uncertainty: Heuristics and biases. *Science*, *185*, 1124–1131.

Tversky, A., & Kahneman, D. (1983). Extensional vs. intuitive reasoning: The conjunction fallacy in probability judgment. *Psychological Review*, *90*, 293–315.

Walkup, J., McAlpine, D., Olfson, M., Labay, L., Boyer, C., & Hansell, S. (2000). Patients with schizophrenia at risk for excessive antipsychotic dosing. *Journal of Clinical Psychiatry*, *61*, 344–348.

Widiger, T. A., & Settle, S. A. (1987). Broverman et al. revisited: An artifactual sex bias. *Journal of Personality and Social Psychology*, *53*, 463–469.

Wilson, T. D. (2002). *Strangers to ourselves: Discovering the adaptive unconscious*. Cambridge, MA: Harvard University Press.

Witteman, C., & Koele, P. (1999). Explaining treatment decisions. *Psychotherapy Research*, *9*, 100–114.

# 17 Sociocultural Issues in the Diagnosis and Assessment of Psychological Disorders

Sopagna Eap
Robyn L. Gobin
Janet Ng
Gordon C. Nagayama Hall

Thomas Szasz (1961) suggested that mental disorders are created by those in power to exert social control over those who do not conform to social norms. History supports this contention. For example, it was a common belief among medical experts in the 19th century that "primitive people," such as Native Americans, would be driven insane if given their freedom (Gamwell & Tomes, 1995). Indeed, this is just one example, among others, that illustrates how past mental health practices have been used as a mechanism for oppression. These instances of diagnostic mistakes by the mental health community can come about when a purely nomothetic approach is taken in understanding psychological processes. A nomothetic perspective seeks out universals in human experiences. Disorders are reified when a set of behaviors is grouped together and labeled without considering the sociocultural context of the individual. Despite past injustices that have been precipitated by the mental health system, a nomothetic approach to assessment and diagnostic procedures is vital for mental health research, collaboration, and proper dissemination of treatment. However, assessment can only be strengthened by also concurrently incorporating an idiographic strategy that emphasizes individual experiences. An idiographic approach incorporates unique individual factors such as cultural background, religious background, and life circumstances into diagnosis. By examining idiographic factors that may affect assessment and diagnosis, we will be able to avoid the kinds of mistakes made by past mental health professionals. Failure to adopt both strategies in our nosological system puts us in danger of perpetuating the situation described by Szasz.

Currently, cultural insensitivity and indirect bias have resulted in a clear pattern of inequitable services and mistreatment for members of ethnic minority groups in the United States. For example, African American persons with schizophrenia are 1.8 times more likely than European American persons with schizophrenia to be prescribed high-potency antipsychotic medication (Diaz & de Leon, 2002). This trend is alarming, given that antipsychotic drugs have the potential to cause extrapyramidal side effects, which can be adverse and permanent. Asian Americans and African Americans are more prone than European Americans to developing these side effects (Binder & Levy, 1981; Pi & Simpson, 2005). Additionally, African Americans are also more likely than other ethnic groups to be involuntarily committed to psychiatric hospitals (Lindsey & Paul, 1989). Thus, the potential of a misdiagnosis can be more detrimental for ethnic minorities than for European Americans.

Dana (2001) contended that "the objective of clinical diagnosis is to reduce emotional distress and suffering by reliable classification of disorders leading toward optimal designation of effective intervention as a consequence of diagnostic procedures" (p. 101). As the cultural fabric of the United States grows increasingly diverse, the recognition of differing cultural frameworks is likely to improve quality of care for a large segment of the population. The *Diagnostic and Statistical Manual of Mental Disorders* (DSM-IV-TR; American Psychiatric Association, 2000), mainly used in the United States, is reflective of mostly Western norms and values (Dana, 2001). Thus, the idiographic experiences of non-Western cultural groups are marginalized in the DSM-IV-TR, compared to the experiences of people from Western cultures, resulting in observed discrepancies in diagnosis. For this reason, mental health professionals need to actively search for and rectify biases present in the current diagnostic system, which may emphasize a nomothetic approach at the cost of an idiographic one.

The purpose of this chapter is to highlight idiographic variables that are associated with each level of a traditionally nomothetic process as a way to dispel the cultural bias inherent in our present diagnostic system (Figure 17.1). The DSM-IV diagnoses an individual on five axes in order to encompass the individual's entire mental health experience. Clinical disorders are coded on Axis I. The DSM-IV considers unique social variables by incorporating idiographic factors on Axis IV on the multiaxial system. This system may misleadingly encourage some to consider sociocultural factors as separate and independent of the psychiatric diagnosis. However, our model of assessment and diagnosis highlights the relationship between these two traditionally dichotomous approaches to understanding mental health categories.

This chapter begins with an examination of client variables relevant for understanding symptoms. Next we discuss how idiographic factors affect DSM-IV-TR definitions of abnormality and the diagnostic process. In particular, idiographic variables are important in understanding the role of clinician bias in influencing assessment and diagnostic procedures. These relevant cultural issues are meant to guide the clinician's framework when assessing clients from diverse cultures. This chapter focuses mainly on ethnic minority groups in the United States, but these issues may also be relevant for a variety of minority groups (e.g., religious or sexual minorities).

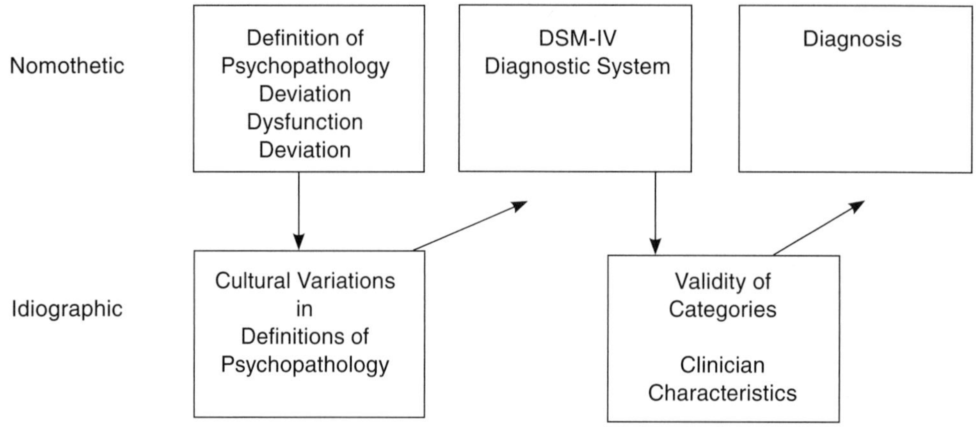


**FIGURE 17.1.** A model of idiographic considerations in a nomethetic process.

## CLIENT CHARACTERISTICS

An idiographic approach to assessment and diagnosis with ethnic minority groups should begin with a flexible framework. Sue (1998) introduced the idea of *dynamic sizing*, which describes the clinical skill of knowing when cultural information is relevant to the client and when it is not, based on client characteristics. Hwang (2006) stressed the importance of dynamic sizing when working with ethnic minority clients in therapy. However, dynamic sizing also has functional relevance during the assessment and diagnostic process. Differences in acculturation and ethnic identity among members of the same ethnic group may result in variability in psychological well-being and psychopathology.

Acculturation is a dynamic process between the minority and majority cultures on a number of dimensions, including language, customs, self-identification, attitudes, and values (Abe-Kim, Okazaki, & Goto, 2001; Felix-Ortiz, Newcomb, & Myers, 1994). Sue, Mak, and Sue (1998) defined acculturation as a change in cultural attitudes, values, and behaviors ensuing from continuous contact between an individual's cultural group and another cultural group. Acculturation to one culture does not necessarily entail the loss of another. Thus, a client may appear to identify with the majority culture but may continue to internalize values of his or her culture of origin.

The relationship between acculturation and psychological well-being and adjustment is complex. Shen and Takeuchi (2001) suggested that the reason for the discrepant findings regarding the role of acculturation in affecting mental health is that acculturation may have an indirect influence on mental health. In their study examining mental health and acculturation status among a sample of Chinese American community members, the influence of acculturation on mental health was moderated by socioeconomic status, social support, stress, and personality characteristics. Thus, clinicians should not assume that the acculturative experience is similar for every ethnic minority client.

For some individuals, acculturation may lead to a loss of important cultural support and exposure to greater antisocial activities. Burnam, Hough, Karno, Escobar, and Telles (1987) found an inverse relationship between acculturation and mental health diagnoses for Mexican Americans. Prevalence rates for alcohol abuse and dependence, drug abuse and dependence, phobia, and antisocial personality disorder increased as level of acculturation increased. Mexican-born immigrants had significantly lower lifetime prevalence rates of mental disorders than U.S.-born Mexican Americans. The researchers attributed the positive mental health profiles of Mexican immigrants to the extended familial support often present in Mexican culture, and the negative mental health profiles of U.S.-born Mexican Americans to greater access to alcohol and drugs in the United States. Thus, acculturation may lead to a loss of social support that contributes to a decrease in mental health functioning.

However, acculturation without the loss of important cultural ties may enhance mental health. Kaplan and Marks (1990) found that increased acculturation was associated with increased depression scores for young Mexican American adults but not for older Mexican Americans. For young Mexican American adults, efforts to adopt the values of the majority culture may isolate them from traditional resources. Acculturated older Mexican American adults may have resolved their ability to retain cultural ties while functioning in mainstream culture. Lafromboise, Coleman, and Gerton (1993) described this bicultural ability as the *alternation model* and contended that this may be the most psychologically optimal acculturative process for ethnic minorities.

Acculturation may also affect symptom patterns that are important for diagnosis. Ying and Miller (1992) found that acculturated Asian Americans were more likely to endorse psychological symptoms than were unacculturated Asian Americans, who were more likely to endorse physical symptoms. Consistent with this finding, Parker, Chan, Tully, and Eisenbruch (2005) found that acculturation was associated with decreased somatic symptoms among a sample of Chinese Australians. Furthermore, degree of acculturation is likely to affect attitudes toward mental illness. In cultures that discourage open emotional expression, physical symptoms may be a more acceptable way of conveying distress. Somatization may occur as a result of stigma attached to mental illness in non-Western cultures; acculturation to Western norms increases the acceptability of psychological distress.

Another cultural variable associated with mental health and psychopathology is ethnic identity. Ethnicity is generally thought to be a component of race, based on the individual's geographic, ancestral origin (Phinney, 2003). For instance, *Asian* is considered a race, whereas Chinese, Korean, and Japanese are considered ethnicities of the Asian race. Ethnic identity, centers around the individual's relationship and sense of self to his or her own ethnic group, which is the extent to which an individual identifies with the values, attitudes, and behaviors of his or her ethnicity. In contrast, *acculturation* evaluates the relationship between the ethnic minority group and the ethnic majority group (e.g., European Americans).

Evidence suggests that a strong ethnic identity may encourage positive mental health outcomes among ethnic minorities. Phinney, Cantu, and Kurtz (1996) found that ethnic identity was a significant predictor of self-esteem for African Americans, Latinos/Latinas, and European American adolescents. Self-esteem is a significant protective factor against depression and hopelessness (Harter, 1993) and thus may promote psychological resilience among adolescents. American identity, however, was significantly related to self-esteem only among the European American students. This study highlights the importance of ethnic identity for ethnic minorities, even for those who are American-born.

Additionally, an individual's ability to manage issues regarding race and ethnicity, coupled with a strong ethnic identification, may be one of the mechanisms that increases well-being among ethnic minorities. Neville and Lilly (2000) examined the relationship between psychological well-being and racial identity profiles among a sample of African American college students. They found five clusters of racial identity among their sample: (1) *dissonance internalization*—individuals who are comfortable with their identity as an African American person but feel conflict over the meaning of being African American in a racially oppressive society; (2) *committed internalization*—individuals who are proud of their African American identity but are less occupied with race and issues of racism; (3) *engaged internalization*—individuals who are comfortable with their racial group and with confronting racial issues; (4) *undifferentiated racial identity*—individuals who are confused over their racial identity; and (5) *dormant racial identity*—individuals that do not consider issues of racial identity. The results indicated that the *engaged internalization* group reported significantly less psychological distress than the *undifferentiated racial identity* group. These results suggest that individuals who have a strong ethnic identity and a willingness to address uncomfortable racial issues may be the most resilient to psychological distress.

These client variables provide an important window into individuals' subjective experience. When individuals from ethnic minorities seek psychological treatment, their multidimensional experience as an individual member of a minority group and their degree of acculturation must be taken into account. This is especially important in assessment and diagnosis because these processes have implications for treatment recommendations and mental health outcomes. By understanding that these idiographic variables can influence symptom presentation and prevalence, the threat of stereotyping based on cultural background is greatly mitigated.

## DEFINING PSYCHOPATHOLOGY

According to the DSM-IV-TR (American Psychiatric Association, 2000), the three components of psychopathology are *distress*, *dysfunction*, and *deviation*. The process of refining a universal definition of psychopathology does not minimize the role of idiographic variables when applying nomothetic categories. Client variables may influence accurate judgments concerning the criteria for mental illness.

### Distress

The process of establishing the presence of distress is contingent on clinician detection and client expression. Thus, this is a reciprocal process in that distress is recognized by the clinician and also verbally or visually expressed by the client. However, a number of variables may complicate the likelihood that distress will be expressed and/or recognized.

The likelihood of disclosure and the preferred recipient of disclosure may be culturally influenced. Certain ethnic groups may be hesitant to express distress to others because of stigmatization or beliefs regarding mental illness. Zhang, Snowden, and Sue (1998) found that Asian Americans were less likely than European Americans to express their distress to mental health professionals, family, or friends. African Americans are also less likely than European Americans to turn to a mental health professional and instead, are more likely to turn to a religious leader during times of personal stress (Neighbors, Musick, & Williams, 1998). These examples are likely associated with cultural values. A fear of losing face or bringing shame to one's in-group is an important cultural value that has implications for behavior among Asian Americans (Zane & Yeh, 2002). For instance, fear of losing face discourages Asian individuals from disclosing personal information in therapy (Zane & Mak, 2003). Spirituality and religiosity also are important for many ethnic minority persons, but especially for African Americans, who may often use religion-based coping strategies (Broman, 1996).

The patterns of nondisclosure to mental health professionals among ethnic minorities suggest that clinicians or physicians may need to rely on nonverbal cues to detect psychological stress. Western clinicians, however, may not always be able to recognize distress in clients from other cultures because of cultural differences in emotional expression. For example, distress cues from members of one cultural group may be less recognizable to an individual from another ethnic group. Okazaki (2002) found that self-reports of depression and social anxiety did not correspond with reports from peer informants for Asian Americans. The relationship between the subject and the peer informant varied and included friends, spouses, and roommates. The majority of the informants were European Americans. Informants consistently underestimated the degree of distress that the Asian Americans were experiencing. Additionally, the greatest mistakes were made for Asian Americans by European American informants. Informants were fairly accurate, however, in judging the emotional states of European Americans.

One reason for this inability to detect distress may be that cultural scripts determine appropriate emotional expression. Kleinman (1988) used the term *cultural idioms of distress* to describe unique cultural patterns of emotional expression. For example, Asian Americans may be less emotive than members of other ethnic groups in their emotional distress. Gross and John (1995) found Asian Americans to be less emotionally expressive than African Americans, European Americans, and Hispanic Americans. Nevertheless, rates of depression among Asian Americans are comparable to those of other ethnic groups (Kessler et al., 1994). Asian Americans who are experiencing depressive symptoms may not express their distress in a way that is familiar or common in the United States, reducing the likelihood that a Western clinician would recognize it.

One idiom of distress that has been studied extensively is somatization, a process by which emotional distress is expressed as physical symptoms and complaints. Indeed, somatization is a frequent indicator of distress among many ethnic minority groups, including African Americans (Brown, Shulberg, & Madonia, 1996), Latino/Latina Americans (Canino, Rubio-Sripec, Canino, & Escobar, 1992), and Asian Americans (Hsu & Folstein, 1997). Le, Berenbaum, and Raghavan (2002) suggested that the tendency to somaticize psychological symptoms among Asian Americans may be related to *alexythymia*, which is characterized by a difficulty in distinguishing emotions from bodily sensations and communicating emotional experiences. In their study, *alexythymia* was more associated with somatization for both Asian American and Malaysian students than for European American students. The Asian groups also reported greater levels of *alexythymia*. This finding may explain the patterns of physical symptoms among Asian Americans. Somatization is also a key feature in a variety of culture-bound syndromes (Guarnaccia & Rogler, 1999). For example, *hwa-byung*, literally "anger-disease" or "fire-disease," is a Korean disorder that includes symptoms of insomnia, fatigue, and heart palpitations (Lin, 1983).

Additionally, subjective experience of distress may be less important in defining pathology for some ethnic groups than definitions of "normal" or "healthy" emotional states. Tsai, Knutson, and Fung (2006) illustrated this complexity by studying how the discrepancy between "ideal affect" and "actual affect" contributed to experiences of depression. They proposed that culture plays a large role in determining ideal affect, the emotional state that people value and would like to feel. They found evidence that ideal affect and emotional affect are distinct constructs. Chinese students from Hong Kong valued low-arousal positive affect ("calm") more than Asian American students, who valued it more than European American students, demonstrating cultural differences in ideal affect. In contrast, European American students valued high-arousal affective states ("excitement") more than Asian American students, who valued it more than Chinese students. Students were then asked to evaluate how they actually feel. The discrepancy between ideal affect and actual affect was significant in explaining depression among Chinese Americans and European Americans, suggesting that individual definitions of ideal affect are as important as actual mood states for conceptualizing well-being. High-arousal emotions, such as anxiety, may be perceived as more distressing for Asian Americans than for European Americans.

## Dysfunction

*Dysfunction* refers to disruptions in social or occupational functioning. Clients may meet this criterion when they experience interpersonal difficulties or job-related problems. However, individuals may differ with respect to which realms of functioning are most important. For example, whereas family conflict may be a mild annoyance for some from a more individualistic culture, the family is a central aspect in Asian cultures (Lee, 1999) and children—even adult children—are expected to respect and obey the wishes of their parents (Kim & Wong, 2002). Asian Americans, in adolescence and into adulthood, often must mediate two conflicting ideals of traditional Asian culture and American culture (Hall & Okazaki, 2002; Sue et al., 1998; Sue & Sue, 1999). Asian American families in which the parents were born in the United States experience less intergenerational conflict than families in which the parents were born in Asia and the children were born in the United States (Chung, 2001). Family conflict may require more attention for Asian Americans or ethnic minorities than for those from Western cultures, because family is a central component of healthy social functioning in some cultures and yet immersion in a different culture may cause increased family conflict.

*Self-construal* is a concept that may explain the significance of behaviors for individual functioning. Self-construal describes the understanding that an individual has about his or her place in the world. Markus and Kitayama (1991) distinguished between *independent* self-construal and *interdependent* self-construal and maintained that these two factors heavily influence behavioral norms and socialization practices. In general, Western cultures encourage an independent self-construal, whereas many other cultures (e.g., Asian, African, Latin American) encourage a more interdependent self-construal. The social goals of interdependent societies emphasize conformity and dependence. This is in contrast to goals from a more independent society, which emphasize uniqueness and self-reliance. Self-construal may influence behaviors that may be considered dysfunctional in the United States. Okazaki (1997) found that self-construal was a significant predictor of social anxiety among a sample of Asian and European American college students. Asian Americans reported higher levels of social anxiety than their European American counterparts did. Okazaki attributed this tendency for Asian Americans to experience concern over negative evaluation to values that emphasize the concerns of the in-group and distrust and fear of the out-group. Although social anxiety may be considered dysfunctional in some contexts, it may be adaptive in cultures that emphasize social harmony. Many collectivistic cultures socialize their children to be dependent and may consider behaviors that violate social harmony to be dysfunctional, whereas a more independent culture may view the same behavior as social competence. For Asian Americans who report symptoms of social anxiety, the symptoms may be impairing in one context but adaptive and necessary in their own cultural context. The incompatibility of the social goals stemming from concepts of self, as illustrated by these examples, demonstrates the nuances underlying constructs of normality and abnormality.

Symptoms may be less predictive of psychopathology among ethnic minorities than among European Americans. Weisz and colleagues (1988) found that Thai parents were less inclined than American parents to judge undercontrolled and overcontrolled behaviors in their children as serious and permanent. For some cultural groups, behavioral problems may be perceived as transient and therefore not as a problem in need of treatment. Coyne and Markus (2006) found that when diagnosis for major depressive disorder was based solely on symptoms, prevalence rates for African Americans and European Americans were equal. However, prevalence was lower for African Americans when the clinician included interference of functioning in the criterion for depression. Many ethnic minorities do not seek out mental health treatment until they are experiencing severe pathology (Lawson, Hepler, Holladay, & Cuffell, 1994), suggesting that they may be functioning adequately during periods of psychological distress. This may be a reflection of African Americans learning to separate the influence of emotional distress from daily obligations, an idea that is not uncommon for many ethnic groups. Indeed in Morita therapy, a Japanese form of psychotherapy, treatment emphasizes fulfilling role obligations in the face of psychological distress (Hedstrom, 1994). Thus, lack of occupational impairment does not mean the absence of psychological distress for members of some ethnic minority groups.

Inherent biases may also influence judgments of functionality. Stereotypes regarding functionality among specific ethnic minority groups may provide an inaccurate baseline for clinicians. For instance, viewing African Americans as hostile (Monteith, 1996) or Asian Americans as a "model minority" (Kitano & Sue, 1973) may hinder clinicians' ability to detect mental health problems because expectations regarding level of functionality may bias some clinicians to identify behaviors in one ethnic group as a problem but not to see it as a problem for a different ethnic group. This phenomenon is illustrated in school settings, where student problem behaviors are evaluated differently based on teachers' stereotypes about specific racial groups (Chang & Sue, 2003). Asian American children who display overcontrolled behaviors such as anxiety and withdrawal may be overlooked because their behavior is viewed as consistent with stereotypes. Although overcontrolled behaviors are less often identified as problematic, in general, these behaviors among Asian American students are considered less of a problem by teachers than among African American and European American students.

For ethnic minorities, deficits in occupational functioning may more often be the cause of depression rather than the result of it. Structural and societal inequalities are pervasive and constant sources of stress that cannot be alleviated by individual efforts (Adebimpe, 2004). The greater economic and social stress experienced by ethnic minorities mediates the relationship between psychopathology and ethnicity, highlighting the presence of persistent daily stress for ethnic minorities (Plant & Sachs-Ericsson, 2004). For a clinician, it is helpful to consider that functioning may not improve with decreased emotional distress for the individual because functionality may depend on societal changes rather than individual changes.

## Deviation

A behavior is considered deviant relative to the behavior of others within the same culture. Thus, individuals who hold social norms from other countries are already more likely to be, or to be viewed as, more deviant. Clinicians working with clients from different cultures must first have knowledge of each individual's social norms before decisions regarding social deviation can be made.

In more collectivistic cultures, deviation may be a more salient predictor than actual affective experience of individual well-being. In a large scale study of 62,446 people in 61 nations, Suh, Diener, Oishi, and Triandis (1998) compared individualistic cultures and collectivistic cultures on predictors of well-being. For people from more individualist cultures, emotions were a stronger predictor of life satisfaction than were social norms (social approval of life satisfaction). Emotions also predicted life satisfaction for people from more collectivistic cultures, but social norms also equally predicted life satisfaction, suggesting that people from collectivistic cultures may put more emphasis on social norms than do people from individualistic cultures. Understanding cultural norms may help predict symptom reports among ethnic minorities. For instance, Okazaki and Kallivayalil (2002) found that reports of depression were associated with cultural norms about depression for Asian American college students but not for European American college students. Asian American college students who judged depression to be more acceptable, more common, and less stigmatizing were more likely to endorse depressive symptoms than Asian Americans who did not hold those views. Asian Americans and European Americans did not differ in their judgments regarding normality of depressive symptoms with respect to their ethnic groups. However, it appears that cultural norms were more salient for Asian Americans than they were for European Americans. Asian American reports of distress are reflective of both their subjective experience and of their cultural norms regarding psychopathology.

Additionally, people of color in the United States also have unique social experiences related to their ethnic minority group membership that may be poorly understood by members from the mainstream culture. For instance, racism is a common experience for many ethnic minorities in the United States. Compared to European Americans, members of ethnic minority groups perceive more lifetime and day-to-day discrimination (Kessler, Mickelson, & Williams, 1999). Ethnic minorities develop cognitive and behavioral adaptations to cope with these experiences. Cultural paranoia (Ridley, 1984) or cultural mistrust (Whaley, 1997) on the part of African Americans has been described as a healthy reaction to chronic experiences of racism and oppression. Cultural mistrust may be normative and adaptive for many ethnic minority groups. Indeed for African Americans racial socialization, which includes preparation for racism, has been shown to promote resiliency among adolescents (Miller, 1999). Nevertheless, its primary feature of mistrust and suspicion of institutional practices may be perceived by mainstream clinicians as delusions of reference or paranoia related to psychopathology. Whaley (2001) suggested that this form of paranoia is not an indicator of pathology. Indeed, more than any other group, African Americans have experienced a long history of abuse by the science and research communities and may have reason to be wary of mainstream care (Harris, Gorelick, Samuels, & Bempong, 1996). A clinician who is less aware of the racist experiences of African Americans may categorize this mistrust as abnormal and indicative of pathology.

## DIAGNOSTIC CATEGORIES, THE CLINICAL INTERVIEW, AND CLINICIAN BIAS

One problem with adopting a purely nomothetic approach rather than considering also an idiographic perspective is that different categorical systems will yield an alternative understanding of a similar phenomenon. A comparison of diagnostic manuals across different nations reveals wide discrepancies in conceptions and categories of mental disorders (Tseng, Xu, Ebata, Hsu, & Cui, 1986). The DSM and the *International Classification of Diseases–10* (ICD-10) are the most widely used psychiatric diagnostic manuals in the world, but there are also many regional systems that exist in different countries, such as the Chinese Classification of Mental Disorders (CCMD), which contains disorders that are not recognized by the DSM-IV-TR (Lee, 2001). These regional systems underscore the importance of social context in understanding emotional distress and behavior. The increasing influence of the DSM, however, is noteworthy. The DSM has been translated into languages other than English, such as Spanish (Grilo, Anez, & McGlashan, 2003) and Chinese (Wilson & Young, 1988), for use with populations outside the United States.

The American Psychiatric Association has made great strides toward incorporating idiographic variables in the DSM in order to increase its validity for multicultural populations (Smart & Smart, 1997). DSM has undergone several revisions, but it was not until 1975 that ethnic minority members were included in the DSM task force. Each DSM revision is reflective of the changing political and social climate of the time. Thus, it is not unreasonable to expect that more changes in the DSM will occur as a result of shifting hegemony.

Smart and Smart (1997) have summarized these recent changes in the DSM, which include (1) a glossary of culture-bound syndromes; (2) an outline for cultural formulations, which takes into account the client's idiographic experience; (3) an expanded definition of Axis IV to include psychosocial and environmental stressors that are more culturally relevant (e.g., discrimination); and (5) an addition of "V codes" that may be culturally significant (e.g., acculturation problems).

Although these efforts are praiseworthy, they are not without significant limitations (Lopez & Guarnaccia, 2000). Because these changes have come about only in the past decade, many mental health professionals may not be familiar with them or may not be incorporating them into their own work. Research has not yet examined if these changes have improved the quality of mental health services for ethnic minority patients. The American Psychiatric Association did not incorporate all suggestions provided by the task force, and more may be added to increase its applicability to diverse populations. For example, Adebimpe (2004) suggests the incorporation of a supplementary diagnostic reasoning criteria for deciphering actual symptoms from normal reactions among members of cultural minority groups in future editions of the DSM to reduce ethnic disparities in mental health diagnosis. Adebimpe discusses how observations of paranoia, auditory hallucinations, visual hallucinations, witchcraft beliefs, somatic complaints, and abnormal speech hostility may not be indicative of mental illness for many African Americans. The supplementary material is intended to inform clinicians of these cultural differences.

One of the more contentious issues resulting from the revision of the DSM is the inclusion of a glossary for *culture-bound syndromes*. (Although we use the term *culture bound* to remain consistent with the DSM, Jilek [2000] suggests using the term *culture-related* because he believes that the notion that these disorders are "bound" to a particular culture is inaccurate.) Including *culture bound* disorders in the appendix but not in the body of DSM-IV-TR suggests that these disorders are outside the scope of formal categories of mental illness and instead constitute "exotic entities" (Alarcon, 1995, p. 454). It also conveys the misconception that these disorders, but not others, are influenced by culture. Indeed, the American Psychiatric Association rejected suggestions by the task force that dissociative and eating disorders should be included in the culture-bound glossary (Lewis-Fernandez & Kleinman, 1995), despite empirical evidence that eating disorders, particularly bulimia nervosa, are more prevalent in Western countries and probably tied to cultural views of beauty (Keel & Klump, 2003).

In addition, culture-bound disorders are listed in the glossary without a systematic way of understanding them (Guarnaccia & Rogler, 1999). For example, the culture-bound disorders are not grouped together in the same way that DSM disorders are (e.g., mood disorders, personality disorders, anxiety disorders). In addition, these disorders may not be as rare as the authors of the DSM seem to assume. For instance, 12% of Korean Americans residing in a Los Angeles community described themselves as suffering from *hwa-byung* (Lin et al., 1992). Lewis-Fernandez (1994) and Liebowitz et al. (1994) observed that 75% of Dominican and Puerto Rican patients in mental health clinics in the United States had experienced an episode of *ataque de nervios*. Neurasthenia is included in the ICD-10 and is commonly diagnosed in China (Young, 1989). Although some believe that the majority of patients diagnosed with neurasthenia may be suffering from major depressive disorder (MDD), there is evidence that it is distinct from MDD. Zheng et al. (1997) found a prevalence rate of 6.7% among a sample of Chinese-Americans living in the Los Angeles area, and only 50% would have met diagnosis for a separate DSM disorder. This percentage is comparable to estimates of comorbidity among people who qualify for a DSM mental disorder (Kessler et al., 1994). The prevalence of these disorders suggests that culture-bound syndromes may warrant a more sophisticated conceptualization than that afforded to mainstream DSM disorders.

Mental health professionals also have idiographic experiences that may influence their clinical judgments. One factor that may affect the type and quality of information gathered for diagnosis is language differences. Malgady and Costantino (1998) found that clinician ethnicity and the language in which the interview is conducted can influence clinical judgments. Latinos/Latinas with a diagnosis of schizophrenia, depression, or anxiety were interviewed by Hispanic or European American clinicians in Spanish, English, or both. Clinicians rated the severity of the symptoms based on two measures: the DSM-IV Global Assessment of Functioning and the Brief Psychiatric Rating Scale. Hispanic clinicians rated symptoms severer than did European American clinicians for all patients, irrespective of client ethnicity. The language in which the interview was conducted also influenced ratings of symptom severity. Judgments of severity were highest during bilingual interviews and lowest during interviews conducted in English. The authors did not explain the reason for this discrepancy. Clinicians should be aware that direct translations do not always ensure reliability of construct.

Clinicians' biases and stereotypes can influence decisions regarding diagnosis (Whaley, 1997; see also, Garb, Chapter 16, this volume). Substantial research evidence indicates a proportionally greater number of diagnoses of schizophrenia and mood disorders for African Americans and European Americans than for any other ethnic group (Adebimpe, 1981, 2004; Neighbors, Jackson, Campbell, & Williams, 1989). However, only recently have researchers attempted to identify reasons for these disparities. Trierweiler, Neighbors, Munday, Thompson, and Binion (2000) examined the influence of patient ethnicity on the application of the diagnostic criteria for schizophrenia to African American and non-African-American psychiatric inpatients who had received a diagnosis of either schizophrenia or major affective disorder. Their findings suggest that clinicians may be giving different weight to their clinical observations based on the patient's ethnic background, which ultimately influences their decisions about diagnoses. For example, negative symptoms (i.e., absence of normal behavior, e.g., flat affect, poverty of speech), which require more clinical interpretation than positive symptoms (overt symptoms, e.g., delusions, paranoia), were associated with a diagnosis of schizophrenia among African American but not for non-African-American patients. Although initial observations may bias clinicians to selectively look for symptoms, the clinical utility of these findings is questionable because rarely do clinicians rely solely on naturalistic observations for diagnosis. (See Garb, Chapter 16, this volume.)

Neighbors, Trierweiler, Ford, and Muroff (2003) expanded their prior work by examining race differences in clinical judgment using a semistructured interview. Although a semistructured interview is intended to reduce clinician bias compared to open-ended interviews, patients' race continued to influence diagnostic decisions. Specific symptoms increased the likelihood of a schizophrenia diagnosis for African Americans but not European Americans. Conversely, specific symptoms were associated with an increased likelihood of a bipolar diagnosis among European Americans but not African Americans. For example, inappropriate affect was associated with a schizophrenia diagnosis for African Americans but not for European Americans. Additionally, auditory hallucinations were more often endorsed for African Americans with a schizophrenia diagnosis than for European Americans with a diagnosis of schizophrenia. Catatonic behavior was associated with an increased likelihood of a bipolar diagnosis for European Americans but not African Americans. However, clinicians' ethnic stereotypes were not measured directly; therefore, it is unclear whether these discrepant findings are a result of true differences or clinician bias.

Arnold et al. (2004) examined blinded ethnicity evaluations to determine whether diagnostic discrepancies in schizophrenia diagnosis among African American and European American patients were the result of true differences in symptoms or clinician bias. The assessors used structured clinical interviews and symptom rating instruments. The psychiatric interview was audiotaped, and information identifying client ethnicity was removed so that client ethnicity could not be determined by the assessors. Both ethnicity-blinded and unblinded assessors rated the African American men as having more first-rank symptoms, symptoms that are most predictive of schizophrenia and more total psychotic symptoms than the European American men. However, ethnically blinded assessors did not find higher rates of schizophrenia among African American men, despite the greater symptomotology. One explanation for this is that when the symptoms are evaluated in the context of other symptoms, specifically affective symptoms, African American males are not judged as being schizophrenic. Although this study does not explain why clinicians evaluate symptoms differently by ethnicity of the client, it does provide further support for the idea that clinicians weigh symptom information differently based on the ethnicity of the client. Reasons for these practices are unknown and may be related to societal stereotypes or cultural misunderstandings. Bias may be recognized and rectified when mental health professionals accept that they also have an idiographic experience relevant to the diagnostic process.

## CONCLUSIONS AND FUTURE DIRECTIONS

The consequences of neglecting unique client variables related to psychopathology are costly. Incorporating an idiographic approach to assessment creates greater precision for nomothetic categories and should be regularly integrated into our current system of assessment and diagnosis, because diagnosis has important implications for effective treatment.

Aklin and Turner (2006) suggested that one way to reduce the impact of clinician bias on assessment and diagnosis is to increase cultural competence among clinicians. Research on culture and psychopathology has elucidated ethnic disparities in mental health prevalence and mental health service utilization. These findings have prompted a series of papers over the past two decades that emphasize the importance of increasing cultural competence among mental health clinicians. These papers discourage adopting a one-size-fits-all model in understanding mental health and emphasize the importance of understanding culture and context. Cultural sensitivity and awareness are important components of clinical skill. Currently, however, cultural competence is mainly a theoretical construct (e.g., Betancourt, Green, Carrillo, & Ananeh-Firempong, 2003; Brach & Fraserirector, 2000; Sue, 1998).

Models for increasing cultural competence are rooted in empirical research findings but have not themselves been tested empirically. Nor are clinicians held responsible for increasing and applying culturally competent knowledge, furthering the divide between nomothetic and idiographic approaches to mental health. Although research has not demonstrated conclusively that these ethnic discrepancies in diagnosis are a result of the mental health system rather than actual differences in psychopathology, Malgady (1996) suggested that the consequence of assuming that mental illness categories are universally experienced and manifested is far more harmful than assuming a culturally specific stance in psychopathology assessment. Low rates of mental health utilization by diverse populations imply that existing services may not be culturally relevant. The assessment and diagnosis process sets the foundation for learning about clients' sociocultural context. When misunderstanding occurs at the onset, individuals may be recommended for treatment without the presence of psychopathology, as illustrated by the overrepresentation of the schizophrenia diagnosis for African Americans. Conversely, individuals may be denied treatment because they do not meet diagnostic criteria, as might occur for Asian Americans who may have cultural scripts regarding open emotional expression. There needs to be a better relationship between empirical science and mental health services to ensure that growing cultural awareness among the research community is informing mental health practices.

## REFERENCES

Abe-Kim, J., Okazaki, S., & Goto, S. (2001). Unidimensional versus multidimensional approaches to the assessment of acculturation for Asian American populations. *Cultural Diversity and Ethnic Minority Psychology*, 7, 232–246.

Adebimpe, V. R. (1981). Overview: White norms and psychiatric diagnosis of black patients. *American Journal of Psychiatry*, *138*, 279–285.

Adebimpe, V. R. (2004). A second opinion on the use of white norms in psychiatric diagnosis of black patients. *Psychiatric Annals*, *34*, 543–551.

Aklin, W. M., & Turner, S. M. (2006). Toward understanding ethnic and cultural factors in the interviewing process. *Psychotherapy*, *43*, 50–64.

Alarcon, R. D. (1995). Culture and psychiatric diagnosis. Impact on DSM-IV and ICD-10. *The Psychiatric Clinics of North America, 18*, 449–465.

American Psychiatric Association. (2000). *Diagnostic and statistical manual of mental disorders* (4th ed., text rev.). Washington, DC: Author.

Arnold, L. M., Keck, P. E., Jr., Collins, J., Wilson, R., Fleck, D. E., Corey, K. B., et al. (2004). Ethnicity and first-rank symptoms in patients with psychosis. *Schizophrenia Research, 67*, 207–212.

Betancourt, J. R., Green, A. R., Carrillo, J. E., & Ananeh-Firempong, O. (2003). Defining cultural competence: A practical framework for addressing racial/ethnic disparities in health and health care. *Public Health Reports, 118*, 293–302.

Binder, R. L., & Levy, R. (1981). Extrapyramidal reactions in Asians. *American Journal of Psychiatry, 138*, 1243–1244.

Brach, C., & Fraserirector, I. (2000). Can cultural competency reduce racial and ethnic disparities? A review and conceptual model. *Medical Care and Research and Review, 57*, 181–217.

Broman, C. L. (1996). Coping with personal problems. In H. W. Neighbors & J. S. Jackson (Eds.) *Mental health in black America* (pp. 117–129). Thousand Oaks, CA: Sage.

Brown, C., Shulberg, H. C., & Madonia, M. J. (1996). Clinical presentations of major depression by African Americans and whites in primary medical care practice. *Journal of Affective Disorders, 41*, 181–191.

Burnam, M. A., Hough, R. L., Karno, M., Escobar, J. I., & Telles, C. A. (1987). Acculturation and lifetime prevalence of psychiatric disorder among Mexican Americans in Los Angeles. *Journal of Health and Social Behavior, 28*, 89–102.

Canino, I. A., Rubio-Sripec, M., Canino, G., & Escobar, J. I. (1992). Functional somatic symptoms: A cross-ethnic comparison. *American Journal of Orthopsychiatry, 62*, 605–612.

Chang, D. F., & Sue, S. (2003). The effects of race and problem type on teachers' assessment of student behavior. *Journal of Consulting and Clinical Psychology, 71*, 235–242.

Chung, R. G. (2001). Gender, ethnicity, and acculturation in intergenerational conflict of Asian American college students. *Cultural Diversity and Ethnic Minority Psychology, 7*, 376–386.

Coyne, J. C., & Marcus, S. C. (2006). Health disparities in care for depression possibly obscured by the clinical significance criterion. *American Journal of American Psychiatry, 163*, 1577–1579.

Dana, R. H. (2001). Clinical diagnosis of multicultural populations in the United States. In L. A. Suzuki, J. G. Ponterotto, & P. J. Meller (Eds.), *Handbook of multicultural assessment* (pp. 101–131). San Francisco: Jossey-Bass/Wiley.

Diaz, F. J., & de Leon, J. (2002). Excessive antipsychotic dosing in 2 U.S. state hospitals. *Journal of Clinical Psychiatry, 63*, 998–1002.

Felix-Ortiz, M., Newcomb, M., & Myers, H. (1994). A multidimensional measure of cultural identity for Latino and Latina adolescents. *Hispanic Journal of Behavioral Sciences, 16*(2), 99–115.

Gamwell, L., & Tomes, N. (1995). *Madness in America: Cultural and medical perceptions of mental illness before 1914*. Ithaca, NY: Cornell University Press.

Grilo, C. M., Anez, L. M., & McGlashan, T. H. (2003). The Spanish language version of the diagnostic interview for DSM-IV personality disorders: Development and initial psychometric evaluation of diagnoses and criteria. *Comprehensive Psychiatry, 44*, 154–161.

Gross, J. J., & John, O. P. (1995). Facets of emotional expressivity: Three self-report factors and their correlates. *Personality and Individual Differences, 19*, 555–568.

Guarnaccia, P. J., & Rogler, L. H. (1999). Research on culture bound syndromes: New directions. *American Journal of Psychiatry, 156*, 1322–1327.

Hall, G., & Okazaki, S. (2002). *Asian American psychology*. Washington, DC: American Psychological Association.

Harris, Y., Gorelick, P. B., Samuels, P., & Bempong, I. (1996). Why African Americans may not be participating in clinical trials. *Journal of National Medical Association, 88*(10), 630–634.

Harter, S. (1993). Causes and consequences of low self-esteem in children and adolescents. In R. Baumeister (Ed.), *Self-esteem: The puzzle of low self-regard* (pp. 87–116). New York: Plenum Press.

Hedstrom, J. L. (1994). Morita and Naikan therapies: American applications. *Psychotherapy: Theory, Research, Practice, and Training*, *31*, 154–160.

Hsu, L. K. G., & Folstein, M. F. (1997). Somatoform disorders in Caucasian and Chinese Americans. *Journal of Nervous and Mental Disease*, *185*, 382–387.

Hwang, W. C. (2006). The psychotherapy adaptation and modification framework: Application to Asian Americans. *American Psychologist*, *61*, 702–715.

Jilek, W. G. (2000). Culture-related syndromes. In M. G. Gelder, J. J. López-Ibor, & N. Andreason (Eds.), *New Oxford textbook of psychiatry* (pp. 1061–1066). New York: Oxford University Press.

Kaplan, M. S., & Marks, G. (1990). Adverse effects of acculturation: Psychological distress among Mexican American young adults. *Social Science and Medicine*, *31*, 1313–1319.

Keel, P. K., & Klump, K. L. (2003). Are eating disorders culture-bound syndromes? Implications for conceptualizing their etiology. *Psychological Bulletin*, *129*, 747–769.

Kessler, R. C., McGonagle, K. A., Zhao, S., Nelson, C. B., Hughes, M., Eshleman, S., et al. (1994). Lifetime and 12-month prevalence of DSM-III-R psychiatric disorders in the United States: Results of the National Comorbidity Study. *Archives of General Psychiatry*, *54*, 313–321.

Kessler, R. C., Mickelson, K. D., & Williams, D. R. (1999). The prevalence, distribution, and mental health correlates of perceived discrimination in the United States. *Journal of Health and Social Behavior*, *40*, 208–230.

Kim, S. Y., & Wong, V. (2002). Assessing Asian and Asian American parenting: A review of the literature. In K. Kurasaki, S. Okazaki, & S. Sue (Eds.), *Asian American mental health: Assessment methods and theories* (pp. 185–203). New York: Kluwer Academic/Plenum Publishers.

Kitano, H., & Sue, S. (1973). The model minorities. *Journal of Social Issues*, *29*, 1–10.

Kleinman, A. (1988). *Rethinking psychiatry*. New York: Free Press.

Lafromboise, T., Coleman, H. L. K., & Gerton, J. (1993). Psychological impact of biculturalism: Evidence and theory. *Psychological Bulletin*, *114*, 395–412.

Lawson, W. B., Hepler, N., Holladay, J., & Cuffell, B. (1994). Race as a factor in inpatient and outpatient admissions and diagnosis. *Hospital and Community Psychiatry*, *45*, 72–74.

Le, H. N., Berenbaum, H., & Raghavan, C. (2002). Culture and alexithymia: Mean levels, correlates, and the role of parental socialization of emotions. *Emotion*, *2*, 341–360.

Lee, S. (1999). "Are you Chinese or what?" Ethnic identity among Asian Americans. In R. Sheets & E. Hollins (Eds.), *Racial and ethnic identity in school practices: Aspects of human development* (pp. 107–121). Mahwah, NJ: Erlbaum.

Lee, S. (2001). From diversity to unity. *Cultural Psychiatry: International Perspectives*, *24*, 421–431.

Lewis-Fernandez, R. (1994). Culture and dissociation: A comparison of ataque de nervios among Puerto Ricans and possession syndrome in India. In D. Speigel (Ed.), *Dissociation: Culture, mind, and body* (pp. 123–167). Washington, DC: American Psychiatric Association.

Lewis-Fernandez, R., & Kleinman, A. (1995). Cultural psychiatry: Theoretical, clinical, and research issues. *The Psychiatric Clinics of North America*, *18*, 433–448.

Liebowitz, M. R., Salmán, E., Jusino, C. M., Garfinkel, R., Street, L., Cárdenas, D. L., et al. (1994). *Ataque de nervios* and panic disorder. *American Journal of Psychiatry*, *151*, 871–875.

Lin, K. M. (1983). Hwa-byung: A Korean culture-bound syndrome? *American Journal of Psychiatry*, *140*, 105–107.

Lin, K. M., Lau, J. K. C., Yamamoto, J., Zheng, Y. P., Kim, H. S., Cho, K. H., et al. (1992). Hwa-byung: A community study of Korean Americans. *Journal of Nervous and Mental Disease*, *180*, 386–391.

Lindsey, K. P., & Paul, G. L. (1989). Involuntary commitments to public mental institutions: Issues involving the overrepresentation of blacks and the assessment of relevant functioning. *Psychological Bulletin*, *106*, 171–183.

Lopez, S. R., & Guarnaccia, P. J. (2000). Cultural psychopathology: Uncovering the social world of mental illness. *Annual Review of Psychology*, *51*, 571–598.

Malgady, R. G. (1996). The question of cultural bias in assessment and diagnosis of ethnic minority clients: Let's reject the null hypothesis. *Professional Psychology: Research and Practice*, *27*, 73–77.

Malgady, R. G., & Costantino, G. (1998). Symptom severity in bilingual Hispanics as a function of clinician ethnicity and language of interview. *Psychological Assessment*, *10*, 120–127.

Markus, H. R., & Kitayama, S. (1991). Culture and the self: Implications for cognition, emotion, and motivation. *Psychological Review*, *98*, 224–253.

Miller, D. B. (1999). Racial socialization and racial identity: Can they promote resiliency for African American adolescents? *Adolescence*, *34*, 493–501.

Monteith, M. J. (1996). Contemporary forms of prejudice-related conflict: In search of a nutshell. *Personality and Social Psychology Bulletin*, *22*, 461–473.

Neighbors, H. W., Jackson, J. S., Campbell, L., & Williams, D. (1989). Racial influences on psychiatric diagnosis: A review and suggestions for research. *Community Mental Health Journal*, *25*, 310–311.

Neighbors, H. W., Musick, M. A., & Williams, D. R. (1998). The African American minister as a source of help for serious personal crises: Bridge or barrier to mental health care? *Health Education and Behavior*, *25*, 759–777.

Neighbors, H. W., Trierweiler, S. J., Ford, B. C., & Muroff, J. R. (2003). Racial differences in DSM diagnosis using semi-structured instrument: The importance of clinical judgment in the diagnosis of African Americans. *Journal of Health and Social Behavior*, *44*, 237–256.

Neville, H., & Lilly, R. L. (2000). The relationship between racial identity cluster profiles and psychological distress among African American college students. *Journal of Multicultural Counseling and Development*, *28*, 194–207.

Okazaki, S. (1997). Sources of ethnic differences between Asian American and white American college students on measures of depression and social anxiety. *Journal of Abnormal Psychology*, *106*, 52–60.

Okazaki, S. (2002). Self–other agreement on affective distress scales in Asian Americans and white Americans. *Journal of Counseling Psychology*, *49*, 428–437.

Okazaki, S., & Kallivayalil, D. (2002). Cultural norms and subjective disability as predictors of symptom reports among Asian Americans and white Americans. *Journal of Cross-Cultural Psychology*, *33*, 482–491.

Parker, G., Chan, B., Tully, L., & Eisenbruch, M. (2005). Depression in the Chinese: The impact of acculturation. *Psychological Medicine*, *35*, 1–9.

Phinney, J. S. (2003). Ethnic identity and acculturation. In K. Chun, P. Organista, & G. Marin (Eds.), *Acculturation: Advances in theory, measurement, and applied research* (pp. 63–82). Washington, DC: American Psychological Association.

Phinney, J. S., Cantu, C. L., & Kurtz, D. A. (1996). Ethnic and American identity as predictors of self-esteem among African American, Latino, and white adolescents. *Journal of Youth and Adolescence*, *26*, 165–185.

Pi, E. H., & Simpson, G. H. (2005). Cross-cultural psychopharmacology: A current clinical perspective. *Psychiatric Services*, *56*, 31–33.

Plant, E. A., & Sachs-Ericsson, N. (2004). Racial and ethnic differences in depression: The roles of social support and meeting basic needs. *Journal of Clinical and Consulting Psychology*, *72*, 41–52.

Ridley, C. R. (1984). Clinical treatment of the nondisclosing black client: A therapeutic paradox. *American Psychologist*, *39*, 1243–1244.

Shen, B., & Takeuchi, D. T. (2001). A structural model of acculturation and mental health status among Chinese Americans. *American Journal of Community Psychology*, *29*, 387–418.

Smart, D. W., & Smart, J. F. (1997). DSM-IV and culturally sensitive diagnosis: Some observations for counselors. *Journal of Consulting and Development*, *75*, 392–398.

Sue, D., Mak, W., & Sue, D. W. (1998). Ethnic identity. In C. Lee & N. Zane (Eds.), *Handbook of Asian American psychology* (pp. 289–323). Thousand Oaks: Sage.

Sue, D. W., & Sue, D. (1999). Counseling Asian Americans. In D. W. Sue & D. Sue (Eds.), *Counseling the culturally different: Theory and practice* (3rd ed., pp. 255–278). New York: Wiley.

Sue, S. (1998). In search of cultural competence in psychotherapy and counseling. *American Psychologist, 59*, 440–448.

Suh, E., Diener, E., Oishi, S., & Triandis, H. C. (1998). The shifting basis of life satisfaction judgements across cultures: Emotions versus norms. *Journal of Personality and Social Psychology, 74*, 482–493.

Szasz, T. S. (1961). *The myth of mental illness: Foundations of a theory of personal conduct.* New York: Harper (Hoeber).

Trierweiler, S. J., Neighbors, H. W., Munday, C., Thompson, E. E., & Binion, V. J. (2000). Clinician attributions associated with the diagnosis of schizophrenia in African American and non-African American patients. *Journal of Consulting and Clinical Psychology, 68*, 171–175.

Tsai, J. L., Knutson, B., & Fung, H. (2006). Cultural variation in affect valuation. *Journal of Personality and Social Psychology, 90*, 288–307.

Tseng, W. S., Xu, N., Ebata, K., Hsu, J., & Cui, Y. (1986). Diagnostic patterns of neurosis among China, Japan, and America. *American Journal of Psychiatry, 143*, 1010–1014.

Weisz, J., Suwanlert, S., Chaiyasit, W., Weiss, B., Walter, B., & Anderson, W. (1988). Thai and American perspectives on over- and undercontrolled child behavior problems: Exploring the threshold model among parents, teachers, and psychologists. *Journal of Consulting and Clinical Psychology, 56*, 601–609.

Whaley, A. L. (1997). Ethnicity/race, paranoia, and psychiatric diagnoses: Clinician bias versus sociocultural differences. *Journal of Psychopathology and Behavioral Assessment, 19*, 1–20.

Whaley, A. L. (2001). Cultural mistrust and mental health services for African Americans: A review and meta-analysis. *Counseling Psychologist, 29*, 513–531.

Wilson, L. G., & Young, D. (1988). Diagnosis of severely ill patients in China: A collaborative project using the structured clinical interview for DSM-III (SCID). *Journal of Nervous Mental Disease, 176*, 585–592.

Ying, Y., & Miller, L. S. (1992). Help-seeking behavior and attitude of Chinese Americans regarding psychological problems. *American Journal of Community Psychology, 20*, 549–556.

Young, D. S. (1989). Neuresthenia and related problems. *Culture, Medicine, and Psychiatry, 13*, 131–138.

Zane, N., & Mak, W. (2003). Major approaches to the measurement of acculturation among ethnic minority populations: A content analysis and an alternative empirical strategy. In K. M. Chun, P. B. Organista, & G. Marin (Eds.), *Acculturation: Advances in theory, measurement, and applied research* (pp. 39–60). Washington, DC: American Psychological Association.

Zane, N., & Yeh, M. (2002). Use of culturally-based variables in assessment: Studies on loss of face. In K. Kurasaki, S. Okazaki, & S. Sue (Eds.), *Asian American mental health: Assessment theories and methods* (pp. 123–138). Dordrecht, Netherlands: Kluwer.

Zhang, A. Y., Snowden, L. R., & Sue, S. (1998). Differences between Asian and white Americans' help seeking and utilization patterns in the Los Angeles area. *Journal of Community Psychology, 26*, 317–326.

Zheng, Y. P., Lin, K. M., Takeuchi, D. T., Kurasaki, K., Wang, Y., & Cheung, F. (1997). An epidemiological study of neurasthenia in Chinese Americans in Los Angeles. *Comprehensive Psychiatry, 38*, 249–259.

# 18 Clinical Assessment of Personality

## *Perspectives from Contemporary Personality Science*

William G. Shadel

Assessment of normal and abnormal behavior and psychological functioning more generally has long been a key professional concern for clinical psychology. Hundreds upon hundreds of standardized psychological tests (e.g., see any addition of the *Mental Measurements Yearbook*) and numerous nontest techniques associated with particular theoretical orientations and specific disorders (e.g., assessment of automatic thoughts in cognitive therapy for depression; see Beck, Rush, Shaw, & Emery, 1979) are used routinely for purposes of clinical assessment. Entire journals are devoted to assessment (e.g., *Assessment, Psychological Assessment*). Professional societies are organized around assessment issues (e.g., Society for Personality Assessment; section 9 of the American Psychological Association's Division 12 [Clinical Psychology]). Clinical psychology doctoral programs must offer training in assessment, and clinical internships must ensure that trainees leave with proficiency across a wide variety of assessment techniques in order to receive accreditation by the American Psychological Association (see *www.apa.org/ed/accreditation*). Nearly 60% of practicing psychologists report that assessment is a core component of their professional activities (Norcross, Hedges, & Castle, 2002). Volumes have been written about what would seem to be every conceivable facet of psychological assessment from the conceptual to the empirical (Hersen, 2004a) to the eminently practical (Hersen, 2004b). One could easily get the impression that there is very little new to contribute in this domain of psychological inquiry.

This impression would not be correct, however. The vast literature on clinical assessment and the vital role that it plays in the day-to-day lives of clinical psychologists stand in contrast to the fact that domains of substantial interest to clinical psychology—domains that have been a core concern for assessment since the early days of the field—are not informed by mature perspectives in other areas of psychology (see also, Hunsley, 2002; Hunsley & Moss, 2007; McFall, 2005). The lack of integration is hardly surprising, given that many of the different subdisciplines and specialties within psychology do not generally "talk" to one another, perhaps to the detriment of clinical psychology in particular (Sechrest, 1992; see also, Strauman, 2001). Developments in the basic psychological sciences are poised to have a significant impact on how clinicians conceptualize, assess, and treat psychological problems (Mischel, 2004; Shadel, 2004; cf. Matarazzo, 1992), but that impact has yet to be fully realized (see Baker, McFall, & Shoham, 2009).

This is nowhere more apparent than in the study and assessment of personality. Personality assessment was a key defining activity in the earliest days of clinical psychology (for a historical overview of the field, see Benjamin, 2005), and understanding and assessing personality are key tasks in contemporary clinical research and practice (Watkins, Campbell, Nieberding, & Hallmark, 1995; see also, Butcher, 2006; Hilsenroth & Segal, 2004). As such, one might assume that conceptual and empirical developments that have emerged from the contemporary field of personality would be routinely drawn upon and carefully applied in the clinical assessment of personality. Unfortunately, this has not happened. How personality is conceptualized and assessed in contemporary clinical psychology bears almost no relation to how it is conceptualized and assessed in the contemporary field that studies it on a day-to-day basis. Moreover, modern-day conceptions of personality that stand a significant chance of uniquely informing clinical assessment (and treatment) are largely ignored. The overall aim of this chapter, then, is to provide an overview of contemporary personality psychology and to discuss how personality may be most profitably conceptualized and assessed in clinical contexts.

## DEFINING PERSONALITY

Open any undergraduate personality text to its introductory pages and a simple definition of personality will be advanced for purposes of orienting the reader: for example, "the distinctive patterns of behavior (including thoughts and emotions) that characterize each individual's adaptation to the situations of his or her life" (Mischel, 1993, p. 5). Such texts are typically quick to point out, though, that the simplicity of such definitions should not be taken as evidence of consensus in the field about the particular theoretical constituents of personality per se. Indeed, defining what is meant by personality has always been a particularly thorny endeavor. The definition has undergone considerable change and debate since the inception of the field, and there has never been a universally accepted definition of personality by the field that has studied it on a day-to-day basis (Allport & Vernon, 1930; Caprara & Cervone, 2000). Efforts to arrive at a clear consensual definition are complicated by several other factors as well. For example, some professional uses of the term seem to equate the definition of personality with the method used to assess it; that is, personality is what is measured by the test (see Shadel, 2004; see also, McFall, 2005). In addition, lay uses of the term often refer to the most dominant descriptive characteristic of an individual, human or nonhuman (see Mischel, 1993)—for example, "My mother-in-law has a strong personality" or "The Irish Setter has a rollicking personality" (see *www.akc.org/breeds/irish_setter/index.cfm*).[1] How, then, can the diversity of definitions that crowds the discipline of personality be reconciled in a way that informs clinical assessment? In arriving at an answer, it is useful to reframe this question (and to somewhat anthropomorphize its content) because the desired use of a concept, in this case, personality, determines the manner in which it is defined (see Garfinkel, 1981): "What would clinical assessment like personality and personality assessment to do for it?" An answer to this question and a definition of personality that can be used to maximum benefit for clinical assessment comes from clearly understanding the purpose of clinical assessment.

## THE PURPOSE OF CLINICAL ASSESSMENT

Clinical psychology is, as a profession, broadly concerned with the identification, remediation, and prevention of psychological maladjustment (Resnick, 1991). Clinical assessment, then, is executed in service of these professional goals and, as such, serves several purposes (see Hersen, 2004b; Persons & Davidson, 2001).

### Diagnosis

One of the most formal and lasting approaches to the diagnosis and classification of abnormal behavior came in 1952 with the introduction of the first *Diagnostic and Statistical Manual of Mental Disorders* (DSM-I). The DSM has undergone several major revisions since this time, and the current version, the DSM-IV-TR (American Psychiatric Association, 2000), is due to be replaced by the DSM-V in 2013 (see *www.dsm5.org*). A key feature of the DSM classification system is that it treats psychological problems as nosological syndromes, that is, as a list of signs and symptoms that cluster more or less meaningfully together to form a given diagnostic classification. For example, to receive a diagnosis of major depression, someone must exhibit either depressed mood or loss of interest in daily activities, and then any four of the following eight symptoms for at least 2 weeks: weight gain or anorexia; insomnia or hypersomnia; psychomotor agitation or retardation; fatigue; feelings of worthlessness; diminished cognitive capacity; and recurrent thoughts of death or suicidal ideation. Other criteria (e.g., significant impairment in daily life) and exclusions (e.g., symptoms cannot be attributed to some other diagnosis) also must be met.

There are strengths (e.g., enhances professional communication) and weaknesses (e.g., negative consequences of diagnostic labeling; validity problems with categorizing complex psychological problems dichotomously) to utilizing diagnostic systems such as the DSM, and it is beyond the scope of this chapter to discuss these issues (for an extended discussion, see Nelson-Gray & Paulson, 2004). Rather, this chapter takes a more pragmatic approach. Classification of behavior that is outside of some proscribed norm has been a part of human discourse for centuries; formal diagnoses have been, are, and probably always will be a key facet of any organized mental health system (e.g., third-party reimbursement all but requires some DSM diagnosis; Pipal, 1995). Thus, diagnosis is a special case of clinical assessment that requires specialized assessment techniques designed to yield a reliable diagnosis (see Barbour & Davidson, 2004). For example, the Structured Clinical Interviews for the DSM (i.e., SCID-I and SCID-II; see First & Gibbon, 2004) is a validated and reliable structured interview that can be used to diagnose Axis I and Axis II DSM-defined pathology.

## Case Conceptualization

Diagnosis provides a very broad descriptive framework of a particular psychological or behavioral problem at a syndromal level. This broad diagnostic classification permits a range of assessment techniques and treatment strategies from a variety of conceptual paradigms to be used for an individual who has been given that particular diagnosis (Nezu, Nezu, Peacock, & Girdwood, 2004). For example, individuals who receive a diagnosis of major depression may have their problem conceptualized within a biomedical model, a cognitive *or* behavioral model, a cognitive-behavioral model, an interpersonal model, a psychodynamic model, or some eclectic amalgam of these models (e.g., see Dobson, 1989). A given conceptual model organizes thinking about the underlying causal mechanisms that drive symptoms of the disorder and, also, the particular assessment techniques that are needed to provide further insight into those mechanisms. Case conceptualization, then, helps the clinician determine how generic theoretical concepts and constructs apply idiographically, at the level of the individual case (Nezu et al., 2004; see also, Matarazzo, 1990; Meyer et al., 2001). Thus, clinical assessment strategies need to permit a conceptual account of those constructs at the level of the individual client.

## Treatment Planning

The number of assessment strategies and/or tests that are available within a given theoretical case conceptualization for a particular diagnosis is substantial (e.g., see Barlow, 2001; Dobson, 2001; McWilliams, 1994; Watchel & Messer, 1997). A key assumption, though, is that the results of assessment during case conceptualization dictate how one proceeds with treatment (Beutler, Kim, Davison, Karno, & Fisher, 1996; Maruish, 1999). In other words, individual differences that are identified through assessments during case conceptualization dictate the different treatment strategies and techniques that then can be applied at the level of the individual. Assessment results are, in effect, used to match clients to treatments.

Formally matching different treatments to different clients is a complex endeavor due to the inherent heterogeneity on any number of characteristics between individuals within a given diagnostic label and the multiple components of a given treatment to which a given client may respond (Haynes, 1993). Although clinicians intuitively match treatments to clients, despite problems with clinical decision making more generally (Garb, Chapter 16, this volume; Garb & Boyle, 2003), the search for empirically supported client-treatment matching algorithms to improve upon this sort of clinically intuitive approach has proven unsuccessful. In other words, assessment has virtually no effect on what one does in treatment (Finn & Tonsager, 1997; Hayes, Nelson, & Jarrett, 1987; Wood, Garb, Lilienfeld, & Nezworski, 2002). For example, Project MATCH (see Project MATCH Research Group, 1997, 1998), the largest and most expensive matching study ever conducted (as of this writing), matched a priori three well-established alcohol/substance abuse treatments (i.e., 12-step, cognitive-behavioral, motivational enhancement) to myriad diverse client characteristics (i.e., severity of alcohol problems, cognitive impairment, conceptual level, gender, meaning seeking, readiness for change, psychiatric severity, social support for drinking, sociopathy, alcohol typology classification [Type A-Type B], alcohol dependence, anger, antisocial personality, assertion of autonomy, psychiatric diagnosis, prior engagement in Alcoholics Anonymous [AA], religiosity, self-efficacy, and social functioning). Over 1,700 alcohol-abusing individuals were randomly assigned to one of the three treatments, and interactions of these individual difference measures with each treatment were investigated a priori. Project MATCH is distinguished by its rigorous design, large sample size, lengthy follow-up, attention to treatment integrity and fidelity, and client adherence. However, the overwhelming majority of a priori and other matching hypotheses failed to generate any support. Thus despite its intuitive promise, client–treatment matching has largely remained in the realm of theory, a "holy grail" of sorts (Shiffman, 1993, p. 721), with multiple heuristic algorithms proposed, but left untested or unsupported in clinical domains as diverse as obesity (Brownell & Wadden, 1991), tobacco smoking (Abrams & Niaura, 2003), headache (Lipchik, Nicholson, & Penzien, 2005), depression (I. W. Miller et al., 2005), and general psychotherapy (Beutler & Harwood, 2000).

The disappointing failure of matching and the inherent complexities of the matching process both suggest that a fundamentally different perspective on matching is needed—one that embraces the complexities of the assessment problem at hand. One of the main complicating factors is the sheer number of client-level variables that must be assessed and related to the particular features of a given set of treatment strategies. At a minimum, individual clients should actually "possess" the psychological construct(s) chosen for matching; those constructs should be organized meaningfully together; and those constructs should causally regulate the problem behavior at hand. Matching paradigms, to date, have relied on the relatively simple strategy of assigning clients to treatment based on responses to a single variable that is more of a surface-level descriptive variable (e.g., gender, severity of the disorder, readiness to change; see Project MATCH discussion above). For matching to work optimally, assessment should identify the organized system of psychological constructs that individual clients actually possess and that regulate their problem behavior.[2]

## Monitoring Treatment Progress

Assessment can be used to monitor treatment progress in three ways. First, assessing treatment outcome is essential for determining the success rates of a given treatment or therapeutic approach. Third-party payers often require that an initially given diagnosis no longer apply as a function of treatment (Braun & Cox, 2001; Butcher & Rouse, 1996), and randomized clinical trials testing different psychological (or pharmacological) treatments against one another often utilize diagnostic categories as key clinical outcomes (Kendall, Flannery-Schroeder, & Ford, 1999). Monitoring treatment progress, then, can be accomplished in this way via diagnostic assessment (as previously described). Second, the presenting complaint of a given client may change during the course of treatment (Sorenson, Gorsuch, & Mintz, 1985). For example, a client who presents initially with panic disorder may suddenly experience a domestic conflict or work-related crisis that needs to be managed acutely. Assessment for this purpose would take two forms: (1) clinical identification of the new problem (e.g., via patient self-report or clinical interview); and (2) case reconceptualization and revised treatment planning to accommodate the new problem (as discussed previously). Finally, once a given treatment plan has been decided upon and executed for a given presenting problem, clinicians are obligated to carefully monitor their client's progress in order to ensure that treatment is being delivered effectively and having its intended effect on the presenting problem (Ey & Hersen, 2004). For example, cognitive therapy for depression requires an ongoing assessment of the depressed client's mood, depressive symptoms, and automatic thoughts

(Beck et al., 1979). This process implies that clinicians assess not only progress toward eliminating the identified problem (e.g., via documented absence of the presenting diagnosis) but also assess change in the mechanisms that the case conceptualization assessment suggested were responsible for regulating the disordered behavior and for which treatment strategies were designed to change.

## PERSPECTIVES FROM CONTEMPORARY PERSONALITY PSYCHOLOGY

The answer to the question that prompted the discussion of the goals of clinical assessment, "What would clinical assessment like personality and personality assessment to do for it?" would seem to be that personality would be especially useful to case conceptualization, treatment planning, and monitoring treatment progress if it could be defined as an organized system of psychological variables that individual clients actually possess and that regulate their problem behavior (see Caprara & Cervone, 2000). Assessment of personality, then, would focus on identifying components of this psychological system. Fortunately, for clinical assessment, the discipline of personality psychology has evolved to the point that it can inform these goals (see Caprara & Cervone, 2000; Carver, 1996; Cervone & Mischel, 2002; Mischel, 2004; Morf, 2002; Swan & Seyle, 2005). Two dominant approaches characterize the contemporary field (Cervone, 1991; Mischel & Shoda, 1994): (1) trait approaches and (2) social cognitive approaches. The latter approach is highly relevant for informing case conceptualization, treatment planning, and treatment monitoring, whereas the former has almost no value for informing these goals. The next sections of this chapter discuss why this is the case.

### Trait Approaches

Trait approaches posit that people differ from one another on any number of global, surface-level dispositional tendencies (i.e., traits) that summarize general trends in cognition, behavior, and affect. The potentially thousands of terms or phrases that have been encoded in the natural language to describe these differences have been subjected to repeated factor analyses in order to reduce them to a more manageable number of traits. A consensus was reached over 15 years ago (see Goldberg, 1993) that the most robust and consistent factor solution yielded five traits: Extraversion, Agreeableness, Conscientiousness, Neuroticism (sometimes termed Emotional Stability), and Openness to Experience (sometimes termed Culture) (reviewed by Digman, 1996; McCrae & Costa, 2003). All persons are presumed to "have" some fixed level on each of the five factors. Across both time and setting, different persons are expected to exhibit different levels or degrees of cognitions, behaviors, and affects and these different levels can be summarized by each of the five factors and measured via questionnaire or observer rating methods. Situations affect trait scores only to the degree that individuals exhibit more or less of the behaviors, cognitions, and affects in some situations versus other situations, although the absolute level of the trait score remains constant across persons. The influence of the situation is viewed as "error variance" that prohibits individuals' true score on the trait from being accurately measured. The factors, then, represent stable between-person differences.

Two camps of five-factor enthusiasts exist. *Big Five* researchers (e.g., Saucier & Goldberg, 1996) adhere to the view that the five factors represent a parsimonious description of population-based individual differences that have been encoded in the natural language. They do not assign explanatory force or causal status to the factors. The factors are phenomena in search of explanation by a theory and are not seen as a substitute for understanding psychological processes that give rise to the decontextualized patterns of affect, behavior, and cognition that are summarized by the factors (Saucier & Goldberg, 1996). Administering a five-factor assessment within this conceptual frame dictates that the resulting scores would be interpreted descriptively, that is, as an overall descriptive summary of how groups of individuals view themselves, in general, based on examples of their behavior, cognitions, and affect. *Five-factor model* adherents (e.g., McCrae & Costa, 1996, 2003), in contrast, make much stronger claims. They assert that the five factors "transcend language" and are "a human universal" (McCrae & Costa, 1997, p. 514); are "influenced not at all by the environment" (McCrae et al., 2000, p. 175); and are "fully developed by age 30" (McCrae & Costa, 1996, p. 72). They also assert that the five factors exert direct causal force on personal strivings, attitudes, and culturally conditioned phenomena; exert direct and indirect causal effects on self-schemas and personal myths; and exert indirect causal effects on emotional reactions, midcareer shifts, behavior, cultural norms, life events, and situations (McCrae & Costa, 2003, Fig. 10). Administering a five-factor assessment within this conceptual frame implies that the resulting scores would be interpreted as having motivational significance for understanding behavior.

Several reliable assessments of the five factors exist—for example, the NEO-Personality Inventory (PI; see Costa & McCrae, 1992) and the international personality item pool (see Goldberg et al., 2006), and there is substantial overlap and shared variance between different scales measuring each of the five factors (Goldberg, 1999).[3] At first blush, then, measuring the five factors and interpreting and using them clinically would seem to be as easy as selecting any one of these self-report measures "off the shelf" and consulting their associated guidebooks and technical manuals. Indeed, this strategy is adopted routinely in clinical contexts; in fact, if one consults only the clinical literature, trait assessments would seem to be meeting the goals of clinical assessment described earlier. In one of the first position papers on the potential clinical use of the five-factor model, Costa (1991, p. 395; see also, Harkness & Lilienfeld, 1997; McCrae, 1991, 2006) suggested that

> [the portrait of five-factor scale scores] can be used in many ways in psychotherapy: to formulate a tentative diagnosis; to aid the clinician's development of empathy; to help select appropriate treatments; to identify the client's strengths; and to anticipate the outcome, duration, and course of therapy.

Clinicians administer the five-factor scales to gauge the degree to which each factor influences a particular client's reactions to treatment (e.g., see McClough & Clarkin, 2004; Miller, 1991; Mutén, 1991). Studies that have assessed the five factors in clinical populations have been variously motivated by a desire to shed light on the genetic etiology of depression (Chopra et al., 2005), to provide conceptual unity to the DSM-IV Axis II personality disorder diagnoses (Bagby, Costa, Widiger, Ryder, & Marshall, 2005; McCrae, Löckenhoff, & Costa, 2005; Widiger, 2005), and to design treatments aimed at stemming hoarding behavior in clients diagnosed with obsessive–compulsive disorder (LaSalle-Ricci et al., 2006), at improving sexual dysfunction and eliminating paraphilias (Fagan et al., 1991), and at reducing the stigma associated with HIV infection (McCrae et al., 2007). Studies have interpreted significant associations between the five factors and features of some clinical problem as evidence that the trait factors affect, cause, or explain the clinical problem in question (Harakeh, Scholte, de Vries, & Engels, 2006; Miller & Lynam, 2003; Sher, Bartholow, & Wood, 2000; Terracciano & Costa, 2004; Williams, Surwit, Babyak, & McCaskill, 1998).

On the surface, then, it would seem that these approaches could be utilized to meet any of the goals of clinical assessment described earlier in this chapter. However, several significant conceptual issues have not been considered in such clinical applications (see also, Cervone, Shadel, Smith, & Fiori, 2006). First, the five trait factors in both models are latent constructs identified through the analysis of populations of persons, *not* individual people. Such population-level constructs cannot be assumed to function at the level of the individual (Borsboom, Mellenbergh, & Heerden, 2003); in other words, the latent variables (e.g., Neuroticism) may account for differences *between* people, but they do not explain *within-person consistency and variation* (Borsboom et al., 2003). In fact, the five factors do not capture much intraindividual variability over time or context (Borkenau & Ostendorf, 1998) and, as such, apply to *hardly anybody* at the level of the individual (Cervone, 2004a; Mischel, 2004). Second, the factors show a very modest level of between-persons predictive utility at a population level (mean $r = .22$; see Pervin, 1994), which necessarily implies much less predictive validity at an individual level (see Lamiel & Trierweiler, 1986) and, as a consequence, implies a very low level of clinical significance (see Kendall et al., 1999). Third, in some perspectives at least (McCrae & Costa, 2003), trait scores are assumed to be stable throughout life; as such, theoretically they are not amenable to interventions or treatments that are, by definition, designed to change some psychological feature of the client. Finally, the five factors summarize decontextualized trends in observable behavior, cognitions, and affect. In the five-factor model the factor summaries of these observables are "internalized" so that they assume a causal role in regulating any number of outcomes at the level of the individual (see McCrae & Costa, 2003). In other words, what the person *does* is used to simultaneously refer to what the person *has*. This conceptual transposition from observed descriptive outcomes to internal causal agents is logically untenable (see Cervone, Shadel, & Jencius, 2001; Cervone et al., 2006, for further discussion). Thus, five-factor assessments may have some descriptive and some modest level of predictive utility at a population level, but they provide no information on internal psychological mechanisms at the level of the individual, which could be the target of change via clinical intervention or therapeutic technique. As such, trait perspectives and assessments *cannot, by definition*, inform treatment planning or case conceptualization, nor can they help with treatment monitoring.

A question might be raised as to why trait perspectives could not be used to descriptively inform or refine the DSM diagnostic classifications, which are themselves atheoretical descriptive classifications of psychological dysfunction. Perspectives have been advanced that argue that personality, however defined and assessed, can be used to inform or to make a clinical diagnosis (e.g., Retzlaff & Dunn, 2003; Weiner, 2004; Widiger & Clark, 2000). Moreover, it might seem a "natural fit" for an assessment of personality to inform an Axis II personality disorder diagnoses; some have even gone so far as to call for a near complete reconceptualization and reclassification of the personality disorders Axis (II) of the DSM within a five-factor framework (e.g., McCrae et al., 2005). Given the well-known conceptual and classificatory problems with the DSM Axis II codes (see Westen & Shedler, 1999), there is clearly merit to rethinking the diagnostic nomenclature. However, over the long term, it is hard to imagine that a system as entrenched as the DSM would be so radically revised (see Kupfer, First, & Reiger, 2002). The practical point, then, is that even if one assumes that five-factor approaches have some utility for informing diagnosis, it seems unlikely that the five-factor paradigm will become a codified reality within the well-established DSM (or other diagnostic) system.[4]

## Social Cognitive Approaches

### *Basic Concepts*

Cognitive structures and processes are the central units of analysis for examining personality in a social cognitive approach. The basic effort is to understand social cognitive mechanisms underlying intraindividual coherence and individual differences in the ways in which people assign meaning to events, reflect upon themselves, and self-regulate their actions and experiences (Bandura, 1999). Mental representations of people, places, situations, and autobiographical events are seen as enduring structures of personality, and the dynamics of cognition, affect, and behavioral execution are the personality processes that mediate the influence of these structures on the flow of thought, affect, and action (Caprara & Cervone, 2000). An overarching principle is that personality develops and functions through reciprocal interactions with the social environment (Bandura, 1999). Knowledge structures and processes are learned as a result of the individual's interaction with the social environment, and different situational and interpersonal contexts shape specific cognitions about those contexts. Cognitive structures and processes, in turn, are linked with different contexts and subsequently come to regulate behavior, affect, and cognition within those contexts. Coherent patterns of cognition, affect, and behavior occur at the level of the individual (Cervone, 1999; Mischel & Shoda, 1995), and situational sources of variability in psychological responding are taken as meaningful indicators of the underlying structure of personality (Mischel & Shoda, 1995).

In a social cognitive approach, then, personality is seen as the product of multiple underlying and interacting cognitive and affective structures and processes, defined explicitly with reference to context. Individual differences can be understood as a consequence of between-subjects variation in these structures and processes and the situations to which they are tied. Understanding intraindividual coherence and variation in response across contexts is seen as a core feature of the social cognitive approach to personality. Overt behaviors are seen as the product of an organized, underlying *system* of cognitive–affective units, such as goals, expectancies, distinct emotions, and mental representations of the situations in which those units come into play (Mischel & Shoda, 1995).

### *Implications for Personality Assessment*

This broad conceptual framework has the following implications for social cognitive personality assessment (Cervone et al., 2001):

- First, underlying psychological structures are distinguished from overt behavioral tendencies in the context of assessment.
- Second, the focus is on assessing personal determinants of action: those underlying knowledge structures, psychological processes, and self-regulatory structures that govern overt behavioral, cognitive, and affective responding.

- Third, different psychological response systems are treated independently, and the reciprocal functional relationships between the response systems are one potential target of assessment.
- Fourth, assessments are employed that preserve the unique qualities of each individual.
- Fifth, assessment of context is a critical source of information about personality functioning.

The number and type of cognitions and affects that individuals may possess are vast (e.g., Mischel, 1973), and conceptualizing and assessing these constructs pose considerable challenges. For example, these constructs include goal systems (e.g., Dweck, 1996; Dweck & Elliott-Moskwa, Chapter 8, this volume), self-regulatory guides (e.g., Doerr & Baumeister, Chapter 5, this volume; Higgins, 1997), cognition and affect (Schwartz & Clore, 1996), and the self-concept (Chandra & Shadel, 2007; Showers & Zeigler-Hill, 2004) (see Caprara & Cervone, 2000, for a more complete review). Fortunately, Cervone (2004b) has developed a conceptual framework that organizes the myriad social cognitive psychological mechanisms in the context of an overarching social cognitive personality system: the Knowledge–Appraisal–Personality–Architecture (KAPA) framework. Among other contributions, the KAPA framework distinguishes between two broad classes of social cognitive personality variables: knowledge and appraisals. *Knowledge* is an enduring structural cognition that can represent features of the self, in addition to features related to others and the social environment. *Appraisals*, in contrast, are evaluative judgments about the relation between the self and some contextualized environmental event. Whereas knowledge is an enduring structural cognition, appraisals are dynamic, changing in response to differing evaluations of environmental events. This distinction is important because appraisals are understood to be a function, in part, of preexisting knowledge (Higgins, 1996). The degree to which knowledge affects appraisals is influenced by the accessibility of that knowledge; knowledge that is more accessible is more likely to influence ongoing appraisals of an environmental event (Higgins & Brendl, 1995). Cervone (2004b; Cervone, 1997) has provided key evidence that aspects of self-knowledge, specifically self-schemas (see Markus, 1977), are important for regulating coherence and variability in self-efficacy appraisals across a variety of contexts.

### *Clinical Implications of a Social Cognitive Approach to Personality Assessment*

Cognitive-behavioral approaches to clinical assessment and treatment, and social cognitive approaches to studying personality plainly share very similar goals and perspectives (Merrill & Strauman, 2004; Mischel, 2004; Shadel, 2004). Both view cognitive–affective processes as key regulators of human behavior (normal and abnormal); both see behavior as having a core functional relationship with situations; and both are focused on identifying within- and between-person sources of variability in cognition, affect, and behavior. The social cognitive approach allows one to move beyond simple description of population-based individual differences, beyond gross prediction of behavioral outcomes on a relatively large scale to a more detailed understanding of the psychological causes of disordered behavior and potentially to matching treatment strategies toward those causes in order to change behavior. What is surprising is that, despite these similarities and potential, social cognitive perspectives on personality have not had any real measurable impact on clinical assessment or treatment.[5]

Part of the reason for this lack of integration might be found by considering the historical relationship between personality and clinical psychology. In the early days of clinical psychology, personality was viewed in broadly psychoanalytic or psychodynamic terms (Benjamin, 2005; Watchel & Messer, 1997). Unconscious drives and forces were seen as the primary ingredients of personality, and an assessment of personality required an assessment of these underlying drives and forces. However, as this approach came under increasing conceptual and empirical scrutiny (see Ollendick, Alvarez, & Greene, 2004; Wood et al., 2002), the empirically more rigorous classical and operant conditioning approaches became dominant and were applied toward understanding and treating problem behavior in the post–World War II era. In these conceptual frameworks there was little tolerance for unobservable, inferred constructs such as *personality* (Ollendick et al., 2004). Although the cognitive-behavioral therapy (CBT) movement of the 1970s refocused clinicians on unobservable but empirically testable constructs such as cognition and affect, conceptions of personality were further pushed aside in many CBT approaches, and this separation has endured to the present day. For example, excellent state-of-the-art texts on CBT (e.g., Dobson, 2001) do not discuss modern social cognitive personality theory or assessment anywhere in their pages.

Part of the problem may also lie with the perception that social cognitive applications are already prevalent in clinical psychology. This perception is only partially true. Many contemporary clinical approaches have been strongly influenced by social cognitive theory (see Ollendick et al., 2004). However, this influence has typically taken the form of assessment and treatment focusing on *single* social cognitive variables, operating in isolation, and *not* as part of an organized psychological system. For example, self-efficacy is a core social cognitive construct in many clinical approaches (Bandura, 1997; Maddux, 1991; Maddux, Chapter 22, this volume) and is typically invoked and assessed in clinical settings in a single-variable format (e.g., What is an alcohol-abusing client's self-efficacy to resist drinking?) or alongside of other social cognitive variables in a multivariate format (e.g., What are this client's cognitive beliefs about drinking alcohol? What were the situational features that characterized the client's relapse?). *Rarely* has self-efficacy been considered part of an integrated and organized cognitive–affective personality system, as is implied when viewing personality from a social cognitive perspective (e.g., How did the client's beliefs about alcohol influence his self-efficacy to maintain abstinence when he was stressed? Why do stressful situations activate his beliefs about alcohol, which, in turn, trigger appraisals of his self-efficacy to remain abstinent?).

Clinical applications of social cognitive personality theory would thus recognize that disordered behavior is a product of an underlying organized *system* of cognitive–affective mechanisms that are inherently tied to specific situations. Assessment, then, would be directed at identifying the within-person variables that comprise this system, the functional relationships between these variables, their functional relationship to the disordered behavior in question, and the situations in which the system operates on behavior (see Cervone et al., 2001). Applications of social cognitive personality theory to clinical assessment exist largely in the domain of theories about anxiety disorders (e.g., Shoda & Smith, 2004) and sport psychology (Smith, 2006), but are starting to be applied both theoretically and empirically in some behavioral health contexts (Cervone, Orom, Aristico, Shadel, & Kassel, 2007; S. M. Miller et al., 2005; Shadel & Cervone, 2006; Shadel, Cervone, Niaura, & Abrams, 2004; Shadel, Niaura, & Abrams, 2000). For example, research with smokers (Cervone et al., 2007; Shadel & Cervone, 2006; Shadel et al., 2004) has adopted an idiographic, social-cognitive approach to personality assessment (Cervone et al., 2001) that taps into organized systems of multiple self-relevant knowledge structures, or self-schemas (Markus, 1977), thought to regulate both cognitive appraisals of self-efficacy to quit smoking and actual quitting behavior in the situations unique to each individual smoker. Interventions designed to facilitate decision making in women receiving genetic biomarker feedback about breast cancer risk have been designed around social cognitive principles in order to match the content of those interventions to the organization of the cognitive–affective systems of individual women (S. M. Miller et al., 2005). Additional research needs to be directed toward applying these conceptions in clinical domains (Shadel, 2004).

## CONCLUDING THOUGHTS

Clinical psychologists continue to use outdated, outmoded, and invalid assessments in service of conceptualizing and assessing personality. Aside from (inappropriately) applying trait perspectives to meet the goals of clinical assessment, many conceptions of personality in 21st-century clinical psychology remain locked in 1940s era conceptions of personality and personality assessment. These assessment strategies (MMPI, Millon Clinical Multiaxial Inventory [MCMI], Thematic Apperception Test [TAT], Rorschach; see Hilsenroth & Segal, 2004) are sometimes referred to as "traditional" clinical assessments (Goldfried & Kent, 1972). Surveys indicate that over 60% clinical psychology internship sites expect incoming clinical trainees to have had graduate training in projective assessments (e.g., Rorschach), and nearly 70% indicate that administration of these devices will occur on a clinical rotation (Clemence & Handler, 2001). Moreover, practicing psychologists devote almost half of their time to administering projective tests (Norcross et al., 2002). Clinical psychology doctoral programs have tended to *de*emphasize training in projective testing in favor of objective assessment (Belter & Piotrowski, 2001; Piotrowski, 1999; Piotrowski & Zalewski, 1993; see McFall, 2006), likely due to several factors, including the abundant evidence pointing to a lack of validity in projective assessments (Hunsley, Lee, & Wood, 2003; Wood et al., 2002). However, even objective personality assessment devices have a number of limitations that makes their clinical use less than optimal (Helmes & Reddon, 1993; Rogers, Salekin, & Sewell, 1999). In any case, perhaps the most telling illustration of the firm hold that such traditional clinical assessments have on the field is found in the recently published, multivolume *Comprehensive Handbook of Psychological Assessment* (Hersen, 2004a). Volume 2 on *Personality Assessment* (Hilsenroth & Segal, 2004) devotes its entire 642 pages to traditional projective assessments, such as the Rorschach, TAT, and "hand test," and traditional objective assessments such as the MMPI and MCMI. *Nowhere* in this volume is there a discussion of modern personality theory or how it could be adapted and applied to problems of clinical importance.

This chapter, then, should be viewed as both an introduction to the contemporary field of personality psychology and a cautionary note for clinicians and clinical researchers to be acutely aware of what they mean when they think of personality, what methods and instruments they are using to assess it, and how they utilize the results of those assessments for clinical or research purposes. There must be a conceptual fit between the clinical goals of personality assessment and the theoretical approach to assessment that is taken. This approach must be testable and supported empirically. Only then will there be a truly meaningful *clinical* assessment of personality.

## ACKNOWLEDGMENTS

The writing of this chapter was supported by Grant No. R01CA12791. Michelle Horner provided invaluable administrative assistance in the preparation of this chapter.

## NOTES

1. Some perspectives within the field suggest that personality can be construed as a cross-species universal and can be found in both humans and animals (see Gosling, 2001). In contrast, other perspectives argue persuasively that personality is a uniquely human characteristic (Cervone, 2004a; p. 116): "Persons share much biological apparatus with other organisms. Yet, they plainly possess psychological qualities unique to our species. If there is to be a science of personality, it must encompass these unique features [such as the capacity to reflect upon themselves, their past, and their future, and to engage in such reflections via language]. ... Otherwise, one is not assessing persons, but mammals." This chapter adheres firmly to the latter perspective: It treats personality as a uniquely human characteristic that is not relevant for understanding the behavior of hyenas (see Gosling, 1998), chimpanzees (see King, Weiss, & Farmer, 2005), or donkeys (see French, 1993).
2. It is not enough to simply identify this organized system in individual clients, though. Treatments or treatment components need to be identified and/or developed that have greater or lesser degrees of efficacy when matched to those psychological systems (Strauman & Merrill, 2004). It is beyond the scope of this chapter to discuss this issue in detail—only to note that assessment of the client is only half the battle.
3. The five factors also account for substantial variance in other trait-like questionnaire measures frequently used in clinical and nonclinical contexts, including the Minnesota Multiphasic Personality Inventory (MMPI), the Eysenck Personality Questionnaire (EPQ), the Interpersonal Adjective Scales (IAS-R), the California Psychological Inventory (CPI), and the 16 Personality Factor Inventory (16-PF) (McCrae & Costa, 2003).
4. Note that my intent is not to become an apologist for the DSM. Rather, my intent is to convey a sense that the current diagnostic system (i.e., a sydromal, multiaxial approach) appears poised to stay with us for the long term for a variety of complex reasons (see Kupfer et al., 2002)—even if the definitions of those syndromes are made more (or less) clear with each subsequent revision of the diagnostic manual itself. As such, I am of the opinion that major efforts designed to radically (or even not so radically) revise the DSM system, while interesting and notable, are not likely to meet with much success.
5. This is not to imply that cognitive-behavioral approaches to assessment and treatment are ineffectual—far from it: Cognitive-behavioral therapy has a lasting ameliorative effect on psychological dysfunction (see Hollon, 2003). Rather, it is to suggest that further improvements in treatments may be realized if social cognitive approaches to the study of personality were integrated into cognitive-behavioral assessment and treatments matched to the results of those assessments (see Strauman et al., 2006, for one example).

## REFERENCES

Abrams, D. B., & Niaura, R. (2003). Planning evidence-based treatment of nicotine dependence. In D. B. Abrams, R. Niaura, R. A. Brown, K. M. Emmons, M. G. Goldstein, & P. M. Monti, *The tobacco dependence treatment handbook* (pp. 1–26). New York: Guilford Press.

Allport, G. W., & Vernon, P. E. (1930). The field of personality. *Psychological Bulletin*, *27*, 677–730.

American Psychiatric Association. (2000). *Diagnostic and statistical manual of mental disorders* (4th ed., text rev.). Washington, DC: Author.

Bagby, R. M., Costa, P. T., Jr., Widiger, T. A., Ryder, A. G., & Marshall, M. (2005). DSM-IV personality disorders and the five-factor model of personality: A multi-method examination of domain- and facet-level predictions. *European Journal of Personality*, *19*, 307–324.

Baker, T. B., McFall, R. M., & Shoham, V. (2009). Current status and future prospects of clinical psychology: Toward a scientifically principled approach to mental and behavioral health care. *Psychological Science in the Public Interest*, *9*, 68–103.

Bandura, A. (1997). *Self-efficacy: The exercise of control.* New York: Freeman.

Bandura, A. (1999). Social-cognitive theory of personality. In D. Cervone & Y. Shoda (Eds.), *The coherence of personality: Social-cognitive bases of personality consistency, variability, and organization* (pp. 185–241). New York: Guilford Press.

Barbour, K. A., & Davison, G. C. (2004). Clinical interviewing. In S. N. Haynes & E. M. Heiby (Eds.), *Comprehensive handbook of psychological assessment: Vol. 3. Behavioral assessment* (pp. 181–193). Hoboken, NJ: Wiley.

Barlow, D. H. (Ed.). (2001). *Clinical handbook of psychological disorders* (3rd ed.). New York: Guilford Press.

Beck, A. T., Rush, A. J., Shaw, B., & Emery, G. (1979). *Cognitive therapy of depression.* New York: Guilford Press.

Belter, R. W., & Piotrowski, C. (2001). Current status of doctoral-level training in psychological testing. *Journal of Clinical Psychology*, *57*, 717–726.

Benjamin, L. T. (2005). A history of clinical psychology as a profession in America (and a glimpse at its future). *Annual Review of Clinical Psychology*, *1*, 1–30.

Beutler, L. E., & Harwood, T. M. (2000). *Prescriptive psychotherapy: A practical guide to systematic treatment selection.* New York: Oxford University Press.

Beutler, L. E., Kim, E. J., Davison, E., Karno, M., & Fisher, D. (1996). Research contributions to improving managed care outcomes. *Psychotherapy*, *33*, 197–206.

Borkenau, P., & Ostendorf, F. (1998). The Big Five as states: How useful is the five-factor model to describe intraindividual variations over time? *Journal of Research in Personality*, *32*, 202–221.

Borsboom, D., Mellenbergh, G., & Heerden, J. (2003). The theoretical status of latent variables. *Psychological Review*, *10*, 203–219.

Braun, S. A., & Cox, C. A. (2001). Managed mental health care: Intentional misdiagnosis of mental disorders. *Journal of Counseling and Development*, *83*, 425–433.

Brownell, K. D., & Wadden, T. A. (1991). The heterogeneity of obesity: Fitting treatments to individuals. *Behavior Therapy*, *22*, 153–177.

Butcher, J. N. (2006). Assessment in clinical psychology: A perspective on the past, present challenges, and future prospects. *Clinical Psychology: Science and Practice*, *13*, 205–209.

Butcher, J. N., & Rouse, S. V. (1996). Personality: Individual differences and clinical assessment. *Annual Review of Psychology*, *47*, 87–111.

Caprara, G. V., & Cervone, D. (2000). *Personality: Determinants, dynamics, and potentials.* New York: Cambridge University Press.

Carver, C. S. (1996). Emergent integration in contemporary personality psychology. *Journal of Research in Personality*, *30*, 319–334.

Cervone, D. (1991). The two disciplines of personality psychology. *Psychological Science*, *2*, 371–377.

Cervone, D. (1997). Social-cognitive mechanisms and personality coherence: Self-knowledge, situational beliefs, and cross-situational coherence in perceived self-efficacy. *Psychological Science*, *8*, 43–50.

Cervone, D. (1999). Bottom-up explanation in personality psychology: The case of cross-situational coherence. In D. Cervone & Y. Shoda (Eds.), *The coherence of personality: Social-cognitive bases of personality consistency, variability, and organization* (pp. 303–341). New York: Guilford Press.

Cervone, D. (2004a). Personality assessment: Tapping the social-cognitive architecture of personality. *Behavior Therapy*, *35*, 113–129.

Cervone, D. (2004b). The architecture of personality. *Psychological Review*, *111*, 183–204.

Cervone, D., & Mischel, W. (2002). Personality science. In D. Cervone & W. Mischel (Eds.), *Advances in personality science* (pp. 1–26). New York: Guilford Press.

Cervone, D., Orom, H., Aristico, D., Shadel, W. G., & Kassel, J. (2007). Using a knowledge-and-appraisal model of personality architecture to understand consistency and variability in smoker's self-efficacy appraisals in high-risk situations. *Psychology of Addictive Behaviors*, *21*, 44–54.

Cervone, D., Shadel, W. G., & Jencius, S. (2001). Social-cognitive theory of personality assessment. *Personality and Social Psychology Review*, *5*, 33–51.

Cervone, D., Shadel, W. G., Smith, R. E., & Fiori, M. (2006). Conceptualizing self-regulation: Reminders and suggestions from personality science. *Applied Psychology: An International Review*, *55*, 333–385.

Chandra, S., & Shadel, W. G. (2007). Crossing disciplinary boundaries: Applying financial portfolio theory to model the organization of the self-concept. *Journal of Research in Personality*, *41*, 346–373.

Chopra, K. K., Bagby, R. M., Dickens, S., Kennedy, S. H., Ravindran, A., & Levitan, R. D. (2005). A dimensional approach to personality in atypical depression. *Psychiatry Research*, *134*, 161–167.

Clemence, A. J., & Handler, L. (2001). Psychological assessment on internship: A survey of training directors and their expectations for students. *Journal of Personality Assessment*, *76*(1), 18–47.

Costa, P. T., Jr. (1991). Clinical use of the five-factor model: An introduction. *Journal of Personality Assessment*, *57*(3), 393–398.

Costa, P. T., Jr., & McCrae, R. R. (1992). *Revised NEO Personality Inventory (NEO-PI) and NEO Five Factor Inventory (NEO-FFI) professional manual.* Odessa, FL: Psychological Assessment Resources.

Digman, J. (1996). The curious history of the five-factor model. In J. Wiggins (Ed.), *The five-factor model of personality: Theoretical perspectives* (pp. 1–20). New York: Guilford Press.

Dobson, K. S. (1989). A meta-analysis of the efficacy of cognitive therapy for depression. *Journal of Consulting and Clinical Psychology*, *57*, 414–419.

Dobson, K. S. (2001). *Handbook of cognitive-behavioral therapies* (2nd ed.). New York: Guilford Press.

Dweck, C. (1996). Capturing the dynamic nature of personality. *Journal of Research in Personality*, *30*, 348–362.

Ey, S., & Hersen, M. (2004). Pragmatic issues of assessment in clinical practice. In M. Hersen (Ed.), *Psychological assessment in clinical practice: A pragmatic guide* (pp. 3–20). New York: Brunner-Routledge.

Fagan, P. J., Wise, T. N., Schmidt, C. W., Ponticas, Y., Marshall, R. D., & Costa, P. T., Jr. (1991). A comparison of five-factor personality dimensions in males with sexual dysfunction and males with paraphilia. *Journal of Personality Assessment*, *57*, 434–448.

Finn, S. E., & Tonsager, M. E. (1997). Information-gathering and therapeutic models of assessment: Complementary paradigms. *Psychological Assessment*, *9*(4), 374–385.

First, M. B., & Gibbon, M. (2004). The Structured Clinical Interview for DSM-IV Axis I Disorders (SCID-I) and the Structured Clinical Interview for DSM-IV Axis II Disorders (SCID-II). In M. J. Hilsenroth & D. L. Segal (Eds.), *Comprehensive handbook of psychological assessment. Vol. 2: Personality assessment* (pp. 134–143). Hoboken, NJ: Wiley.

French, J. M. (1993). Assessment of donkey temperament and the influence of home environment. *Applied Animal Behaviour Science*, *36*, 249–257.

Garb, H. N., & Boyle, P. A. (2003). Understanding why some clinicians use pseudoscientific methods: Findings from research on clinical judgment. In S. O. Lilienfeld, S. J. Lynn, & J. M. Lohr (Eds.), *Science and pseudoscience in clinical psychology* (pp. 17–38). New York: Guilford Press.

Garfinkel, A. (1981). *Forms of explanation*. New Haven, CT: Yale University Press.

Goldberg, L. R. (1993). The structure of phenotypic personality traits. *American Psychologist*, *48*, 33–44.

Goldberg, L. R. (1999). A broad-bandwidth, public domain, personality inventory measuring the lower-level facets of several five-factor models. In I. Mervielde, I. Deary, F. De Fruyt, & F. Ostendorf (Eds.), *Personality psychology in Europe* (Vol. 7, pp. 7–28). Tilburg, The Netherlands: Tilburg University Press.

Goldberg, L. R., Johnson, J. A., Eber, H. W., Hogan, R., Ashton, M. C., Cloninger, C. R., et al. (2006). The International Personality Item Pool and the future of public-domain personality measures. *Journal of Research in Personality*, *40*, 84–96.

Goldfried, M. R., & Kent, R. N. (1972). Traditional versus behavioral assessment: A comparison of methodological and theoretical assumptions. *Psychological Bulletin*, *77*, 409–420.

Gosling, S. (1998). Personality dimensions in spotted hyenas (*Crocuta crocuta*). *Journal of Comparative Psychology*, *112*, 107–118.

Gosling, S. (2001). From mice to men: What can we learn about personality from animal research? *Psychological Bulletin*, *127*, 45–86.

Harakeh, Z., Scholte, R. H. J., de Vries, H., & Engels, R. C. M. E. (2006). Association between personality and adolescent smoking. *Addictive Behaviors*, *31*, 232–245.

Harkness, A. R., & Lilienfeld, S. O. (1997). Individual differences science for treatment planning: Personality traits. *Psychological Assessment*, *9*(4), 349–360.

Hayes, S. C., Nelson, R. O., & Jarrett, R. B. (1987). The treatment utility of assessment: Functional approach to evaluating assessment quality. *American Psychologist*, *42*, 963–974.

Haynes, S. N. (1993). Treatment implications of psychological assessment. *Psychological Assessment*, *5*(3), 251–253.

Helmes, E., & Reddon, J. R. (1993). A perspective on developments in assessing psychopathology: A critical review of the MMPI and MMPI-2. *Psychological Bulletin*, *113*, 453–471.

Hersen, M. (Ed.). (2004a). *Comprehensive handbook of psychological assessment.* Hoboken, NJ: Wiley.

Hersen, M. (2004b). *Psychological assessment in clinical practice: A pragmatic guide.* New York: Taylor & Francis.

Higgins, E. T. (1996). Knowledge activation: Accessibility, applicability, and salience. In E. T. Higgins & A. W. Kruglanski (Eds.), *Social psychology: Handbook of basic principles* (pp. 133–168). New York: Guilford Press.

Higgins, E. T. (1997). Beyond pleasure and pain. *American Psychologist*, *52*, 1280–1300.

Higgins, E. T., & Brendl, C. M. (1995). Accessibility and applicability: Some "activation rules" influencing judgment. *Journal of Experimental Social Psychology*, *31*, 218–243.

Hilsenroth, M. J., & Segal, D. L. (Eds.). (2004). *Comprehensive handbook of psychological assessment. Vol. 2. Personality assessment.* Hoboken, NJ: Wiley.

Hollon, S. D. (2003). Does cognitive therapy have an enduring effect? *Cognitive Therapy and Research*, *27*, 71–76.

Hunsley, J. (2002). Psychological testing and psychological assessment: A closer examination. *American Psychologist*, *56*(2), 139–140.

Hunsley, J., Lee, C. M., & Wood, J. M. (2003). Controversial and questionable assessment techniques. In S. O. Lilienfeld, S. J. Lynn, & J. M. Lohr (Eds.), *Science and pseudoscience in clinical psychology* (pp. 39–76). New York: Guilford Press.

Hunsley, J., & Moss, E. J. (2007). Evidence-based assessment. *Annual Review of Clinical Psychology*, *3*, 29–51.

Kendall, P. C., Flannery-Schroeder, E. C., & Ford, J. D. (1999). Therapy outcome research methods. In P. C. Kendall, J. N. Butcher, & G. N. Holmbeck (Eds.), *Handbook of research methods in clinical psychology* (2nd ed., pp. 330–363). New York: Wiley.

King, J. E., Weiss, A., & Farmer, K. H. (2005). A chimpanzee (*Pan troglodytes*) analogue of cross-national generalization of personality structure: Zoological parks and an African sanctuary. *Journal of Personality*, *73*, 389–410.

Kupfer, D. J., First, M. B., & Reiger, D. A. (Eds.). (2002). *A research agenda for DSM-V.* Washington, DC: American Psychiatric Association.

Lamiel, J. T., & Trierweiler, S. J. (1986). Personality measurement and intuitive personality judgments from an idiothetic point of view. *Clinical Psychology Review*, *6*, 471–491.

LaSalle-Ricci, V. H., Arnkoff, D. B., Glass, C. R., Crawley, S. A., Ronquillo, J. G., & Murphy, D. L. (2006). The hoarding dimension of OCD: Psychological comorbidity and the five-factor personality model. *Behaviour Research and Therapy*, *44*(10), 1503–1512.

Lipchik, G. L., Nicholson, R. A., & Penzien, D. B. (2006). Allocation of patients to conditions in headache clinical trials: Randomization, stratification, and treatment matching. *Headache*, *45*, 419–428.

Maddux, J. E. (1991). Self-efficacy. In C. R. Snyder & D. R. Forsyth (Eds.), *Handbook of social and clinical psychology* (pp. 57–78). New York: Pergamon Press.

Markus, H. (1977). Self-schemata and processing information about the self. *Journal of Personality and Social Psychology*, *35*, 63–78.

Maruish, M. E. (Ed.). (1999). *The use of psychological testing and treatment planning* (2nd ed.). Mahwah, NJ: Erlbaum.

Matarazzo, J. D. (1990). Psychological assessment versus psychological testing: Validation from Binet to the school, clinic, and courtroom. *American Psychologist*, *45*(9), 999–1017.

Matarazzo, J. D. (1992). Psychological testing and assessment in the 21st century. *American Psychologist*, *47*, 1007–1018.

McClough, J. F., & Clarkin, J. F. (2004). Personality disorders. In M. Hersen (Ed.), *Psychological assessment in clinical practice: A pragmatic guide* (pp. 117–146). New York: Taylor & Francis.

McCrae, R. R. (1991). The five-factor model and its assessment in clinical settings. *Journal of Personality Assessment*, *57*(3), 399–414.

McCrae, R. R. (2006). Psychopathology from the perspective of the five-factor model. In S. Strack (Ed.), *Differentiating normal and abnormal personality* (2nd ed., pp. 51–64). New York: Springer.

McCrae, R. R., & Costa, P. T., Jr. (1996). Toward a new generation of personality theories: Theoretical context for the five-factor model. In J. S. Wiggins (Ed.), *The five-factor model of personality: Theoretical perspectives* (pp. 51–87). New York: Guilford Press.

McCrae, R. R., & Costa, P. T., Jr. (1997). Personality trait structure as a human universal. *American Psychologist*, *52*, 509–516.

McCrae, R. R., & Costa, P. T., Jr. (2003). *Personality in adulthood: A five-factor theory perspective.* New York: Guilford Press.

McCrae, R. R., Costa, P. T., Jr., Martin, T. A., Oryol, V. E., Senin, I. G., & O'Cleirish, C. O. (2007). Personality correlates of HIV stigmatization in Russia and the United States. *Journal of Research in Personality*, *41*, 190–196.

McCrae, R. R., Costa, P. T., Jr., Ostendorf, F., Angleitner, A., Hrebickova, M., Avia, M. D., et al. (2000). Nature over nurture: Temperament, personality, and lifespan development. *Journal of Personality and Social Psychology*, *78*, 173–186.

McCrae, R. R., Löckenhoff, C. E., & Costa, P. T., Jr. (2005). A step toward DSM-V: Cataloguing personality-related problems in living. *European Journal of Personality*, *19*, 269–286.

McFall, R. M. (2005). Theory and utility: Key themes in evidence-based assessment: Comment on the special section. *Psychological Assessment*, *17*, 312–323.

McFall, R. M. (2006). Doctoral training in clinical psychology. *Annual Review of Clinical Psychology*, *2*, 21–49.

McWilliams, N. (1994). *Psychoanalytic diagnosis: Understanding personality structure in the clinical process.* New York: Guilford Press.

Merrill, K., & Strauman, T. (2004). The role of personality in cognitive-behavioral therapies. *Behavior Therapy*, *35*, 131–146.

Meyer, G. J., Finn, S. E., Eyde, L. D., Kay, G. G., Moreland, K. L., Dies, R. R., et al. (2001). Psychological testing and psychological assessment: A review of evidence and issues. *American Psychologist*, *56*(2), 128–165.

Miller, I. W., Keitner, G. I., Ryan, C. E., Solomon, D. A., Cardemil, E. V., & Beevers, C. G. (2005).

Treatment matching in the posthospital care of depressed patients. *American Journal of Psychiatry, 162*(11), 2131–2138.

Miller, J. D., & Lynam, D. R. (2003). Psychopathy and the five-factor model of personality: A replication and extension. *Journal of Personality Assessment, 81*, 168–178.

Miller, S. M., Roussi, M., Daly, M. B., Buzaglo, J. S., Sherman, K., Godwin, A. K., et al. (2005). Enhanced counseling for women undergoing BRCA1/2 testing: Impact on subsequent decision making about risk reduction behaviors. *Health Education and Behavior, 32*, 654–667.

Miller, T. R. (1991). The psychotherapeutic utility of the five-factor model of personality: A clinician's experience. *Journal of Personality Assessment, 57*(3), 415–433.

Mischel, W. (1973). Toward a cognitive social learning reconceptualization of personality. *Psychological Review, 80*, 252–283.

Mischel, W. (1993). *Introduction to personality* (5th ed.). New York: Harcourt, Brace, Jovanovich.

Mischel, W. (2004). Encompassing behavior, cognition, affect, and process: Toward an integrative model for CBT. *Behavior Therapy, 35*, 185–203.

Mischel, W., & Shoda, Y. (1994). Personality psychology has two goals: Must it be two fields? *Psychological Inquiry, 5*, 156–158.

Mischel, W., & Shoda, Y. (1995). A cognitive-affective system theory of personality: Reconceptualizing situations, dispositions, dynamics, and invariance in personality structure. *Psychological Review, 102*, 246–286.

Morf, C. (2002). Personality at the hub: Extending the conception of personality psychology. *Journal of Research in Personality, 36*, 249–660.

Mutén, E. (1991). Self-reports, spouse ratings, and psychophysiological assessment in a behavioral medicine program: An application of the five-factor model. *Journal of Personality Assessment, 57*(3), 449–464.

Nelson-Gray, R. O., & Paulson, J. F. (2004). Behavioral assessment and the DSM system. In S. N. Haynes & E. M. Heiby (Eds.), *Comprehensive handbook of psychological assessment. Vol. 3. Behavioral assessment* (pp. 470–486). Hoboken, NJ: Wiley.

Nezu, A. M., Nezu, C. M., Peacock, M. A., & Girdwood, C. P. (2004). Case formulation in cognitive-behavioral therapy. In S. N. Haynes & E. M. Heiby (Eds.), *Comprehensive handbook of psychological assessment. Vol. 3. Behavioral assessment* (pp. 402–426). Hoboken, NJ: Wiley.

Norcross, J. C., Hedges, M., & Castle, P. H. (2002). Psychologists conducting psychotherapy in 2001: A study of the Division 29 membership. *Psychotherapy: Theory, Research, Practice, Training, 39*, 97–102.

Ollendick, T. H., Alvarez, H. K., & Greene, R. W. (2004). Behavioral assessment: History of underlying concepts and methods. In S. N. Haynes & E. M. Heiby (Eds.), *Comprehensive handbook of psychological assessment. Vol. 3. Behavioral assessment* (pp. 19–34). Hoboken, NJ: Wiley.

Persons, J. B., & Davidson, J. (2001). Cognitive-behavioral case formulation. In K. S. Dobson (Ed.), *Handbook of cognitive-behavioral therapies* (2nd ed., pp. 86–110). New York: Guilford Press.

Pervin, L. A. (1994). A critical analysis of trait theory. *Psychological Inquiry, 38*, 103–113.

Piotrowski, C. (1999). Assessment practices in the era of managed care: Current status and future directions. *Journal of Clinical Psychology, 55*(7), 787–796.

Piotrowski, C., & Zalewski, C. (1993). Training in psychodiagnostic testing in APA-approved PSYD and PhD clinical psychology programs. *Journal of Personality Assessment, 61*, 394–405.

Pipal, J. E. (1995). Managed care: Is it the corpse in the living room? An expose. *Psychotherapy, 32*(2), 323–332.

Project MATCH Research Group. (1997). Matching alcoholism treatments to client heterogeneity: Project MATCH posttreatment drinking outcomes. *Journal of Studies on Alcohol, 58*, 7–29.

Project MATCH Research Group. (1998). Matching alcoholism treatments to client heterogeneity: Treatment main effects and matching effects on drinking during treatment. *Journal of Studies on Alcohol, 59*, 631–639.

Resnick, J. (1991). Finally, a definition of clinical psychology: A message from the president of Division 12. *Clinical Psychologist, 44*, 3–11.

Retzlaff, P. D., & Dunn, T. (2003). The Millon Clinical Multiaxial Inventory–III. In L. E. Beutler & G. Groth-Marnat (Eds.), *Integrative assessment of adult personality* (pp. 192–226). New York: Guilford Press.

Rogers, R., Salekin, R. T., & Sewell, K. W. (1999). Validation of the Millon Multiaxial Inventory for Axis II disorders: Does it meet the *Daubert* standard? *Law and Human Behavior*, *23*, 425–443.

Saucier, G., & Goldberg, L. R. (1996). The language of personality: Lexical perspectives on the five-factor model. In J. S. Wiggins (Eds.), *The five-factor model of personality: Theoretical perspectives* (pp. 21–50). New York: Guilford Press.

Schwartz, N., & Clore, G. L. (1996). Feelings and phenomenological experiences. In E. T. Higgins & A. W. Kruglanski (Eds.), *Social psychology: Handbook of basic principles* (pp. 433–465). New York: Guilford Press.

Sechrest, L. (1992). The past future of clinical psychology: A reflection of Woodworth (1937). *Journal of Consulting and Clinical Psychology*, *60*, 18–23.

Shadel, W. G. (2004). Introduction to the special series: What can personality science offer cognitive-behavioral therapy and research? *Behavior Therapy*, *35*, 101–111.

Shadel, W. G., & Cervone, D. (2006). Evaluating social-cognitive mechanisms that regulate self-efficacy in response to provocative smoking cues: An experimental investigation. *Psychology of Addictive Behaviors*, *20*, 91–96.

Shadel, W. G., Cervone, D., Niaura, R., & Abrams, D. B. (2004). Developing an integrative social-cognitive strategy for personality assessment at the level of the individual: An illustration with regular cigarette smokers. *Journal of Research in Personality*, *38*, 394–419.

Shadel, W. G., Niaura, R., & Abrams, D. B. (2000). An idiographic approach to understanding personality structure and individual differences among smokers. *Cognitive Therapy and Research*, *24*, 345–359.

Sher, K. J., Bartholow, B. D., & Wood, M. D. (2000). Personality and substance use disorders: A prospective study. *Journal of Consulting and Clinical Psychology*, *68*(5), 818–829.

Shiffman, S. (1993). Smoking cessation treatment: Any progress? *Journal of Consulting and Clinical Psychology*, *61*, 718–722.

Shoda, Y., & Smith, R. E. (2004). Conceptualizing personality as a cognitive-affective processing system: A framework for models of maladaptive behavior patterns and change. *Behavior Therapy*, *35*, 147–166.

Showers, C. J., & Zeigler-Hill, V. (2004). Organization of partner knowledge: Relationship outcomes and longitudinal change. *Personality and Social Psychology Bulletin*, *30*, 1198–1210.

Smith, R. E. (2006). Understanding sport behavior: A cognitive-affective processing systems approach. *Journal of Applied Sport Psychology*, *18*, 1–27.

Sorenson, R. L., Gorsuch, R. L., & Mintz, J. (1985). Moving targets: Patients' changing complaints during psychotherapy. *Journal of Consulting and Clinical Psychology*, *53*(1), 49–54.

Strauman, T. J. (2001). Paradigms, promises, and the potential of clinical psychology. *Journal of Clinical Psychology*, *57*, 1125–1132.

Strauman, T. J., & Merrill, K. A. (2004). The basic science/clinical science interface and treatment development. *Clinical Psychology: Science and Practice*, *11*, 263–266.

Strauman, T. J., Vieth, A. Z., Merrill, K. A., Kolden, G. G., Woods, T. E., Klein, M. H., et al. (2006). Self-system therapy as an intervention for self-regulatory dysfunction in depression: A randomized comparison with cognitive therapy. *Journal of Consulting and Clinical Psychology*, *74*, 367–376.

Swan, W. B., & Seyle, C. (2005). Personality psychology's comeback and its emerging symbiosis with social psychology. *Personality and Social Psychology Bulletin*, *31*, 155–165.

Terracciano, A., & Costa, P. T., Jr. (2004). Smoking and the five-factor model of personality. *Addiction*, *99*, 472–481.

Watchel, P. L., & Messer, S. B. (1997). *Theories of psychotherapy: Origins and evolution*. Washington, DC: American Psychological Association.

Watkins, C. E., Campbell, V. L., Nieberding, R., & Hallmark, R. (1995). Contemporary practice of psychological assessment by clinical psychologists. *Professional Psychology: Research and Practice*, 26, 54–60.

Weiner, I. B. (2004). Rorschach assessment: Current status. In M. J. Hilsenroth & D. L. Segal (Eds.), *Comprehensive handbook of psychological assessment. Vol. 2. Personality assessment* (pp. 343–355). Hoboken, NJ: Wiley.

Westen, D., & Shedler, J. (1999). Revising and assessing Axis II, part II: Toward an empirically-based and clinically useful classification of personality disorders. *American Journal of Psychiatry*, *156*, 273–286.

Widiger, T. A. (2005). Five-factor model of personality disorder: Integrating science and practice. *Journal of Research in Personality*, *39*, 67–83.

Widiger, T. A., & Clark, L. A. (2000). Toward DSM-V and the classification of psychopathology. *Psychological Bulletin*, *126*(6), 946–963.

Williams, P. G., Surwit, R. S., Babyak, M. A., & McCaskill, C. C. (1998). Personality predictors of mood related to dieting. *Journal of Consulting and Clinical Psychology*, *66*(6), 994–1004.

Wood, J. M., Garb, H. N., Lilienfeld, S. O., & Nezworski, M. T. (2002). Clinical assessment. *Annual Review of Psychology*, *53*, 519–543.

# 19 Interpersonal Assessment and Treatment of Personality Disorders

Lorna Smith Benjamin

This chapter is concerned with personality and personality disorders from an interpersonal, clinically oriented perspective. It presents a review of clinicians' definitions of personality disorder and problems with those definitions; describes personality trait profiles based on factor analysis; and reviews in greater depth some definitions of personality based on a single circumplex. The emphasis is on the description of personality using an alternative circumplex model, the Structural Analysis of Social Behavior (SASB; Benjamin, 1979, 1996b), which derives from observations of primate social behavior. These various approaches to personality, aspects of which can be considered representative of social psychology, are illustrated by applying them to a pattern that is highly problematic for clinicians: borderline personality disorder (BPD). The different methodologies are assessed in light of clinical goals of identifying what has gone wrong when a patient comes for treatment and determining what to do about it. It is likely that clinicians ultimately will be most responsive to contributions from social psychology that credibly address their fundamental concerns about the causes and treatments of psychological problems.

## INTERPERSONAL APPROACHES TO UNDERSTANDING PERSONALITY

### The Sullivanian Tradition

Harry Stack Sullivan declared that "personality is made manifest in interpersonal situations, and not otherwise" (Greenberg & Mitchell, 1983, p. 90). A clinically gifted psychiatrist, Sullivan made it very clear that *social interactions* are fundamental in the development of personality, starting with the neonate. For example, he theorized that the *self system* (Sullivan, 1953, pp. 164–171) is, in part, formed by incorporation or *introjection* of the "bad" mother's forbidding gestures that appear as the infant tries to meet his or her "zonal needs." Introjection (treating the self as the mother did) is one of many methods the infant uses to avoid anxiety arising from, as Sullivan says, the need to live with this significant other person. His theory of the developmental sequence emphasizes social interaction at every phase. Sullivan's view of personality as interactional was applied even to the severest of disorders in his *Schizophrenia as a Human Process* (1963). His interpersonal emphasis had a major effect on psychodynamic versions of psychiatric theory, though he appears not to have been an inside member of the conceptually related British school of object relations. Most importantly, there was little or no empirical data to support or refute his theories about social development.

### The Single Circumplex Tradition: The Interpersonal Circle

The interpersonal and empirical emphases by Sullivan and others (e.g., Murray) were antecedents to the interpersonal circumplex (IPC), which seeks to measure personality empirically. The IPC model is build on two axes: the horizontal runs from Hate to Love, and the vertical, from Control to Submit. Successive points around the interpersonal circle theoretically are comprised of balanced proportions of these underlying axes. The first version, described by Freedman, Leary, Ossorio, and Coffey (1951), included (1) Managerial–autocratic, (2) Responsible–hypernormal, (3) Cooperative–overconventional, (4) Docile–dependent, (5) Self-effacing–masochistic, (6) Rebellious–distrustful, (7) Aggressive–sadistic, (8) Competitive–narcissistic. In the early 1960s Guttman developed a clear mathematical rationale for plotting complex spaces in simpler forms, such as a circle.

Clinical implications of the IPC were developed at the Kaiser Foundation Hospital during the 1950s, and in 1957, Timothy Leary published *Interpersonal Diagnosis of Personality*, which described particular personality types that could be identified by their characteristic positions on the IPC. Following the publication of Leary's book, there have been at least 21 variations of the IPC (Wiggins, 1982). Wiggins (1982) offered his own version of the IPC, and, updating Leary's lead in relating the IPC to personality types, proposed the following mapping of the single circumplex onto the DSM-III: (1) PA, Ambitious, dominant = compulsive personality; (2) NO, Gregarious, extroverted = chronic hypomanic personality; (3) LM, Warm, agreeable = histrionic personality; (4) JK, Unassuming, ingenuous = dependent personality; (5) HI, Lazy, submissive = passive–aggressive personality; (6) FG, Aloof, introverted = schizoid personality; (7) DE, Cold, quarrelsome = paranoid personality; (8) BC, Arrogant, calculating = narcissistic personality. BPD was not mentioned in this proposal. Wiggins concluded that his Interpersonal Adjective Scale (IAS) represents a useful taxonomic framework within which to view personality from a variety of traditions. Later, he refined his measure, and presently it is called the Interpersonal Adjective Scale—Revised (IAS-R; Wiggins, Trapnell, & Phillips, 1988).

Sim and Romney (1990) used interpersonal ratings of personality disorders on the Leary Interpersonal Checklist (ICL) and the Millon Multi Axial Clinical Inventory (MMCI-I) to test Wiggins's predictions in a sample of 90 patients and 90 students. There was modest support for the predictions when the reconstructed models were compared to predictions in terms of quadrants rather than octants (p. 338). According to O'Connor and Dyce (1998), factor analyses of data from eight published studies of assessments for personality disorders by a variety of measures found very little support for circumplex ordering, whereas there was moderate support for multifactorial descriptions such as the NEO-Personality Inventory (NEO-PI) (Costa & McCrae, 1992).

The single circumplex has been used primarily within select research traditions of social psychology, but samples from clinical populations are rarely studied, and the work has had little impact on clinical practice. An important exception is Horowitz's Inventory of Interpersonal Problems Inventory (IIP, 1988), based on collation of the interpersonal complaints of persons presenting for outpatient treatment, which were factor-analyzed and projected onto the Wiggins Interpersonal Adjective scale—Revised (IAS-R). The IIP is a popular research measure that can compare pre- to posttreatment changes during psychotherapy (Gurtman, 1996). For such IPC-based measures, and for factorial measures such as the NEO-PI,[1] assessments are reliable and orderly, but there are no clear causal or treatment implications.

## STRUCTURAL ANALYSIS OF SOCIAL BEHAVIOR: SASB

Virtually all circumplex models of personality include some aspect of a love (friendliness)–hate (hostility) dimension. The various versions of the Leary IPC all add a vertical dimension that runs from *dominate* to *submit*. Schaefer (1965) created a different circumplex model of parenting behavior that had the usual horizontal axis, but used control–emancipate (rather than control–submit) on the vertical axis. Benjamin (1974, 1979, 1987, 1996b) proposed SASB, which introduced multiple surfaces (circumplexes) reflecting differences in attentional focus and corresponding differences in the definitions of poles on the vertical axes. A simplified version of the SASB model appears in Figure 19.1.[2]

The SASB model includes Shaefer's (1965) version of **CONTROL** and **EMANCIPATE** as opposites on the vertical axis (located 180 degrees apart on the model). This can be seen on Figure 19.1. Rather than appearing opposite **CONTROL**, SUBMIT is located at the same point in interpersonal space as is **CONTROL**. They are in geometrically identical locations

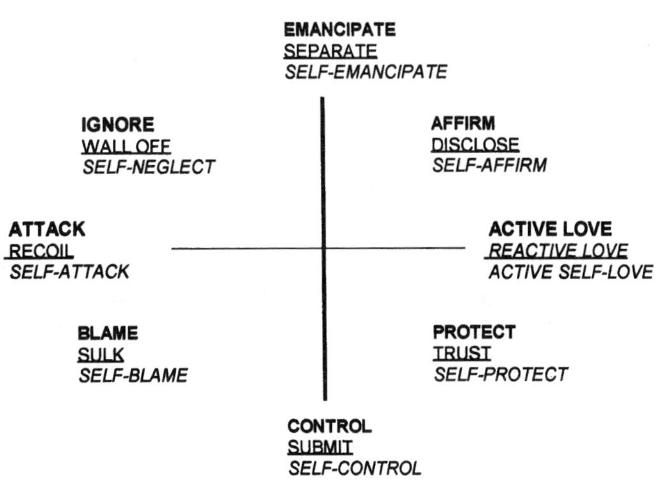


**FIGURE 19.1.** Simplified cluster version of the SASB model. From Benjamin (1996b). Copyright 1996 by The Guilford Press. Reprinted by permission.

on the underlying axes and differ only in interpersonal focus (explained below and represented in Figure 19.1 by different types of font).

## Dimensions of the SASB Model

The SASB model has three, rather than two, dimensions. The added dimension, attentional focus, is shown only as three discrete planes, but might eventually be developed as a continuum.[3]

### *Focus*

The first surface (**BOLD** print) describes prototypic parentlike behavior (*transitive* focus on other), and its vertical axis runs from **CONTROL** to **EMANCIPATE.** The second surface (<u>UNDERLINED</u> print) describes prototypic childlike behavior (*intransitive* focus on self), and its vertical axis runs from <u>SUBMIT</u> to <u>SEPARATE</u>. The third surface (*ITALICIZED* print) describes introjective focus (transitive focus on other, with self as the direct object). Across all three surfaces, the lower part of the vertical axis describes enmeshment, while the upper part describes differentiation. The concept of focus is very important in clinical applications because it explicitly calls the clinician's attention to whether the patient is talking about taking transitive action in relation to someone or something else, or about his or her own intransitive state of being in interpersonal reaction to someone or something else. If a client frequently focuses on another individual in the therapy narrative, it can be interpreted as a form of external orientation that precludes personal growth. There has to be some focus on self during psychotherapy for the self (the personality) to change. The dimension of focus is not represented in any version of the IPC, and yet this aspect of interpersonal transaction is clearly very important to clinicians. Trying to help someone change who has an external orientation will result in what I have called the "wrong patient syndrome" (Benjamin, 1996b). A person with this "disorder" assumes that other people have to be different for him or her to feel better. Another clinical advantage of SASB is its ability to define enmeshment and differentiation, with differentiated space having many clinically relevant variations. The most vital subspace is the region of friendly differentiation (being separate but still warm), which defines an important part of therapy goal behaviors.

Points located between the axes within each surface are made up of proportionate amounts of the underlying axes. Content validity for points on the SASB is easy to see by inspection: For example, **PROTECT** is comprised of about equal amounts of **LOVE** and **CONTROL,** while **AFFIRM** is comprised of about equal amounts of **LOVE** and **EMANCIPATE. BLAME** is composed of **CONTROL** and **ATTACK,** while **IGNORE** is made up of **ATTACK** and **EMANCIPATE.** These geometric features for focus-on-other also apply to the second and third surfaces. One of the methods of validating names and placements of points on the model is to obtain content ratings by psychology undergraduates unfamiliar with the model (Benjamin, 2000). The full SASB model (Benjamin, 1979) adds many subdivisions to each quadrant and thereby provides even greater resolution and precision in its interpersonal descriptions.

Interactions can be coded by objective observers using the dimensional ratings method, which, among other things, helps observers develop precise language to describe the quintessence of complex events. Consider the incestually abusing father saying to his 5-year-old daughter: "You are so beautiful, you made me do this." The transaction process is from father (*X*) to daughter (*Y*); codes are made of the initiator of the message (*X*) in relation to the receiver (*Y*). He is focusing on other and giving two discernible messages. "You are so beautiful" is coded focus-on-other, friendly, and acknowledging of a separate self. On Figure 19.1, that coding places this message at **AFFRIM**. "You made me do this" is focus-on-other, unfriendly, and definitely exerts influence. That places it in the region of **BLAME** on Figure 19.1. The sentence has two parts that are inextricably related, and so it is called a complex message. The components of a complex message are joined by a plus, so the final code of the process between father and daughter is **AFFIRM + BLAME**. Complex messaging cannot be identified by questionnaires. They only can be generated by objective observer ratings, usually of videotapes of interactions.

SASB coding also can describe the content of a message separately from its process. Both are important, and both need to be tracked carefully in both practice as well as research. In therapy, for example, there is an active process between therapist and patient, and the content presumably is mostly about narratives in the patient's stories. In the incest example just coded as **AFFIRM + BLAME**, the abusive father's focus is on himself; it is unfriendly toward his daughter; and he speaks of being submissive. His hostile (resentful) submission places the content code in the region of <u>SULK</u> in Figure 19.1. Since the father was actually in control by virtue of size, role, and authority, his claim to have been helpless represents a jarring departure from reality (**IGNORE**). Add the fact that he both affirms and denigrates his daughter when he claims he was helpless when he overwhelmed her, it is no wonder that incest victims so frequently have a shattered sense of self.

## SASB Predictive Principles

Because the SASB model provides a way to describe personality in interactional terms, it can generate hypotheses about causal aspects of developmental experience (or any other important social input) in relation to adult personality. The model also can suggest corrective experiences (treatment implications) for current problem personality patterns; this was detailed in Benjamin, 1996b.

### *Introjection*

This predictive principle (derived directly from Sullivan) specifies that people will treat themselves as they have been treated. It is shown on the model by the relationship between the first and third surfaces (**BOLD** and *ITALICIZED* points at the same locus). For example, an **IGNORED** child will likely *SELF-NEGLECT* (not take care of, protect) him- or herself. A **BLAMED** child likely will engage in extensive *SELF-BLAME*. An **AFFIRMED** client is more likely to learn how to *AFFIRM SELF*. The folk wisdom holds that "children learn what they live." The SASB model provides a way to track that principle. Many studies in different contexts have shown that introjections do correspond, as predicted, to memories of early parenting. Moreover, introject data correlate powerfully with different measures of psychopathology (Benjamin, 1996a; Benjamin, Rothweiler, & Critchfield, 2006). I am working on developing parsimonious ways of expanding the concept of introject that goes beyond turning the other's focus inward on the self and includes all possible aspects of the relationship with the internalized representations (e.g., reacting to the internalization; focusing on internalization).

### *Complementarity*

The SASB model describes natural matches in terms of points that are comprised of the same underlying components (of horizontal and vertical axes) but differ in interpersonal focus (transitive and intransitive). **CONTROL** and SUBMIT are natural complements. So are **PROTECT** and TRUST. These relations between points at the same geometric location, differing only in focus, hold everywhere on the model. The SASB version of the vertical axes was strongly supported by Lorr (1991) and probably is responsible for the fact that evidence in support of complementarity, as defined by the SASB model, is strong, even when adjusting statistically for base rates (Critchfield & Benjamin, 2008; Gurtman, 2001).

### *Opposition*

The SASB model defines natural incompatibilities in terms of opposites that have the same interpersonal focus. Opposite points on the model have opposite values on the affiliation (horizontal) and interdependence (vertical) axes. Using vector notation of the form (Horizontal, Vertical), the 180-degree opposites of **PROTECT** and **IGNORE** have the respective vector values of (+4.5, –4.5) and (–4.5, +4.5); the complements of TRUST and WALL-OFF also are opposite in sign and they have the same vector values and the same attentional focus. *BLAME SELF* and *AFFIRM SELF* are opposites as well. They both describe introjective focus, but their vectors are (–4.5, –4.5) and (+4.5, +4.5).

These relations hold everywhere on the model. The validity of SASB's definitions of opposites is well established by factor-analytic reconstructions of the SASB model (e.g., Benjamin, 1974; Benjamin et al., 2006; Lorr & Strack, 1999). Moreover, SASB assessments do not use negation (*not*, *un-*) to define opposites (in contrast to the IAS-R, which uses many *not* and *un-* prefixes to define opposites).

There has been argument over whether the SASB model is an ellipse (data) or a circle (e.g., Pincus, Newes, Dickinson, & Ruiz, 1998). No arguments have been put forward to explain why IAS advocates take the perfect circle as the correct version. Their items were chosen to create a perfect circle when items are applied by raters to themselves, and results are factor-analyzed. If reconstructions of the IAS model were not a perfect circle, items (eight per model point) were rewritten. SASB items, by contrast, were constructed by dimensional ratings of the items themselves. A symmetric model was generated by this method (one or two or five items per model point, depending on which version was being validated). Then, when raters applied the items to themselves (as distinct from rating the items for content), factor analysis yielded the ellipses. I have suggested that if factor analyses of SASB data of self-descriptions reconstruct an ellipse rather than a circle, perhaps attachment (love–hate axis on the horizontal) carries more variance than interdependence (enmeshment–differentiation on the vertical). From an evolutionary perspective, it is reasonable to postulate that the interpersonal programming of a herd animal would emphasize attachment (horizontal affiliation axis) even more than allocation of space and supplies within and between herds. According to SASB theory, anger is used in service of control or distancing. If the affiliation pole represents keeping the herd together, then greater length in the horizontal axis could suggest that maintaining herd togetherness is more important than allocating space and supplies within and for the herd. Warmth, affiliation, and positivity (represented on the horizontal axis) always show very strong inverse associations with psychopathology, and they virtually always are the first factor to emerge when analyzing measures of social interaction.

### *Antithesis*

Antithetical relations are defined as the opposite of the complement. For example, the opposite of WALL-OFF is TRUST; the complement of TRUST is **PROTECT**. This principle suggests that if a client is WALLED OFF, he or she feels unsafe (not protected), and the treatment implication would be to provide friendly and credible structure to the therapy process. The principle of antithesis seems useful clinically, but it has not been formally tested in research.

## The Predictive Principles Are Consistent with the Developmental Literature

SASB predictive principles are consistent with many findings in the developmental literature, even though the developmental data in the clinic and in SASB questionnaire ratings usually are based on retrospective ratings of childhood by adults. The predictive principles also have been reliably validated in clinical use, as described in *Interpersonal Reconstructive Therapy (IRT): An Integrative, Personality-Based approach to Complex Cases* (Benjamin, 2003/2006). IRT proposes that psychopathology derives from "attachment gone awry," and a sequel to the book includes a chapter that integrates research findings on the epigenetics of attachment-based stress and mechanisms of depression, anxiety and anger in adults. The main principles of IRT are illustrated later in this chapter.

### *Assessment of Perception Can Be More Effective in Predicting Behavior than Objective Observation*

The reliance on self-narratives and self-ratings is sometimes challenged by social psychologists, who place more trust in objective observer ratings. Research that consistently shows that there can be large discrepancies between objective observer ratings and self-ratings usually is interpreted as showing that the self-ratings are invalid. According to IRT theory and practice, however, the rule when trying to predict the behavior of a patient is first to understand how the patient sees things. Assessment begins with input from the patient ("What is going on in your life now?"). The guiding principle is that people act on their perceptions, which may or may not be consistent with an objective observer's opinion. For example, if a paranoid individual hears God tell him or her to kill everybody in church because they are sinners, she or he becomes a real danger. For the clinician, *the client's view* is a better predictor of behavior, not the lack of reality in the client's view. This primacy of perception is not limited to psychotic individuals. In general, from a clinical point of view, Murray's (1938) beta press (perception) is a better predictor of the individual's behavior than is alpha press (objective reality).

### *Assessment of Objective Reality Is Required When Intervening*

Nonetheless, assessment of reality becomes vital when it comes to treatment. One should not try to change behavior without having a consensual view of where things actually are now[4] and without presenting a very concrete explanation of the treatment goals. The mantra of IRT treatment is "Reality is my best friend." Because perception and objective observer ratings have different advantages and disadvantages depending on context, optimal SASB research includes both. Discrepancies often are focal points for determining where and how to intervene in a family system. Assessing everyone's point of view along with observer-rated reality is the best way to plan and implement interventions.

### Validity of the SASB Model

As noted in the previous section, content validity is established by naïve raters' assignments of dimensions to items assessing the model points. Concurrent construct and predictive validity have been generally supported by others' tests of the model using factor analysis, and by using SASB data to compare various clinical groups and measures and obtaining clinically meaningful results (Illustrative reviews appear in Benjamin, 1995; Benjamin et al., 2006; Constantino, 2000).

### SASB Invokes Trait × Situation × State View of Personality

SASB assessments and treatment applications are primarily interactional. They are contextualized to relationship, state, and situation. Experienced clinicians know that patients will behave differently in different situations and states. For example, even severely personality-disordered individuals can be profoundly kind, effective, and generative in certain relationships and states. The SASB seeks to assess those differences and link them to their antecedents in social learning. That information, combined with clear theory, makes it possible, for example, to account for why an extremely competent executive or professional can at times be lethally suicidal or very dysfunctional in his or her relationships with spouse or children.

Situations or relationships that are most often useful for clinical assessment by SASB Intrex (Benjamin, 2000) are the introject at best and worst; a spouse in best and worst states; parents as remembered from ages 5 to 10; and the current person of interest, such as a problem child or a difficult boss. Data are generated via ratings by self (or sometimes by others). The same items[5] are applied to the same person in different states and in different relationships. Figures 19.2 and 19.3, which appear later in this chapter on pp. 360–361, show that these different perspectives do yield differential and informative descriptions. The parallel SASB objective observer coding system yields identical parameters. It is extremely important that observers use the dimensional rating system to describe interactions in terms of SASB; they need to identify focus and location on the love–hate dimension and on the control–submit versus emancipate–separate dimension of whatever is being coded. Material must include specific quotes representing concrete descriptions of behavior (e.g., "Mother locked me in a dark closet several times a week") rather than general evaluative statement (e.g., "Mother did not love me").

### Application of the SASB to Personality Disorders

For clinicians, assessment of personality ideally should have implications for both cause and treatment of personality problems. Their focus is on psychopathology and on problematic personality patterns. Contemporary practice defines personality disorder via the American Psychiatric Association's (1994) fourth edition of the *Diagnostic and Statistical Manual of*

*Mental Disorders* (DSM-IV). Personality disorders are labeled according to lists of symptoms on Axis II of the DSM-IV, while lists of symptoms for clinical syndromes (e.g., depression, anxiety) appear on Axis I.

### *Defining BPD*

The DSM-IV details 10 officially defined personality disorders, one of which is the ubiquitous BPD. An individual can be diagnosed with BPD if he or she has five or more of the following characteristics, identified by clinical interview or by Structured Clinical Interviews for DSM (SCID-II; First, Spitzer, Gibbon, Williams, & Benjamin, 1997).

1. Frantic efforts to avoid real or imagined abandonment.
2. A pattern of instability in the intense interpersonal relationships characterized by alternating between extremes of idealization and evaluation.
3. Identity disturbance: markedly and persistently unstable self image or sense of self.
4. Impulsivity in at least two areas that are potentially self-damaging (e.g., spending, sex, substance abuse, reckless driving, binge eating).
5. Recurrent suicidal behavior, gestures, or threats, or self-defeating behavior.
6. Affective instability due to a marked reactivity of mood.
7. Chronic feelings of emptiness.
8. Inappropriate, intense anger or difficulty controlling anger (e.g., frequent displays of temper, constant anger, recurrent physical fights).
9. Transient, stress-related paranoid ideation or severe dissociative symptoms (American Psychiatric Association, 1994, p. 654).

BPD has been the subject of so much interest because it often involves unrelenting depression accompanied by self-mutilating and suicidal behaviors that are dangerous and very difficult for clinicians to manage. Bender et al. (2001) note:

> Patients with personality disorders had more extensive histories of psychiatric outpatient, inpatient, and psychopharmacologic treatment than patients with major depressive disorder. Compared to the depression group, patients with borderline personality disorder were significantly more likely to have received every type of psychosocial treatment except self-help groups. Patients with borderline personality disorder were also more likely to have used anti-anxiety, antidepressant, and mood stabilizer medications, and those with borderline or schizotypal personality disorder had a greater likelihood of having received antipsychotic medications. Patients with borderline personality disorder had received greater amounts of treatment, except for family/couples therapy and self-help, than the depressed patients and patients with other personality disorders. (p. 295)

Because they require frequent sessions and are likely to need multiple hospitalizations, people with BPD utilize a disproportionate number of health care resources. Their personality patterns lead to extended suffering for themselves and their loved ones, friends, coworkers, and health care providers. Self-mutilation and suicide attempts are the target of most treatment interventions. A number of treatment approaches has been shown empirically to be successful in addressing these high-priority features of BPD. Effectiveness is established according to rules favored by journal editors, granting agencies, training program certifiers, some insurance companies, and others. Those rules provide that a given treatment group must be shown superior to a control condition in randomized control trials (RCTs) before that treatment is considered to be effective. Impressive recent examples of studies that establish efficacy with BPD are best illustrated by Linehan et al. (2006).

### *SASB-Based Interpersonal Translations of BPD*

My analysis of the DSM-IV personality disorders by coding DSM items in terms of SASB dimensions yielded interpersonal descriptions of each of the DSM personality disorders (Benjamin, 1996b). SASB predictive principles and clinical experience were used to link the resulting codes to generate likely developmental histories. My interpersonal translation of BPD (with SASB codes in brackets) follows:

> There is a morbid fear of abandonment [**IGNORE**] and a wish for protective nurturance [**PROTECT**], preferably received by constant physical proximity [TRUST] to the rescuer (lover or caregiver). The baseline position is friendly dependency on a nurturer [TRUST], which becomes hostile control [**BLAME**] if the caregiver or lover fails to deliver [**IGNORE**] enough (and there never is enough). There is a belief that the provider secretly if not overtly likes dependency and neediness [TRUST], and a vicious introject attacks the self [*SELF-ATTACK; SELF-BLAME*] if there are signs of happiness or success [*SELF-AFFIRM*]. (Benjamin, 1996b, p. 117)

The predicted developmental history and links to this interpersonal description appear in my earlier publication (Benjamin, 1996b, 2003). The idea of self-sabotage is at variance with most social psychologist's views of personality. Rather than seeking to thrive and enhance the self, as is normative, individuals with BPD (and, it turns out, most others with severe psychopathology) actively undermine themselves for reasons that are detailed in the IRT book. Naturally, self-sabotaging individuals are difficult to treat and likely to vex clinicians and theorists alike. The phenomenon of self-sabotage is so visible to the observer using SASB to organize interpersonal detail and explore phenomenology that severe mental disorder is better characterized in terms of an autoimmune version of the medical model than in terms of the broken brain model (Benjamin, 2009).

The SASB-based interpersonal descriptors of BPD behaviors seem to compare reasonably to the DSM definition of BPD presented earlier in this chapter. Many clinicians have reported that they find the SASB conceptualization of the personality disorders to be very helpful. I (Benjamin, 1996b) included testable hypotheses about likely interpersonal histories that lead to BPD (and other personality disorder patterns) as well as related treatment suggestions. Clinician and patient reactions also have confirmed the developmental predictions, but much remains to be done to test them as well as the related treatment suggestions. Large *N* research studies using structured interviews and, ultimately, observations and self-ratings from childhood through adulthood, would be ideal.

### *Empirical Tests of SASB Descriptions of BPD*

One research-based check of my interpersonal translation of the DSM descriptions of personality disorders was offered by Klein, Wonderlich, and Crosby (2001). They compared scores on the Wisconsin Personality Disorders Inventory (WISPI)[6] to SASB Intrex ratings of self-concept and examined the correlations between SASB and WISPI scores, controlling for comorbidities on each measure by using partial *r*. They reported: "Although there was some overlap between DSM categories, most were associated with fairly distinct patterns of self-concept" (p. 150). Inspection of their Table 1 (p. 153) shows the significant partial *r* very often corresponded to the predicted features of self concept for the respective disorders. For example, as can be seen in the interpersonal description for BPD, the predicted introject features, based on SASB codes of the DSM description of BPD, are *SELF-AFFIRM*, *SELF BLAME* and *SELF ATTACK*. Subjects scoring higher on the BPD scale from the WISPI endorsed these SASB features to a greater extent than other raters, even after partialing out associations between the SASB measures of introject and the respective scale scores for the remaining 10 personality disorder categories.

Smith (2002) studied 83 psychiatric inpatients and compared their SASB Intrex ratings to the percent of items for the respective categories of DSM personality disorder endorsed during the SCID-II (First et al., 1997). She found modest correlations between the predictions for BPD and the diagnosis based on DSM interviews.

## New Analysis of BPD and SASB Intrex Measures

### *Inpatients' BPD Scores*

Using a database of 136 psychiatric inpatients[7] rating themselves and their loved ones on the SASB Intrex (Long Form), predictions for interpersonal behavior and antecedent developmental factors associated with BPD are explored here. The method is to correlate SASB Intrex ratings of various relationships for each point on Figure 19.1, with the personality disorder scores for BPD derived from each patient's Minnesota Multiphasic Personality Inventory (MMPI-I; the original MMPI) ratings, as determined by Morey, Waugh, and Blashfield (1985). For a sample this size, correlations of about .23 are significant at the .01 two-tailed level. There are correlations involved in Figures 19.2 and 19.3, and because of multiple comparisons, "significance" here is taken only to mark a cutoff point indicating that a trend likely is "present." A Bonferonni standard might be set, but that is vulnerable to arbitrary decisions about how to group results. The level .01 is chosen for discussion rather than .05 to make a minimal adjustment for multiple-comparison error. Replication using other measures of personality disorder, including the DSM itself, is desirable. Ideally, longitudinal predictions that include data from objective observers making prospective ratings, as well as sequential self-descriptions, would test these causal hypotheses about connections between patterns that evolve with loved ones and adult patterns of personality.

### *Patterns of Correlations in the Inpatient Sample*

The top panel of Figure 19.2 shows, as predicted for a BPD introject, that BPD dimensional scores on the MMPI-I, as generated by the Morey et al. (1985) method, are associated with *SELF-BLAME*, *SELF-ATTACK*, *SELF-NEGLECT*, rated for the worst state ($p < .01$). The figure shows that *SELF-EMANCIPATE* also is significant, and that was not predicted. However, it is only one step away from *SELF-NEGLECT* on the model in Figure 19.1. Endorsement of that region does indirectly indicate lack of its opposite, *SELF-CONTROL*, a clinically recognized marker of BPD. Inspection of a focus-on-other, shown in the middle panel of Figure 19.2, shows that BPD scores have higher associations with **BLAME**, **ATTACK**,

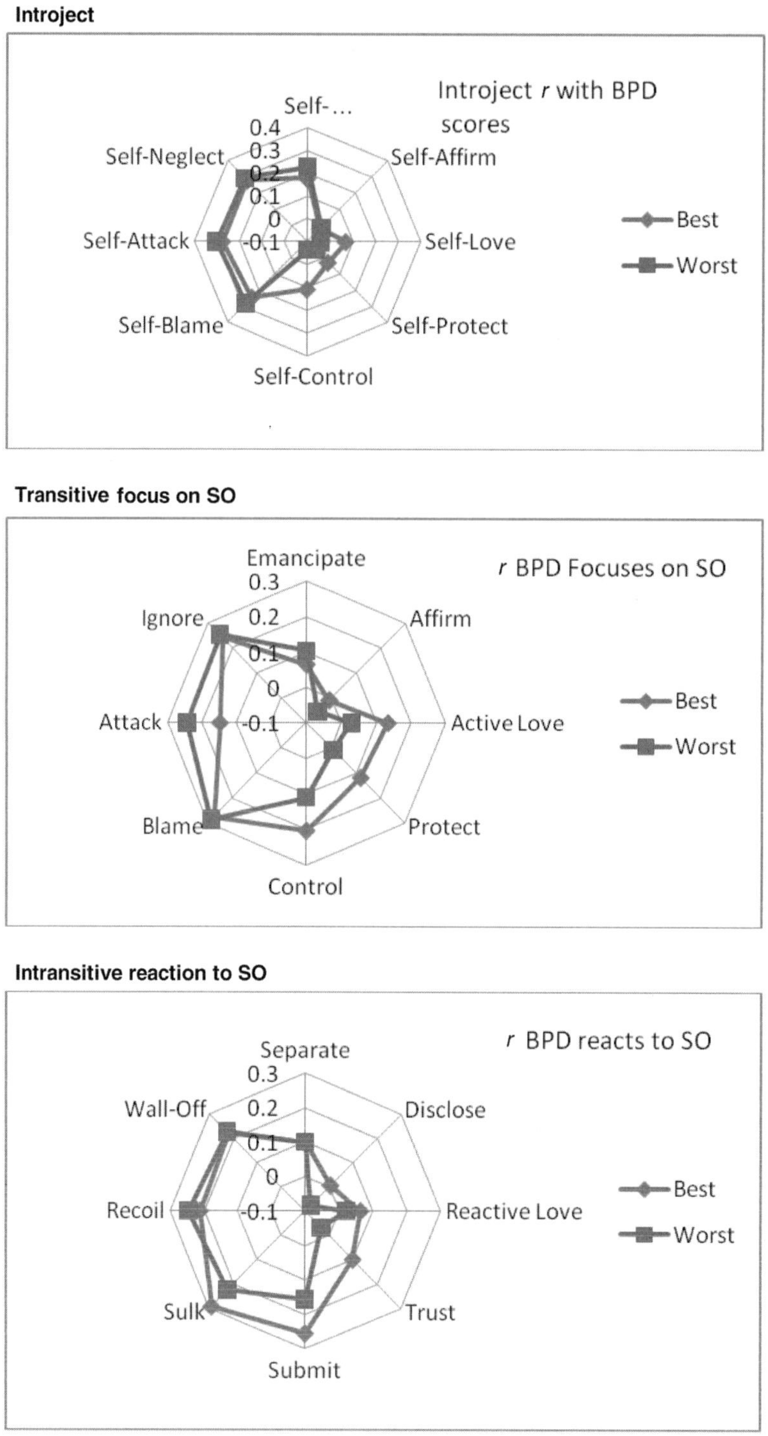


**FIGURE 19.2.** Correlations between BPD scores and SASB Intrex ratings for introject and relations with a significant other person at best and worst. BPD, borderline personality disorder; SO, significant other.

Norms introject

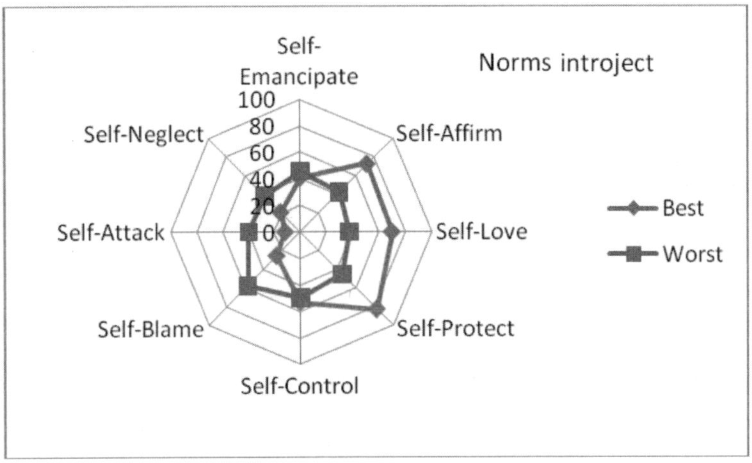


Norms transitive focus on SO

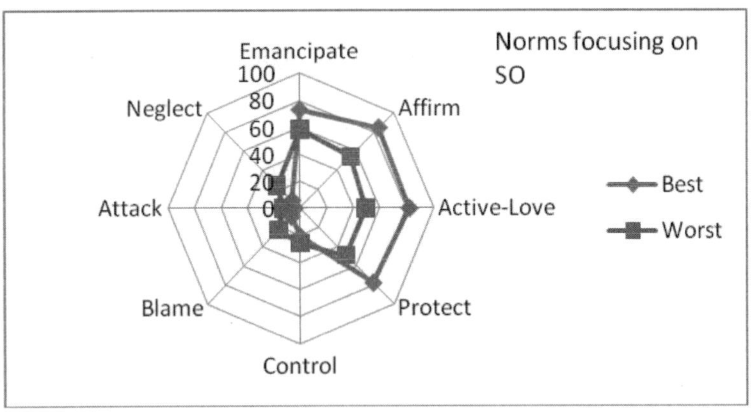


Norms intransitive reaction to SO

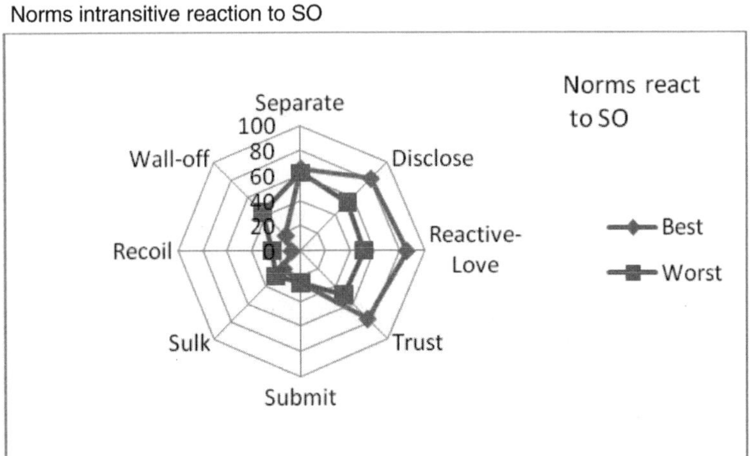


**FIGURE 19.3.** Norms for introject and relations with significant other person at best and worst. SO, significant other.

and **IGNORE** their significant other, especially when in their worst state. In their best state, **CONTROL**, **ACTIVE LOVE**, and **PROTECT** are more salient, but hostile points remain associated with higher BPD scores. Inspection of focus-on-self, shown in the bottom panel of Figure 19.2, marks correlations between BPD scores and hostility at worst; at best, higher correlations can be seen between BPD and tendencies toward submission (SUBMIT) in hostile (SULK) and friendly ways (TRUST).

### *Patterns of Means in a Normal Sample*

The top panel of Figure 19.3 presents mean endorsements for a sample of 133 nonclinical participants rating the same relationships studied in Figure 19.2. Data in Figures 19.2 and 19.3 can be compared in terms of patterns, even though the parameters are different. Figure 19.2 shows correlations between BPD scores and Intrex self-ratings. Figure 19.3 shows levels of endorsement of those same Intrex items by normal volunteers. Comparisons of Figure 19.2 with Figure 19.3 involve the assumption that if BPD scores in the inpatient sample correlated more with a given Intrex parameter (e.g., **BLAME**), while the nonclinical participants do not endorse that parameter very highly, then one could conclude that BPD in the inpatient sample would endorse BLAME more than would nonclinical participants. Unfortunately, the obvious check on this assumption cannot be performed because BPD in the inpatient sample is defined only by Morey et al.'s (1985) scores based on the MMPI-I. One could rank the inpatients on the basis of their BPD score and create an arbitrary cutoff to define a BPD group. Then group means on the SASB scores for the "BPD Group" could be compared to the normal group. However, nonarbitrary guidelines for choosing a proper cutoff point (e.g., median or top quartile?) do not exist. Moreover, since the two samples were gathered under such different conditions, it might be inappropriate to compare them by statistical testing. The present pattern analysis using the entire inpatient sample is chosen as a better way to perform an exploratory analysis of trends in the available data sets.

### *Non-Normative Inpatient Patterns Compared to DSM*

In general, normal subjects tend to rate everything on the attachment side of the SASB model higher than items representing the hostile side of the model. Low endorsement of hostile items is not observed in BPD correlational patterns. On the contrary, Figure 19.2, which shows associations between higher BPD scores on the MMPI and SASB self-ratings, shows that hostile tendencies are more salient for patients having higher scores on the Morey et al. (1985) BPD scale. More specifically, the higher scores on BPD in the inpatient sample were likely to be associated with more *SELF-NEGLECT*, *SELF-ATTACK*, and *SELF-BLAME*. Salience of *SELF-NEGLECT* is consistent with DSM item 4—"impulsivity in at least two areas that are potentially self-damaging (e.g., spending, sex, substance abuse, reckless driving, binge eating)"—and DSM item 7—"chronic feelings of emptiness" (p. 654). *SELF-ATTACK* is consistent with DSM item 5: "recurrent suicidal behavior, gestures, or threats, or self-mutilating behavior" (p. 654). *SELF-BLAME* also is consistent with DSM item 5. These results are also consistent with the Klein et al. (2001) findings cited above.

Inspection of analyses of self-ratings of focus on significant other (SO), in the middle panel of Figure 19.2, shows that higher BPD scores are associated with **BLAME**, **ATTACK**, and **IGNORE** of their SO, especially at worst. This is consistent with DSM item 8: "inappropriate, intense anger or difficulty controlling anger (e.g., frequent displays of temper, constant anger, recurrent physical fights)" (p. 654). Anger also is suggested by hostile focus-on-self in reaction to SO trends by individuals scoring higher on the BPD scale are shown at the bottom of Figure 19.2. Not predicted, but of clinical interest, is the tendency for higher BPD self-descriptive scores to be associated with more submission (SUBMIT) in both hostile (SULK) and friendly ways (TRUST).

In addition to the implied endorsements of submissiveness when at best for those scoring higher on BPD, there are other interesting surprises in this SASB dataset. For example, there were noteworthy (> .23) correlations between participants' BPD personality scores and participants' ratings of themselves as engaging in **BLAME**, **ATTACK**, and **NEGLECT** of mothers and fathers during childhood, as well as vice versa. In other words, higher participants' BPD scores are associated with (in participants' view) hostility toward, and control of, parents *and* of having been subjected to more hostility and control from parents. Submission also went both ways. Seeing the association between BPD scores and the various forms of hostile enmeshment (attack, control, and submit by everyone toward everyone) helps makes it clear why health care providers have such difficulty working with this population. Health care providers are not accustomed to being attacked, controlled, or expected to submit (at least not while in their professional roles).

It is important to know that the ratings of various versions of hostility delineated by the left-hand side of the SASB model are not unique to individuals with BPD tendencies. Other personality disorders, and for that matter, people scoring high on measures of symptoms on Axis I, such as anxiety and depression, likewise score high on hostility—the hostility, however, appears in different places on the vertical axis and/or focus dimension. Some are hostile and withdrawn; some are hostile and enmeshed; some attack others; some attack themselves. Some do all the above. If one sees hostility as the opposite of attachment, as suggested by the geometry of SASB and other interpersonal models, then hostility is a marker of disrupted attachment. According to IRT, disrupted attachment is the basis of much psychopathology, not just BPD. The general association between hostility and psychopathology may mean that, rather than speak of categories of personality disorder, an emphasis on variation within symptom clusters (e.g., anxiety, depression, anger) in relation to interpersonal variation in expression of hostility might prove useful in the upcoming DSM-V. At least one group of influential writers (Kupfer, First, & Reiger, 2002) has suggested that categories of the DSM (Axes I and II) be replaced by a study of groups of similar symptoms as defined by their mechanisms.

## INTERPERSONAL RECONSTRUCTIVE THERAPY

Interpersonal reconstructive therapy (IRT; Benjamin, 2003/2006) emerged from decades of research and clinical observations guided by SASB. By clearly and consistently attending to patterns in relationships in a sharply focused and reliable manner (i.e., by identifying interactants, focus, position on the love–hate and the enmeshment–differentiation dimensions), it became apparent that the predictive principles hold with simplicity and generality. An IRT case formulation for an individual with BPD is presented and a proposed change in the paradigm (autoimmune disease) for understanding cause and treatment intervention is described.

## IRT Case Formulation for an Individual with BPD

A brief description of a clinical case illustrates IRT theory about connections between early social learning and problem personality patterns and associated symptoms. Implications for psychosocial treatment are sketched.

### *Rules for IRT Case Formulation*

Presenting symptoms are linked via "copy process" to problem patterns that evolved in relation to loved ones. These evolved from the SASB predictive principles. The main three copy processes are (1) *identification* (be like him or her), (2) *recapitulation* (act as if he or she were still present and in control), and (3) *introjection* (treat yourself as you were treated). When copy processes link to problem patterns (e.g., suicidality), they are called Red (Regressive Loyalist). Normal patterns are Green (Growth Collaborator) and are defined by SASB theory and data as composed of a baseline of friendliness, moderate enmeshment, moderate differentiation, and balance of focus.[8] If the presenting problems are highlighted, and the patient is asked to track his or her history, "key figures" will naturally emerge. Copy processes are maintained by loyalty to key (attachment) figures. This loyalty is supported by hopes and wishes that if the rules are followed well enough, love, protection, and affirmation will follow. Those wishes are called Gifts of Love (GOL).

Copy processes and GOLs are detailed and illustrated in the case that follows. This is a one-time case consultation that illustrates the IRT case formulation method. Sometimes we have resources to follow-up with treatment, but that was not possible for many.

### *Presentation at the Hospital*

Mary is a 30-year-old married mother (one daughter) with a long history of depression. She reports that she has tried "every medication" and that nothing works. Her husband had urged her to try psychotherapy, but her mother was opposed to the idea, so she never tried it. She came to the hospital with dozens of significant razor cuts on her chest and abdomen and then overdosed on pain killers. Her first suicide attempt was at the age of 11. Since then, she has found relief by cutting herself about twice a month every year until the present hospitalization. She explains that she goes numb and feels out of her body and that "cutting brings me back to myself." For many years, she had requisite symptoms for the diagnosis of major depressive disorder. When referred for the IRT consultation, in addition to major depression, she had been diagnosed with social anxiety disorder, chronic fatigue syndrome, and migraine headaches. Axis II diagnosis was deferred and was one of the reasons for the consultation. She has had several surgeries. My consultative interview supported the Axis II (personality disorder) labels of obsessive–compulsive personality disorder (OCD-PD) and avoidant personality disorder. She also met criteria for BPD. During the interview, Mary explained that she had been fired from her job for frequent absences "due to depression," but upon detailed inquiry, it became clear she had a recently increased Herculean work schedule. Because she was depressed, her husband had taken over many household duties, and Mary had concluded that her husband and daughter would be better off if she were dead. Shortly before hospitalization, a neighbor verbally abused her, calling her stupid. In addition, her abusive mother wanted to move in, declaring that she was owed this for raising the patient. Her mother has a history of depression and her father of alcoholism. Her brother was addicted to street drugs.

### *Key Figure: Mother*

Mary reports that she was "never wanted." Her mother declares that Mary's life is a punishment for her and that she told Mary that she was conceived to become a playmate for her older brother. Unfortunately, the brother never liked Mary, and so the mother did not like her either. When the patient was 4, she was hurt in a playground accident and required some special care for 2 years. Mary's mother called her stupid for having the accident and complained about the burden of having to take care of her, by, for example, getting a baby sitter. Over the years, unlike her older brother, who was regarded as special, Mary was saddled with many chores such as cleaning the house, mowing the lawn, weeding the garden, and making dinner. She often was yelled at and called "stupid, a dumb bitch, no good, a horrible person." She was beaten with a leather belt for not getting home on time, upsetting her brother, or not doing what she was supposed to do. Crying was met with more beating ("I will give you something to cry about"). Mary responded: "I tried to do my jobs very well. I still do. I am so meticulous, I don't do it all. I make it so perfect, I don't finish." Because of these attitudes and behaviors, Mary also met the criteria for OCD-PD.

Copy processes linking Mary's mother to her symptoms included *introjection* (Mary now feels that she is a burden to her husband and daughter, and that she is stupid, lazy, and should not be around) and *recapitulation* (Mary is shy, fears humiliation, is also a perfectionistic who works very hard). Axis I symptoms are linked to personality patterns by "parallelism" logic (Benjamin, 2003/2006). For example, depression is likely to accompany feelings of being helpless and without recourse, habitual self-criticism, and a sense of loss. Anxiety is likely to be triggered by similar situations, but with a response disposition to cope rather than to give up. It is easy to see why Mary might feel these ways.

### *Key Figure: Older Brother*

Mary reports that her brother pushed her down the stairs when she started to walk and claims that her brother stole from her aunt, her mother, and Mary herself. But according to her mother, the brother could do no wrong. When Mary and her brother were home alone, the brother chased her with knives. Mary said: "I do not know what I did that made him so mad." The patient and sometimes the neighbors telephoned her mother at work for help in dealing with the attacking brother. On the day of her first suicide attempt, Mary's mother said that she had been threatened with loss of her job because of another distress call. Mary concluded: "I had better not be here." She took a dull knife and cut herself. She received no psychiatric attention and no hospitalization.

## Presenting Problems in Personality Derive Directly from Patterns with Earlier Loved Ones

Mary recognized that she was more concerned with her childhood memories (i.e., representations of her mother and brother) than she was with her own life and current family. She understood that when she overwhelmed herself by complying with unreasonable demands, attacked herself as stupid, lazy, etc., she was repeating her mother's words and implementing her mother's rules and values. When she attacks herself with blades, she is replicating her brother's recurrent attacks with knives. When she calls herself a burden and says that she should not exist, she is repeating her mother's very words. Mary agreed with the interviewer's summary of her experience: "It is as if she possesses you" and "You want to do something, anything, to please her, make her love you." This was a summary of the GOL that supported the destructive copy processes. But she then puzzled over why she still let mother affect her in this way. Providing the answer herself, she said: "It is hard to let go of that dream that mother will finally love me." This was confirmation that the GOL was operating to support her self-sabotage.

Mary's Red (Regressive Loyalist) personality derived from her devotion to the destructive patterns, rules, and values just described. Her Green (Growth Collaborator) personality was the highly functional aspect that had been a reliable and much valued worker, wife, and mother. The Green "crashed and burned" with exhaustion and the reactivation of old states when the neighbor called her "stupid" and by her mother's recent intrusive attempts to live with her. The conflict between Red and Green can be operationalized by separate ratings on the SASB Intrex of her views of herself and others in the two states. (Patients willingly do this in our clinic protocol.)

### Treatment Implications Specific to Presenting Problems

Treatment involves containing and reducing the Red states (patterns associated with the rules and values of the Regressive Loyalist representations), and enhancing the Green states (patterns associated with rules and values of the Growth Collaborator representations that stem from constructive aspect of parents, siblings, teachers, grandparents, and other important persons). After understanding that her reluctance to try psychotherapy was a derivative of her mother's wish that she not do so and that treatment would be good for her "Green self," Mary became willing to do so. Her belief that she must not accept affirmation and love from her husband and daughter had not been resolved by the cognitive-behavioral treatment offered by the hospital staff before the IRT consultation. Logic could not override loyalty to Mother's rules and values for Mary (her GOLs). The key to successful treatment would lie in helping her make different decisions about the perceived Red rules. Mary was very responsive to the remark, "When you try to kill yourself, you are making your mother's and brother's rules and values more important than your relationship with your husband and daughter." Although she agreed, she found this thought to be very offensive. Emotional as well as cognitive understanding of this dynamic could decrease the likelihood that she would turn to suicide again.

### Preliminary Data on Effectiveness of IRT

In our IRT clinic at the University of Utah Neuropsychiatric Institute, Ken Critchfield and I are gathering data from such severely disordered patients with personality disorders as they progress through treatment. We are slowly cumulating self-ratings and objective observer ratings of clinical interviews that can be used to test predictions as well as the effectiveness of the IRT treatment model.

Significant personality change requires longer outpatient treatment that continues through five steps in IRT: (1) collaborate to achieve change, (2) learn about patterns and where they came from; (3) block problem patterns, (4) engage the will to change, and (5) learn new patterns. This sounds simple, but engaging a patient's will to change is very difficult. Mary explained why—that it is hard to give up the dream of affirmation from her mother (and other figures associated with Red patterns). It is at least as hard as giving up a chemical addiction. But giving it up and grieving all the losses are vital to the ability to become open to learning new, healthier patterns. Additional detail appears in past publications (Benjamin, 2003, 2006, 2009).

Pre–post data show that for a sample of over 40 patients, IRT consultation followed by a brief inpatient therapy yielded significant reductions in suicide attempts and rehospitalization days for the year following the hospitalization during which the consultation occurred, compared to the year preceding it (Critchfield, Benjamin, Hawley, & Dillinger, 2006). Pre–post comparisons are necessarily compromised by lack of a control comparison. It is noteworthy that these individuals are referred to us because of treatment resistance manifest by frequent rehospitalizations; this could mean that our sample is less likely than average to improve after any given hospitalization. If so, the pre–post comparisons for this group are more remarkable than they would be for an unselected group of hospitalized patients.

We regard our data on associations between outcome and high adherence to critical aspects of the IRT treatment model (using a reliable and unusually specific adherence scale) to be the strongest test of the IRT concepts and methods. The outpatient treatments that follow hospitalization of these difficult cases are lengthy. Usually they last two or more years. Given the length of the treatment and the time that it takes to train graduate student therapists to become skilled in IRT, our sample is very small. Results so far on seven cases show a very strong, highly significant linear association between focus on a key aspect of the IRT treatment model (GOL) and symptom reduction (Davis, Critchfield, MacKenzie, & Benjamin, 2008). The sample is small, but the results are dramatically clear and wholly consistent with supervisory impressions.

## Paradigm Shift

Kupfer et al. (2002) noted that a simple model of psychiatric disease that defines categories of disorder deriving from genetically based deficits has not been supported by data. They call for paradigm shift. I suggest (Benjamin, 2009) that if the copy process, supported by attachment-based Gifts of Love, is valid in the way just illustrated for Mary, then psychiatric disease might better be modeled by an autoimmune version of medical disease. Clinical data show that the Red aspects of personality lead to self-sabotage, whereas feeling happy and doing well is experienced as an "internal crime." This, of course, means the "disorder" is intractable. Change can follow only if people are helped to give up the dream of being affirmed by loved ones for complying with their perceived maladaptive rules and values (GOL). After being freed from the ideology that they deserve to be punished or suffer or must be the world's "greatest," and so on, these individuals become less "allergic" to becoming realistically happy, balanced, and functional. When they have permission to thrive, ordinary principles of learning can prevail and instructive therapies can become truly effective. Such a provocative theory regarding developmental contributions to problem personality patterns can be tested by subjective and objective measures of interactive patterns and internalized representations of loved ones along with measures of parallel psychiatric symptoms. SASB measures, organized by IRT theory, offer one attempt to develop this line of thinking that was marked so well by Sullivan (1953).

## SUMMARY AND METHODOLOGICAL SUGGESTIONS FOR CLINICALLY RELEVANT ASSESSMENT OF PERSONALITY

After touching on the IPC literature and trait profiles developed via factor analysis, the discussion focused in more detail on the DSM definition of BPD, as translated into interpersonal terms by my SASB codes of DSM-III-R items. Although the IPC and NEO-5 approaches are neat methodologically, they do not have the causal or treatment implications that are so important to clinicians. Application of SASB to clinical material and in research study has resulted in the development of IRT, an attachment-based theory of psychopathology that is accompanied by very specific motivational as well as instructional treatment implications. IRT was illustrated by the case of a woman who had been diagnosed with BPD, followed by an attachment-based alternative diagnosis and interpretation of the patient's personality disorder. Whether or not the reader is interested in SASB or IRT, the discussion of concerns here is intended to raise methodological issues that should be addressed regardless of the content of the measures if social psychological concepts are to be relevant to clinicians who work with severely disordered individuals. The following principles provide a framework for conducting clinically relevant social psychological research:

1. Measure personality in interactive terms as well as in terms of baseline traits. At a minimum, interaction can be considered by including views of others as well as views of self.
2. Recognize that assessment from the perspective of the client is useful in understanding deviant behavior because, as Murray emphasized in his definition of beta press, perception drives behavior. Of course, assessment by objective observers is relevant too, especially when planning treatment interventions.
3. Assess persons in different states and situations to account for the fact that people, whether in the region of normal or abnormal interpersonal patterns, are not the same in different roles (e.g., parent, child; lover, friend; boss, employee; teacher, student; health and sickness). Trait theory is not consistent with this suggestion.
4. Offer specific testable, refutable, theory that helps us to identify and understand specific connections between social learning and patterns of personality.
5. If social psychologists wish to contribute to treatment suggestions that derive from assessment, then the suggestions much go beyond tautological formulations that amount to recommending that identified problems be replaced. Changing personality is like changing an addiction; some kind of functional analysis is needed to lead to changes in motivation. For example, telling someone to stop being so self-critical or critical of others is about as likely to be successful as telling someone to stop using drugs. Personality change is more likely if the assessment and treatment help the individual access compelling reasons to give up problem habits and replace them with constructive ones. (See also, Kross, Mischel, & Shoda, Chapter 20, and Shadel, Chapter 18, this volume.)

## NOTES

1. Hoffman, Buteau, and Fruzzetti (2007) used the NEO to assess individuals with BPD and their families. The findings of greatest relevance to BPD are: "Patients and family members agree that patients were high on N(neuroticism), average on E (extroversion) and O (openness) and low on A (Agreeableness) and C (conscientiousness)" (p. 204). They were above the 50th percentile on all facets of the Neuroticism factor: vulnerability, impulsiveness, self-consciousness, depression, hostility, and anxiety. Clinicians have not been very receptive to diagnosis based on factor-analytic profiles that have been proposed for use in the DSM-V so far, mainly because it is not clear how such profiles would be used.
2. The SASB model appears in a diamond shape, and yet the discussions here and elsewhere refer to it as a "circle." The difference, of course, is that the diamond shape represents positions on the underling axes as simple numbers (ordinary geometry), whereas circles are plotted in terms of squares of those underlying components. That tradition of circles stems from the theory of factor analysis, which, for convenience uses squares to avoid having to track sign. Benjamin (1974) prefers the diamond shape because it marks the axes as distinct "primitive basics," more intense and qualitatively different from all other points. By contrast, circles imply arbitrary choices in axial definitions. Nonetheless, Benjamin uses factor analysis in validity tests because the technology for that is available, and the differences are functionally unimportant when testing structure and predictive principles in terms of percent of variance accounted for and statistical significance.
3. Since 1974, I (Benjamin, 1974) have maintained that the SASB model might be represented as a Riemann surface, and if focus is redefined as a continuous variable, the various present surfaces might be represented by different coils. Along with considering that, I have recently explored the possibility of using projective geometry to link full "interpersonal" codes of internalized representations (family in the head) to objective codes of current interactions. Much work remains to finish exploring that approach and to establish whether it can be done reliably, with good fits between data and model.
4. Reality is defined as the consensual view of normal individuals. SASB theory and data provide a clear standard for defining normal. This is discussed in a later section on IRT.
5. There are three forms of the questionnaires: short, medium, and long. They differ in number of items and in the degree of resolution of the space covered on the model. For example, the short-form item for the region signifying **CONTROL** is: "To keep things in good order, *X* takes charge of everything and makes *Y* follow *X*'s rules." The medium form adds a second item: "To make sure things turn out right, *X* tells *Y* exactly what to do and how to do it." The medium and short forms are written at the sixth-grade level of reading skill. The long form has five items for the region of **CONTROL**. It starts on the controlling edge of **PROTECT**, where there are friendlier versions of control, moves through neutral control, and ends with hostile control just short of **BLAME**. The long-form items, from the friendliest version through neutral control to the most hostile version of control, are: "For *O*'s own good, *S* checks on and reminds *O* of what to do." "For *O*'s own good, *S* tells *O* exactly what to do, be, think." "*S* controls *O* in a matter-of-fact way." "*S* takes charge of everything." "*S* makes *O* follow *S*'s rules and ideas of what is right and proper." "*S* butts in and takes over. *S* blocks and restricts *O*."
6. The WISPI provides 2 items per DSM item for each personality disorder. They are written from a SASB-based interpersonal perspective of the rater. Diagnosis by WISPI corresponds quite well to diagnosis by the SCID-II (Smith, Klein, & Benjamin, 2003).
7. Supported by Grant No. MH-33604 from the National Institute of Mental Health. This is one of many publications by me and by others independently using this database.
8. This is the region between about 1:30 to 4:30 o'clock on Figure 19.1. Those points correlate inversely with psychopathology, and they are endorsed positively by normal populations.

## REFERENCES

American Psychiatric Association. (1994). *Diagnostic and statistical manual of mental disorders* (4th ed.). Washington, DC: Author.

Bender, D. S., Dolan, R. T., Skodol, A. E., Sanislow, C. A., Dyck, I. R., McGlashan, T. H., et al. (2001). Treatment utilization by patients with personality disorders. *American Journal of Psychiatry, 158*, 295–302.

Benjamin, L. S. (1974). Structural analysis of social behavior (SASB). *Psychological Review, 81*, 392–425.

Benjamin, L. S. (1979). Structural analysis of differentiation failure. *Psychiatry: Journal for the Study of Interpersonal Processes, 42*, 1–23.

Benjamin, L. S. (1987). Use of the SASB dimensional model to develop treatment plans for personality disorders, I: Narcissism. *Journal of Personality Disorders, 1*, 43–70.

Benjamin, L. S. (1996a). Introduction to the special section on structural analysis of social behavior (SASB). *Journal of Consulting and Clinical Psychology, 64*, 1203–1212.

Benjamin, L. S. (1996b). *Interpersonal diagnosis and treatment of personality disorders* (2nd ed.). New York: Guilford Press.

Benjamin, L. S. (2000). *SASB Intrex user's manual.* Salt Lake City: University of Utah.

Benjamin, L. S. (2003). *Interpersonal reconstructive therapy: Promoting change in nonresponders.* New York: Guilford Press. (Paperback edition, 2006, with subtitle: *An integrative, personality-based treatment for complex cases*)

Benjamin, L. S. (2008). What is functional about functional autonomy? *Journal of Personality Assessment, 90*(5), 412–420.

Benjamin, L. S. (2009). *Interpersonal reconstructive therapy for anger, anxiety and depression.* Manuscript in preparation.

Benjamin, L. S., Rothweiler, J. R., & Critchfield, K. L. (2006). Use of structural analysis of social behavior as an assessment tool. *Annual Review of Clinical Psychology, 2*, 83–109.

Constantino, M. J. (2000). Interpersonal process in psychotherapy through the lens of the structural analysis of social behavior. *Applied and Preventive Psychology: Current Scientific Perspectives, 9*, 153–172.

Costa, P. T., Jr., & McCrae, R. R. (1992). Normal personality assessment in clinical practice: The NEO Personality Inventory. *Psychological Assessment, 4*, 5–13.

Critchfield, K. L., & Benjamin, L. S. (2008). Internalized representations of early interpersonal experience and adult relationships: A test of copy process theory in clinical and nonclinical populations. *Psychiatry: Interpersonal and Biological Processes, 71*, 71–92.

Critchfield, K. L., Benjamin, L. S., Hawley, N., & Dillinger, R. (2006, June). *Attempted replication of effectiveness for interpersonal reconstructive therapy to reduce hospitalizations and suicide attempts in "nonresponder" populations.* Paper presented at the 38th annual meeting of the International Society of Psychotherapy Research, Edinburgh, Scotland.

Davis, M. J., Critchfield, K. L., MacKenzie, J., & Benjamin, L. S. (2008, June). *Conceptualizing and illustrating stages of change in interpersonal reconstructive therapy (IRT).* Paper presented at the 39th annual meeting of the International Society of Psychotherapy Research, Barcelona, Spain.

First, M. B., Spitzer, R. L., Gibbon, M., Williams, J. B. W., & Benjamin, L. S. (1997). *Structured clinical interview for DSM-IV Axis II personality disorders (SCID-II).* Washington, DC: American Psychiatric Association.

Freedman, M. B., Leary, T. F., Ossorio, A. G., & Coffey, H. S. (1951). The interpersonal dimensions of personality. *Journal of Personality, 20*, 143–161.

Greenberg, J. R., & Mitchell, S. (1983). *Object relations in psychoanalytic theory.* Cambridge, MA: Harvard University Press.

Gurtman, M. (1996). Interpersonal problems and the psychotherapy context: The construct validity of the Inventory of Interpersonal Problems. *Psychological Assessment, 8*, 241–255.

Gurtman, M. (2001). Interpersonal complementarity: Integrating interpersonal measurement with interpersonal models. *Journal of Counseling Psychology*, *48*, 97–110.

Hoffman, P. D., Buteau, E., & Fruzzetti, A. E. (2007). Borderline personality disorder: NEO-Personality ratings of patients and their family members. *International Journal of Social Psychiatry*, *53*, 204–215.

Horowitz, L. M. (1988). Inventory of Interpersonal Problems: Psychometric properties and clinical applications. *Journal of Clinical and Consulting Psychology*, *56*, 885–892.

Klein, M. H., Wonderlich, S. A., & Crosby, R. (2001). Self-concept correlates of the personality disorders. *Journal of Personality Disorders*, *15*, 150–156.

Kupfer, D. J., First, M., & Reiger, D. (2002). *A research agenda for DSM-V*. Washington, DC: American Psychiatric Press.

Leary, T. (1957). *Interpersonal diagnosis of personality: A functional theory and methodology for personality evaluation*. New York: Ronald Press.

Linehan, M. M., Comtois, K. A., Murray, A. M., Brown, M. Z., Gallop, R. J., Heard, H. L., et al. (2006). Two-year randomized controlled trial and follow up of dialectical behavioral therapy versus therapy by experts for suicidal behavior and borderline personality disorder. *Archives of General Psychiatry*, *63*, 756–766.

Lorr, M. (1991). A redefinition of dominance. *Personality and Individual Differences*, *12*, 877–979.

Lorr, M., & Strack, S. (1999). A study of Benjamin's eight facet structural analysis of social behavior (SASB) model. *Journal of Clinical Psychology*, *55*, 207–215.

Morey, L. C., Waugh, M. H., & Blashfield, R. K. (1985). MMPI scales for DSM-IIII personality disorders: Their derivation and correlates. *Journal of Personality Assessment*, *49*, 245–251.

Murray, H. A. (1938). *Explorations in personality*. New York: Oxford University Press.

O'Connor, B. P., & Dyce, J. A. (1998). A test of models of personality disorder configuration. *Journal of Abnormal Psychology*, *107*, 3–16.

Pincus, A. L., Newes, S. L., Dickinson, K. A., & Ruiz, M. A. (1998). A comparison of three indexes to assess the dimensions of structural analysis of social behavior. *Journal of Personality Assessment*, *70*, 145–170.

Schaefer, E. S. (1965). Configurational analysis of children's reports of parent behavior. *Journal of Consulting Psychology*, *29*, 552–557.

Sim, J. P., & Romney, D. M. (1990). The relationship between a circumplex model of interpersonal behavior and personality disorders. *Journal of Personality Disorders*, *4*, 329–341.

Smith, T. L. (2002). *Specific psychosocial perceptions and specific symptoms of personality and other psychiatric symptoms*. PhD dissertation, University of Utah, Salt Lake City.

Smith, T. L., Klein, M. H., & Benjamin, L. S. (2003). Validation of the Wisconsin Personality Disorders Inventory–IV with the SCID-II. *Journal of Personality Disorders*, *17*, 173–187.

Sullivan, H. S. (1953). *The interpersonal theory of psychiatry*. New York: Norton.

Sullivan, H. S. (1963). *Schizophrenia as a human process*. With introduction and commentary by Helen Swick Perry. New York: Norton.

Wiggins, J. S. (1982). Circumplex models of interpersonal behavior in clinical psychology. In P. C. Kendall & J. N. Butcher (Eds.), *Handbook of research methods in clinical psychology* (pp. 183–221). New York: Wiley.

Wiggins, J. S., Trapnell, P., & Phillips, N. (1988). Psychometric and geometric characteristics of the Revised Interpersonal Adjective Scales (IAS-R). *Multivariate Behavioral Research*, *23*, 517–530.

# PART IV

# SOCIAL PSYCHOLOGY OF BEHAVIORAL CHANGE AND CLINICAL INTERACTIONS

# 20 Enabling Self-Control

## *A Cognitive–Affective Processing System Approach to Problematic Behavior*

Ethan Kross
Walter Mischel
Yuichi Shoda

For four decades (1925–1964) social/personality and clinical psychologists reported their most novel findings in the *Journal of Abnormal and Social Psychology* (*JASP*). The mission of the journal was to publish work that illuminated "basic" and "fundamental" knowledge concerning the "pathology, dynamics and development of personality or individual behavior" (1964, p. 591). It thus reflected the zeitgeist of the time—that people's experiences and behaviors, whether normal or abnormal, were the product of a common set of underlying processes, and that knowledge of such basic processes could shed light on people's cognitive and affective reactions.

In 1965, *JASP* split into two separate publications. Research focusing on the basic processes underlying normal human behavior and group interactions went to what became the *Journal of Personality and Social Psychology*, whereas work examining the processes underlying dysfunctional behavior went to the *Journal of Abnormal Psychology*. For this and many other reasons, cross talk between the two areas slowed and the belief that both areas could be profitably integrated eroded. Nevertheless, many clinical psychologists, especially those working within cognitive and behavioral therapy frameworks, remained committed to basing their practice choices on relevant research findings and theoretical advances (e.g., Linehan, 1993; Shadel, 2004). To facilitate that goal, it is encouraging to see a volume that seeks to embrace the original mission of *JASP*, providing a capsule for examining how current social and personality psychology can contribute to advances in clinical psychology. For us, the key questions to address in such a volume are: How does the mind generate important individual differences in diverse types of problematic behaviors of clinical relevance? And how can people be helped to enhance their ability to exert self-control when they sorely need to do so? (See Maddux, Chapter 22, this volume, for more information on the history of the social–clinical interface.)

We begin with the assumption that in order to make sense of the psychological processes that underlie problematic behaviors and enable self-control, it is first necessary to understand how they operate within the larger model of how personality is organized. Over the last 40 years, this conception has undergone dramatic change, with substantial implications for the assessment and treatment of problematic behaviors. For centuries, in a tradition dating to the ancient Greeks and their Big Four humors of personality, trait-dispositional models assumed that personality was to be found in a person's consistent behavior across diverse situations. For example, the person who is high in neuroticism should be more neurotic than most people in many different kinds of situations (home, school, with boss, with friends). Challenging these convictions, Mischel's 1968 monograph, *Personality and Assessment*, showed that rigorous study after study failed to support these classic assumptions. Instead, the findings revealed that the aggressive child at home may be less aggressive than most when in school; the man exceptionally hostile when rejected in love may be unusually tolerant about criticism of his work; the one who shakes with anxiety in the doctor's office may be a calm mountain climber; and the business entrepreneur may take few social risks.

These discrepancies between what theories and intuition predicted and what was actually observed were glaring, creating a paradigm crisis for personality psychology. In the following decades, new research discoveries have enabled a reconceptualization of the structure and organization of personality, its links to situations, and the consistencies and variability that characterize the individual. This model, and the findings that led to it, speak directly to many of the diagnostic and treatment challenges faced in clinical psychology and psychiatry. We begin by describing this reconceptualization and the model to which it has led, called the Cognitive–Affective Processing System (CAPS; Mischel & Shoda, 1995, 1998; Mischel, 2004a). Drawing from research on self-regulation in both children and adults, we then discuss how this model can shed light on the psychological processes that underlie various forms of problematic behaviors, focusing specifically on the critical role that "hot" and "cool" mental representations play in self-control. We conclude by discussing how a CAPS approach can be readily integrated into clinical treatment and assessment.

## THE CAPS

The CAPS was developed to take account of findings about two different types of consistency in the behavior of individuals across situations and over time. Each type has its distinctive uses, advantages, and limitations.

- *Type 1: Average overall levels of behavior tendencies.* The first or "classic" form of consistency is seen in the overall average differences in the levels of typical behavior of different kinds (e.g., aggressiveness, sociability, neuroticism) that may characterize the individual. The trait level of analysis captures these by aggregating ratings of what the individual seems like on the whole, as when people are described on the Big Five, on dimensions such as "conscientiousness" and "agreeableness" (e.g., Goldberg, 1993; John, 1990; McCrae & Costa,

1990). While consistency across diverse situations is not zero, it accounts for only a small percent of the variance in actual behavior in different types of situations (e.g., Mischel & Peake, 1982).

• *Type 2: If ... then ... (situation–behavior) signatures.* These consistencies are seen in patterns of stable links between types of situations and types of characteristic behavior. Such patterns have been demonstrated in the signatures of the aggressive behavior and withdrawn behavior characterizing different individuals (Shoda, Mischel, & Wright, 1993b, 1994), and in extensive related research (e.g., Borkenau, Riemann, Spinath, & Angleitner, 2006; Fournier, Moskowitz, & Zuroff, 2008; Moskowitz, Suh, & Desaulniers, 1994).

## Uses of the Two Types of Consistency

Is it more useful to try to infer broad traits or situation-specific *if ... then ...* behavioral signatures of personality? The answer, of course, always depends on the particular purpose. Inferences about global traits have limited value for the practical prediction of a person's future behavior in specific situations or for the design of specific psychological treatment programs to help facilitate constructive change. But broad trait ratings have many other uses. Indeed, they have value for everyday inferences about what other people seem like on the whole. With people we know well and who are important to us, and surely in clinical practice, one wants to understand "what makes them tick." Therefore, one needs to understand each person's goals, motivations, and feelings in order to make sense of the *if ... then ...* patterns—the personality signatures—that characterize him or her (Chen-Idson & Mischel, 2001).

To go beyond broad trait descriptions to in-depth assessments of individuals, the CAPS approach incorporates the situation into the measurement of individual differences. It shifts the unit of study from global traits inferred from behavioral signs to the person's cognitions, affects, and actions assessed in relation to the particular psychological conditions in which they occur (Mischel, 1973). The focus thus changes from describing situation-free people with broad trait adjectives to analyzing the interactions between conditions and the cognitions and behaviors of interest. (See also Shadel, Chapter 18, this volume, and Maddux, Chapter 22, this volume.)

## Basic Features of the CAPS Framework

CAPS conceptualizes the human mind as a network (using the metaphor of a neural network) of mental representations whose distinctive pattern of activation determines the thoughts and feelings that people experience and the behaviors they display (e.g., Higgins, 1990; see also, Shoda & Smith, 2004). At a molar level of analysis, these mental representations, or *cognitive–affective units* (CAUs), can be thought of in terms of such person variables as encodings, goals, expectations, beliefs, and affects, as well as self-regulatory standards, competencies, plans, and strategies (for description of CAUs, see Table 20.1).

In this framework, different CAUs are interconnected within a stable associative network that guides and constrains the activation of different mental representations with pathways of activation and deactivation. A visual example of this network is illustrated in Figure 20.1. The larger circle in the middle represents the individual's mind; the smaller interconnected set of circles within it represent the CAUs that give rise to the mental representations

**TABLE 20.1. Types of Cognitive–Affective Units in the CAPS**

1. ENCODINGS: Categories (constructs) for the self, people, events, and situations (external and internal).
2. EXPECTATIONS AND BELIEFS: About the social world, about outcomes for behavior in particular situations, about one's self-efficacy.
3. AFFECTS: Feelings, emotions, and affective responses (including physiological reactions).
4. GOALS: Desirable outcomes and affective states, aversive outcomes and affective states, goals and life projects.
5. COMPETENCIES AND SELF-REGULATORY PLANS: Potential behaviors and scripts that one can do and plans and strategies for organizing action and for affecting outcomes and one's own behavior and internal states.

*Note.* From Mischel and Shoda (1995, p. 253). Copyright 1995 by the American Psychological Association. Reprinted by permission.

that become activated in response to specific environmental triggers. Each time a person encounters a situation, a subset of these units becomes activated. Once a given unit becomes active, the activation then spreads to other units, following the stable associative links in the individual's network. The sum total of these activations and deactivations gives rise to the behaviors people display.

In this model, individual differences reflect differences in both the chronic accessibility of CAUs and the distinctive organization of interrelationships among them. As the person experiences situations that contain different psychological features, different CAUs become activated in relation to these features. Consequently, the activation of CAUs changes from one time to another and from one situation to another. However, although cognitions and affects that are activated at a given time change, *how* they change—that is, the sequence and pattern of their activation—remains stable, reflecting the stable structure of the organization within the system (Mischel & Shoda, 1995; Shoda & Mischel, 1998). It is this organization that guides and constrains the activation in stable ways, although it is modifiable by new learning experiences and cognitive transformations (e.g., as in therapy). The result is a distinctive pattern of *if . . . then . . .* relations that are expressed in predictable patterns of behavior as the individual moves across different situations (e.g., Shoda & LeeTiernan, 2002).

## The Contextualized If . . . Then . . . Expressions of Personality Coherence

In CAPS, different situations acquire different meanings for the same person as a function of social learning and biological (e.g., temperament) predispositions. Consequently the kinds of appraisals, expectations, beliefs, affects, goals, and behavioral scripts that are likely to become activated in relation to particular situations will vary. Theoretically, as well as empirically, there is no reason, therefore, to expect the individual to manifest similar behavior in relation to different psychological situations unless these situations are functionally equivalent in meaning. Thus to find the coherence in personality, we have to take into account the situation and its meaning for the individual, which is seen in the stable interactions—the *if . . . then . . .* relationships—that distinctively characterize the individual (e.g., Cervone & Shoda, 1999; Kunda, 1999; Magnusson & Endler, 1977; Mischel, 1973; Mischel & Shoda, 1995).

To demonstrate the stability and meaningfulness of such *if . . . then . . .* situation–behavior patterns, the behavior of children was observed in vivo over the course of a summer within a residential camp setting (Mischel & Shoda, 1995). The data collection effort yielded an

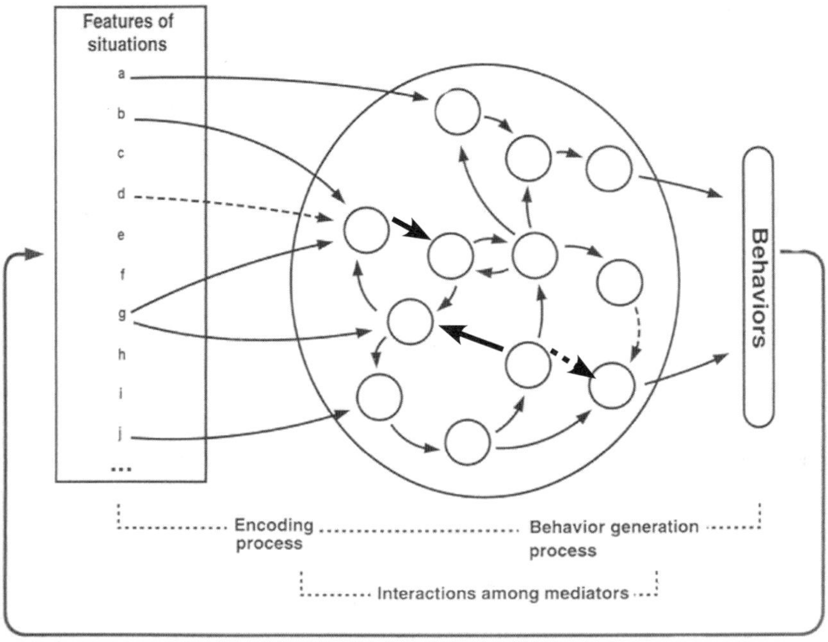


**FIGURE 20.1.** The CAPS network is illustrated by the large circle, and the smaller circles within it represent the cognitive–affective units (CAUs). The CAUs are interconnected either through excitatory (solid lines) or inhibitory (broken lines); the thickness of a line indicates the strength of the association between any two CAUs. As illustrated, situational features are encoded by CAUs, which, in turn, activates a subset of mediating units that are interconnected through a stable activation network. The dynamics of this network guide and constrain the individual's behavior in relation to particular situation features.

archival database that allowed systematic analyses of coherence in behavior as it unfolded across naturalistic situations and over many occasions (Shoda, Mischel, & Wright, 1989; Shoda et al., 1993a, 1993b, 1994; Wright & Mischel, 1987, 1988). The children's social behavior (e.g., verbal aggression, withdrawal, friendly, or prosocial behavior) was unobtrusively observed and recorded as it occurred in each of the selected interpersonal situations, with an average of 167 hours of observation per child over the course of the 6-week camp.

With this data archive, it was possible to assess the stability of the hypothesized situation–behavior relationships for each person. The frequencies of behavior were first converted to standardized *Z*-scores within each situation to indicate how much a given person's behavior deviated from normative levels in that situation. This standardization removes situational main effects, so that the remaining intra-individual variance in the profile reflects the unique way a person's behavior varies distinctively and stably across situations in characteristic, meaningful patterns. These patterns are found above and beyond what is expected from the differences in the normative levels of behavior across situations. If personality is conceptualized in terms of stable cross-situational behavioral dispositions, then the mean stability of the intra-individual pattern of variation after standardization should be zero, reflecting no change across situations (Mischel & Shoda, 1995). Alternatively, if the observed situation–behavior relationships reflect enduring coherence in personality, they should show some significant stability despite the noise, as they in fact do. (For a more elaborate discussion, see Mischel, 2004a; Mischel & Shoda, 1995.)

The findings revealed that individuals who have similar average levels of a type of behavior (e.g., their overall aggression) nevertheless differ predictably and meaningfully in the types of situations in which their aggressiveness occurs (Mischel & Shoda, 1995). It is obvious that people will become more aggressive in situations in which they are provoked or teased than when they are approached positively or praised. But the new finding of theoretical importance was that the person's rank order in relation to others changes systematically and predictably in different situations. The same person who is one of the least aggressive when teased may be well known for his or her characteristically high level of anger and irritation when flattered and praised. As every clinician knows, even if two children have similar overall levels of total aggressive behavior, the one characterized by a consistent pattern of becoming exceptionally aggressive when peers approach him or her to play, but less aggressive than most other children when chastised by an adult for misbehaving, is different psychologically from the one who shows the opposite pattern. Thus, overall, these results showed unequivocally that individuals are characterized by stable, distinctive patterns of variability in their actions, thoughts, and feelings across different types of situations. These behavioral signatures of personality, like psychological fingerprints, identify what is distinctive about the individual (Shoda et al., 1993a, 1994).

### From the Individual to Personality Types: Similar Distinctive Processing Dynamics and Behavioral Signatures

One may want to go from considering the unique patterns that characterize the individual to considering groups of people who have similar behavioral signatures, as in different psychiatric diagnostic categories. In CAPS, a personality type consists of people who share a common organization of relations among mediating units in the processing of certain situational features—that is, who have similar "processing dynamics." The types are defined in terms of distinctive social cognitive and affective processing dynamics that generate characteristic *if ... then ...* patterns of thoughts, feelings, and behavior visible in particular types of situations. To illustrate, the *high rejection sensitivity* individual (Downey & Feldman, 1996; Downey, Feldman, & Ayduk, 2000; Feldman & Downey, 1994) describes individuals who have intense anxieties about interpersonal rejection and abandonment that become evident if they encounter what could be construed as uncaring behavior in their intimate relationships —for example, their partner is attentive to someone else. They scan interpersonal situations for possible cues of rejection and appraise them in terms of their potential rejection threats, anxiously expecting to find them and vigilantly ready to see them (Downey, Mougios, Ayduk, London, & Shoda, 2004). Then they tend to become excessively concerned about whether or not they are loved. Their own ruminations then trigger further a cascade of feelings of anger, resentment, and rage as their fears of abandonment escalate (Ayduk, Downey, & Kim, 2001; Kross, Egner, Ochsner, Hirsch, & Downey, 2007). In reaction, they may engage in coercive and controlling behaviors, often blaming such behaviors on the partner's actions. They readily create a self-fulfilling prophecy in which fears of abandonment become validated by the rejections that they, in part, generate for themselves through their attempts to control (Downey, Freitas, Michealis, & Khouri, 1998). Nevertheless, on average, across a multitude of situations, they may not be more likely than others to express anger, disapproval, and coercive behaviors, and under some conditions can be exceptionally caring, tender, and thoughtful toward their partners. Diagnostic personality signatures like this (e.g., rejection sensitivity) offer new ways to explore the psychological processes and the social and biological histories that underlie them. A key challenge for future research is to articulate the mechanisms through which these patterns are maintained and can be changed through therapeutic interventions—a topic to which we return later.

### Specifying the Active Ingredients of Situations

To develop typologies of processing dynamics and structures that incorporate situations into personality assessment, one has to go beyond their surface features or nominal characteristics of situations (e.g., "in the dining room," "in group therapy") to capture their specific psychologically active ingredients (Shoda et al., 1994). These are the features of the situation that have significant meaning for a given individual and that are related to the experienced psychological situation—the thoughts and affects and goals that become activated within the personality system and that activate the behavior patterns that are expressed. This is seen, for example, in the rejection cues in intimate relations that activate the fears and defensive maneuvers of highly rejection-sensitive people. The importance of finding these features and elaborating their meaning for the individual has long been recognized (e.g., Kelly, 1955), as clinicians who employ functional analyses know, and recent conceptual and analytic developments (e.g., computer simulations) within the social cognitive approach to personality are rapidly facilitating the analyses of such active ingredients of situations (e.g., Cervone, 2004; LeeTiernan, 2002; Shoda & LeeTiernan, 2002; Shadel, Chapter 18, this volume). These innovations make it possible to go beyond the single case to identify types of individuals (e.g., high-rejection-sensitive individuals) for whom particular sets of features have common meanings and activate similar processing dynamics (Ayduk, Downey, Testa, Yen, & Shoda, 1999; Cervone & Shoda, 1999; Shoda & Smith, 2004; Wright & Mischel, 1987).

### Summary

The CAPS framework allows researchers to move beyond broad trait-level descriptions of behavior and focus instead on the processes that underlie the way people respond to different kinds of psychological trigger situations. This type of understanding can be particularly useful for clinicians who are interested in facilitating adaptive changes in the way people respond to situations that trigger destructive responses, because it provides a window into the psychological processes that generate them. In the next section we illustrate how this model can shed light on the specific patterns of mental representations that undermine versus facilitate peoples' ability to exert self-control adaptively.

## HOT VERSUS COOL MENTAL REPRESENTATIONS IN THE CAPS FRAMEWORK

Assuming that the specific types of situations that elicit problematic responses are known (e.g., the dieter when faced with the desert tray; the alcoholic at cocktail hour; the abusive husband when receiving criticism from his wife), according to the CAPS framework the next step for facilitating self-control involves identifying the specific types of mental representations that become automatically activated in these situations and determining how to deactivate them. In this sense, the ability to control problematic responses depends on the interaction between automatic and controlled processes that influence the types of mental representations that become active in the individual.

To account for the role that automatic and controlled processes play in the CAPS framework, Metcalfe and Mischel (1999) proposed two fundamentally different types of mental representations—one cognitive or "cool" and the other affective or "hot"—that are controlled by two different subsystems within the broader CAPS framework under situations that require self-control. Briefly, the hot system is an automatic system that responds reflexively to trigger features in the environment, both positive and negative, and elicits automatic, aversive, fight-or-flight reactions as well as appetitive and sexual approach reactions. The hot system consists of relatively few representations, which, when activated by trigger stimuli, elicit virtually reflexive avoidance and approach reactions. The cool system, on the other hand, is conceptualized as a controlled system that is attuned to the informational, cognitive, and spatial aspects of stimuli. It consists of a network of informational *cool nodes* that are elaborately interconnected to each other and generate rational, reflective, and strategic behavior. Whereas the hot system is conceptualized as the basis of emotionality, the cool system is viewed as the basis of self-control.

Although the regions of neural activity underlying these different systems currently remain a vigorously pursued topic of research (for review, see Kross & Ochsner, 2010; also see Lieberman, 2007; Ochsner & Gross, 2005), collectively the findings thus far suggest that the amygdala—a small, almond-shaped region in the forebrain thought to enable fight-or-flight responses—is critically involved in hot system processing (Gray, 1982, 1987; LeDoux, 2000; Metcalfe & Jacobs, 1996, 1998). This brain structure reacts almost instantly to stimuli that individuals encode as arousing (Adolphs et al., 1999; LeDoux, 1996, 2000; Phelps et al., 2001; Winston, Strange, O'Doherty, & Dolan, 2002), immediately cueing behavioral, physiological (autonomic), and endocrine responses. The cool system, in contrast, seems to be associated with prefrontal and cingulate systems involved in cognitive control and executive function (e.g., Jackson et al., 2003; Ochsner & Gross, 2005).

The hot and cool systems operate in continuous interaction with each other to produce phenomenological experiences and behavioral responses (see also, Epstein, 1994; Lieberman, Gaunt, Gilbert, & Trope, 2002). Hot representations and cool representations that have the same external referent are directly connected to one another and thus link the two systems (Metcalfe & Mischel, 1999; see also, Metcalfe & Jacobs, 1996, 1998). Thus hot representations can be evoked by the activation of corresponding cool representations. For example, an abusive husband can become filled with rage by merely conjuring up a fantasy in which he finds his wife cheating on him with another man. Alternatively, hot representations can be cooled through cool-system cognitive processes (e.g., attention switching, reconstrual). Thus the same abusive husband can calm himself down by distracting himself or by recognizing that his fantasy is nothing more than a mental fiction with no real implications for his relationship. Self-control becomes possible to the extent that cooling strategies generated by the cognitive cool system circumvent hot-system activation.

Several factors that influence the balance of hot–cool system processing are relevant for clinicians trying to determine how to aid people in their attempts to exert self-control over problematic behaviors and emotions. In the context of the impulsive responses and emotional reactions that fully developed adults commonly face, perhaps the most important determinant of hot–cool system balance is stress. At high levels, stress deactivates the cool system and creates hot-system dominance. At lower levels of stress, complex thinking, planning, and remembering are possible. When stress levels jump from low to very high, as in life-threatening emergency conditions, responding tends to be reflexive and automatic. Under conditions in which an animal's life is threatened, quick responses driven by innately determined stimuli may be essential. For humans, however, such automatic reactions may undo rational efforts at constructive self-control.

A second factor is the developmental level of the individual. The hot system develops and dominates early in life, whereas the cool system begins to develop later (at age 4) and becomes increasingly dominant over the course of development. These developmental differences in the balance of hot–cool systems are consistent with research on the differential rates of development of the relevant brain areas for these two systems (for reviews, see Eisenberg, Smith, Sadovsky, & Spinrad, 2004; Rothbart, Ellis, & Posner, 2004). Consequently, early in development young children are primarily under stimulus control, as they have not yet developed the cool-system structures needed to regulate hot-system processing. As the cool system develops over time, it becomes increasingly possible for children to generate cooling strategies as a way to regulate impulses (Mischel, Shoda, & Rodriguez, 1989).

In sum, the hot–cool model helps specify the types of mental representations within the CAPS system that are relevant to understanding the interactions between cognition and emotion that enable self-regulation under highly arousing conditions. In the following sections we describe how this framework can shed light on the psychological processes that underlie people's ability to cope adaptively with a range of problematic behaviors.

## Hot–Cool Processes Involved in Coping with Impulsive Tendencies

A key challenge at the heart of many self-regulatory dilemmas involves making the decision to forgo engaging in an immediately rewarding behavior in order to obtain a more desirable long-term goal—for example, the struggling addict's inability to refrain from shooting up in order to achieve his or her long-term goals of professional success and sobriety, or the dieter who desperately wants to lose weight but cannot abstain from consuming the chocolate cake. Understanding how people can adaptively forgo immediately tempting rewards in the service of long-term goal pursuit requires identifying the specific cooling operations that can be used to deactivate hot representations that become activated when people are exposed to psychological trigger situations.

Research from our lab has addressed this issue using a simple laboratory paradigm called the delay-of-gratification task, or the "marshmallow test" in the media. In this task, a young child is presented with a desired treat (e.g., pretzel sticks or little marshmallows) and then posed with a dilemma: The child can wait until the experimenter returns and get two of the desired treats *or* ring a bell to summon the experimenter immediately but receive only one treat. The child prefers the larger outcome and typically commits him- or herself to wait for it. However, as waiting for the chosen goal drags on, the child becomes increasingly tempted to ring the bell and take the immediately available treat.

Although this kind of choice conflict may seem trivial when compared to the problems of self-control that clients suffering from clinical disorders face, this task provides a powerful conflict for young children and an experimental analogue for many of the more difficult conflicts that people encounter in their everyday lives. Indeed, performance on this task has been shown to predict a number of consequential life outcomes, such as self-regulation in goal pursuit decades later, suggesting that this paradigm is capable of tapping into the processes that are needed to exert self-control in a variety of domains (e.g., Ayduk et al., 2000; Eigsti et al., 2006; Kross & Mischel, 2010; Mischel, Shoda, & Peake, 1988; Shoda, Mischel, & Peake, 1990). The question is: What strategies can a child use to resist the temptation of the immediately available reward? How can he or she replace hot mental representations of the rewards with cooler ones?

Collectively, the findings suggest that there are two primary ways in which delay of gratification can be facilitated in young children. One way is by diverting children's attention from focusing on the appetitive features of the rewards they are trying to delay gratification in order to receive. For example, making the rewards available for children to look at as they attempt to wait for the larger reward leads them to ring the bell more quickly and delay gratification for shorter periods of time, compared to children who wait with the rewards concealed from attention (Mischel & Ebbesen, 1970). In a similar vein, distracting children from focusing on the rewards by giving them a fun toy with which to play (Mischel, Ebbesen, & Zeiss, 1972) or by cueing them to think fun thoughts (e.g., "Think about Mommy pushing you on a swing") as they wait for the larger reward has also been shown to enhance delay time. In contrast, when children are waiting with the rewards exposed without receiving distraction instructions, or when they are cued to focus on sad thoughts, delay reliably decreases (Mischel et al., 1972).

Changing the way children cognitively construe the outcomes for which they are waiting or for which they are working can also enhance impulse control. Here the goal is to modify how children mentally represent the stimulus they are trying to delay gratification in order to receive rather than directing their attention away from the appetitive stimulus. For example, Mischel and colleagues have shown that cueing children to think about the rewards in terms of their concrete, motivating, "hot" features (i.e., "You can think about how gooey and yummy marshmallows taste") undermines children's ability to delay gratification. In contrast, cueing children to focus on the more abstract, informational, "cool" features of desired treats (i.e., "You can think about how round and puffy marshmallows are like cotton balls or clouds") enhances their ability to delay (Mischel & Baker, 1975; Mischel & Moore, 1973; Moore, Mischel, & Zeiss, 1976; for review, see Mischel et al., 1989).

In short, voluntary delay of reward can be aided by attentional and cognitive reconstrual strategies that function to replace mental representations of rewards that are emotionally "hot" and difficult to resist with alternative representations that are "cool" and do not elicit impulsive trigger reactions. Through such distraction and mental rerepresentation, it is possible to convert the frustrating delay-of-reward situation into a psychologically less aversive condition. When considering how people can be helped to self-regulate adaptively, however, there is an important caveat: In the real world, situations that require individuals to exert self-control often involve both strategic cooling processes that enable them to remain calm and reflective in the face of temptation, as well as strategic heating processes to maintain commitment to pursuing the goals rather than quitting. For example, Peake, Hebl, and Mischel (2002) investigated second-by-second attention deployment during efforts at sustained delay of gratification. Self-regulation depended not just on cooling strategies but on flexible deployment of attention—delay in working situations was facilitated most when attention was intermittently shifted to the rewards, as if the children tried to strategically enhance their motivation to abstain from immediately taking the reward by reminding themselves about them, but then quickly shifted away to prevent excessive arousal (Peake et al., 2002). Such flexibility in attention deployment is consistent with the idea that it is the balanced interactions between the hot and cool systems that sustain delay of gratification, as people exert their motivating and cooling effects in tandem (see also, Bonanno, Papa, Lalande, Westphal, & Coifman, 2004; Cheng, 2001, 2003; Mischel et al., 1989).

## From Marshmallow to Melancholy: Hot–Cool Processes in Coping with Negative Emotions

Our research has shown that the processes involved in delaying gratification also help people regulate automatically triggered defensive emotional reactions (e.g., angry outbursts, hostile responses). According to the hot–cool model, effective coping in threatening contexts should involve using the same type of strategic attention deployment and cognitive reconstrual strategies to cool the "hot" emotional features associated with threatening situations that children use in the delay-of-gratification task to control their appetitive responses. One study exploring this prediction was an adult follow-up of participants from the original delay-of-gratification studies (Ayduk et al., 2000). This study showed that the number of seconds that high-rejection-sensitive participants were able to wait as preschoolers in the delay situation protected them against the destructive interpersonal effects of rejection sensitivity. Thus, high-rejection-sensitive adults who had high-delay ability in preschool displayed more positive functioning (high self-esteem, self-worth, and coping ability) compared to similarly high-rejection-sensitive adults who were not able to delay in preschool. They also showed lower levels of cocaine/crack use and higher levels of education than high-rejection-sensitive individuals who had low-delay ability in preschool, and in these respects were similar to low-rejection-sensitive individuals (see also, Ayduk et al., 2007).

A similar pattern of results was found in a second study with middle school children. Specifically, whereas high-rejection-sensitive children with low-delay ability were more aggressive toward their peers and had less positive peer relationships than children low in rejection sensitivity, high-rejection-sensitive children who were able to delay longer were even less aggressive and more liked than low-rejection-sensitive children (Ayduk et al., 2000). Similarly, in a cross-sectional study of preadolescent boys with behavioral problems characterized by heightened hostile reactivity to interpersonal threats, the spontaneous use of cooling strategies in the delay task (i.e., looking away from the rewards and self-distraction) predicted reduced verbal and physical aggression (Rodriguez, Mischel, & Shoda, 1989).

We are also conducting research using the hot–cool framework to reconcile a paradox in the coping literature. The paradox is that, on the one hand, abundant findings indicate that it is helpful for people to express and analyze negative past experiences in order to "work through" them (Pennebaker & Graybeal, 2001). On the other hand, their attempts to do so often lead to rumination and brooding, which have been associated with a variety of negative physical and mental health consequences (Nolen-Hoeksema, Wisco, & Lyubomirsky, 2008). Thus the question is: How can people adaptively focus on negative experiences in order to work through them in a cool way, but without spiraling into rumination and becoming overwhelmed with hot-system activation and negative feelings?

To address this question, Kross, Ayduk, and Mischel (2005) proposed that a critical factor determining whether people's attempts to adaptively work through negative experiences lead to the activation of hot or cool mental representations is the type of self-perspective they adopt. Prior research indicates that when people focus on negative past experiences, they typically do so from a self-immersed perspective in which self-relevant events and emotions are experienced in the first-person through their own eyes (Nigro & Neisser, 1983). Drawing from this literature, Kross et al. (2005) hypothesized that when individuals focus on negative feelings from a self-immersed perspective, "hot," episodic information concerning the specific chain of events (i.e., "What happened?") and emotions experienced (i.e., "What did I feel?") would become accessible (cf. McIsaac & Eich, 2004), serving to increase negative affect. In contrast, they predicted that focusing on negative feelings in order to analyze them from a self-distanced perspective in which the individual adopts the vantage point of an observer (e.g., James, 1890; see also, e.g., Leary, 2002; Libby & Eibach, 2002; McIsaac & Eich, 2004; Nigro & Neisser, 1983) should have the opposite effect. Namely, it should reduce people's tendency to reflexively recount what happened to them and instead allow them to reconstrue their experience in cool ways that reduce its aversiveness (Metcalfe & Mischel, 1999; Mischel, 1974; see also, Gross, 2001; Lazarus, 1991).

These hypotheses were supported in a set of studies that manipulated the type of self-perspective (self-immersed vs. self-distanced) participants adopted as they analyzed the reasons they felt angry in an interpersonal conflict (Kross et al., 2005). Specifically, when participants analyzed their feelings from a self-immersed perspective (*immersed analysis* from hereon), episodic information concerning the specific chain of events (e.g., "He told me to back off; I remember watching her cheat on me ... ") and emotions experienced (e.g., "I was so angry ... ") became more accessible. In contrast, participants who analyzed their feelings from a self-distanced perspective (*distanced analysis* from hereon) focused relatively less on what happened to them (i.e., recounting) and relatively more on reconstruing the event (e.g., "I understand why the fight happened; it might have been irrational but I understand his motivation now"). This shift in the content of peoples' thoughts about their past experience (less recounting, more reconstruing) mediated the effect of the perspective manipulations on negative affect (see also, Strack, Schwarz, & Gschneidinger, 1985). Thus the more reconstruing and less recounting participants engaged in, the less negative affect they displayed. This finding is consistent with research indicating that strategies and interventions that direct individuals to construct narratives about distressing events leads to a variety of physical and mental health benefits (for reviews, see Grossmann & Kross, in press; Pennenbaker & Graybeal, 2001; Smyth, 1998), presumably by leading people to assign meaning, coherence, and structure to their emotions (Chung & Pennebaker, 2007).

This work has been replicated, and the initial findings are being extended in multiple directions. In one study, for example, Kross and Ayduk (2008) demonstrated that distanced analysis leads not only to reductions in short-term negative affect but also buffers individuals against future negative affect assessed 1 day and 1 week after the initial experiment, and reduces people's tendencies to ruminate over time (see also, Ayduk & Kross, 2010; Kross, Davidson, Weber, & Ochsner, 2009). In another study, Ayduk and Kross (2008) demonstrated that instructing participants to analyze anger experiences from a self-distanced perspective leads not only to reductions in levels of self-reported anger, but also to reductions in autonomic nervous system reactivity as well.

### Summary

The findings reviewed in this section help clarify the psychological processes that underlie people's ability to cope adaptively with a range of situations that require self-control and highlight the role that hot and cool mental representations play in determining the outcomes of self-regulatory efforts. One question that emerges from this work is how the CAPS approach can be integrated into psychotherapy to help clients cope with serious problems of living and dysfunction. In the next section we review recent work that has begun to tackle this question.

## CLINICAL IMPLICATIONS

The research reviewed thus far indicates that the stable patterns of *if* ... *then* ... relations displayed by people are not isolated, functional relations between single situations and responses. Instead, they constitute stable and predictable patterns. Thus the individual who is high in rejection sensitivity may consistently respond to situations in which rejection by an intimate partner is possible with intense aggression and hostility, but may be relatively undisturbed when receiving rejection feedback from a colleague in a nonintimate relationship. The challenge for the clinician is to identify the specific types of psychological situations that trigger problematic behavioral signatures in their clients, and the modifications needed in the mental representations and processing dynamics to make those signatures less automatic and more open to constructive modification.

Although obtaining this kind of information may seem simple in the lab under tightly controlled conditions, in the real world, when people are confronted with many types of complicated experiences, eliciting and identifying this kind of information poses major methodological challenges. Fortunately, a number of research groups are rapidly developing new techniques to overcome these obstacles. For example, Van Mechelen and colleagues have recently developed procedures for performing CAPS-based clinical assessments (Claes, Van Mechelen, & Vertommen, 2004; Vansteelandt & Van Mechelen, 1998). In the first step of their approach the clinician generates a list of psychological situations that a given client encounters on a semiregular basis. This list can be generated either using normative data on the frequency of certain kinds of situations and behaviors or through the use of idiographic interview methods. Subsequently, a list of potentially relevant behaviors and cognitive–affective variables that capture how an individual may respond to different psychological situations must be specified. As with the specification of a list of psychological situations, constructing a list of these behaviors and cognitive–affective variables may be done using both idiographic (i.e., collected from the client through some construct-eliciting procedure) and nomothetic (i.e., derived from a priori clinical theories or previous empirical research) methods.

Once these lists of situations, behaviors, and cognitive–affective variables have been generated, the therapist places them in the form of a grid, the rows of which refer to different situations as experienced by the client in the recent past, and the columns of which refer to the manifest behaviors and underlying cognitive–affective variables (see Figure 20.2; for general guidelines regarding the collection and processing of such data, see Claes et al., 2004). This grid is then presented to the client (or a family member or friend of the client) with the instruction that he or she indicates whether each behavior and cognitive–affective variable

| | *Encoding*: "coalition against me"<br>*Affect*: anxiety | *Behavior*: urge to binge<br>*Expectancy*: exclusion | *Behavior*: urge to self-injury | *Behavior*: urge to physical aggression |
|---|---|---|---|---|
| *Situation Cluster 1*: rejection by significant others | | | | |
| *Situation Cluster 2*: blocking in relation with significant others | | | | |
| *Situation Cluster 3*: aggression by other | | | | |

**FIGURE 20.2.** Linkage structure between situation clustering and behavior/CAU clustering as derived from data of eating-disordered patient. A dark cell indicates that the situation cluster, as represented by the corresponding row, elicits the behavioral and cognitive–affective variables included in the corresponding column cluster.

listed across the top row becomes activated (yes or no) in each situation. Once this grid of data is obtained, the main goal of subsequent analysis is to identify the most significant situation–behavior signatures through the use of clustering methods (Van Mechelen, Bock, & De Boeck, 2004, 2005) that are capable of highlighting (1) clusters of functionally equivalent situations (potentially reflecting the most prominent active psychological features of the situations); (2) clusters of co-occurring behaviors and/or CAUs; and (3) a linkage structure between both types of clustering, which can be read as a summary description of the most significant behavioral signatures of the client, along with his or her underlying cognitive–affective process basis.

To illustrate, Claes et al. (2004) presented a case regarding a 20-year-old female client who came to therapy suffering from an eating disorder along with self-injurious behavior. The primary goal of the CAPS assessment was to help the therapist identify the specific types of psychological situations that were triggering maladaptive behaviors and to identify what mental representations were driving these behaviors in order to focus subsequent cognitive-behavioral treatment. To do this, the therapist worked with the client to construct a list of 36 situations that she commonly experienced in her everyday life. The client was then asked to indicate whether she engaged in bingeing and purging behavior and/or self-injurious behavior, along with several forms of aggression, in each one of these 36 situations. In addition, the client was asked to indicate the extent to which she experienced certain kinds of cognitive–affective variables, which were identified on the basis of existing theories and from interviews with the client. Subsequently, the client was asked to indicate whether each behavioral and process variable was present or absent in each situation. These data were then subjected to clustering analysis, which revealed three types of situation–behavior clusters.

One cluster contained situations such as "The parents of my boyfriend hurt me by hiding my diabetes from their family" and "My mother says that I am an unwanted child." These situations had in common rejection by significant others. A second cluster contained situations such as "A friend ignores me because she has to deal with her own divorce problems" and "My mother says that I am an unwanted child" (note that the latter situation reflects an instance of cluster overlap). These situations have in common that they reflect some kind of blocking in a relationship with significant others. A third cluster included situations such as "A friend of my father grips me and pushes his body against mine" and "During a teaching internship one of the pupils calls me a blond whore." The authors interpreted this cluster as involving aggression displayed by someone other than the client.

Figure 20.2 presents a partial representation of the specific cognitive–affective and behavioral processes (e.g., urge to binge; urge to aggress; expectations of exclusion) that become active in specific types of psychological situations (e.g., rejection by significant other vs. blocked relationship by significant other vs. aggression by other) that the client experiences. Dark cells indicate that a cognitive–affective and/or behavioral process is reliably activated in response to a particular type of psychological situation. For example, the left upper dark cell denotes that rejection by significant others gives rise to the encoding "There is a coalition against me" as well as an anxious affect. As this figure illustrates, the first target symptom behavior, urge to binge, appears to show up in the case of relational problems with significant others. Moreover, in terms of the CAUs that are related to this behavior, the urge to binge co-occurs with the expectancy of being excluded. Second, the behavioral signature of self-injury reveals a close link between this target symptom behavior and direct negative actions (i.e., rejection or aggression) of others.

The results of this analysis provided clear guidelines for subsequent cognitive-behavioral therapy, specifying how clinical intervention could be maximally effective. For example, given the relational nature of the situations driving the client's maladaptive responses, the authors determined that a primary task in therapy was to guide the client in actively selecting and creating more rewarding social situations involving significant others. An example of a concrete plan that might be effective toward accomplishing this involves reestablishing connections with former good friends that were lost. Second, regarding the client's urge to inflict self-injurious behavior in response to the situations listed in Figure 20.2, recommendations were made for teaching the client alternative forms of self-regulatory strategies in order to deal with the negative actions of other people.

The approach described here offers a route to integrating data-driven theory into clinical practice to help clinicians tailor therapy by targeting specific psychological situations and CAUS that trigger and perpetuate problematic responses. In this vein, it offers a potential bridge between the research lab and the clinician's practice. Of course, as an evolving approach to clinical assessment and practice, it raises a host of self-evident questions that, in turn, call for research on its translational value and limits, which we hope will follow in the future.

## CONCLUDING COMMENTS

In the 1921 editorial accompanying the first issue of the *JASP*, its editors wrote: "The definition of a science is always an arbitrary matter. Quibbling over what should be included or excluded is futile" (Prince & Allport, 1921, p. 2). Reflecting on this statement now, it seems to apply equally well today. Clearly, important substantive differences exist between "normal" and "abnormal" behavior that warrant the existence of different areas of study, each with its own focus and concerns. While recognizing the need for specialization, in this chapter we have pointed to some of the basic psychological processes that underlie behavior of interest to both specialties, focusing on the cognitive–affective dynamics that enable—or undermine—adaptive self-control and self-regulation. Consistent with the goals Prince and Allport had for JASP almost a century ago, we hope it is a step toward psychology's becoming an increasingly integrative science of human behavior, in which clinical and social psychology recognize their common ground and build on each other's efforts, ideas, and findings.

## ACKNOWLEDGMENTS

Preparation of this chapter was supported by grants from the National Institute of Mental Health (No. MH39349) and the National Science Foundation (No. BCS-0624262). Portions of this chapter were based on an article written for a special issue of *Behavior Therapy* (Mischel, 2004). We thank Iven Van Mechelen for providing materials relevant to the "Clinical Implications" section of this chapter.

## REFERENCES

Adolphs, R., Tranel, D., Hamann, S., Young, A. W., Calder, A. J., Phelps, E. A., et al. (1999). Recognition of facial emotion in nine individuals with bilateral amygdala damage. *Neuropsychologia*, 37, 1111–1117.

Ayduk, O., Downey, G., & Kim, M. (2001). Rejection sensitivity and depressive symptoms in women. *Personality and Social Psychology Bulletin*, *27*, 868–877.

Ayduk, O., Downey, G., Testa, A., Yen, Y., & Shoda, Y. (1999). Does rejection sensitivity elicit hostility in rejection sensitive women? *Social Cognition*, *17*, 245–271.

Ayduk, O., & Kross, E. (2008). Enhancing the pace of recovery: Differential effects of analyzing negative experiences from a self-distanced vs. self-immersed perspective on blood pressure reactivity. *Psychological Science*, *19*, 229–231.

Ayduk, O., & Kross, E. (2009). Asking "why" from a self-distanced perspective facilitates adaptive emotional processing: A reanalysis of Wimalaweera & Moulds (2008). *Behaviour Research and Therapy, 47*(1), 88–92.

Ayduk, O., & Kross, E. (2010). From a distance: Implications of spontaneous self-distancing for adaptive self-reflection. *Journal of Personality and Social Psychology, 98*, 809–829.

Ayduk, O., Mendoza-Denton, R., Mischel, W., Downey, G., Peake, P., & Rodriguez, M. L. (2000). Regulating the interpersonal self: Strategic self-regulation for coping with rejection sensitivity. *Journal of Personality and Social Psychology*, *79*(5), 776–792.

Ayduk, O., Zayas, V., Downey, G., Cole, A. B., Shoda, Y., & Mischel, W. (2007). Rejection sensitivity and executive control: Joint predictors of borderline personality features. *Journal of Research in Personality*, *42*, 151–168.

Bonanno, G. A., Papa, A., Lalande, K., Westphal, M., & Coifman, K. (2004). The importance of being flexible: The ability to enhance *and* suppress emotional expression predicts long-term adjustment. *Psychological Science*, *157*, 482–487.

Borkenau, P., Riemann, R., Spinath, F. M., & Angleitner, A. (2006). Genetic and environmental influences on person × situation profiles. *Journal of Personality and Social Psychology*, *74*, 1451–1480.

Cervone, D. (2004). The architecture of personality. *Psychological Review*, *111*, 183–204.

Cervone, D., & Shoda, Y. (Eds.). (1999). *The coherence of personality: Social–cognitive bases of consistency, variability, and organization*. New York: Guilford Press.

Cheng, C. (2001). Assessing coping flexibility in real-life and laboratory settings: A multimethod approach. *Journal of Personality and Social Psychology*, *80*, 814–833.

Cheng, C. (2003). Cognitive and motivational processes underlying coping flexibility: A dual-process model. *Journal of Personality and Social Psychology*, *84*, 425–438.

Chen-Idson, L., & Mischel, W. (2001). The personality of familiar and significant people: The lay perceiver as a social–cognitive theorist. *Journal of Personality and Social Psychology*, *80*, 585–596.

Chung, C. K., & Pennebaker, J. W. (2007). The psychological function of function words. In K. Fiedler (Ed.), *Social communication: Frontiers of social psychology* (pp. 343–359). New York: Psychology Press.

Claes, L., Van Mechelen, I., & Vertommen, H. (2004). Assessment of situation–behavior profiles and their guiding cognitive and affective processes: A case study from the domain of aggressive behaviors. *European Journal of Psychological Assessment*, *20*, 216–226.

Downey, G., & Feldman, S. (1996). Implications of rejection sensitivity for intimate relationships. *Journal of Personality and Social Psychology*, *70*(6), 1327–1343.

Downey, G., Feldman, S., & Ayduk, O. (2000). Rejection sensitivity and male violence in romantic relationships. *Personal Relationships*, *7*, 45–61.

Downey, G., Freitas, A., Michealis, B., & Khouri, H. (1998). The self-fulfilling prophecy in close relationships: Do rejection sensitive women get rejected by romantic partners? *Journal of Personality and Social Psychology*, *75*(2), 545–560.

Downey, G., Mougios, V., Ayduk, O., London, B. E., & Shoda, Y. (2004). Rejection sensitivity and the defensive motivational system: Insights from the startle response to rejection cues. *Psychological Science*, *15*, 668–673.

Eigsti, I., Zayas, V., Mischel, W., Shoda, Y., Ayduk, O., Dadlani, M. B., et al. (2006). Predictive cognitive control from preschool to late adolescence and young adulthood. *Psychological Science*, *17*, 478–484.

Eisenberg, N., Smith, C. L., Sadovsky, A., & Spinrad, T. L. (2004). Effortful control: Reactions with emotion regulation, adjustment, and socialization in childhood. In R. F. Baumeister & K. D. Vohs (Eds.), *Handbook of self-regulation* (pp. 259–283). New York: Guilford Press.

Epstein, S. (1994). Integration of the cognitive and psychodynamic unconscious. *American Psychologist*, *49*, 709–724.

Feldman, S. I., & Downey, G. (1994). Rejection sensitivity as a mediator of the impact of childhood exposure to family violence on adult attachment behavior. *Development and Psychopathology*, *6*, 231–247.

Fournier, M. A., Moskowitz, D. S., & Zuroff, D. C. (2008). Integrating dispositions, signatures, and the interpersonal domain. *Journal of Personality and Social Psychology*, *94*, 531–545.

Goldberg, L. R. (1993). The structure of phenotypic personality traits. *American Psychologist*, *48*, 26–34.

Gray, J. A. (1982). *The neuropsychology of anxiety.* London: Oxford University Press.

Gray, J. A. (1987). *The psychology of fear and stress* (2nd ed.). New York: McGraw-Hill.

Gross, J. J. (2001). Emotion regulation in adulthood: Timing is everything. *Current Directions in Psychological Science*, *10*, 214–219.

Grossmann, I., & Kross, E. (in press). The impact of culture on adaptive vs. maladaptive self-reflection. *Psychological Science*.

Higgins, E. T. (1990). Personality, social psychology, and person–situation relations: Standards and knowledge activation as a common language. In L. A. Pervin (Ed.), *Handbook of personality: Theory and research* (pp. 301–338). New York: Guilford Press.

Jackson, D. C., Muller, C. J., Dolski, I., Dalton, K. M., Nitschke, J. B., Urry, H. L., et al. (2003). Now you feel it, now you don't: Frontal brain electrical asymmetry and individual differences in emotion regulation. *Psychological Science*, *14*, 612–617.

James, W. (1981). *The principles of psychology* (Vol. 2). Cambridge, MA: Harvard University Press. (Original work published 1890)

John, O. P. (1990). The "Big Five" factor taxonomy: Dimensions of personality in the natural language and in questionnaires. In L. A. Pervin (Ed.), *Handbook of personality: Theory and research* (pp. 66–100). New York: Guilford Press.

Kelly, G. A. (1955). *The psychology of personal constructs.* New York: Norton. Reprinted by Routledge (London), 1991.

Kross, E., & Ayduk, O. (2008). Facilitating adaptive emotional analysis: Short-term and long-term outcomes distinguishing *distanced*-analysis of depressive experiences from *immersed*-analysis and distraction. *Personality and Social Psychology Bulletin, 34*, 924–938.

Kross, E., Ayduk, O., & Mischel, W. (2005). When asking "why" does not hurt: Distinguishing rumination from reflective processing of negative emotions. *Psychological Science, 16*, 709–715.

Kross, E., Davidson, M., Weber, J., & Ochsner, K. (2009). Coping with emotions past: The neural bases of regulating affect associated with negative autobiographical experiences. *Biological Psychiatry, 65*(5), 361–366.

Kross, E., Egner, T., Ochsner, K., Hirsch, J., & Downey, G. (2007). Neural dynamics of rejection sensitivity. *Journal of Cognitive Neuroscience, 19*(6), 945–956.

Kross, E., & Mischel, W. (2010). From stimulus control to self-control: Towards an integrative understanding of the processes underlying willpower. In Y. Trope, R. Hassin, & K. Ochsner (Eds.), *Self-control in society, mind, and brain* (pp. 428–448). New York: Oxford University Press.

Kross, E., & Ochsner, K. N. (2010). Integrating research on self-control across multiple levels of analysis: Insights from social cognitive and affective neuroscience. In Y. Trope, R. Hassin, & K. Ochsner (Eds.), *Self-control in society, mind, and brain* (pp. 76–92). New York: Oxford University Press.

Kunda, Z. (1999). *Social cognition: Making sense of people.* Cambridge, MA: MIT Press.

Lazarus, R. S. (1991). *Emotion and adaptation.* New York: Oxford University Press.

Leary, M. (2002). The self and emotion: The role of self-reflection in the generation and regulation of affective experience. In R. Davidson, K. Scherer, & H. Goldsmith (Eds.), *Handbook of affective sciences* (pp. 773–786). New York: Oxford University Press.

LeDoux, J. (1996). *The emotional brain.* New York: Simon & Schuster.

LeDoux, J. (2000). Emotion circuits in the brain. *Annual Review Neuroscience, 23*, 155–184.

LeeTiernan, S. J. (2002). *Modeling and predicting stable response variation across situations.* Unpublished doctoral dissertation, University of Washington, Seattle.

Libby, L., & Eibach, R. (2002). Looking back in time: Self-concept change affects visual perspective in autobiographical memory. *Journal of Personality and Social Psychology, 82*, 167–179.

Lieberman, M. D. (2007). The X- and C-systems: The neural basis of automatic and controlled social cognition. In E. Harmon-Jones & P. Winkelman (Eds.), *Fundamentals of social neuroscience* (pp. 290–315). New York: Guilford Press.

Lieberman, M. D., Gaunt, R., Gilbert, D. T., & Trope, Y. (2002). Reflection and reflexion: A social cognitive neuroscience approach to attributional inference. In M. Zanna (Ed.), *Advances in experimental social psychology* (pp. 199–249). New York: Academic Press.

Linehan, M. M. (1993). *Cognitive-behavioral treatment of borderline personality disorder.* New York: Guilford Press.

Magnusson, D., & Endler, N. S. (1977). Interactional psychology: Present status and future prospects. In D. Magnusson & N. S. Endler (Eds.), *Personality at the crossroads: Current issues in interactional psychology* (pp. 3–36). Hillsdale, NJ: Erlbaum.

McCrae, R. R., & Costa, P. T., Jr. (1990). *Personality in adulthood.* New York: Guilford Press.

McIsaac, H. K., & Eich, E. (2004). Vantage point in traumatic memory. *Psychological Science, 15*, 248–253.

Metcalfe, J., & Jacobs, J. W. (1996). A "hot/cool-system" view of memory under stress. *PTSD Research Quarterly, 7*, 1–6.

Metcalfe, J., & Jacobs, J. W. (1998). Emotional memory: The effects of stress on "cool" and "hot" memory systems. In D. L. Medin (Ed.), *Psychology of learning and motivation* (pp. 188–222). San Diego, CA: Academic Press.

Metcalfe, J., & Mischel, W. (1999). A hot/cool system analysis of delay of gratification: Dynamics of willpower. *Psychological Review, 106*, 3–19.

Mischel, W. (1968). *Personality and assessment.* New York: Wiley.

Mischel, W. (1973). Toward a cognitive social learning reconceptualization of personality. *Psychological Review*, *80*, 252–283.

Mischel, W. (1974). Cognitive appraisals and transformations in self-control. In B. Weiner (Ed.), *Cognitive views of human motivation* (pp. 33–49). New York: Academic Press.

Mischel, W. (2004a). Toward an integrative science of the person. *Annual Review of Psychology*, *55*, 1–22.

Mischel, W. (2004b). Toward an integrative model for CBT: Encompassing behavior, cognition, affect, and process. *Behavior Therapy*, *35*, 185–203.

Mischel, W., & Baker, N. (1975). Cognitive appraisals and transformations in delay behavior. *Journal of Personality and Social Psychology*, *31*(2), 254–261.

Mischel, W., & Ebbesen, E. B. (1970). Attention in delay of gratification. *Journal of Personality and Social Psychology*, *16*(2), 239–337.

Mischel, W., Ebbesen, E. B., & Zeiss, A. R. (1972). Cognitive and attentional mechanisms in delay of gratification. *Journal of Personality and Social Psychology*, *21*(2), 204–218.

Mischel, W., & Moore, B. (1973). Effects of attention to symbolically-presented rewards on self-control. *Journal of Personality and Social Psychology*, *28*(2), 172–179.

Mischel, W., & Peake, P. K. (1982). In search of consistency: Measure for measure. In M. P. Zanna, E. T. Higgins, & C. P. Herman (Eds.), *Consistency in social behavior: The Ontario symposium* (Vol. 2, pp. 187–207). Hillsdale, NJ: Erlbaum.

Mischel, W., & Shoda, Y. (1995). A cognitive–affective system theory of personality: Reconceptualizing situations, dispositions, dynamics and invariance in personality structure. *Psychological Review*, *102*(2), 246–268.

Mischel, W., & Shoda, Y. (1998). Reconciling processing dynamics and personality dispositions. *Annual Review of Psychology*, *49*, 229–258

Mischel, W., Shoda, Y., & Peake, P. (1988). The nature of adolescent competencies predicted by preschool delay of gratification. *Journal of Personality and Social Psychology*, *54*(4), 687–696.

Mischel, W., Shoda, Y., & Rodriguez, M. L. (1989). Delay of gratification in children. *Science*, *244*, 933–938.

Moore, B., Mischel, W., & Zeiss, A. (1976). Comparative effects of the reward stimulus and its cognitive representation in voluntary delay. *Journal of Personality and Social Psychology*, *34*, 419–424.

Moskowitz, D. S., Suh, E. J., & Desaulniers, J. (1994). Situational influences on gender differences in agency and communion. *Journal of Personality and Social Psychology*, *66*, 753–761.

Nigro, G., & Neisser, U. (1983). Point of view in personal memories. *Cognitive Psychology*, *15*, 467–482.

Nolen-Hoeksema, S., Wisco, B., & Lyubomirsky, S. (2008). Rethinking rumination. *Perspectives on Psychological Science*, *3*(5), 400–424.

Ochsner, K. N., & Gross, J. J. (2005). The cognitive control of emotion. *Trends in Cognitive Science*, *27*, 26–36.

Peake, P., Hebl, M., & Mischel, W. (2002). Strategic attention deployment for delay of gratification in waiting and working situations. *Developmental Psychology*, *38*(2), 313–326.

Pennebaker, J., & Graybeal, A. (2001). Patterns of natural language use: Disclosure, personality, and social integration. *Current Directions in Psychological Science*, *10*, 90–93.

Phelps, E. A., O'Connor, K. J., Gatenby, J. C., Gore, J. C., Grillon, C., & Davis, M. (2001). Activation of the left amygdala to a cognitive representation of fear. *Nature Neuroscience*, *4*, 437–441.

Prince, M., & Allport, F. H. (1921). Editorial announcement. *Journal of Abnormal Psychology and Social Psychology*, *16*, 1–5.

Rodriguez, M. L., Mischel, W., & Shoda, Y. (1989). Cognitive person variables in the delay of gratification of older children at risk. *Journal of Personality and Social Psychology*, *57*(2), 358–367.

Rothbart, M. K., Ellis, L. K., & Posner, M. I. (2004). Temperament and self-regulation. In R. F. Baumeister & K. D. Vohs (Eds.), *Handbook of self-regulation*. New York: Guilford Press.

Shadel, W. G. (2004). Introduction to the special series: What can personality science offer cognitive-behavioral therapy and research [Special issue]? *Behavior Therapy*, *35*, 101–111.

Shoda, Y., & LeeTiernan, S. J. (2002). What remains invariant? Finding order within a person's thoughts, feelings, and behaviors across situations. In D. Cervone & W. Mischel (Eds.), *Advances in personality science* (pp. 241–270). New York: Guilford Press.

Shoda, Y., LeeTiernan, S. J., & Mischel, W. (2002). Personality as a dynamical system: Emergence of stability and consistency in intra- and inter-personal interactions. *Personality and Social Psychology Review*, *6*, 316–325.

Shoda, Y., & Mischel, W. (1998). Personality as a stable cognitive-affective activation network: Characteristic patterns of behavior variation emerge from a stable personality structure. In L. C. Miller (Ed.), *Connectionist models of social reasoning and social behavior* (pp. 175–210). Mahwah, NJ: Erlbaum.

Shoda, Y., Mischel, W., & Peake, P. (1990). Predicting adolescent cognitive and self-regulatory competencies from preschool delay of gratification: Identifying diagnostic conditions. *Developmental Psychology*, *26*(6), 978–986.

Shoda, Y., Mischel, W., & Wright, J. C. (1989). Intuitive interactionism in person perception: Effects of situation–behavior relations on dispositional judgments. *Journal of Personality and Social Psychology*, *56*, 41–53.

Shoda, Y., Mischel, W., & Wright, J. C. (1993a). Links between personality judgments and contextualized behavior patterns: Situation–behavior profiles of personality prototypes. *Social Cognition*, *4*, 399–429.

Shoda, Y., Mischel, W., & Wright, J. C. (1993b). The role of situational demands and cognitive competencies in behavior organization and personality coherence. *Journal of Personality and Social Psychology*, *65*, 1023–1035.

Shoda, Y., Mischel, W., & Wright, J. C. (1994). Intraindividual stability in the organization and patterning of behavior: Incorporating psychological situations into the ideographic analysis of personality. *Journal of Personality and Social Psychology*, *67*, 674–687.

Shoda, Y., & Smith, R. (2004). Conceptualizing personality as a cognitive affective processing system: A framework for maladaptive behavior patterns and change. *Behavior Therapy*, *35*, 147–165.

Strack, F., Schwarz, N., & Gschneidinger, E. (1985). Happiness and reminiscing: The role of time perspective, affect, and mode of thinking. *Journal of Personality and Social Psychology*, *49*, 1460–1469.

Van Mechelen, I., Bock, H.-H., & De Boeck, P. (2004). Two-mode clustering methods: A structural overview. *Statistical Methods in Medical Research*, *13*, 363–394.

Van Mechelen, I., Bock, H.-H., & De Boeck, P. (2005). Two-mode clustering methods. In B. Everitt & D. Howell (Eds.), *Encyclopedia of behavioral statistics* (pp. 2081–2086). Chichester, UK: Wiley.

Vansteelandt, K., & Van Mechelen, I. (1998). Individual differences in situation–behavior profiles: A triple typology model. *Journal of Personality and Social Psychology*, *75*, 751–765.

Winston, J. S., Strange, B. A., O'Doherty, J., & Dolan, R. J. (2002). Automatic and intentional brain responses during evaluation of trustworthiness of faces. *Nature Neuroscience*, *5*, 277–283.

Wright, J. C., & Mischel, W. (1987). A conditional approach to dispositional constructs: The local predictability of social behavior. *Journal of Personality and Social Psychology*, *53*, 1159–1177.

Wright, J. C., & Mischel, W. (1988). Conditional hedges and the intuitive psychology of traits. *Journal of Personality and Social Psychology*, *55*, 454–469.

# 21 The Social Psychology of Help Seeking

Ronda L. Dearing
Cheryl Twaragowski

This chapter concerns the social psychology of help seeking for mental health problems (including substance abuse) among adults. Before delving into the heart of the chapter, we first offer clarification regarding the scope of our discussion. For the most part, we have limited our coverage to formal/professional help seeking for a specific problem (or problems). We acknowledge that a broader definition of help seeking could include other topics, such as help for *other types of problems* (e.g., medical problems, interpersonal problems) or more detailed information about help seeking from sources other than medical or mental health professionals at *other levels* (e.g., from family, friends, clergy). Because those who study (and describe) help seeking may choose to limit their coverage differently, and because there is no single, universally accepted definition of help seeking, we draw from information on other aspects of help seeking when it could add to the readers' understanding.

Throughout our discussion, we use the term *help seeking* interchangeably with terms such as *health service use* and *treatment entry*. Often (although not always) the term *help seeking* is used to describe the process from the viewpoint of the individual (i.e., the individual differences perspective), whereas the term *health service use* often refers to a systems-level investigation of how people use existing sources of care (i.e., the health services research perspective). Our primary focus is at the level of individual differences; however, we include aspects of the health services perspective, in terms of how it can inform understanding of the behavior of *individuals within the system*.

Person-related variables and treatment-related variables are both important when studying help seeking at the individual level. Person-related variables include static characteristics (e.g., gender, race/ethnicity) and dynamic characteristics (e.g., attitudes, social networks). Treatment-related variables include aspects of treatment that affect the individual's decision about seeking help, such as cost, location, and characteristics of the treatment provider. Treatment-related variables should not be confused with the systems level of investigation that we mentioned earlier, which includes factors such as the number of treatment facilities in a given city, the average waiting time to schedule a first appointment, or the no-show rate at a specific clinic. When referring to treatment-related variables at the individual level, we are referring to how these variables come into play *for the specific person seeking help*. For example, individual-level considerations might include concerns such as whether the person can afford the cost of services or whether is it relevant that the most readily accessible treatment providers in the area are European American and the potential client is African American. Rather than viewing person-related and treatment-related variables as separate, it is probably more informative to consider the reciprocal associations between them. This interplay is consistent with a social psychological perspective on the bidirectional relations between a person and his or her environmental context. In fact, the types of variables that are relevant to help seeking—thoughts, feelings, behaviors, attitudes, and actions—are central to social psychology.

Help seeking is not limited to the moment that a person decides to seek help nor to the instant that he or she schedules an appointment; rather, help seeking is best understood as a process that encompasses all of the events related to recognizing the need for help, making a decision to change, deciding to get outside help, and obtaining needed treatment (Saunders, Zygowicz, & D'Angelo, 2006; see also, Prochaska & Prochaska, Chapter 23, this volume). Most of our discussion is limited to single episodes of help seeking (whether it is the person's first time in treatment or a subsequent episode), but we acknowledge that any treatment episode is likely to influence subsequent help-seeking events. We focus our discussion on events leading up to the first appointment, except when discussing service use models that include factors beyond the first appointment and when presenting the clinical implications of help-seeking research. For readers interested in treatment engagement (Horvath & Symonds, 1991; Meier, Barrowclough, & Donmall, 2005) and treatment retention (Bornovalova & Daughters, 2007; Stark, 1992; Wierzbicki & Pekarik, 1993), useful information can be found in the sources cited here.

Models of help seeking usually can be applied equally well to mental health and substance abuse services, although some models have been more commonly applied to one or the other (e.g., the stages-of-change model has more often been used to investigate help seeking for substance abuse). Although there are many similarities between help seeking for mental health problems and help seeking for substance abuse problems, there are also some notable differences. We have attempted to highlight these differences throughout the chapter.

Because of space limitations, we cannot give full coverage to all of the many topics that are potentially relevant to help seeking. For example, we acknowledge that our distinction between mental health problems and medical health problems is somewhat arbitrary, especially because mental health and medical health are both better understood as interrelated biopsychosocial processes. Furthermore, although out-of-pocket cost, managed care, and insurance coverage (or lack thereof) are likely to influence help-seeking decisions, we have opted to mostly disregard these topics because any attempt to cover them would be superficial.

## SPECIFIC VARIABLES RELEVANT TO HELP SEEKING

Because many of the variables we discuss are interrelated, investigation of the relationships of specific variables to treatment entry is of limited benefit without taking into account other variables known to influence help seeking. For example, it is inadequate to state that women are more likely than men to seek help for major depressive disorder without noting the higher prevalence of the disorder among women. The models of help seeking that we present later in the chapter are more informative than the specific variables because they integrate the variables in ways that can enhance our understanding of the broader picture of the help-seeking process. As we show, *attitude* toward obtaining help for problems can affect the tendency to seek mental health services, with positive attitudes predicting a greater tendency to seek help (Cramer, 1999; Diala et al., 2000). Because attitude often is dependent upon other variables (e.g., problem severity, gender, age, race/ethnicity), we present findings concerning attitude toward seeking help in the sections for each specific variable rather than in a separate section.

### Problem Severity, Perceived Need, and Treatment Delay

Perhaps the most important predictors of help seeking are level of distress and perceived need (Pescosolido & Boyer, 1999). The worse people feel, the more likely they are to seek help. For example, in a nationwide household survey of mental illness, severity of diagnosis and having multiple diagnoses were associated with greater likelihood of service use and greater number of appointments (Kessler et al., 1999). Similarly, self-reports of a high level of distress in a sample of college students were positively related to intention to seek help (Cramer, 1999). Moreover, a commonly cited reason for not seeking therapy is lack of perceived need (Wells, Robins, Bushnell, Jarosz, & Oakley-Browne, 1994).

However, a perceived need for treatment does not necessarily result in immediate help seeking. There are often lengthy delays between acknowledging a need for help and seeking services. For example, in one study of individuals entering treatment at a community mental health center (Saunders, 1993), 48% of participants indicated that they had been distressed for more than 2 years by the problem for which they were seeking help. Furthermore, after deciding that therapy would help, 50% of individuals waited at least a month to decide to enter therapy. Individuals with addiction problems often wait even longer to seek help, with up to a decade being the typical amount of time from problem recognition to entering treatment (e.g., Hasin, Stinson, Ogburn, & Grant, 2007; Simpson & Tucker, 2002).

### Gender

Research has demonstrated that women are more likely than men to seek professional help for medical care (Green & Pope, 1999), mental health problems (Diala et al., 2000; Kushner & Sher, 1989), and preventive services (Galdas, Cheater, & Marshall, 2005). Women use more health services overall (including services that are not sex-specific), even when controlling for age, education, self-reported health status, reported mental and physical health symptoms, and health-related concerns (Green & Pope, 1999). Women are more likely to report having mental health symptoms (Green & Pope, 1999), to perceive a need for mental health assistance (Rabinowitz, Gross, & Feldman, 1999), and to have more favorable attitudes toward psychological help seeking (Kelly & Achter, 1995; Leong & Zachar, 1999). However, when experiencing emotional distress, women are more likely than men to visit a general practitioner, whereas men are more likely than women to turn to a mental health care professional (Leaf et al., 1988; Tijhuis, Peters, & Foets, 1990; Wang et al., 2005). Findings have been mixed regarding help seeking for alcohol and substance abuse problems, with some studies showing that men are more likely to use services (Kaskutas, Weisner, & Caetano, 1997), and other studies not finding differences by gender (Hser, Maglione, Polinsky, & Anglin, 1998).

In a review of health-related help-seeking behavior, Galdas and colleagues (2005) outlined several explanations for differences between men's and women's use of services. The authors suggested that gender differences in help-seeking behavior cannot be fully understood without also investigating other variables such as socialization, socioeconomic status, and specific career and lifestyle choices of men and women. For example, men are traditionally discouraged from acknowledging that they are experiencing any type of pain and even more so from admitting to emotional distress and needing help. Consequently, men may be more likely than women to try to normalize and minimize their discomfort, whereas women may be more comfortable than men asking for help or seeking treatment (Galdas et al., 2005).

## Age

The relation between age and mental health help seeking is not well understood. People over 65 years of age describe themselves as less informed about mental health and less knowledgeable about when to contact a mental health professional, as compared to people younger than 65 (Robb, Haley, Becker, Polivka, & Chwa, 2003). However, a study contrasting younger (ages 17–26) and older adults (ages 60–95) found that the two groups did not differ in their self-reported *willingness* to seek help for a mental health problem (Segal, Coolidge, Mincic, & O'Riley, 2005). There have been mixed findings regarding age-related perceived need for mental health care. In one study, Rabinowitz and colleagues (1999) found that older age was related to a greater perceived need for mental health services. In contrast, Klap, Unroe, and Unützer (2003) found that individuals over 65 reported lower perceived need compared to younger and middle-age adults, even when comparing among those diagnosed with a mental health disorder.

Some early studies found a curvilinear relationship between age and mental health service use and attitudes. Older and younger individuals reported more negative attitudes (Surgenor, 1985) toward seeking mental health services and were less likely to seek help (Shapiro et al., 1984), whereas individuals in the middle range (roughly 25–64) had more positive attitudes and were more likely to seek services. However, more recent studies show that younger people are more likely to use mental health services than are older people (Kessler, Olfson, & Berglund, 1998; Robb et al., 2003). Individuals under 65 were twice as likely (43%) to have seen a mental health practitioner in their lifetime than individuals over 65 (21.5%; Robb et al., 2003).

Although the available data are not definitive, two possible interpretations of differing use patterns by age include cohort effects and the influence of financial resources on help seeking. The age-related findings suggest that people born in the first half of the 20th century are less likely to seek specialty mental health services than people born in the latter half of the 20th century. Reasons for this discontinuity may include differing attitudes about the implications of admitting a need for help with problems, differing levels of knowledge about available services, and differing levels of perceived stigma regarding mental health issues. In addition to the probable cohort effect, few studies account for whether availability of financial resources influences help-seeking patterns by age. Individuals in their middle years are more likely to be well established in the workforce, giving them greater financial freedom than individuals in their early 20s or older retired individuals. Two other areas warranting further investigation are that older people may be more likely to seek out mental health care from a primary care physician than from a mental health specialist, and older people may have greater concerns about whether mental health services would be covered by their insurance plan or by Medicare (Robb et al., 2003).

## Race and Ethnicity

Patterns of help seeking among various racial and ethnic groups are complex and must be interpreted in light of potential underlying differences in socioeconomic status and differing prevalence, by group, of various disorders. Many studies of help seeking do not account for these potentially confounding variables. Although a comprehensive portrayal of the various ethnic/racial trends in help seeking is beyond the scope of this chapter, a few findings are worth noting. More detailed information can be found in Harris, Edlund, and Larson (2005).

Harris and colleagues (2005) used a large national survey dataset to investigate racial and ethnic differences in the occurrence of mental health problems and service use. Determination of problems was derived from participant reports of one or more symptoms based on the fourth edition of the *Diagnostic and Statistical Manual of Mental Disorders* (DSM-IV; American Psychiatric Association, 1994) criteria and a screening for serious mental illness (SMI). We focus our attention on the three (of nine) most prevalent groups in the sample: non-Hispanic European Americans (hereafter referred to as European Americans), African Americans, and Mexican Americans. African Americans and Mexican Americans reported a lower likelihood of having at least one mental health symptom, a lower likelihood of meeting criteria for SMI, and lower overall use of services than did European Americans. Considering only those individuals with one or more mental health symptoms, African Americans and Mexican Americans reported lower use of mental health services than European Americans. This difference was also found when restricting the sample to only those participants diagnosed with SMI. Self-reported unmet need did not differ among the three groups. These findings generally persisted (but were sometimes attenuated) when controlling for an assortment of variables, including sociodemographic characteristics, physical health status, and drug or alcohol dependence.

Consistent with the above findings, research has repeatedly demonstrated lower prevalence of mental health disorders and less usage of mental health services among African Americans than among European Americans (e.g., Kessler et al., 1994). Another large nationally-representative sample was used to further explore differences between European Americans and African Americans on mental health care attitudes and usage patterns (Diala et al., 2000). African Americans were less likely to use mental health services overall and when diagnosed with major depressive episode (MDE) than were European Americans (despite similar prevalence of MDE). Among individuals who *had not* received mental health services in the past 12 months, African Americans reported more positive attitudes in terms of comfort with seeking care and inclination to seek care than their European American counterparts. However, among individuals who *had* sought any mental health treatment in the past 12 months, African Americans reported more negative attitudes than did European Americans. These findings are not well understood, but they suggest that negative attitudes do not account for lower use of services among African Americans, and they imply that African Americans are less satisfied with the mental health services they receive than are European Americans (Diala et al., 2000).

### History of Prior Service Use

Prior treatment is assumed to influence help seeking in a positive direction; indeed, research has demonstrated a positive relationship between prior mental health services and favorable attitudes toward therapy (Fischer & Farina, 1995; Tijhuis et al., 1990). However, Saunders (1993) found that a history of mental health treatment was not related to the difficulty (or elapsed time) of recognizing a problem, deciding that therapy might be helpful, deciding to seek therapy, or making an appointment to begin therapy. These findings are somewhat surprising because it would seem likely that if an individual had previously been through the process of deciding to seek therapy (especially for a related problem), he or she might recognize the problem and the need for help more quickly. However, Saunders's results suggest that the difficulty of each step is similar for a first or a subsequent help-seeking event. In contrast to seeking help for mental health problems, when considering seeking help for alcohol problems, prior treatment was found to be a strong positive predictor of subsequent use of outpatient services and self-help groups (Freyer et al., 2007).

### Social Networks

Social networks were first identified as contributing to help-seeking attitudes and behaviors in classic studies by Andersen (as cited in Andersen, 1995) and Kadushin (as cited in Saunders, 1993), and most subsequent models have attempted to account for social influences. Pescosolido (1991) aptly summarizes the relevance of social networks as follows: "The importance of understanding a particular medical care decision [is] embedded in a social process where individuals' network ties not only provide support and advice during illness episodes but are the sources of beliefs, attitudes and knowledge about medical options, their availability, and the seriousness of the medical condition" (p. 162). Pescosolido, Wright, Alegría, and Vera (1998) cite research demonstrating that social network influences sometimes facilitate and other times impede help seeking. Pescosolido and colleagues suggest that in addition to measuring the size and density of an individual's social network, studies should also evaluate whether, when a need arises, the social network steps in to provide informal help (if the social norm is to be wary of professional help) or whether the social network encourages help seeking (if the social norm includes positive beliefs about professional help).

Other explanations for the differing effects of social networks on help seeking may be that social networks serve different functions at different points in the help-seeking process, or that social networks function differently depending on level of distress. For example, Saunders (1993) found that efforts to obtain help from one's informal network resulted in a longer time to recognize a problem. Conversely, individuals who sought informal help took less time to decide to seek therapy (Saunders, 1993). Cramer (1999) speculated that at low levels of distress, the support of an informal network may be sufficient to preclude formal help seeking, whereas if distress is high, one's social support network may encourage formal help seeking.

## Coercion

*Individual choice* and *coercion* can be conceptualized as being at opposite ends of a continuum. Coerced treatment includes treatment entry that is "influenced" or "controlled" by someone other than the patient (Gardner et al., 1993). Entering treatment may be based on the choice of the individual or may be attributable to some form of coercion. Most treatment "choices" fall somewhere between these two extremes. When discussing coercion, the term *treatment entry* may be more appropriate, because *help seeking* implies individual choice. Coercion is often characterized as legal (also referred to as *formal* or *hard* coercion) versus extralegal (also referred to as *informal* or *soft* coercion; Gardner et al., 1993; Pescosolido, Brooks Gardner, & Lubell, 1998). *Legal coercion* can include involuntary hospitalization (such as in cases of suicidality or homicidality), court-mandated treatment, and recommendations by an attorney (e.g., as a means of getting a lesser sentence). Sources of *extralegal coercion* may include employers, family members, and friends. In many cases, the distinction between individual choice and coercion is somewhat ambiguous. Pescosolido, Brooks Gardner, and colleagues (1998) suggest two other possible paths into treatment: "muddling through" and "supported choice." In cases of *muddling through*, the individual does not make an active choice to enter treatment, but he or she does not refuse or resist either. Such individuals might be thought of as acquiescing to treatment. This type of treatment entry sometimes occurs when the patient's family becomes concerned and makes arrangements for the patient to enter treatment. *Supported choice* includes decisions that are assisted by the patient's social network. For example, the patient's family may encourage him or her to enter treatment and may offer to help find appropriate services.

Coercion frequently plays a role in treatment entry for mental health or substance abuse problems, whereas it is less likely to be a factor when obtaining medical care (especially acute medical care). Coercion is seldom considered in the commonly used models of help seeking because of the medical origin of such models (Pescosolido, Brooks Gardner et al., 1998). As we have demonstrated in our review of specific contributing factors to entering treatment, the help-seeking literature has some inconsistencies (e.g., some studies find effects whereas others do not). Although methodological differences likely account for some of these conflicting findings, Pescosolido and colleagues (1998) point out that most studies do not account for voluntary versus coerced paths to service entry. These two paths may involve very different individual-level processes, yet differences may "wash out" in analyses that do not allow for the possibility of coercion. Therefore, Pescosolido and colleagues suggest that models that include coercion would more accurately portray the help-seeking process.

## Stigma

Stigma is another contributing factor that prevents people from seeking treatment. In a review of how stigma interferes with mental health care, Corrigan (2004; Corrigan, Larson, & Kuwabara, Chapter 4, this volume) describes how both public stigma and self-stigma can negatively affect a person who is experiencing symptoms of emotional distress. *Public stigma* involves being pejoratively labeled as mentally ill, which can result in prejudice, stereotypes, and discrimination. Common public stereotypic views include false beliefs that people with mental illnesses are violent, are incompetent, or are to blame for their illness. These mistaken views can result in discrimination in the everyday lives of people with mental illnesses, such as when applying for jobs or renting property. Furthermore, individuals with a mental health diagnosis may receive fewer medical services and less insurance benefits than people who are not labeled as mentally ill. Concerns about public stigma may interfere with help seeking if the perceived benefits of treatment do not outweigh the potential costs of disclosing mental distress and obtaining help (Corrigan, 2004; Corrigan, Larson, & Kuwabara, Chapter 4, this volume). *Self-stigma* occurs when the individual internalizes the stereotypic and prejudicial beliefs of society. These internalized beliefs can have a negative effect on one's sense of self, including a diminished sense of self-esteem and decreased feelings of self-efficacy. Individuals with self-stigma concerning mental illness may view themselves as worthless and incapable of successfully performing certain tasks or behaviors. These feelings can interfere with a person's goals and quality of life and, as with public stigma, concerns about viewing oneself as mentally ill can interfere with help seeking (Corrigan, 2004).

## THEORIES AND MODELS OF HELP SEEKING

Now that we have presented a few of the specific concepts that are important to understanding help seeking, we turn to an introduction of the commonly used theories and models of entering treatment. Each of these theories and models offers a unique framework for integrating an assortment of factors contributing to help-seeking behavior.

### Behavioral Model

Andersen's early work (as discussed in Andersen, 1995) on health care utilization was instrumental in identifying the role of social context in health care decision making. Andersen's behavioral model (also called the socio-behavioral model) has gone through multiple iterations and has had a profound influence on more recent models of health care utilization (Aday & Awe, 1997). Original elements of the model included *predisposing characteristics* (e.g., demographics, social structure, health beliefs), *enabling resources* of the individual and the community (e.g., personal knowledge, financial resources, insurance coverage, availability of health care facilities), and *need* (perceived and evaluated), as they relate to the use of health services. Subsequent revisions of the model have incorporated aspects of the health care system (policy, resources, organization), services used (type, purpose, time interval; Andersen & Newman, as cited in Andersen, 1995), consumer satisfaction, site of services (Aday & Andersen, 1974), and, later, outcome of treatment (Andersen, 1995).

Various versions of the behavioral model have been applied to an array of help-seeking contexts (e.g., dental care, prescription drug use, mental health, substance abuse), to the help-seeking behaviors of many specific populations (e.g., the homeless, various minority groups, the elderly, veterans), and to cross-national comparisons of help seeking (Aday & Awe, 1997). The initial and later behavioral models have been used in the evaluation of equitable access to care, both in terms of whether those who need care obtain it and in terms of fair distribution of limited health care resources (Aday & Awe, 1997). Andersen's most recent model (1995), deemed the "emerging model," includes feedback loops to represent how treatment outcome influences later health behavior, predisposing factors, and perceived need for services. Concurrent research has proposed a more complex model, the expanded access framework, that also incorporates the elements of quality of life, equity, efficiency, and effectiveness (Aday & Awe, 1997).

A few concerns about the behavioral model have been noted. In particular, the model includes the independent effects of a large number of variables (which require large datasets and complex statistics), but does not account for how the variables may interact with one another to affect decision making. Furthermore, some critics of the behavioral model have indicated that it places too much emphasis on perceived need as a predictor of help seeking. Finally, as with many health behavior models, the behavioral model is limited in its ability to accurately predict help-seeking behavior (Aday & Awe, 1997; Andersen, 1995).

## Health Belief Model

The health belief model (HBM) was initially conceptualized in the 1950s and has remained one of the most influential conceptual models of health behavior. It was originally created to better understand people's behavior with regard to participation in prevention and early detection programs, but the model quickly evolved to investigate people's actions in response to symptoms or to being diagnosed with an illness. Protection motivation theory (PMT; see Rogers & Prentice-Dunn, 1997) is very similar to the HBM; however, we were not able to find any studies that used PMT to investigate help-seeking behavior. Our coverage of the HBM is based on a chapter by Strecher, Champion, and Rosenstock (1997), all of whom have been actively involved in the development and/or evolution of the model.

The HBM framework is perhaps best understood in terms of *value-expectancy theory*. When applied to health behaviors, value-expectancy theory includes the *value* of preventing illness (or recovering from illness) combined with the *expectancy* that one can take specific action to avoid becoming ill (or to recover). Additional factors relevant to the HBM include the individual's perception of personal *susceptibility*, the perceived *severity* (or potential severity) of the condition, the perceived *benefits* of personal action to prevent or avoid the condition, and *self-efficacy*, which is the belief that one can effectively engage in the desired action. In many cases, health actions have associated *perceived barriers* (i.e., negative consequences), such as cost, time, unpleasant side effects, and inconvenience. In the context of the HBM, any individual decision to take health action occurs when perceived benefits outweigh perceived barriers.

The current version of the HBM would predict that people will engage in a specific health behavior if they believe that they are susceptible to the specific illness, that the consequences of having the illness are severe, and that the specific health behavior will lessen their susceptibility or lessen the severity of the condition. With regard to help seeking, in order to take action an individual must believe (or acknowledge) that he or she has an illness (perceived susceptibility), that leaving the illness untreated has potential consequences, that obtaining help will result in a positive outcome, and that he or she is capable of engaging in the necessary action (e.g., participating in therapy, reducing drinking, complying with a medication regimen).

The HBM has considerable empirical support as applied to a wide array of health behaviors. The greatest limitation of research pertaining to the HBM concerns inconsistencies in the measurement of relevant concepts. Effective testing of the model requires that assessment instruments be specific to the behavior of interest (e.g., a study of help seeking for depression would need to measure whether the individual thinks that therapy can be useful *for reducing symptoms of depression*); however, various studies have used differing operational definitions of the relevant constructs, which makes it difficult to compare across studies. Another concern about the model (and most models of health behavior) is that it is limited in its ability to predict actual health behaviors, help seeking or otherwise (Strecher et al., 1997).

### Theory of Reasoned Action and Theory of Planned Behavior

The theory of reasoned action (TRA; Fishbein & Ajzen, as cited in Maddux & DuCharme, 1997) and its successor, the theory of planned behavior (TPB; Ajzen, 1991), are not specific to health behaviors, but were developed to study the general relations between attitudes and behaviors. However, because the TRA and the TPB are often mentioned with regard to help-seeking behaviors, we provide a brief overview of these theories. Our discussion is based primarily on a summary by Maddux and DuCharme (1997).

The basis for the TRA is that *intentions* are the most accurate predictor of whether an individual will perform a specific behavior. Because intentions may not be known (or may be difficult to measure accurately), they can be evaluated as a function of the individual's *attitude toward the behavior* in combination with *perceived social norms*. Attitudes about a specific behavior are formed based on the *expected outcome* of engaging in the behavior and the *subjective value* of that outcome. Social norms can be understood as a combination of *normative beliefs* (i.e., whether important social contacts believe that the individual should perform the behavior) and *motivation to comply* (i.e., the importance the individual places on the reactions of important social contacts). To sum up the TRA, "People will perform behaviors that they value highly and that are popular with others and will refrain from behaviors that they do not regard favorably and that are unpopular with others" (Petty & Cacioppo, 1996, p. 193). According to the TRA, variables other than attitude and social norms, such as demographic variables, are only relevant to the extent that specific variables result in differing attitudes. For example, men and women may hold different attitudes about the importance of seeking help for anxiety, which in turn may affect intention and behavior.

The TPB is identical to the TRA with the added dimension of *perceived behavioral control*, which is conceptually similar to *self-efficacy*. Specifically, perceived behavioral control is the individual's belief that he or she can control (or execute) the behavior of interest. Whereas the TRA assumes that the individual has full volitional control over the behavior, the construct of perceived behavioral control allows the TPB to extend to behaviors that involve varying degrees of choice.

With relation to help seeking from the perspective of the TRA, whether an individual seeks psychotherapy (for example) depends on (1) the expectation that therapy will result in an improvement of symptoms (expected outcome), (2) the value of having an improvement in symptoms (value of the outcome), (3) the belief that important others think he or she should enter therapy (normative beliefs), and (4) the value the individual places on what important others think (motivation to comply). From the perspective of the TPB, it would also be important to know whether the individual believes that he or she has the necessary resources (e.g., monetary and psychological resources) to participate in, and benefit from, therapy.

The TRA and the TPB are applicable to a wide range of behaviors and have withstood rigorous testing. The addition of behavioral intention in the TPB has resulted in enhanced prediction of behavior, as compared to the TRA. Limitations of these theories are mostly related to measurement. In particular, measurement of intention and behavior must be close in time, must be defined similarly, and must be equally precise (Sutton, 1998). Another concern is that measurement of behavioral intention may influence subsequent behavior (Ogden, 2003).

## Network-Episode Model

The network-episode model (NEM; Pescosolido, 1991) is based on the central premise that health care decisions involve a dynamic social process influenced by an individual's social network, his or her community ties, and the services that are available. Pescosolido suggests that although most decision-making models focus on individual choice (often referred to as *rational choice models*), health care decisions are probably more accurately viewed as a combination of individual choice and social influence. The NEM is dynamic in that the focus includes patterns of help seeking within an illness episode and the reciprocal interactions among four broad constructs: social content, social support system, the "illness career" (i.e., all help-seeking events related to a particular illness), and the treatment system.

*Social content* includes demographic characteristics, personal health history, nature of the illness, and organizational constraints such as financing and accessibility. The *social support system* is highly individualized and can include close contacts (e.g., family, friends), community resources (e.g., clergy), and existing relationships with health care providers. Important aspects of the social support system that can influence help seeking include the number, closeness, and reciprocity of network ties; the beliefs and attitudes held by the social support network; and the types of information, advice, and support offered by the network. The *illness career* not only includes timing and sequence of help sought for the specific episode of illness (e.g., the individual might seek help from family members, then a primary care physician, and finally a psychologist for a specific episode of depression), but also the associated roles related to the illness (e.g., patient role, chronic illness role). The *treatment system* includes types of care available, location of services, who has access to services, and characteristics of the providers.

The main assets of the NEM include its unique focus on social (rather than individual) decision making and its inclusion of multiple help-seeking behaviors within a given illness episode. Because the NEM includes such a comprehensive set of factors that can influence help seeking, it is a useful heuristic model. However, these conceptual strengths also add a level of analytic complexity that make the model difficult to test, as the developer of the model acknowledges in her statement: "Clearly, no multivariate technique could deal with the long list of possibilities and the 'thin cells' that result in many of the pathways" (Pescosolido, 2000, p. 192). This practical limitation may explain why relatively few studies have attempted to investigate help seeking from a network episode perspective. However, the results of these studies have offered unique insights about pathways to care (Bussing, Koro-Ljungberg, Gary, Mason, & Garvan, 2005; Lindsey et al., 2006; Pescosolido, 2000; Pescosolido, Wright, et al., 1998).

## Process of Seeking Treatment Model

The process of seeking treatment model (PSTM; S. Saunders, personal communication, March 28, 2007) was developed to help explain decisions to enter psychotherapy and substance abuse treatment (Saunders, 1993, 1996; Saunders et al., 2006). The PSTM proposes that once a problem develops, the process of seeking help can be characterized by four sequential steps: (1) recognizing the problem, (2) deciding that change is needed (and/or that treatment might help), (3) deciding to seek formal treatment, and (4) contacting the mental health system. An individual may encounter barriers at any of the steps, which can derail the process from proceeding further (Saunders et al., 2006). For example, denial (or lack of awareness) that a problem exists will result in failure to recognize a problem. Downplaying the severity of the problem or attributing the problem to external factors can result in a failure to decide that change is needed. Deciding to work on the problem without formal help would negate the decision to get professional help. Many factors can disrupt the process before the individual contacts the mental health system, such as a belief that the barriers to entering treatment are too great, ongoing efforts to change the problem without assistance, or resolution of the problem prior to seeking services. Saunders's test of the PSTM among individuals entering a community mental health center demonstrated that the problem recognition step took the most time to achieve and was perceived as the most difficult (1993).

The PSTM is well suited to the idea of help seeking as a socially influenced process, and Saunders's work has demonstrated that seeking help from informal sources influences each of the four steps. Receiving help from others was endorsed by over 50% of individuals for each of the steps in the process of entering therapy; nearly 75% of individuals entering treatment indicated that they had sought informal help related to at least two of the steps (Saunders, 1996). The PSTM shows promise, but will require further testing to evaluate its usefulness.

### Stages-of-Change Model

One relevant model that has been applied infrequently to help-seeking behaviors is the stages-of-change (SOC) or transtheoretical model (Prochaska & DiClemente, 1982; Prochaska, DiClemente, & Norcross, 1992; Prochaska & Prochaska, Chapter 23, this volume). This model was developed to explain people's decisions and actions related to changing addictive and maladaptive behaviors (Prochaska et al., 1992; Prochaska, Norcross, & DiClemente, 1994). The five stages of change include precontemplation, contemplation, preparation, action, and maintenance. (A four-stage variation of the model does not include the preparation stage.) These stages are not mutually exclusive; with regard to a particular targeted behavior (e.g., drug addiction), an individual may exhibit behaviors characteristic of more than one stage. Individuals use different combinations of coping strategies at each stage of the change process, and certain coping strategies are more effective depending on the individual's current motivational level (Prochaska et al., 1994).

Three studies have demonstrated that readiness to change and readiness to seek treatment are related yet distinct variables among problem drinkers (Freyer et al., 2004), alcohol-dependent individuals (Freyer et al., 2005), and dually diagnosed individuals (Heesch, Velasquez, & von Sternberg, 2005). Furthermore, in a study of medical hospital admissions among people with alcohol problems, individuals in the preparation stage (with regard to alcohol-related treatment) were five to six times more likely to enter inpatient treatment for their alcohol problem in the year following the initial assessment, as compared to individuals in the precontemplation or contemplation stages (Freyer et al., 2007). These findings suggest that the SOC model might be useful for conceptualizing the differences between those who "need help" but do not acknowledge a problem (precontemplators), as compared to those who perceive a need for help and are considering entering therapy (contemplators). The preparation stage may relate to deciding to seek therapy and researching what services are available. The action stage seems akin to entering treatment, and the maintenance stage may relate to deciding to remain in therapy (or to sustaining a successful outcome). The SOC model, although often useful clinically, can be difficult to test because the stages may not be mutually exclusive. The development of assessment instruments that conceptualize motivational readiness as a continuous construct, rather than as discrete stages, may need to be explored (see Carey, Purnine, Maisto, & Carey, 1999).

## OVERVIEW AND ANALYSIS

All of the models presented lend unique insight into our understanding of the help-seeking process. However, some of the models have become increasingly complex in an attempt to incorporate every aspect of health care utilization, such as individual choice, coercion, satisfaction, outcome, health policy, illness career, and so forth. It is unlikely that any model could account for all aspects of help seeking, and it is our belief that some of these constructs (e.g., outcome and satisfaction) go beyond the realm of help seeking per se. From the standpoint of simplicity, we found the NEM and the recent revisions of the behavioral model to be a bit overwhelming. Furthermore, in our presentation of the various models, we noted some measurement concerns that have yet to be resolved concerning the HBM, the TRA, the TPB, and the SOC model. In particular, the HBM, the TRA, and the TPB lack uniformly agreed-upon operationalization of relevant constructs. The SOC model is problematic because current assessment instruments tend to measure motivation in terms of discrete stages, rather than as a continuous construct. We think that the PSTM is commendable in that it includes the most salient constructs, depicts help seeking as a dynamic process that may or may not end in a help-seeking event, allows for the influence of external forces (e.g., social network, courts, coercion), and appears practical from a measurement standpoint. However, as previously mentioned, the PSTM requires more rigorous empirical testing.

Scientific inquiry into help seeking has most often focused on individuals *who enter treatment*. Unquestionably, information gathered from such investigations is useful for understanding the factors that lead to treatment entry. However, some studies have suggested that as few as 20% of individuals with a major mental disorder seek professional help (Kessler et al., 1994; Kushner & Sher, 1991), despite considerable evidence that treatment is beneficial (e.g., Miller, Walters, & Bennett, 2001; Seligman, 1995). Therefore, it is also important to study people who need but do not seek treatment for their problems—individuals who constitute the "service gap" (Stefl & Prosperi, 1985) of unmet mental health need. Considering the point of view of help seekers *and* individuals in the service gap will lead to a more comprehensive understanding of the facilitating factors and obstacles related to help seeking. We are not trying to suggest that everyone with a mental health problem *should* seek help. There are instances when help seeking may not be the best course of action for a given individual—self-change, for many people, results in successful outcomes (see Sobell, Ellingstad, & Sobell, 2000).

## BROAD APPLICATIONS

Findings from help-seeking research can be used to enhance mental health service access and to encourage treatment (or earlier treatment) for those in need. For instance, information concerning groups who seek help at lower rates (e.g., men, African Americans) should lead to more detailed investigations of why this is the case. Results of these studies could be used to implement policies, information campaigns, and treatment programs that facilitate access, decrease barriers, and appeal to a range of differing needs and preferences.

Corrigan (2004; Corrigan, Larson, & Kuwabara, Chapter 4, this volume) asserts that stigma and related negative attitudes concerning mental health problems and mental health treatment act as obstacles to use of existing services. He proposes the use of public education to reduce stigma as a means of increasing help seeking. Vogel, Wade, and Hackler (2007) suggest that in addition to a focus on education, such campaigns should attempt to reduce the shame, self-blame, and stigma that may be experienced by people suffering from a mental illness. Various media sources can be used to decrease stigma and to provide educational information regarding mental health problems and the effectiveness and availability of treatments. Public information campaigns can be delivered using television, radio, billboards, the Internet, mass mailings, and pamphlets in primary care settings and emergency rooms. Because of the social influences on help seeking, such campaigns should be directed not only toward the intended client but also toward "important others" who may influence help-seeking decisions. At the public policy level, it is essential to implement guidelines that eliminate discriminatory disparities in access to services (e.g., related to race/ethnicity, sex, age). Similarly, policies should ensure parity of the mental health services that insurance plans are required to cover and that public assistance programs are obligated to provide.

Individual clinics and practitioners should consider whether the services offered by their practice are likely to meet the needs of specific underserved groups. Practices might consider bolstering the range of services offered and might consider implementing "low-threshold" services, such as walk-in clinics, when feasible. Front-line practitioners (e.g., primary care and emergency room physicians) can also help in the effort to destigmatize and normalize mental health treatment services. They should have readily available referral networks that include a variety of specialty mental health practitioners to meet the needs of those clients who raise concerns about mental health problems (or who are identified as having a mental heath problem based on routine screening procedures). Referrals should include routine follow-up to inquire whether the client scheduled and attended an appointment in the specialty sector. These and other efforts should help to increase help seeking at the individual and societal level.

## CLINICAL IMPLICATIONS

We suspect that our review of the various variables, theories, and models relevant to seeking help may seem overwhelming from the perspective of practical clinical implications. However, the take-home message is relatively straightforward: Seeking help for a mental health problem is a difficult and individualized decision that is influenced by a host of internal and external contributing factors. Therefore, when working with clients, it is important to keep in mind several factors. Namely, (1) the client entering treatment is likely to have struggled with his or her decision to seek help; (2) each individual comes to treatment with a unique set of factors that contributed to his or her decision to enter treatment; (3) external influences, such as social network and societal factors, likely played a role in the individual's decision to seek services and are likely to play a role in the client's decisions to continue in treatment. Keeping these considerations in mind, the clinician should attempt to gain an understanding of the multiplicity of competing forces that contributed to the client's decision to enter treatment and should attempt to reinforce the client's decision to seek help and to remain in treatment. In particular, the clinician should emphasize the potential benefits of treatment in order to retain the client in therapy and to enhance the client's self-efficacy for achieving a successful outcome. Furthermore, the clinician could attempt to gather information regarding the client's difficulties when deciding to seek treatment. This information concerning the client's struggles to initiate change could then be used to inform the process of treatment. Even if the client does not return to treatment after the first appointment, a single clinical encounter is likely to influence the client's future help-seeking behavior. Therefore, every client contact can be an opportunity for the therapist to demonstrate the potential benefits of treatment. If the client has a positive help-seeking experience, his or her future decisions to enter treatment are likely to be easier. As a way of illustrating these clinical implications, we present a clinical vignette in the next section of the process of deciding to seek help for a woman with problems related to drinking.

## Clinical Vignette

Although she had been a social drinker since her late teens, Mary began drinking heavily after she was laid off from her job as a pharmaceutical sales representative at age 28. Her unsuccessful attempts to find work resulted in feelings of depression, and she often tried to dull the pain by drinking in the evenings. Many nights she drank a half gallon bottle of wine before passing out on her couch. Mary woke up most mornings feeling miserable, and the only way she could get her hands to stop shaking was to have an early morning drink. As this pattern continued and she became more and more socially isolated, Mary's family began to worry. When family members tried to talk to Mary about her drinking, she shrugged off their concerns. However, despite wanting to put up a good front for her family, Mary knew she had a problem. She was uncertain about whether treatment was the right answer because she had a cousin who had been through numerous treatment programs with limited success. She was also concerned about how she would afford a treatment program. The last few times Mary had seen her primary care physician, the doctor had cautioned her about the potential long-term health consequences associated with heavy drinking. In addition to concerns about her health, Mary realized that she would never be able to find a stable job if her drinking continued. The final straw occurred when Mary had a near miss while driving to the liquor store after running out of wine. She ran her car off the side of the road in order to avoid hitting another car. Although there was no damage to the car and Mary was not hurt, she was very shaken up by what could have happened. For several weeks, Mary tried to cut back on her drinking, but she soon realized that she was not going to be able to make the necessary changes on her own. She attended an Alcoholics Anonymous (AA) meeting, but she was reluctant to label herself as an alcoholic, and she decided that the meetings just weren't for her. Mary finally shared her concerns with her best friend, JoAnne. Mary acknowledged that she needed help to change her drinking, but she confided that she was afraid of what people would think of her if she entered a treatment program. JoAnne was supportive of Mary's decision to change, and she offered to help Mary find a suitable treatment program. JoAnne also related a story of a friend who had a similar problem and who had turned his life around by entering treatment. After they researched and found a nearby sliding-fee-scale treatment facility, JoAnne handed Mary the phone to call and schedule her first appointment.

## Conceptualization of Mary's Help Seeking Using the PSTM

Readers may find it useful to consider Mary's help-seeking process from the perspective of the various theories and models of help seeking that have been presented in this chapter. We will provide one such interpretation using the PSTM. Recall that the PSTM consists of four sequential steps: (1) recognizing the problem, (2) deciding that change is needed, (3) deciding to seek help in therapy or formal treatment, and (4) contacting the mental health system (Saunders et al., 2006).

After a prolonged period of unemployment and daily heavy alcohol consumption, Mary's drinking was interfering in numerous areas of her life. Mary *recognized that she had a problem* well before she acknowledged that she might need help in order to change. During the recognition phase, Mary vaguely considered treatment as a means of changing her drinking, but she had doubts about whether treatment was the right answer. She made the conscious *decision that she needed to change* her behavior subsequent to a frightening experience while driving under the influence. Mary's initial attempts to change her drinking on her own were unsuccessful. She eventually *decided that she was going to need outside help*, at which point she attended an AA meeting. AA did not seem to be a good fit for Mary, but she then reached out to her friend, JoAnne, who helped to allay some of Mary's concerns about treatment. With JoAnne's help and support, Mary *scheduled her first treatment appointment* at an affordable facility. It is evident at each of the steps that Mary's help-seeking process was socially influenced: Her family expressed concern, her doctor warned her about the potential health risks, others' experiences in therapy influenced her views of the benefits (and potential drawbacks) of treatment, she was concerned about how others would react to her being in treatment, and her friend ultimately helped her find an appropriate source of formal help.

For the purpose of this chapter, Mary's help-seeking trajectory was created to be fairly straightforward. In real life, the process of deciding to seek help usually occurs over a prolonged period of time (often years) and may be accompanied by numerous false starts (e.g., Mary's brief attendance at AA). Mary's case should be thought of as illustrative of some of the decisional processes and behaviors relevant to deciding to seek help, but should not be considered to be an exhaustive example of the variety of factors that constitutes this decision process.

### *Clinician's Response*

The clinician's first meeting with Mary will be critical to her engagement in the process of treatment. The clinician should acknowledge that Mary has obviously struggled with her decision to reach out for help with her drinking problem; the clinician should gather additional information about the aspects of the decision that made entering treatment more difficult. Gaining a better understanding of the potential obstacles to treatment can offer useful clinical information regarding possible barriers to behavior change. The therapist should be empathic and try to normalize this struggle by saying something like "Most people have a really difficult time deciding to seek treatment" and should reinforce her decision by stating "It is a really positive step that you decided to come in today." The therapist could commend Mary for her courage and persistence in taking this step and could emphasize that entering treatment is an indication of Mary's apparent desire for a healthier lifestyle. Although Mary has indicated that the main reason she decided to enter therapy concerns her drinking, the therapist should make note of the other clinical concerns (e.g., depression, social isolation) and try to instill hope about how therapy can help with these issues as well. In addition, the clinician should make an effort to recognize the specific factors that contributed to Mary's help-seeking decision. For example, the therapist could say: "It sounds like your drinking has been interfering with your life and that you have some concerns about how it may be affecting your health. That close call when you were driving must have been really scary." In addition, the clinician should attempt to encourage the client to use existing sources of social support. For example: "I know that you have some concerns about what people will think about your being in treatment, but from what you've told me, it sounds like your family is just concerned about you. And it sounds like your friend JoAnne has been really supportive about helping you get into treatment." The clinician should attempt to educate the client about the potential benefits of therapy in a way that will increase the likelihood that she will return and that will enhance her self-efficacy for success. The clinician might say: "I think that your determination to make some changes will really work in your favor. Most clients who enter treatment are able to make substantial reductions in their drinking. Let's come up with some specific goals that we can work on together over the next couple of weeks." These types of statements will offer reinforcement to the client and will convey that the client and the clinician will be working as a team toward positive change.

## CONCLUDING REMARKS

Regardless of the theory or model used to explain help-seeking decisions, entering treatment is undoubtedly a socially influenced process. Whereas theories and models are helpful for conceptualizing and studying the process, for the practicing clinician, a full understanding of help seeking can best be gained by understanding the specific factors that come into play for the individual client who is seeking services. These individual factors depend on the client's social context and include variables that range from his or her age to pressures from the legal system. To ignore any of these contributing factors would be to assume that every help-seeking decision is commonplace and predictable. On a broader level, knowledge about help seeking can be used to ensure that needed services are available and to initiate large-scale efforts to reduce stigma and encourage the use of mental health services.

As we have shown, even the most complex models of help seeking are limited in their ability to accurately predict treatment decisions. Help-seeking behavior is influenced by many factors, some of which may never be ascertained. However, ongoing communication between researchers and practitioners can lead to a better understanding of the help-seeking process from the clients' perspective. This dialogue can be used to maximize the likelihood that clients will enter, remain in, and make the best use of treatment.

## REFERENCES

Aday, L. A., & Andersen, R. (1974). A framework for the study of access to medical care. *Health Services Research*, 9, 208–220.

Aday, L. A., & Awe, W. C. (1997). Health services utilization models. In D. S. Gochman (Ed.), *Handbook of health behavior research* (pp. 153–172). New York: Plenum Press.

Ajzen, I. (1991). The theory of planned behavior. *Organizational Behavior and Human Decision Processes, 50*, 179–211.

American Psychiatric Association. (1994). *Diagnostic and statistical manual of mental disorders* (4th ed.). Washington, DC: Author.

Andersen, R. M. (1995). Revisiting the behavioral model and access to medical care: Does it matter? *Journal of Health and Social Behavior, 36*, 1–10.

Bornovalova, M. A., & Daughters, S. B. (2007). How does dialectical behavior therapy facilitate treatment retention among individuals with comorbid borderline personality disorder and substance use disorders? *Clinical Psychology Review, 27*, 923–943.

Bussing, R., Koro-Ljungberg, M. E., Gary, F., Mason, D. M., & Garvan, C. W. (2005). Exploring help-seeking for ADHD symptoms: A mixed-methods approach. *Harvard Review of Psychiatry, 13*, 85–101.

Carey, K. B., Purnine, D. M., Maisto, S. A., & Carey, M. P. (1999). Assessing readiness to change substance abuse: A critical review of instruments. *Clinical Psychology: Science and Practice, 6*, 245–266.

Corrigan, P. (2004). How stigma interferes with mental health care. *American Psychologist, 59*, 614–625.

Cramer, K. M. (1999). Psychological antecedents to help-seeking behavior: A reanalysis using path modeling structures. *Journal of Counseling Psychology, 46*, 381–387.

Diala, C., Muntaner, C., Walrath, C., Nickerson, K. J., LaVeist, T. A., & Leaf, P. J. (2000). Racial differences in attitudes toward professional mental health care and in the use of services. *American Journal of Orthopsychiatry, 70*, 455–464.

Fischer, E. H., & Farina, A. (1995). Attitudes toward seeking professional psychological help: A shortened form and considerations for research. *Journal of College Student Development, 36*, 368–373.

Freyer, J., Coder, B., Bischof, G., Baumeister, S. E., Rumpf, H.-J., John, U., et al. (2007). Intention to utilize formal help in a sample with alcohol problems: A prospective study. *Drug and Alcohol Dependence, 87*, 210–216.

Freyer, J., Tonigan, J. S., Keller, S., John, U., Rumpf, H.-J., & Hapke, U. (2004). Readiness to change versus readiness to seek help for alcohol problems: The development of the Treatment Readiness Tool (TReaT). *Journal of Studies on Alcohol, 65*, 801–809.

Freyer, J., Tonigan, J. S., Keller, S., Rumpf, H.-J., John, U., & Hapke, U. (2005). Readiness for change and readiness for help-seeking: A composite assessment of client motivation. *Alcohol and Alcoholism, 40*, 540–544.

Galdas, P. M., Cheater, F., & Marshall, P. (2005). Men and health help-seeking behaviour: Literature review. *Journal of Advanced Nursing, 49*, 616–623.

Gardner, W., Hoge, S. K., Bennett, N., Roth, L. H., Lidz, C. W., Monahan, J., et al. (1993). Two scales for measuring patients' perceptions for coercion during mental hospital admission. *Behavioral Sciences and the Law, 11*, 307–321.

Green, C. A., & Pope, C. R. (1999). Gender, psychosocial factors and the use of medical services: A longitudinal analysis. *Social Science and Medicine, 48*, 1363–1372.

Harris, K. M., Edlund, M. J., & Larson, S. (2005). Racial and ethnic differences in the mental health problems and use of mental health care. *Medical Care, 43*, 775–784.

Hasin, D. S., Stinson, F. S., Ogburn, E., & Grant, B. F. (2007). Prevalence, correlates, disability, and comorbidity of DSM-IV alcohol abuse and dependence in the United States: Results from the National Epidemiologic Survey on Alcohol and Related Conditions. *Archives of General Psychiatry, 64*, 830–842.

Heesch, K. C., Velasquez, M. M., & von Sternberg, K. (2005). Readiness for mental health treatment and for changing alcohol use in patients with comorbid psychiatric and alcohol disorders: Are they congruent? *Addictive Behaviors, 30*, 531–543.

Horvath, A. O., & Symonds, B. D. (1991). Relation between working alliance and outcome in psychotherapy: A meta-analysis. *Journal of Counseling Psychology, 38*, 139–149.

Hser, Y.-I., Maglione, M., Polinsky, M. L., & Anglin, M. D. (1998). Predicting drug treatment entry among treatment-seeking individuals. *Journal of Substance Abuse Treatment, 15,* 213–220.

Kaskutas, L. A., Weisner, C., & Caetano, R. (1997). Predictors of help seeking among a longitudinal sample of the general population, 1984–1992. *Journal of Studies on Alcohol, 58,* 155–161.

Kelly, A. E., & Achter, J. A. (1995). Self-concealment and attitudes toward counseling in university students. *Journal of Counseling Psychology, 42,* 40–46.

Kessler, R. C., McGonagle, K. A., Zhao, S., Nelson, C. B., Hughes, M., Eshleman, S., et al. (1994). Lifetime and 12-month prevalence of DSM-III-R psychiatric disorders in the United States. *Archives of General Psychiatry, 51,* 8–19.

Kessler, R. C., Olfson, M., & Berglund, P. A. (1998). Patterns and predictors of treatment contact after first onset of psychiatric disorders. *American Journal of Psychiatry, 155,* 62–69.

Kessler, R. C., Zhao, S., Katz, S. J., Kouzis, A. C., Frank, R. G., Edlund, M., et al. (1999). Past-year use of outpatient services for psychiatric problems in the National Comorbidity Survey. *American Journal of Psychiatry, 156,* 115–123.

Klap, R., Unroe, K. T., & Unützer, J. (2003). Caring for mental illness in the United States: A focus on older adults. *American Journal of Geriatric Psychiatry, 11,* 517–524.

Kushner, M. G., & Sher, K. J. (1989). Fear of psychological treatment and its relation to mental health service avoidance. *Professional Psychology: Research and Practice, 20,* 251–257.

Kushner, M. G., & Sher, K. J. (1991). The relation of treatment fearfulness and psychological service utilization: An overview. *Professional Psychology: Research and Practice, 22,* 196–203.

Leaf, P. J., Bruce, M. L., Tischler, G. L., Freeman, D. H., Weissman, M. M., & Myers, J. K. (1988). Factors affecting the utilization of specialty and general medical mental health services. *Medical Care, 26,* 9–26.

Leong, F. T. L., & Zachar, P. (1999). Gender and opinions about mental illness as predictors of attitudes toward seeking professional psychological help. *British Journal of Guidance and Counselling, 27,* 123–132.

Lindsey, M. A., Korr, W. S., Broitman, M., Bone, L., Green, A., & Leaf, P. J. (2006). Help-seeking behaviors and depression among African American adolescent boys. *Social Work, 51,* 49–58.

Maddux, J. E., & DuCharme, K. A. (1997). Behavioral intentions in theories of health behavior. In D. S. Gochman (Ed.), *Handbook of health behavior: Personal and social determinants* (pp. 133–151). New York: Plenum Press.

Meier, P. S., Barrowclough, C., & Donmall, M. C. (2005). The role of the therapeutic alliance in the treatment of substance misuse: A critical review of the literature. *Addiction, 100,* 304–316.

Miller, W. R., Walters, S. T., & Bennett, M. E. (2001). How effective is alcoholism treatment in the United States? *Journal of Studies on Alcohol, 62,* 211–220.

Ogden, J. (2003). Some problems with social cognition models: A pragmatic and conceptual analysis. *Health Psychology, 22,* 424–428.

Pescosolido, B. A. (1991). Illness careers and network ties: A conceptual model of utilization and compliance. *Advances in Medical Sociology, 2,* 161–184.

Pescosolido, B. A. (2000). Rethinking models of health and illness behaviour. In M. Kelner, B. Wellman, M. Saks, & B. A. Pescosolido (Eds.), *Complementary and alternative medicine* (pp. 175–193). Amsterdam: the Netherlands: Harwood Academic.

Pescosolido, B. A., & Boyer, C. A. (1999). How do people come to use mental health services? Current knowledge and changing perspectives. In A. V. Horwitz & T. L. Scheid (Eds.), *A handbook for the study of mental health: Social contexts, theories, and systems* (pp. 392–411). New York: Cambridge University Press.

Pescosolido, B. A., Brooks Gardner, C., & Lubell, K. M. (1998). How people get into mental health services: Stories of choice, coercion and "muddling through" from "first-timers." *Social Science and Medicine, 46,* 275–286.

Pescosolido, B. A., Wright, E. R., Alegría, M., & Vera, M. (1998). Social networks and patterns of use among the poor with mental health problems in Puerto Rico. *Medical Care, 36,* 1057–1072.

Petty, R. E., & Cacioppo, J. T. (1996). *Attitudes and persuasion: Classic and contemporary approaches.* Boulder, CO: Westview Press.

Prochaska, J. O., & DiClemente, C. C. (1982). Transtheoretical therapy: Toward a more integrative model of change. *Psychotherapy: Theory, Research, and Practice, 19*, 276–288.

Prochaska, J. O., DiClemente, C. C., & Norcross, J. C. (1992). In search of how people change: Applications to addictive behaviors. *American Psychologist, 47*, 1102–1114.

Prochaska, J. O., Norcross, J. C., & DiClemente, C. C. (1994). *Changing for good: A revolutionary six-stage program for overcoming bad habits and moving your life positively forward.* New York: Avon Books.

Rabinowitz, J., Gross, R., & Feldman, D. (1999). Correlates of a perceived need for mental health assistance and differences between those who do and do not seek help. *Social Psychiatry and Psychiatric Epidemiology, 34*, 141–146.

Robb, C., Haley, W. E., Becker, M. A., Polivka, L. A., & Chwa, H.-J. (2003). Attitudes towards mental health care in younger and older adults: Similarities and differences. *Aging and Mental Health, 7*, 142–152.

Rogers, R. W., & Prentice-Dunn, S. (1997). Protection motivation theory. In D. S. Gochman (Ed.), *Handbook of health behavior research: I. Personal and social determinants* (pp. 113–132). New York: Plenum Press.

Saunders, S. M. (1993). Applicants' experience of the process of seeking therapy. *Psychotherapy, 30*, 554–564.

Saunders, S. M. (1996). Applicants' experience of social support in the process of seeking psychotherapy. *Psychotherapy, 33*, 617–627.

Saunders, S. M., Zygowicz, K. M., & D'Angelo, B. R. (2006). Person-related and treatment-related barriers to alcohol treatment. *Journal of Substance Abuse Treatment, 30*, 261–270.

Segal, D. L., Coolidge, F. L., Mincic, M. S., & O'Riley, A. (2005). Beliefs about mental illness and willingness to seek help: A cross-sectional study. *Aging and Mental Health, 9*, 363–367.

Seligman, M. E. P. (1995). The effectiveness of psychotherapy: The Consumer Reports study. *American Psychologist, 50*, 965–974.

Shapiro, S., Skinner, E. A., Kessler, L. G., Von Korff, M., German, P. S., Tischler, G. L., et al. (1984). Utilization of health and mental health services: Three Epidemiologic Catchment Area sites. *Archives of General Psychiatry, 41*, 971–978.

Simpson, C. A., & Tucker, J. A. (2002). Temporal sequencing of alcohol-related problems, problem recognition, and help-seeking episodes. *Addictive Behaviors, 27*, 659–674.

Sobell, L. C., Ellingstad, T. P., & Sobell, M. B. (2000). Natural recovery from alcohol and drug problems: Methodological review of the research with suggestions for future directions. *Addiction, 95*, 749–764.

Stark, M. J. (1992). Dropping out of substance abuse treatment: A clinically oriented review. *Clinical Psychology Review, 12*, 93–116.

Stefl, M. E., & Prosperi, D. C. (1985). Barriers to mental health service utilization. *Community Mental Health Journal, 21*, 167–177.

Strecher, V. J., Champion, V. L., & Rosenstock, I. M. (1997). The health belief model and health behavior. In D. S. Gochman (Ed.), *Handbook of health behavior research: I. Personal and social determinants* (pp. 71–91). New York: Plenum Press.

Surgenor, L. J. (1985). Attitudes toward seeking professional psychological help. *New Zealand Journal of Psychology, 14*, 27–33.

Sutton, S. (1998). Predicting and explaining intentions and behavior: How well are we doing? *Journal of Applied Social Psychology, 28*, 1317–1338.

Tijhuis, M. A. R., Peters, L., & Foets, M. (1990). An orientation toward help-seeking for emotional problems. *Social Science and Medicine, 31*, 989–995.

Vogel, D. L., Wade, N. G., & Hackler, A. H. (2007). Perceived public stigma and the willingness to seek counseling: The mediating roles of self-stigma and attitudes toward counseling. *Journal of Counseling Psychology, 54*, 40–50.

Wang, P. S., Lane, M., Olfson, M., Pincus, H. A., Wells, K. B., & Kessler, R. C. (2005). Twelve-month use of mental health services in the United States. *Archives of General Psychiatry*, *62*, 629–640.

Wells, J. E., Robins, L. N., Bushnell, J. A., Jarosz, D., & Oakley-Browne, M. A. (1994). Perceived barriers to care in St. Louis (USA) and Christchurch (NZ): Reasons for not seeking professional help for psychological distress. *Social Psychiatry and Psychiatric Epidemiology*, *29*, 155–164.

Wierzbicki, M., & Pekarik, G. (1993). A meta-analysis of psychotherapy dropout. *Professional Psychology: Research and Practice*, *24*, 190–195.

# 22 Social Cognitive Theories and Clinical Interventions

## *Basic Principles and Guidelines*

James E. Maddux

One of the most important subfields of social psychology is the study of *social cognition*, which is concerned with what people think about other people, and how what people think about other people influences how they themselves feel and behave (Barone, Maddux, & Snyder, 1997; Fiske & Taylor, 2008). The study of social cognition includes, but is not limited to, what are often referred to as *social cognitive theories*.

Social cognitive theories are extensions of *social learning theory*, as originally developed by Rotter (1954; see also, Woodward, 1982). One of the most important differences between social learning theory and traditional behavioral learning theory is that social learning theory allows for vicarious learning or observational learning (i.e., learning by watching other people), which occurs in the absence of direct reinforcement or punishment of the learner. The most important psychological information that people learn is *about* other people and *from* other people, hence the term *social* learning theory. Learning about and from other people requires the ability to *think*. Because social learning theory presumed that thinking, particularly symbolic thought, plays an important role in learning, it was both *social* and *cognitive* from the beginning.

As social learning theory evolved, however, it became more explicitly cognitive. For example, Bandura's (1986) *social cognitive theory* and Mischel's (1973) *cognitive social learning theory* both emphasized the important role of people's interpretations of, and predictions about, events on learning, behavior, and personality development, as does Mischel's more recent *Cognitive–Affective Processing Systems* (CAPS) approach (Kross, Mischel, & Shoda,

Chapter 20, this volume). Both of these theorist-researchers added much to our understanding of the role of *social cognition*—what people think about other people and their relationships with other people—in the acquisition and change of behavioral and affective patterns and in people's conceptions of "self" and "personality."

A number of other models from social and personality psychology might also be called *social cognitive*. Personal construct theory (Kelly, 1955), the theories of reasoned action (Fishbein & Ajzen, 1975) and planned behavior (Ajzen, 1988), goal-setting theory (Locke & Latham, 1990), and various goal-based theories of personality (e.g., Cantor, 1990; Dweck & Elliott-Moskwa, Chapter 8, this volume) are all concerned, to some extent, with the role of cognitive and interpersonal processes in behavior.

The social cognitive theories that have had the greatest impact on clinical psychology in general and clinical practice in particular are the various *cognitive* and *cognitive-behavioral* theories of psychological disorders and psychotherapy (e.g., Hollon & Beck, 1994; Dobson, 2002). In fact, social cognitive theories find their greatest expression in clinical work in cognitive and cognitive-behavioral therapies, which are perfectly compatible with a broad social cognitive approach to human behavior and personality.

Despite some differences, the various social cognitive theories have much in common. First, they share a set of basic principles or assumptions about human psychological processes and activities. Second, they share a set of basic conceptual elements, units, or variables from which their principles and processes are built.

## BASIC PRINCIPLES, PROCESSES, AND VARIABLES

### The Primacy of Cognitive Construals

People have powerful *cognitive* or *symbolizing* capabilities that allow for the creation of internal models of experience, the development of innovative courses of action, the hypothetical testing of such courses of action through the prediction of outcomes, and the communication of complex ideas and experiences to others. Because of this capacity, people can engage in *self-observation* and can analyze and evaluate their own behavior, thoughts, and emotions. These self-reflective activities set the stage for *self-regulation* (to be discussed below). People also are "meaning makers." They strive to understand their worlds, especially their social worlds, and continually give meaning to or interpret events, especially the behavior of self and others. These meanings and interpretations greatly influence behavior. People also use their interpretations of events to make predictions about future events. In social cognitive terms, people generate *causal attributions* (or explanations) for their own behavior and for the behavior of others and *expectancies* (predictions) about future events (especially the behavior of self and others) based partly on these attributions. Perhaps the most influential of expectancies are *self-efficacy expectancies* (beliefs about one's ability to coordinate one's personal resources to attain desired goals; Bandura, 1997) and *response expectancies* (expectations about one's emotional reactions to anticipated events; Kirsch, 1999). These attributions and expectancies, regardless of their accuracy, influence cognitive, emotional, and behavioral reactions to events, as demonstrated by research on the influence of spouses' attributions for each others' behavior on marital satisfaction (Bradbury & Fincham, 1990), self-efficacy beliefs in anxiety and depression (Bandura, 1997), and response expectancies in a variety of psychological problems (Kirsch, 1999).

## Reciprocal Influences of Person and Situation

The social cognitive view assumes three interacting and reciprocal person-centered influences: cognition, emotion, and behavior. These influences are interdependent; change in one usually produces change in the other two. In addition, the person influences and is influenced by environmental or situational events. People respond cognitively, emotionally, and behaviorally to situational events. Also, through cognition people exercise control over their own feelings and actions. Their actions then influence not only the environment but also their own cognitive and affective states. When the situation involves ongoing interactions with another person or other people, as is so often the case in life, the interactions of these influences can become extremely complex. Each person is continually attempting to explain (generate causal attributions) and predict (generate expectancies) for the behavior of him- or herself and others, responding emotionally to these explanations and predictions, and adjusting his or her behavior in an attempt to influence the other person or persons. These expectancies often concern the immediate future, as when a person anticipates another person's immediate behavior in an ongoing interaction. These expectancies often become *self-fulfilling prophecies* because people often experience the emotions that they expect to experience, perform those behaviors that they expect will be successful, and behave in ways that elicit from others the behavior expected from them. (See Kross, Mischel, & Shoda, Chapter 20, and Shadel, Chapter 18, this volume.)

## The Social Nature of Self and Personality

Despite tremendous individual differences in social motives and goals (e.g., introversion–extraversion), people are essentially social animals. The need to develop relationships with other people seems innate to our species (Baumeister & Leary, 1995; Guisinger & Blatt, 1994). Therefore, from the social cognitive view, *self* and *personality* are perceptions (accurate or not) of the individual's own and others' patterns of social cognition, emotion, and action as they occur in patterns of situations. People define themselves largely by what they think about, how they feel about, and how they behave toward other people. Their behavior is influenced not only by the behavior of other people but also by what they expect other people to think, feel, and behave. Thus, *self* and *personality* are inextricably embedded in social contexts, and understanding an individual cannot be accomplished without understanding how he or she thinks, feels, and behaves in specific situations, especially social interactions (Bandura, 1986; Kross, Mischel, & Shoda, Chapter 20, this volume; Shadel, Chapter 18, this volume).

Because they are socially embedded, personality and self are not simply what people *bring* to their interactions with others; they are *created* in these interactions, and they are *changed by* these interactions.

## Self-Regulation

The ability to think symbolically provides people with the tools for *self-regulation*—that is, the self-management of behaviors, cognitions, and emotions (see also, Doerr & Baumeister, Chapter 5, this volume; Strauman, McCrudden, & Jones, Chapter 6, this volume; Oettingen & Gollwitzer, Chapter 7, this volume). People choose *goals*, develop *plans* for achieving these goals, and regulate their behavior in the pursuit of these goals. People observe the influence of their behavior on situational events (especially the behavior of other people) and the influence of the situation (again, especially the behavior of other people) on their own thoughts, feelings, and behavior. People also use experience gleaned from past events to anticipate or develop expectancies about possible future events such as the possible reactions of themselves and others.

The ability to set goals allows people to create incentives that motivate and guide behavior. People set *standards* for their progress toward their goals (immediate, short-term, and long-term) and then continually gather and evaluate information about their progress, usually referred to as *performance feedback*. These evaluations lead to emotional reactions and to the reevaluation of the effectiveness of goal-related behavior. People then adjust their behavior accordingly. People's evaluations and emotional reactions can either facilitate or interfere with self-regulation. For example, feeling pleased with one's progress usually encourages one to continue, whereas disappointment may lead to disengagement from a goal. (See Dweck & Elliott-Moskwa, Chapter 8, this volume, for a more complete and complex discussions of the impact of negative feedback on goal pursuit.)

People also choose to enter or avoid certain situations based on their perceptions of the relevance of those situations to their goals. These choices can either facilitate or hinder the development of competencies, as when the socially anxious individual avoids the very situations that might help him or her develop the skills and beliefs important in alleviating the social anxiety.

### Biological Bases of Cognition and Behavior

The ability to engage in complex cognitive activities such as symbolization, self-reflection, and self-regulation is rooted in complex neuropsychological structures and processes. The social cognitive theories acknowledge the biological bases of human thought, affect, and behavior, but they are concerned with understanding the social and interpersonal influences on and manifestations of the basic processes rather than the basic processes themselves, the understanding of which is the goal of neuroscience. Thus, a social cognitive approach acknowledges biological influences on psychological phenomena, the effectiveness of certain biological interventions (particularly pharmacological interventions) that have been shown to influence cognition and affect, and the neurological changes that can result from psychological interventions (Smith, 2008).

## GENERAL IMPLICATIONS FOR CLINICAL INTERVENTIONS

A social cognitive approach to the practice of clinical psychology is concerned with understanding how people are actors as well as reactors in life. More specifically, it strives to understand how cognition, emotion, and behavior in specific situations sometimes interact in ways that facilitate psychological well-being and how they so often operate ineffectively and counterproductively. It also is concerned with understanding how people unwittingly contribute to the development and maintenance of dysfunctional and maladaptive patterns through their own choices and behaviors.

## The Situational Nature of Psychological Adaptation and Adjustment

Psychological adjustment and maladjustment are not properties of persons but of the complex interaction of person (cognition, emotion, and behavior) and situation. For this reason, understanding difficulties in psychological adjustment and designing effective interventions to enhance adjustment (e.g., psychotherapy) require knowledge of the specific problematic aspects of cognition, emotion, and action and their interactions in and with specific situations (see also, Kross, Mischel, & Shoda, Chapter 20, this volume; Shadel, Chapter 18, this volume). Generic conceptions and descriptions of problems that lack details about the specific situations in which problems occur and about the complex interactions of cognition, emotion, behavior, and situational events can lead only to vague and generic suggestions for change rather than to specific suggestions for thinking, feeling, and behaving more adaptively. The best way to gather this information is to ask people to provide recent examples of situations in which their problem has occurred (e.g., "Can you describe a recent situation in which you've felt particularly anxious?") and then to probe relentlessly for the details about the situations ("What? When? Where? Who?") and for the client's explanations and predictions of situational events, his or her emotional reactions, his or her behavior, the impact of those behaviors on the situation (particularly the behavior of other people), the reactions of other people, the client's reactions to their reactions, and so on. The clinician needs to gather information about a sufficient number of situational examples to allow the identification of patterns of situations, client thoughts, client emotions, and client behaviors, and especially the effectiveness of the client's effort to solve or cope with the problem (e.g., "What have you tried to do about this? How well has it worked?").

The clinician should gather this kind of information not only about situations in which the problem occurs (or occurs with greater severity) but also about situations in which the problem does not occur (or occurs with less severity). This involves asking questions such as "Can you give some examples of situations recently in which you've felt less anxious/depressed/angry?" By comparing information on the situations in which the problem is better or worse and by comparing differences in the client's thoughts, feelings, and behaviors across the contrasting situations—including strategies the client is already using that appear to be successful in certain situations—the clinician and the client can begin to identify what specifically can be changed to alleviate the problem or the client's distress about it.

## Psychological Problems Are Interpersonal Problems

The most important aspects of psychological adaptation and adjustment are social or interpersonal, and most adjustment difficulties either arise from, or are manifested in, our relationships with others and in specific interactions (conversations) with others. Most people who seek psychological services do so either because they are distressed about their relationships with others or find other people to be impediments to their goals (or both). Depression, anxiety, marital discord, loneliness, and hostility consist primarily of interpersonal beliefs and behaviors that are expressed in interpersonal settings and make little sense when examined outside of an interpersonal context. Even sexual dysfunction and substance abuse and addiction occur in the context of relationships and are greatly influenced, for better or worse, by other people.

Thus, the social cognitive perspective assumes that "maladjusted behavior resides in a person's recurrent transactions with others ... [and] results from ... an individual's failure to attend to and correct the self-defeating, interpersonally unsuccessful aspects of his or her interpersonal acts" (Kiesler, 1991, pp. 443–444). It focuses not on the behavior of individuals but on the behavior of individuals interacting in a system with others (Benjamin, Chapter 19, this volume; Kross, Mischel, & Shoda, Chapter 20, this volume; Shadel, Chapter 18, this volume; Kiesler, 1991).

Therefore, clinicians need to explore carefully with clients the ways in which their relationships are both a cause of their dysfunction and distress and are affected (usually for the worse) by their dysfunction and distress. Because relationships are acted out in specific *conversations* between people, the clinician needs to explore the ways in which the client and important people in his or her life *talk* to each other—or avoid talking to each other (e.g., avoidance of certain topics of conversations, avoidance of conversation altogether)—and how the client feels about the way he or she talks to others. This discussion should include *what* the client talks about with other people, *how* he or she talks about it (Calmly? Angrily?), the client's specific *goals* in specific conversations ("What were you trying/hoping to accomplish in this conversation?"), how well the client believes he or she accomplished these goals, and the ways in which the client believes these conversations could be changed for the better.

## Psychological Adjustment Requires Self-Regulation

Psychological adaptation and adjustment, as well as a general sense of happiness or subjective well-being, depend to a large extent on people's ability to set goals and regulate behavior effectively and efficiently in pursuit of those goals. Conversely, psychological maladjustment and unhappiness can be viewed as the result of self-regulatory dysfunction or self-regulation failure (Doerr & Baumeister, Chapter 5, this volume; Strauman, McCrudden, & Jones, Chapter 6, this volume; Oettingen & Gollwitzer, Chapter 7, this volume; Dweck & Elliott-Moskwa, Chapter 8, this volume). Indeed, the vast majority of people who seek the help of mental health professionals do so because they are distressed about their failure (real or perceived) to achieve, or make sufficient progress toward, important goals or because they believe that they have encountered an insurmountable barrier to an important life goal. Therefore, understanding a client's problems requires understanding his or her long-term life goals, more immediate and short-term goals (plans), attempts to attain those goals, perceived success of those attempts, and the perceived barriers to those goals. In addition, it requires understanding how the client gathers and interprets information about progress toward goals (feedback), how he or she evaluates that progress, his or her emotional reactions to those evaluations, and the effect of those emotions on goal-directed behavior.

People usually are more satisfied with their lives when they believe that they are making good progress in moving toward valued goals. For this reason, effective self-regulation is crucial to psychological adjustment and well-being. In addition, ineffective self-regulation can lead to serious psychological problems, including depression and anxiety disorders. This is not to say, however, that the happy and psychologically healthy person is one who is capable of exerting perfect control over his or her behavior, feelings, and thoughts at all times. Self-regulation in the pursuit of perfectionistic, unrealistic, or unhealthy goals can lead to unhappiness and dissatisfaction with life, as when the pursuit of the "perfect" body leads to eating disorders or to excessive worry about normal physical imperfections.

Many important life goals are either interpersonal goals (e.g., developing and maintaining relationships) or require the cooperation and collaboration of other people (e.g., work and career goals). Likewise, many, if not most, psychological problems can be understood as difficulties in self-regulation in interpersonal contexts. For these reasons, effective self-regulation in interpersonal situations (e.g., managing and expressing emotions effectively) is particularly important for psychological adjustment and well-being.

From a social cognitive perspective, self-regulation is viewed not as a fixed and unchanging property of the person but as a set of skills that can be learned, can be improved through practice, and can be adapted from one situation to another. Numerous models of self-regulation have been proposed over the past several decades. Taken together, these models identify nine components of self-regulation:

1. Goals—what a person is either trying to accomplish or trying to avoid.
2. Plans—the person's strategy for accomplishing the goals.
3. Self-efficacy beliefs—the person's confidence in his or ability to implement specific aspects of the plan.
4. Goal-directed action—actual attempts to implement specific aspects of the plan.
5. Standards of evaluation—the person's "yardstick" for measuring progress along the way.
6. Feedback—information about progress toward a goal (as compared to standards of performance) that people either gather themselves through self-monitoring or that is provided by other people or automatically by the situations (e.g., a computer video game).
7. Self-evaluation—judgments about oneself and one's ability to attain the goal as a result of feedback about progress toward the goal.
8. Emotion—emotional reactions to these evaluations.
9. Corrective action—attempts to changes one's behavior to move oneself toward one's goal more efficiently, based on feedback, self-evaluation, and emotional reactions.

Self-regulation does not, of course, consist of an invariable sequence of nine steps, beginning with a goal and ending with corrective action. Instead, self-regulation consists of a number of *components* that interact continually in complex feedback loops. In attempting to understand a client's problems, the clinician needs to gain an understanding of the client's ability to employ these specific self-regulatory skills in specific situations and in the service of specific goals. This understanding can lead to an identification of the specific ways in which the client's attempts to self-regulate in the pursuit of goals are unsuccessful and to specific suggestions for improvement.

As does the exercise of any set of skills, self-regulation requires effort and can be emotionally taxing. Self-regulatory efforts in one situation (e.g., not eating those additional cookies) can leave the person temporarily depleted or less able to exert his or her self-regulatory skills in a new situation (e.g., studying for an exam) (Doerr & Baumeister, Chapter 5, this volume). In addition, self-regulation can be viewed as a "muscle" that can be strengthened by practicing the various components (e.g., setting goals, developing plans, monitoring progress) (Doerr & Baumester, Chapter 5, this volume).

## Maladaptive = Ineffective

Effective psychological adaptation is characterized by cognitive, emotional, and behavioral responses that comprise relatively effective and efficient strategies for achieving specific goals in specific situations and for coping with specific challenges and problems in these specific situations. Likewise, psychological dysfunction consists of behavioral, cognitive, and affective responses that are inefficient, ineffective, or counterproductive in the pursuit of specific goals in specific situations. Thus efforts to understand and change psychological difficulties should be directed toward identifying and changing patterns of effective and ineffective behaving, thinking, and feeling as they occur in specific situations in clients' lives.

## Psychological Problems as Vicious Cycles

The social cognitive principle of the reciprocal interaction of person and situation includes that notion that people are active participants in, and contributors to, their own life stories and to their problems in living (see Shadel, Chapter 18, this volume; McAdams & Adler, Chapter 3, this volume). The choices people make can facilitate personal growth and psychological well-being or can contribute to personal decline and to the development and maintenance of problematic psychological patterns. People's patterns of thinking, feeling, and behavior and their interactions with situations often develop into self-maintaining systems that achieve a kind of equilibrium that can be highly resistant to change. A social cognitive approach to personality views personality not as a fixed, internal entity that determines behavior but as a dynamic, self-maintaining system (Kross, Mischel, & Shoda, Chapter 20, this volume; Shadel, Chapter 18, this volume; Riskind, Alloy, & Iacoviello, Chapter 15, this volume.)

When these self-maintaining patterns or systems are maladaptive, we might refer to them as *negative feedback loops* or *vicious cycles*. A vicious cycle is a situation that starts out bad and gets worse the more a person tries to cope with it or resolve it. Vicious cycles are the result of ineffective and rigid coping strategies. Often people's basic beliefs about themselves and other people—their social cognitions—lead them to attempt to cope with stress, resolve interpersonal problems, protect themselves from expected harm, or avoid unpleasant feelings in ways that not only do not solve the problem but make the problem worse.

An example of a common vicious cycle is social anxiety. Social anxiety is a common experience, and many normal, healthy people are at times anxious in social situations. Even mildly socially anxious people create for themselves a kind of vicious cycle, but it can be seen most vividly in chronically socially anxious people. People who experience frequent and debilitating social anxiety usually believe that other people will not like them or will reject them. For this reason, they often experience anxiety in social situations or even while thinking about an upcoming social situation. Too often the socially anxious person copes with this anxiety by avoiding situations in which he or she feels anxious, such as parties and other social gatherings. If a socially anxious person enters a social situation, he or she may stand around waiting for others to initiate conversation, or, seeing a group of people talking, not make an attempt to enter the conversation. Also because the anxious person looks uncomfortable, other people may be reluctant to talk to him or her, since people tend to experience anxiety in the presence of an anxious person. Thus, because of the socially anxious person's own passive behavior and discomfort, no one talks to that person. The anxious person may then conclude that other people really are unfriendly or that he or she is not attractive to the others. If someone does attempt to engage the person in conversation, he or she may feel and appear anxious, avoid eye contact, and give minimal responses to the other person's attempts to engage him or her. As a result, the otherwise friendly person who initiated the conversation is apt to move on to someone else. The socially anxious person then uses this failed interaction as evidence that people will indeed reject him or her. (See Kross, Mischel, & Shoda, Chapter 20, this volume for additional examples.)

By avoiding social situations, socially anxious people also deprive themselves of opportunities to work on overcoming their anxiety by learning a few social skills and by learning to manage their anxiety around other people. In addition, the more the socially anxious person avoids and otherwise "acts shy," the more the person and others will label him or her as a "shy" person. Such labels, of course, tend to be self-fulfilling prophecies, because people treat us in ways that bring out the behavior they expect from us. Our labels for ourselves have the same effect. In this way, the socially anxious person's avoidance, which is a strategy for coping with anxiety, not only fails to reduce the anxiety but helps maintain it and may even make it worse over time.

A thorough social cognitive case formulation must consist of an analysis of clients' particular vicious cycles—the ways in which clients' attempts to solves their problems, including attempts to avoid or reduce painful emotions, make those problems worse. This analysis can be accomplished only by asking clients detailed questions about what they think, feel, and do in specific problematic life situations, especially problematic interactions with others. In particular, the clinician must ask specifically what the client has tried to do to resolve the problem and how those attempted solutions have not only not worked but also have either made the problem worse or contributed to its continuation.

## The Continuity of Normal and Abnormal

Because psychological dysfunction is identified by behavioral, emotional, and cognitive maladjustment and because adjustment and maladjustment are situation-dependent, the distinctions between adaptive and maladaptive, normal and abnormal, and psychological "order" and "disorder" are elusive. Adaptive and maladaptive psychological phenomena differ not in kind but in degree. Normal and abnormal are relative points on a continuum, not different types or categories. The explanations for the problems of people who present themselves to mental health professionals ("clinical populations") also apply to the problems of people who, for a variety of reasons, do not seek professional assistance. The vast body of research documenting the continuities between so-called "clinical" and "nonclinical" populations and problems undermines the validity and utility of the distinction between normal problems in living and "mental disorders" (Maddux, 2009; Maddux, Gosselin, & Winstead, 2008; Widiger, 2008).

Social cognitive theories reject the categorization of people and behavior and endorse a *dimensional model* that assumes that normality and abnormality, wellness and illness, and effective and ineffective psychological functioning all lie along a continuum. In the dimensional model, so-called psychological "disorders" are simply extreme variants of normal psychological phenomena and ordinary problems in living (Keyes & Lopez, 2002; Widiger, 2008). The dimensional model is concerned not with classifying people or disorders but with identifying and measuring individual differences in psychological phenomena such as emotion, mood, intelligence, and personal styles (e.g., Lubinski, 2000). Great differences among individuals on the dimensions of interest are expected, such as the differences we find on formal tests of intelligence. As with intelligence, divisions made between normality and abnormality may be demarcated for convenience or efficiency but are not to be viewed as indicative of true discontinuity among "types" of phenomena or "types" of people.

Empirical evidence for the validity of a dimensional approach to psychological adjustment can be found in research on personality disorders (Costello, 1996; Lowe & Widiger, 2008; Maddux & Mundell, 2005), the variations in normal emotional experiences (e.g., Oatley & Jenkins, 1992), adult attachment patterns in relationships (Fraley & Waller, 1998), self-defeating behaviors (Baumeister & Scher, 1988), children's reading problems or "dyslexia," (Shaywitz, Escobar, Shaywitz, Fletcher, & Makuch, 1992), attention-deficit/hyperactivity disorder (Barkley, 1997), posttraumatic stress disorder (Anthony, Lonigan, & Hecht, 1999), depression (Costello, 1993a) and schizophrenia (Claridge, 1995; Costello, 1993a, 1993b; Persons, 1986).

This dimensional view is not unique to a social cognitive approach, nor is it new. Freud and other psychoanalytic theorists assumed that normal and abnormal were on a continuum. Shapiro (1965) made the same assumption in his theory of "neurotic styles." In addition, a number of longstanding assessment techniques, such as the Rorschach and Minnesota Multiphasic Personality Inventory (MMPI) have used a dimensional approach.

Although largely a compendium of categories, the DSM does employ dimensional thinking to some extent. Its introduction cautions clinicians against taking a purely categorical view of mental disorder in general and against viewing the specific diagnostic categories as having hard and fast boundaries. In addition, a dimensional view of severity is employed in the classification of some disorders (e.g., mood disorders) and the inclusion of global adjustment ratings in a complete formal diagnosis. Finally, underway are plans to incorporate research on dimensions in the diagnosis of personality disorders. In this way, a DSM diagnosis and a social cognitive "diagnosis" may become more similar.

## Continuity of Clinical and Nonclinical Situations

In the social cognitive view, interactions between clinicians and clients are more similar to than different from everyday nonclinical interpersonal encounters. Psychotherapy, counseling, and other interventions (whether with an individual client, a couple, or a group) are first and foremost, social situations. Thus, the theories and research findings that explain interpersonal behavior in everyday social encounters and everyday close relationships apply also to encounters between the clinician and his or her clients. For this reason, understanding clinical interactions and clinical interventions requires an understanding of everyday social cognition, interpersonal behavior, and close relationships, including theory and research on attachment, interpersonal attraction, relationship development, self-disclosure, persuasion, person perception, and errors and biases in social perception and judgment.

Clinicians' perceptions and judgments of their clients—and clients' perceptions and judgment of their clinicians—involve the same processes as everyday social perception and judgment. The way clinicians gather and process information about their clients and the way they form impressions of their clients, especially the errors and biases that they display in these processes, are more similar to than different from those displayed by laypersons in everyday social encounters and relationships. (See also Garb, Chapter 16, this volume.)

For example, social cognitive research on the psychodynamic concept of *transference*—the assumption that clients superimpose old feelings, expectations, and patterns of behavior learned with a past significant other onto the psychotherapist—has revealed that transference is not unique to the client–therapist relationship but occurs regularly in everyday life. This research shows that "mental representations of significant others are stored in memory and can be activated and applied in new social encounters, with consequences for cognition, evaluation, affect, motivation, expectancies, and self-evaluations" (Andersen & Berk, 1998, p. 81). We can say the same about the reciprocal notion of *countertransference*. These are not mysterious processes unique to the client–clinician relationship but common interpersonal phenomena.

## The Focus of Clinical Interventions on Social Cognitions

Because most psychological problems are either interpersonal problems in some form or another or affect interpersonal behavior, most clinical psychological interventions focus to some extent on changing what people think about, how people feel about, and how people behave toward other people. Even disorders with largely biological causes, such as bipolar disorder and schizophrenia, are viewed as disorders because they result in disturbed and disturbing interpersonal behaviors. Likewise, strategies targeted primarily toward the reduction of painful emotional states such as anxiety and depression must take into consideration the influence of such emotions on people's relationships and the influence of relationships on people's emotions. People are continually generating causal attributions to explain and expectancies to predict the behavior of self and others. These explanations and predictions figure prominently in the development and maintenance of maladaptive patterns of affect and behavior in interactions with others. Thus, the design of effective clinical interventions depends on the therapist's and client's clear understanding of how the client's social cognitions lead to maladaptive patterns of feeling about and behaving toward other people.

## The Limitations of Diagnostic Categories

Because the distinction between normal psychological phenomena and everyday problems in living and maladaptive functioning is fuzzy, at best, patterns of maladaptive psychological responses are not easily classified into discrete categories of "disorders" that have specific "symptoms." Diagnostic categories obscure individual differences among people with apparently similar psychological difficulties and may lead to error and bias in the clinician's information gathering and decision making (Garb, Chapter 16, this volume). A classification scheme that is, by design, *atheoretical* and therefore *nonconceptual* (e.g., the DSM) cannot provide a conceptual framework for gathering information about a client's problems, making sense of that information, and subsequently developing guidelines for interventions. A system of categories based purely on descriptions of problems (and generic descriptions, at that) may suggest somewhat vaguely *what* needs to be changed but cannot possibly provide guidelines for *how* that change is to be effected. Thus, assignment of clients and their problems to such categories does not by itself, provide the kind of conceptual understanding of an individual's problems that guides the design of intervention strategies, unless the clinician has an understanding of the research on the causes and treatment of the construct being categorized (e.g., depression).

Finally, diagnostic labels are easily interpreted by clients as implying that there is an internal condition that must somehow be eradicated before they can make changes for the better. Thus diagnostic labels can make it more difficult for clients to believe that change is possible and even likely.

To note the limitations of diagnostic categories is not to say that they do not have their uses. Categorical language is more efficient and convenient in some ways than dimensional language. It is particularly more efficient and convenient when conducting research on the causes and treatments of psychological problems. For example, the vast majority of the researchers who have developed and refined empirically supported clinical interventions have used diagnostic categories in their research. Yet the vast majority of these researchers also acknowledge that a dimensional view of the problems they deal with is more accurate than a categorical view.

### Focus on Healthy Functioning and Client Strengths

The social cognitive emphasis on person-in-situation interactions; the variability of behavior, thought, and emotion across situations; and a dimensional (noncategorical) view of human adaptation and adjustment all lead logically to an emphasis on understanding what the client is doing well in addition to what he or she is doing poorly. In other words, the social cognitive approach easily leads to a shift in focus from an exclusive analysis of maladaptive functioning to an analysis of adaptive and maladaptive functioning. Understanding the conditions under which a depressed client finds joy can be as useful, if not more so, than understanding the conditions under which the client is more depressed. Likewise, understanding the topics that a couple in therapy can discuss with relatively little acrimony can be as useful as understanding the topics that lead to major disagreements and fights. What can be learned from these examples of adaptive functioning are the strategies and skills that people employ that actually work at least some of the time. Once fully understood, these strategies and skills might be enhanced and employed in the more problematic situations that are causing the client so much distress.

In addition, the clinician might shift his or her own emphasis from one of alleviating pathology and solving problems to finding ways to enhance happiness and subjective well-being. The research on happiness and subjective well-being indicates some very strong relationships between happiness and certain cognitive and behavioral patterns of habits, such as developing close relationships, actively pursuing valued life goals, and developing a religious or spiritual outlook on life (e.g., Lyubomirksky & Dickerhoof, Chapter 13, this volume).

## SUMMARY

The social cognitive models offer a comprehensive approach to understanding human psychological functioning and adaptation and a practical set of general strategies for clinical psychologists and other mental health professionals. This approach assumes that people are active participants in, and shapers of, the environments they inhabit and the lives they lead. It views people as strategic and motivated observers, thinkers, and planners who set goals and attempt to achieve them, although not always efficiently and effectively. It views psychological adjustment and maladjustment not as properties of people but as properties of the complex interactions among behavior, cognition, emotion, and the situations in which these are played out.

The goal of psychological interventions or "treatments" is not to eliminate "disorders" inside of clients but to facilitate the learning and maintenance of more effective and satisfying ways of thinking, feeling, and behaving in response to specific situational challenges and demands. The social cognitive perspective is concerned not with what people *have* (e.g., traits, disorders) or what people *are* (e.g., "addictive personalities") but with what people *do* (including what they think and feel) and under what conditions they do it. Likewise, a social cognitive approach to clinical psychology is concerned not with diagnosing "mental disorders" but with understanding and trying to modify the maladaptive aspects of clients' patterns of thoughts, feelings, and behaviors as they occur in specific life situations and to enhance clients' strengths and well-being.

## ACKNOWLEDGMENTS

I am grateful to June Tangney and John Riskind for their very helpful comments and suggestions on this chapter and to Jennifer Kane for her help constructing the reference section.

## REFERENCES

Ajzen, I. (1988). *Attitudes, personality, and behavior.* Chicago: Dorsey Press.

Andersen, S. M., & Berk, M. S. (1998). Transference in everyday experience: Implications of experimental research for relevant clinical phenomena. *Review of General Psychology, 2,* 81–120.

Anthony, J. L., Lonigan, C. J., & Hecht, S. A. (1999). Dimensionality of post-traumatic stress disorder symptoms in children exposed to disaster: Results from a confirmatory factor analysis. *Journal of Abnormal Psychology, 108,* 315–325.

Bandura, A. (1986). *Social foundations of thought and action.* New York: Prentice-Hall.

Bandura, A. (1997). *Self-efficacy: The exercise of control.* New York: Freeman.

Barkley, R. A. (1997). *ADHD and the nature of self-control.* New York: Guilford Press.

Barone, D., Maddux, J. E., & Snyder, C. R. (1997). *Social cognitive psychology: History and current domains.* New York: Plenum Press.

Baumeister, R. F., & Leary, M. R. (1995). The need to belong: Desire for interpersonal attachments as a fundamental human motivation. *Psychological Bulletin, 117,* 497–529.

Baumeister, R. F., & Scher, S. J. (1988). Self-defeating behavior patterns among normal individuals: Review and analysis of common self-destructive tendencies. *Psychological Bulletin, 104,* 3–22.

Bradbury, T. N., & Fincham, F. D. (1990). Preventing marital dysfunction: Review and analysis. In F. D. Fincham & T. N. Bradbury (Eds.), *The psychology of marriage* (pp. 375–401). New York: Guilford Press.

Cantor, N. (1990). From thought to behavior: "Having" and "doing" in the study of personality and cognition. *American Psychologist, 45,* 735–750.

Claridge, G. (1995). *The origins of mental illness.* Cambridge, MA: Malor Books.

Costello, C. G. (1993a). *Symptoms of depression.* New York: Wiley.

Costello, C. G. (1993b). *Symptoms of schizophrenia.* New York: Wiley.

Costello, C. G. (1996). *Personality characteristics of the personality disordered.* New York: Wiley.

Dobson, K. S. (Ed.). (2002). *Handbook of cognitive-behavioral therapy* (2nd ed.). New York: Guilford Press.

Fishbein, M., & Ajzen, I. (1975). *Belief, attitude, intention, and behavior: An introduction to theory and research*. Reading, MA: Addison-Wesley.

Fiske, S. T., & Taylor, S. E. (2008). *Social cognition: From brains to culture*. New York: McGraw-Hill.

Fraley, R. C., & Waller, N. G. (1998). Adult attachment patterns: A test of the typological model. In J. A. Simpson & W. S. Rholes (Eds.), *Attachment theory and close relationships* (pp. 77–114). New York: Guilford Press.

Guisinger, S., & Blatt, S. J. (1994). Individuality and relatedness: Evolution of a fundamental dialectic. *American Psychologist*, *49*, 104–111.

Hollon, S. D., & Beck, A. T. (1994). Cognitive and cognitive-behavioral therapies. In A. E. Bergin & S. L. Garfield (Eds.), *Handbook of psychotherapy and behavior change* (4th ed., pp. 428–466). New York: Wiley.

Kelly, G. A. (1955). *The psychology of personal constructs: A theory of personality* (2 vols.). New York: Norton.

Keyes, C. L. M., & Lopez, S. (2002). Toward a science of mental health: Positive directions in diagnosis and interventions. In C. R. Snyder & S. Lopez (Eds.), *Handbook of positive psychology* (pp. 45–59). New York: Oxford University Press.

Kiesler, D. J. (1991). Interpersonal methods of assessment and diagnosis. In C. R. Snyder & D. R. Forsyth (Eds.), *Handbook of social and clinical psychology* (pp. 438–468). New York: Pergamon.

Kirsch, I. (Ed.). (1999). *How expectancies shape behavior.* Washington, DC: American Psychological Association.

Locke, E. A., & Latham, G. P. (1990). *A theory of goal setting and task performance.* Englewood Cliffs, NJ: Prentice-Hall.

Lowe, J. R., & Widiger, T. A. (2008). Personality disorders. In J. E. Maddux & B. A. Winstead (Eds.), *Psychopathology: Foundations for a contemporary understanding* (2nd ed., pp. 223–250). New York: Taylor & Francis.

Lubinski, D. (2000). Scientific and social significance of assessing individual differences: "Sinking shafts at a few critical points." *Annual Review of Psychology*, *51*, 405–444.

Maddux, J. E. (2009). Stopping the madness: Positive psychology and the deconstruction of the illness ideology and the DSM. In C. R. Snyder & S. J. Lopez (Eds.), *Oxford handbook of positive psychology* (2nd ed., pp. 61–70). New York: Oxford University Press.

Maddux, J. E., Gosselin, J. T., & Winstead, B. A. (2008). Conceptions of psychopathology: A social constructionist perspective. In J. E. Maddux & B. A. Winstead (Eds.), *Psychopathology: Foundations for a contemporary understanding* (pp. 3–18). New York: Taylor & Francis.

Maddux, J. E., & Mundell, C. E. (2005). Disorders of personality: Diseases or individual differences? In V. J. Derlega, B. A. Winstead, & W. H. Jones (Eds.), *Personality: Contemporary theory and research* (3rd ed., pp. 541–571). Chicago: Nelson-Hall.

Mischel, W. (1973). Toward a cognitive social learning reconceptualization of personality. *Psychological Review*, *80*, 252–284.

Oatley, K., & Jenkins, J. M. (1992). Human emotion: Function and dysfunction. *Annual Review of Psychology*, *43*, 55–86.

Persons, J. (1986). The advantages of studying psychological phenomena rather than psychiatric diagnosis. *American Psychologist*, *41*, 1252–1260.

Rotter, J. B. (1954). *Social learning and clinical psychology*. Englewood Cliffs, NJ: Prentice-Hall.

Shapiro, D. (1965). *Neurotic styles*. New York: Basic Books.

Shaywitz, S. E., Escobar, M. D., Shaywitz, B. A., Fletcher, J. M., & Makuch, R. (1992). Evidence that dyslexia may represent the lower tail of normal distribution of reading ability. *New England Journal of Medicine*, *326*, 145–150.

Smith, R. (2008). Biological bases of psychopathology. In J. E. Maddux & B. A. Winstead (Eds.), *Psychopathology: Foundations for a contemporary understanding* (2nd ed., pp. 67–82). New York: Taylor & Francis.

Widiger, T. A. (2008). Classification and diagnosis: Historical development and contemporary issues. In J. E. Maddux & B. A. Winstead (Eds.), *Psychopathology: Foundations for contemporary understanding* (2nd ed., pp. 83–102). New York: Taylor & Francis.

Woodward, W. R. (1982). The "discovery" of social behaviorism and social learning theory, 1870–1980. *American Psychologist*, *37*, 396–410.

# 23 Self-Directed Change

## *A Transtheoretical Model*

James O. Prochaska
Janice M. Prochaska

Our search for how people change on their own—self-directed change—actually began with trying to solve the mystery of how very different treatments can produce very common outcomes. How is it that in the large National Institute of Mental Health Depression Treatment Study (Elkin et al., 1989), cognitive therapy, interpersonal therapy, and antidepressants produced comparable outcomes? How is it that in the large Project MATCH study on alcohol disorders (Project Match Research Group, 1997), cognitive-behavioral therapy, motivational interviewing, and 12-step programs produced comparable outcomes?

The most popular hypothesis focuses on common factors such as the therapeutic relationship that are part of all effective therapies. These common factors are believed to produce common outcomes (Hubble, Duncan, & Miller, 1999). Our search for common factors began with a comparative analysis of 25 leading psychotherapies (Prochaska & Norcross, 1979/2009). This theoretical analysis focused on the processes of change that were used most often across the leading therapies. The first discovery was that the theories of psychotherapy had much more to say about why people do *not* change than how people *can* change. They were largely theories of personality and psychopathology.

We identified 10 processes of change based on our comparative analysis. One example of a process is consciousness raising, the most broadly used process, which has its roots in the Freudian theory of making unconscious processes conscious in order to facilitate change and enhance self-control. Psychotherapies differed in the techniques used to facilitate this process: from observations, interpretations, and confrontations to education, information, and feedback. The fact that these 10 processes were derived from many different theories led to the transtheoretical model of therapy and behavior change. One of the goals of this model was to provide a theoretical, empirical, and practical framework for integrating processes of change from across leading theories of therapy.

The next step in our search was to empirically validate the processes of change. Our assumption was that if these are fundamental processes common to change, then they should be applied when people change on their own without the help of therapy. So we began to study people struggling to change on their own, as well as people changing via therapy. From qualitative interviews these people taught us something that we had not learned from any of the 300 systems of psychotherapy we had studied: that behavior change is a *process* that unfolds *over time* and involves progress through a *series of stages*.

## STAGES OF CHANGE

*Precontemplation* is the stage in which people have no intention to take action in the foreseeable future, usually measured as the next 6 months. People may be in this stage because they are uninformed or underinformed about the consequences of their behavior, or they may have tried to change a number of times and have become demoralized about their abilities to change. Both the uninformed and underinformed tend to avoid reading, talking, or thinking about their high-risk behaviors. Other theories often characterize them as resistant or unmotivated clients or as not ready for therapy or health promotion programs. We suspect that traditional health promotion programs are not ready for such individuals and are not motivated to match their needs. As a group, people in precontemplation view the cons (costs) of changing their behavior as clearly outweighing the pros (benefits).

*Contemplation* is the stage in which people intend to change within the next 6 months. They are now aware of the pros of changing but are also acutely aware of the cons of changing. This balance between the costs and benefits of changing can produce profound ambivalence that can keep people stuck in this stage for long periods of time. We often characterize this phenomenon as chronic contemplation or behavioral procrastination. These people are also not ready for traditional action-oriented programs. Given the intense ambivalence that can characterize the contemplation stage, people in it often end up not wanting to take action. At least, they do not want to change enough to risk taking action and to risk giving up the immediate benefits of their problem behavior. They often go on thinking about changing and telling themselves that "some day" they will take action.

*Preparation* is the stage in which people intend to take action in the immediate future, usually measured as within the next month. As the name of the stage indicates, they see themselves as preparing for action. They are more confident than contemplators that they can control their problem behavior. They view the pros of changing as clearly outweighing the cons. They also have a concrete plan for changing and may be taking small steps to reduce their problem behaviors (DiClemente et al., 1991). The large majority of people identified as being in the preparation stage ultimately take action to change (Prochaska, Velicer, Prochaska, & Johnson, 2004). As with many problems, however, a majority of people who take action will fail, either quickly or eventually relapsing back to their old patterns.

*Action* is the stage in which people must apply more existential processes such as self-liberation, more humanistic processes such as helping relationships, and more behavioral processes such as counterconditioning, stimulus control, and reinforcement management (Prochaska & DiClemente, 1983). In the action stage, people use these processes to overtly modify their problem behavior to at least some minimum criterion of success.

The action stage lasts longer than most people expect; it usually takes about 6 months of concentrated effort before risks for relapse are greatly reduced. If people move from preparation to action and continue to rely on processes such as consciousness raising and self-reevaluation, they are more likely to fail because they are not matching the appropriate processes of change to their stage of change. These people do not know how to change.

*Maintenance* is the stage in which people are working to consolidate the gains they made during action in order to minimize risks for relapse. In the transtheoretical model, maintenance begins after 6 months of concerted action. Maintenance used to be viewed as a stable stage in which people do not have to work at changing. We now know that people continue to apply particular processes of change, such as counterconditioning and stimulus control, to keep from relapsing (Prochasksa & DiClemente, 1983).

How long does maintenance last? For some problems (e.g., obesity), it may last a lifetime. For other problems (e.g., smoking and certain anxiety and mood disorders), people may be able to entirely eliminate their problems and not have to do anything to prevent relapse.

The criteria we use for termination is that people attain maximum self-efficacy or confidence and minimum temptation to engage in their problem behavior across all previously risky situations. Many smokers get to the point at which they experience no desire to smoke, are fully confident that they will never smoke again, and report having to do nothing to keep from smoking. How long does it take to complete the maintenance stage? We used to think that for smokers, 12 months of continuous abstinence meant that they were home free. We now know that even after a year of never smoking, 37% of adults will relapse back to regular smoking over the course of their lifetimes. After 5 years of continuous abstinence the risks for relapse finally drop to 7%. Therefore, maintenance lasts from 6 months to 5 years after action is taken.

In our research on how people change, we have discovered that one of the secrets of success is using appropriate processes of change to progress through particular stages of change. Progressing from precontemplation to contemplation involves the application of affective and cognitive processes, such as dramatic relief (catharsis) and consciousness raising (DiClemente et al., 1991; Prochaska & DiClemente, 1983). Movement from contemplation to preparation involves the use of evaluative processes such as self-reevaluation and environmental reevaluation.

Table 23.1 summarizes the relationship between the stages of changes and the processes of change people must apply to progress to the next stage, as observed in previous research (DiClemente et al., 1991; Prochaska & DiClemente, 1983, 1984).

With the discovery of the stages of change, we believed that we had found the missing link that could lead to the integration of processes of change derived from many different theories. To our original 10 processes we also added the pros and cons of changing derived from Janis and Mann's (1977) decision-making theory and self-efficacy from Bandura's (1977) self-efficacy theory. What follows are principles for progressing through the stages of change that were discovered in this initial study and from decades of research since on both self-changers and therapy-changers. These principles can help individuals and entire populations progress from one stage of change to the next.

**TABLE 23.1. Stages by Processes and Principles of Change**

| Precontemplation | Contemplation | Preparation | Action | Maintenance |
|---|---|---|---|---|
| Consciousness raising | | | | |
| Dramatic relief | | | | |
| Environmental reevaluation | | | | |
| | Self-reevaluation | | | |
| | | Self-liberation | | |
| | | | Reinforcement management | |
| | | | Helping relationships | |
| | | | Counterconditioning | |
| | | | Stimulus control | |
| Pros of changing increasing | | | | |
| | Cons of changing decreasing | | | |
| | | Self-efficacy increasing | | |

*Note.* Social liberation has been found to not have differentiated emphasis across all five stages. Copyright by James O. Prochaska. Reprinted by permission.

## Principle 1

*The pros of changing must increase for people to progress out of precontemplation.* We found that in 12 out of 12 studies, the mean pros were higher in contemplation than in precontemplation (Prochaska et al., 1994). This pattern held true across 12 behaviors: cocaine abuse, smoking, delinquency, obesity, condom use, safe-sex practices, sedentary lifestyles, high-fat diets, sun exposure, radon testing, mammography screening, and physicians practicing behavioral medicine. The pattern also held true for patients' views of psychotherapy. Those in precontemplation for changing their problems perceived the cons of psychotherapy as outweighing the pros. Those in contemplation perceived the pros and cons as about equal, reflecting their ambivalence. Those in action or maintenance were convinced that the pros of therapy clearly outweighed the cons. Meta-analyses (Hall & Rossi, 2008) revealed a consistent pattern of the pros and cons across stage of change for 48 problem behaviors.

An example of an intervention that we have found useful involves asking persons in precontemplation to name the benefits or pros of changing, such as addressing a weight problem by starting to exercise. They typically can list four or five reasons. We tell them that there are 8–10 times that many and challenge them to double or triple their list. If their list of pros for exercising starts to indicate more motives, such as a healthier heart, healthier lungs, more energy, healthier immune system, better moods, less stress, better sex life, and enhanced self-esteem, they will be more motivated to begin to seriously contemplate change.

## Principle 2

Through intervention, *the cons of changing must decrease for people to progress from contemplation to action.* In 12 out of 12 studies, we found that the cons of changing were lower in action than in the contemplation stage (Prochaska et al., 1994).

### Principle 3

*The pros and cons must cross over for people to be prepared to take action.* In 12 out of 12 studies, the cons of changing were higher than the pros in precontemplation, but in 11 out of 12, the pros were higher than the cons in the action stage. The one exception was with people trying to quit using cocaine, which was the only population where we had a large percentage of people as inpatients. We interpret this exception to mean that among these inpatient addicts, their action may have been more under the control of residential care than under self-control (Rosenbloom, 1991).

### Principle 4

*The pros of changing must increase twice as much as the cons decrease.* Therefore, we place twice as much emphasis on the benefits of changing than on the costs. The ratio of pros and cons is important, as is a higher threshold of pros.

### Principle 5

*Processes of change are differentially linked to specific stages of change.* Table 23.1 presents the integration that we have found between processes and stages of change in our empirical research.

### Ten Processes

*Consciousness raising* involves increasing people's awareness about the causes, consequences, and cures for a particular problem. Interventions that can increase awareness include observations, confrontations, interpretations, feedback, and education. Some techniques (e.g., confrontation) involve high risk in terms of retention and are not recommended as strongly as motivational enhancement methods such as personal feedback about the current and long-term consequences of continuing with the problem. Increasing the cons of not changing is the corollary of raising the pros of changing. Therefore, one goal of consciousness raising is to increase the pros of changing.

*Dramatic relief* involves emotional arousal about one's current behavior and the sense of relief that can come from changing. Fear, inspiration, guilt, and hope are some of the emotions that can move people to contemplate changing. Journaling, role playing, grieving, and giving personal testimonies are examples of techniques that can produce emotional arousal.

*Environmental reevaluation* combines affective and cognitive assessments of how a behavior affects one's social environment and how changing would impact that environment. Empathy training, values clarification, and family or network interventions can facilitate such reevaluation. For example, in a brief media intervention aimed at smokers in the precontemplation stage, a man clearly in grief says, "I always feared that my smoking would lead to an early death. I always worried that my smoking would cause lung cancer. But I never imagined it would happen to my wife." Beneath his grieving face appears this statistic: 50,000 deaths per year are caused by passive smoking. In 30 seconds, we have consciousness raising, dramatic relief, and environmental reevaluation. Such media interventions have been an important part of the California Department of Health's programs aimed at reducing smoking for self-changers (Prochaska, personal communication, 2009).

*Self-reevaluation* combines cognitive and affective assessments of one's self-image free from the problem. Using imagery, identifying healthier role models, and clarifying values are techniques that can produce self-image reevaluations.

*Self-liberation* is the belief that one can change, coupled with the commitment and recommitment to act on that belief. Techniques that can enhance self-liberation include having individuals make public commitments (rather than private commitments). Motivational research also suggests that if people only have one choice, they are less motivated than if they have two choices; three is better still, but four does not enhance motivation (Miller, 1987). Accordingly, we try to provide people with three of the best choices for applying each process, such as choosing Alcoholics Anonymous, cognitive-behavioral theory or motivational interviewing for help with alcohol problems.

*Reinforcement management* involves the systematic use of reinforcements for taking steps in the right direction. Contingency contracts, overt and covert reinforcements, and group recognition are procedures for increasing reinforcement; such incentives increase the probability that healthier responses will be repeated. To prepare people for the longer term, we teach them to rely more on self-reinforcements than social reinforcements. In our clinical work we have found that many clients expect much more reinforcement and recognition from others than those others actually provide. Too many relatives and friends can take the action stage for granted too quickly. Average acquaintances typically generate only a few positive consequences early in the action stage. Self-reinforcements are obviously much more under self-control and can be given more quickly and consistently when dealing with temptations to lapse or relapse.

*Helping relationships* combine caring, openness, trust, acceptance, and support for changing. Rapport building, a therapeutic alliance, counselor calls, buddy systems, sponsors, and self-help groups can be excellent resources for the social support that comes from helping relationships.

*Counterconditioning* requires the learning of healthier behaviors that can substitute for unhealthy behaviors. Counterconditioning techniques tend to be quite specific to a particular behavior and include desensitization, assertion, and cognitive counters to irrational self-statements that can elicit distress.

*Stimulus control* involves modifying the environment to increase cues that prompt healthier responses and decrease cues that are tempting. Avoidance, environmental reengineering (e.g., removing addictive substances and paraphernalia), and attending self-help groups can provide stimuli that elicit healthier responses and reduce risks for relapse.

*Social liberation* involves increases in social opportunities or alternatives. Advocacy, empowerment procedures, and public policies can produce increased opportunities for health promotion. For example, smoke-free zones, salad bars in school lunchrooms, and easy access to condoms and other contraceptives can be used to help people make difficult health-promoting changes.

## Common Pathways to Change

Most recently we have been working on research (funded by the National Institute on Aging) designed to study factors in the successful maintenance of change across 10 different behaviors: smoking, diet, exercise, sun exposure, stress, alcohol abuse, obesity, medication adherence, depression, and domestic violence. This collaborative project is a secondary data analysis of about 35 studies funded by the National Institutes of Health in the Cancer Prevention Research Center at the University of Rhode Island.

In an analysis of smoking, we compared three *dynatypes* (patterns of change) over time in both therapy changers (those in treatment) and self-changers (those not in treatment). The dynatypes studied were (1) stable smokers who were smoking at each of the 6-month follow-ups over 24 months; (2) maintainers who quit at one of the follow-ups and remained abstinent at subsequent follow-ups; and (3) relapsers who quit at one follow-up but were back to smoking at a subsequent follow-up (Sun, Prochaska, & Velicer, 2007). The six groups (three dynatypes for self-changers and three for therapy changers) were compared on their frequency of use of the transtheoretical model (TTM) processes and principles of change.

The stable smokers showed very little change over 2 years in their use of the change processes and principles. Paralleling their smoking behavior, stable smokers' use of the processes and principles of change exhibited high test–retest reliability at 6-month intervals over a 2-year period. The maintainers, on the other hand, showed dramatic changes in their use of the change variables. Some variables, such as the pros of changing, increased dramatically. Other variables, such as temptations to smoke, decreased dramatically. Still other variables, such as self-reevaluation, initially increased in use and then decreased as the individuals progressed further into the maintenance stage. The relapsers initially paralleled the maintainers in their profile of change variables, but then shifted in the direction of the stable smokers. Relapsers typically ended up somewhere between the maintainers and the stable smokers. They appeared to still engage in the change processes to some degree as they contemplated action or prepared to take action again.

In all three dynatypes, the therapy changers and self-changers essentially followed the same pathways in their applications of the principles and processes of change. The therapy changer group produced a higher percentage of successful maintainers, but the self-changer group followed the same pathways to change. Our interpretation of this finding is that the expert guidance available in the treatment group helped a higher percentage of smokers to follow the successful pathways, but both the therapy changers and the self-changers followed parallel pathways.

These findings may help us understand how very different therapies can produce the same outcome. By definition, two different types of effective treatments are more similar to each other than to a no-treatment group. Yet our secondary analysis of several dozens of treatment studies demonstrates that *treatment and self-changer groups follow common pathways of change*.

Individuals in psychotherapy typically spend more than 99% of their waking hours outside of therapy. What they do during the 99% of their week will account for more of their change than what they do in the 1% of their time spent in the therapy room. Helping clients follow the more successful pathways to change between sessions should increase the effectiveness of therapy.

## Clinical Examples

### *Stress Management*

As part of a national study of stress, 1,200 individuals suffering from stress symptoms were recruited to participate in a stress-management intervention program based on the TTM (Evers et al., 2006). The program involved three computerized tailored interventions (CTIs) over 6 months and a stage-matched self-help manual. At 6 months, substantial success was observed in the TTM group (about 60%), and this outcome was maintained over the next 12 months. At the 18-month follow-up, over 60% of the TTM group had reached the action or maintenance stage, compared to 40% of the proactive assessment-alone control group.

### *Depression Prevention*

Levesque et al. (in press) recruited 902 adults at risk for depression from primary care waiting rooms and by telephone. The treatment group received a stage-matched manual and an individualized printed report in the mail at baseline, and additional individualized reports at 1- and 3-month follow-ups. The treatment and control groups were assessed by phone at baseline and at 9 months. At 9 months, among individuals who were in a pre-action stage for depression prevention at baseline, treatment group participants were significantly more likely than control group participants to experience a clinically significant reduction in depression (37 vs. 17%). The treatment group was more likely than the control group to be in the action or maintenance stage for depression prevention (70 vs. 55%) and to be taking antidepressant medication, if prescribed (71 vs. 50%). Among study participants who were in the action or maintenance stage at baseline, the intervention was more likely to prevent the onset of depression; only 11% of treatment group participants (vs. 19% of control group participants) experienced a new episode of major depression during the follow-up period.

### *Computerized Tailored Interventions Plus Counselors*

In a large study of smokers recruited from a managed care setting, counselor enhancements through proactive telephone counseling were added to our TTM CTI. Four interventions were compared: (1) the CTI; (2) the CTI plus counselor calls; (3) the CTI plus a stimulus control computer designed to produce nicotine fading; and (4) an assessment-only condition. We employed a 4 (intervention) × 4 (occasions; 0, 6, 12, and 18 months) design. Smokers were contacted at home via telephone or mail.

Of the 4,653 smokers who were contacted, 85.3% enrolled in the study. At baseline, 38% were in the precontemplation stage, 45% in the contemplation stage, and 17% in the preparation stage. At 18 months, 23.3% of those in the CTI group were no longer smoking, a rate of abstinence that was 33% greater than that of the assessment-only group. The counselor enhancement produced increased smoking cessation at 12 months but not at 18 months. The stimulus control computer produced no improvement, resulting in a 20% worse cessation rate than the assessment-only condition. The enhanced conditions failed to outperform the CTI alone (Prochaska et al., 2001).

### *Counselor Plus CTI*

There is considerable evidence that standard protocols for coaching and counseling can have substantial impact on behavior. There is also growing evidence that enhancing these protocols by adding TTM-tailored communications results in substantially larger treatment effects. For example, adding TTM-tailored communications to proactive coaching with pregnant smokers produced more than eight times as much behavior change as the standard protocol alone (Lawrence, Aveyard, Evans, & Cheng, 2003). In the domain of domestic violence, adding tailored communications to weekly group counseling reduced partner violence by more than seven times that observed in response to standard group counseling (Levesque, 2007). Adding tailored communications to counseling for violent partners who were not progressing, reduced partner violence by about 50% and more than doubled other clinically significant outcomes. Adding CTI feedback to counseling for clients can increase treatment effects on problems such as partner violence and prenatal smoking. In addition, adding CTI feedback to counseling for counselors can increase treatment effectiveness across a broad range of mental health problems. Findings across multiple studies consistently indicate that CTI feedback enhances performance of *both* professionals and patients.

## CLINICAL IMPLICATIONS

Research on the TTM indicates that people are more likely to change their behavior in healthy, adaptive, and desired directions when:

1. They progress one stage at a time rather than taking action before they are prepared.
2. They apply processes that are appropriate to their current stage of change.
3. They learn from their relapses rather than becoming demoralized.
4. They understand the complexities of change rather than reducing it all to one process, such as consciousness raising or stimulus control.
5. They understand that resistance to change is often due to mismatches between the client's stage of change and therapists or others trying to pressure them to take action when they are not ready.
6. They have better road maps to help guide them through the stages of change.

That these strategies can enhance the effectiveness of both professionally assisted change (e.g., psychotherapy and counseling) and self-directed change underscores one of the basic assumptions of this volume: that clinical and nonclinical problems, populations, and interventions are more similar than they are different.

## REFERENCES


Bandura, A. (1977). Self-efficacy: Toward a unifying theory of behavior change. *Psychological Review*, *84*, 191–215.

DiClemente, C. C., Prochaska, J. O., Fairhurst, S., Velicer, W. F., Velasquez, M., & Rossi, J. S. (1991). The process of smoking cessation: An analysis of precontemplation, contemplation and preparation stages of change. *Journal of Consulting and Clinical Psychology*, *59*, 259–304.

Elkin, I. E., Shea, M. T., Watkins, J. T., Imber, S. D., Sotsky, S. M., Collins, J. F., et al. (1989). National Institute of Mental Health Treatment of Depression Collaborative Research Program: General effectiveness of treatment. *Archives of General Psychiatry*, *46*, 974–982.

Evers, K. E., Prochaska, J. O., Johnson, J. L., Mauriello, L. M., Padula, J. A., & Prochaska, J. M. (2006). A randomized clinical trial of a population- and transtheoretical model-based stress-management intervention. *Health Psychology*, *25*, 521–529.

Hall, K., & Rossi, J. S. (2008). Meta-analytic examination off the strong and weak principles across 48 health behaviors. *Preventive Medicine*, *46*, 266–274.

Hubble, M. A., Duncan, B. L., & Miller, S. D. (1999). *The heart and soul of change*. Washington, DC: American Psychological Association.

Janis, I. L., & Mann, L. (1977). *Decision making: A psychological analysis of conflict, chance, and commitment*. New York: Free Press.

Lawrence, T., Aveyard, P., Evans, O., & Cheng, K. K. (2003). A cluster randomized controlled trial of smoking cessation in pregnant women comparing interventions based on the transtheoretical (stages of change) model to standard care. *Tobacco Control, 12*, 168–177.

Levesque, D. A. (2007). *Expert system intervention for domestic violence offenders*. Final report to the National Institute of Mental Health (Grant No. R44MH62858).

Levesque, D. A., Van Marter, D. F., Schneider, R. J., Bauer, M. R., Goldberg, D. N., Prochaska, J. O., et al. (in press). Randomized trial of a Transtheoretical Model Intervention for depression in primary care. *American Journal of Health Promotion*.

Miller, W. R. (1987). Motivation and treatment goals. *Drugs and Society, 1*, 133–151.

Prochaska, J. O., & DiClemente, C. C. (1983). Stages and processes of self-change of smoking: Toward an integrative model of change. *Journal of Consulting and Clinical Psychology, 51*, 390–395.

Prochaska, J. O., & DiClemente, C. C. (1984). *The transtheoretical approach: Crossing the traditional boundaries of therapy*. Melbourne, FL: Krieger.

Prochaska, J. O., & Norcross, J. C. (2009). *Systems of psychotherapy: A transtheoretical analysis* (7th ed.). Pacific Grove, CA: Brooks-Cole. (Original work published 1979)

Prochaska, J. O., Velicer, W. F., Fava, J., Ruggiero, L., Laforge, R., Rossi, J. S., et al. (2001). Counselor and stimulus control enhancements of a stage matched expert system for smokers in a managed care setting. *Preventive Medicine, 32*, 23–32.

Prochaska, J. O., Velicer, W. F., Prochaska, J. M., & Johnson, J. L. (2004). Size, consistency and stability of stage effects for smoking cessation. *Addictive Behaviors, 29*, 207–213.

Prochaska, J. O., Velicer, W. F., Rossi, J. S., Goldstein, M. G., Marcus, B. H., Rakowski, W., et al. (1994). Stages of change and decisional balance for 12 problem behaviors. *Health Psychology, 13*, 39–46.

Project MATCH Research Group. (1997). Matching alcoholism treatments to client heterogeneity: Project MATCH post treatment drinking outcome. *Journal of Studies on Alcohol, 58*, 7–29.

Rosenbloom, D. (1991). *A transtheorertical analysis of change among cocaine users*. Unpublished doctoral dissertation, University of Rhode Island, Kingston, RI.

Sun, X., Prochaska, J. O., & Velicer, W. F. (2007). Transtheoretical principles and processes for quitting smoking: A 24-month comparison of a representative sample of quitters, relapsers, and nonquitters. *Addictive Behaviors, 32*, 2707–2726.

# 24 Social Influence Processes and Persuasion in Psychotherapy and Counseling

Paul B. Perrin
Martin Heesacker
Chandylen Pendley
Mary B. Smith

Suave Power of Persuasion,
help me to persuade you
to help me be
persuasive.

May I be as profound as a bass drum,
without the emptiness

and as clever as Oscar Wilde
before he went to jail.

—Kenneth Burke

This chapter presents a brief overview of the history of the interface between the social influence and psychotherapy fields before the early 1990s, and then more thoroughly addresses the scholarly literature at this interface published over the past 15 years. The results of our review suggest that there have been relatively few publications at this interface since the early 1990s. We advance the possibility that this small number of publications is, at least in part, the result of the recent flourishing of multiculturalism in psychotherapy and psychotherapy research. This chapter details some of the tenets of multiculturalism that may put it at odds with research advocating the use of social influence and attitude change processes in counseling and psychotherapy. The chapter then identifies pathways by which this interface can thrive in both practice and scholarship, as part of this new, more multiculturally aware era. The chapter concludes by presenting a new perspective on therapeutic attitude change that we call the *route-shift* approach. This approach asserts that, at its core, effective psychological functioning—at least in part—involves a directed, dynamic, and two-way interplay between effortful and automatic cognitive processing. We believe that an approach to psychotherapy that incorporates depth-of-processing models of attitude change into this route-shift perspective holds promise for wedding multicultural competence with effective social influence in counseling and psychotherapy.

## A BRIEF HISTORY OF SOCIAL INFLUENCE AND PSYCHOTHERAPY

### Attitudes

Most of the social influence theory applied to counseling and psychotherapy focuses on attitudes and attitude change.[1] For our purposes, *attitudes* are defined as "general and enduring positive or negative feelings about some person, object, or issue" (Petty & Cacioppo, 1981, p. 7). People's attitudes organize their perceptions of the world and ultimately affect their behavior (Cacioppo, Claiborn, Petty, & Heesacker, 1991), so addressing attitudes within the context of counseling and psychotherapy is vital. Hoyt and Janis (1975), for example, found that a clinical attitude change treatment produced nearly twice the participant adherence to a health regimen as a no-treatment control group. In other words, attitude change regarding adherence to the health regimen led to corresponding behavior change (see Ajzen & Fishbein, 1977, 1980, and Crano & Prislin, 2006, for reviews of the literature on the prediction of behavior from attitude change).

Not only can attitudinal change improve adherence to health regimens, but it can also alter maladaptive beliefs. Clients' beliefs may be maladaptive if they constitute racism, sexism, or pessimism toward changing a dysfunctional behavior pattern (Heppner & Frazier, 1992). One of the goals of psychotherapy is to facilitate client realization of the maladaptive consequences of certain beliefs, as well as the dysfunctional inconsistencies that may exist in one's beliefs (Cacioppo et al., 1991). This goal is typically in line with clients' own desires because people generally want to have consistent (Abelson et al., 1968) and accurate (Petty & Cacioppo, 1986) beliefs. Therefore, clients' attitudinal inconsistencies can result in psychotherapeutic attitude change, though achieving this change is often difficult.

Two well-known and widely researched theories regarding the mechanisms by which attitudinal inconsistencies result in change are Leon Festinger's *dissonance theory* (1957) and E. Tori Higgins's *self-discrepancy theory* (e.g., Higgins, Klein, & Strauman, 1985). Both theories posit that holding inconsistent attitudes leads to an uncomfortable internal state. The discomfort of this state results in an openness to attitudinal change that might not otherwise exist. Therapists can use this client discomfort to facilitate change, but there are many pathways by which clients can reduce their discomfort, only some of which are likely to fit therapeutic goals. One factor that makes attitudinal change challenging, even for clients experiencing the discomfort of inconsistent attitudes, is a strong attitudinal inertia. For example, Lord, Ross, and Lepper (1979) demonstrated that people are motivated to retain their beliefs and attitudes even in the face of conflicting or contradictory evidence. They presented to two groups of participants—one that favored capital punishment and one that did not—evidence that both discredited and credited, respectively, the success of capital punishment in preventing crime. Results indicated that even when given credible, contradictory evidence, participants retained their original beliefs. The section that follows describes a dissonance-based model of attitudinal change in psychotherapy.

## Interpersonal Influence in Psychotherapy

Strong's two-stage model (1968) of interpersonal influence in psychotherapy was derived from Festinger's cognitive dissonance theory (1957) and the work of Hovland, Janis, and Kelley (1953). In the first stage of Strong's model the therapist gains credibility in the eyes of the client by exhibiting expertise, trustworthiness, and attractiveness. This credibility then enables the therapist to enter the second stage, where he or she makes recommendations to the client that are dissonant from the client's attitudes and behaviors. The therapist attempts to influence the client's attitudes, opinions, and/or behaviors by using his or her personal credibility to create client attitude change. The client's attitude change ostensibly results in a reduction in the dissonance between his or her attitudes and the therapist's (Bochner & Insko, 1966).

Therapists' responsive nonverbal behaviors (e.g., smiling, nodding head, learning forward) have been consistently shown to enhance clients' opinions of their therapists (Corrigan, Dell, Lewis, & Schmidt, 1980; Heppner & Claiborn, 1989; Heppner & Dixon, 1981). However, such verbal behaviors as self-disclosure, psychological jargon, and profanity can either positively or negatively affect clients' perception of a therapist (Corrigan et al., 1980; Heppner & Claiborn, 1989; Heppner & Dixon, 1981). Research on the influence of therapist credibility on client change has been mixed and suggests that, compared to therapists with low credibility, therapists with high credibility sometimes are *better at* changing the attitudes of their clients (Heppner & Dixon, 1978; Strong & Schmidt, 1970), sometimes are *just as good* at changing attitudes (Greenberg, 1969; Sprafkin, 1970), and sometimes are *worse at* changing attitudes (Heesacker, 1986). In short, evidence is lacking that therapist credibility is a major influence in facilitating therapeutic change (see review by Heppner & Claiborn, 1989, as well as a meta-analytic review by Hoyt, 1996).

Frank (1963) took a different approach to client behavior change, suggesting that the therapist's verbal and nonverbal *communications* are the underlying causes of change. Levy (1963) similarly suggested a link between clients' interpretations of the therapist's message and client attitude change. Frank's and Levy's insights paved the way for models that explicitly distinguish source factors from message content factors, such as the elaboration likelihood model (Petty & Cacioppo, 1986).

## The Elaboration Likelihood Model

Because of the mixed evidence regarding the effectiveness of therapist credibility on client attitude change, research and theory began to focus more on depth-of-processing models, in which the client is viewed as an active participant in the attitude change process. One of the more notable theories in this regard is the elaboration likelihood model (ELM), a depth-of-processing theory of attitude change that posits both a *deep processing* route and a *shallow processing* route to attitude change. This model predicts specific interactions among source, subject, and message variables (Heppner & Frazier, 1992).

The ELM explains how persuasive communications—such as comments by a counselor or psychotherapist—result in attitude change (Cacioppo et al., 1991) and posits that attitude change has two sources: the *central route* and the *peripheral route*. The central route results from careful, systematic, and reasoned deliberation, whereas the peripheral route results from the use of heuristics (simple decision rules), such as a speech with big words, and associative cues, such as the level of attractiveness or authority of the communicator (Cacioppo et al., 1991). If a message is perceived as irrelevant, as too difficult to comprehend, or as too discrepant from one's initial attitude, message recipients are less likely to engage in central-route processing and more likely to engage in peripheral-route processing (Cacioppo et al., 1991). With the large amount of sensory information people typically have to process on a daily basis and the finite capacity to engage in thoughtful analysis, people are generally miserly in their allocation of effortful thought (Langer, Blank, & Chanowiu, 1978). Hence a great deal of attitude change results from peripheral-route processing rather than central. However, attitude changes resulting from the peripheral route are less likely to last, more likely to be changed by subsequent communications, and less likely to influence subsequent behavior than attitude changes resulting from the central route (Petty & Cacioppo, 1986).

The ELM has been quite informative for psychotherapy. For example, it has helped therapists understand that different kinds of attitudes (thought-based vs. cue-based) have different levels of influence on clients' subsequent behavior. Factors that had been emphasized to therapists in earlier work on persuasion in psychotherapy as important in changing client attitudes are, according to the ELM, associated mostly with attitudes that only weakly influence subsequent behavior. Factors that had not been a focus of therapists before the advent of the ELM, such as facilitating a preponderance of client thoughts supportive of the target attitudes and behaviors, were highlighted as critically important to behavior change, as a result of the ELM. Yet, like other theories, the ELM can be challenging to apply to particular psychotherapy clients (Cacioppo et al., 1991; Heppner & Frazier, 1992). Many studies have applied the ELM to psychotherapy (e.g., McNeil & Stoltenberg, 1988), though some of these studies have been criticized (see Cacioppo et al., 1991). For example, some of these studies made ostensibly ELM-based predictions that were not, in fact, correctly derived from the model, according to the authors of the model. Also, a number of ELM-related constructs have been operationalized in ways that the model's authors have questioned (Cacioppo et al., 1991). Cacioppo et al. (1991) have observed that studies applying the ELM sometimes ignore the important practical implications of *moderate* elaboration likelihood, which is when initial elaboration likelihood is neither high nor low. In these cases, multiple factors operate to determine whether people will or will not effortfully process a communication.

### The Input/Output Matrix

One of the other major frameworks for understanding attitude change is McGuire's (1985) input/output matrix, which attempts to account for the complexity of persuasion processes. The matrix consists of five sets of *input* factors: source variables, message variables, channel variables, receiver variables, and target variables. These input variables are, in turn, crossed with a dozen *output* steps that begin with tuning in to the communication and end with consolidation of the new behavior pattern. The resulting 60-cell matrix is unrivaled in its comprehensiveness, and yet this comprehensiveness is both the model's greatest virtue and its greatest vice. McGuire's model may be too complicated to render straightforward, practical, and user-friendly guidance to practitioners. Our concern about this complexity is magnified when contemplating the challenges facing practitioners who are new to adopting social influence perspectives in their clinical work. For this reason, this chapter focuses on more accessible models and perspectives.

## SOCIAL INFLUENCE AND PSYCHOTHERAPY BEFORE THE EARLY 1990s

The long history of the interface between social influence and psychotherapy fields produced two major reviews in the early 1990s (Cacioppo et al., 1991; Heppner & Frazier, 1992). These articles provided important suggestions for practice and practice-related research, as well as for projected directions of the field. Cacioppo et al. (1991) suggested that research should focus both on the effects of attitude change via different psychotherapy interventions as well as on other unexamined influence variables that are relevant to psychotherapy but not incorporated into the ELM. Cacioppo et al. (1991) also predicted that research on the ELM would transition from highly controlled laboratory environments using relatively homogeneous samples to more diverse and ecologically valid psychotherapy settings. They suggested that, as this transition unfolds, practitioners and practice researchers need to consider several critical aspects of the ELM that can easily be overlooked. For example, persuasion can predictably operate across three distinct dimensions: message arguments, peripheral cues, and the elaboration-likelihood continuum. The influence of variables is not always simple and linear. For example, message repetition has differing effects on cognitive responding, depending on the frequency of repetition. In addition, attitude changes resulting from peripheral-route processing, though ephemeral, can create a platform from which the therapist can affect more central and enduring attitude change. Finally, they pointed out that clients process many of therapists' recommendations using moderate elaboration likelihood rather than high or low elaboration likelihood. What is important about this point is that other factors in the therapy context, such as the credibility of the therapist, may not simply alter attitudes directly but instead may trigger high or low elaboration likelihood.

Heppner and Frazier (1992) broadly reviewed social psychological processes in counseling and psychotherapy. They advocated that research and theory be based on both inhibitory and facilitative motivational factors related to client attitude change, on contextual and message variables influencing client attitude change, and on long-term effects of client attitude change on behavior.

## SOCIAL INFLUENCE AND PSYCHOTHERAPY OVER THE LAST 15 YEARS

Most of the theory and research at the interface of social influence and psychotherapy fields over the past 15 years fall into one of the following three categories: (1) prevention/psychoeducation with a *health* emphasis, (2) prevention/psychoeducation with a *psychological* emphasis, and (3) persuasion in *psychotherapy*.

## Prevention/Psychoeducation with a Health Emphasis

Without question, the most vigorous line of research at the interface of social influence and psychotherapy over the past 15 years has been in the area of prevention/psychoeducation with a health emphasis. Much of the focus has been on matching clinicians' health-related messages to personal characteristics of clients or patients. Probably the oldest system for matching health-related messages to client characteristics is the *health belief model* (HBM), which was originally developed in the 1950s (Hochbaum, 1956) by public health officials attempting to understand and facilitate patient use of X-rays in the wake of a tuberculosis threat (Becker, 1974). Such factors as the client's beliefs about his or her risk of illness, seriousness of the illness, costs versus benefits of doing what health care professionals advocate, and some behavioral triggers were all important elements of the original model. Empirical support for the HBM can be characterized as modest.

Shifting now to more recent approaches to matching health-related messages to client personal characteristics, Slater (1999) has suggested that myriad theories of persuasion and attitude change are complementary, not contradictory, and can often be used in concert because they typically address different types of problems. Slater suggested the use of Prochaska, DiClemente, and Norcross's (1992) *stages-of-change model* (reminiscent of McGuire's, 1985, outcome steps) as a template to map, organize, and synthesize a variety of potentially complementary theories of attitude and behavior change. One approach is to use an ELM framework to develop messages that allow an audience/recipient to move from a precontemplation to a contemplation stage. In the precontemplation stage clients have no intention of changing, often because they do not see a need for change. Cognitive involvement during this stage is often low, and message details may be less important than peripheral cues. Therefore, in this stage, messages intended to build initial awareness should be very simple, delivered by credible sources, and engaging enough to draw attention. According to Slater, the next move from contemplation (in which clients recognize a problem exists and consider taking action) to preparation (in which the balance shifts toward action) is most analogous to persuasion because preparation implies the acceptance of the message arguments and a willingness to consider acting on them. Slater's theory generally suggests the importance of applying stage-appropriate communication, persuasion, and behavior change theories to health-promoting communications (see also Prochaska & Prochaska, Chapter 23, this volume).

Social influence theory has been applied to a number of psychoeducation and prevention initiatives, including communication about cancer (Brinol & Petty, 2006; Dillard & Nabi, 2006); heart disease awareness (Lira et al., 2006); HIV prevention (Albarracin et al., 2003; Albarracin, Kumkale, & Johnson, 2004; Durantini, Albarracin, Mitchell, Earl, & Gillette, 2006); adolescent drug, alcohol, or tobacco use (Brown, D'Emidio-Caston, & Pollard, 1997; Donaldson, Graham, & Hansen, 1994; Donaldson, Graham, Piccinin, & Hansen, 1995; Hwang, Yeagley, & Petosa, 2004); diet (Shepherd, 1999); and contraception (Visser & Vanbilsen, 1994).

Some prevention-focused initiatives attempt to change people's attitudes and behaviors by triggering fear in them. An example of research on these so-called fear appeals comes from work by Floyd, Prentice-Dunn, and Rogers (2000), who found that increases in the threat severity and threat vulnerability of fear appeals changed both message recipients' behavioral intentions and their actual behaviors. However, specific personal characteristics of the message recipients were necessary for fear appeals to work, such as an openness to prevention and detection behaviors, as well as believing in one's own ability to perform the suggested threat-reducing response (Girandola, 2000). The combination of high personal self-efficacy and a strong fear appeal resulted in much larger attitude and behavioral changes than did the combinations of low self-efficacy and either high or low fear appeals (Witte & Allen, 2000). Intense fear appeals were better at inspiring health *prevention* behaviors, whereas less intense fear appeals were better at creating health *detection* behaviors (Girandola & Atkinson, 2003).

There is now solid evidence that the amount and directionality of client thinking are the key mediators of the effect of fear appeals on attitudes. Fear appeals arouse thinking. Increased thinking can lead to enduring attitude change. On the other hand, very frightening fear appeals or fear appeals that do not readily suggest an effective action are apt to trigger *biased* thinking—thinking that serves to protect the self by undermining some aspect of the fear appeal. Such self-protective cognitions can actually result in a *worse* outcome than no fear appeal (e.g., Janis & Feshbach, 1953).

In addition to self-efficacy, another important personal characteristic to take into account in persuasion is client emotionality. Dillard and Nabi (2006) suggested that health-related messages can arouse one or more emotions, and that the type and intensity of emotional reactions to health-related messages vary across individuals based on their cognitive appraisals. To arouse emotions effectively, the emotional theme should match the persuasive goals. Emotions can enhance, inhibit, or be unrelated to the persuasive effectiveness of health-related messages (Dillard & Nabi, 2006). Finally, for an emotional response to exert persuasive force, it must be perceived as both caused by the message and relevant to the advocacy. Because of the importance of the message receiver's personal characteristics, such as emotionality, it is important that communicators of health-related information understand the basic mechanisms of persuasion and that they can apply them in a variety of social contexts (Brinol & Petty, 2006).

What is important for clinicians to draw from this work is that emotion can serve *multiple* roles in therapeutic attitude change. Emotion can (1) enhance or retard the *amount* of cognitive processing in which clients engage, (2) trigger *bias* or directionality in client cognition, (3) constitute an argument for or against an attitude position, (4) lead to positive or negative associations with an attitude object, and (5) influence the degree of confidence one has about one's attitude. Making things more complex, these roles can co-occur. For example, a public service announcement on television that advocates annual mammograms can create increased confidence in one's positive attitudes regarding getting a mammogram while at the same time creating a more positive association about mammograms generally. Moreover, these different roles for emotion can work at cross purposes. For example, a fear appeal might motivate more cognitive processing, which could be therapeutic if it led to enduring and behavior-influencing attitude change. On the other hand, that same fear appeal may lead the client to associate more negative feelings with the therapist who gave the fear appeal and may lead to biased cognitive processing that systematically discounts real but threatening information, thus thwarting treatment goals.

It is also important to focus on message characteristics. In reviewing this literature, Albarracin, Durantini, and Earl (2006) made five evidence-based assertions regarding health prevention initiatives. They reported that interventions are better at influencing knowledge and motivational change than at creating immediate behavioral change. The research suggests that motivational change decays across time, but behavioral change increases. Activity-based interventions have been shown to be more effective than passive presentations of information. Likewise, interventions based on the theories of reasoned action and planned behavior, self-efficacy models, and behavioral skills models are more effective than exclusively fear-based interventions. Finally, the research indicates that experts in intervention are more effective than nonexperts in almost all cases, especially with disempowered populations.

Practitioners seeking to develop effective health-promoting messages should think broadly about the kinds of theories from which to draw. For example, practitioners should consider information-processing theories pertinent to behavior change (e.g., Brinol & Petty, 2006), but they should not stop there. Practitioners developing health-promoting messages also should not ignore message–effect theories that predict the format and content of messages that produce effects on cognitive, attitudinal, and emotional outcomes (e.g., Dillard & Nabi, 2006). Finally, theories of behavior change that focus on rational, emotional, social, and personal predictors of healthy and risky behavior are also worthy of the attention of those developing health-promoting behaviors (e.g., Krosnick, Chang, Sherman, Chassin, & Presson, 2006; see Cappella, 2006, for more details on using these different kinds of theories).

## Prevention/Psychoeducation with a Psychological Emphasis

A number of recent studies has explored a middle ground between psychoeducation and psychotherapy by attempting to examine various treatment modalities in changing clients' attitudes. For example, Brooks-Harris, Heesacker, and Mejia-Millan (1996) attempted to change men's attitudes about traditional male gender roles through videotaped interventions that encouraged central-route processing. Results, however, showed that participants' attitudes about gender roles were unaltered, and that their fear of femininity and resistance to help seeking were especially resistant to change. Withers, Twigg, Wertheim, and Paxton (2002) also used a videotaped intervention meant to change attitudes, but theirs was intended to affect early adolescent girls' attitudes toward eating disorders. The authors specifically examined whether receiver characteristics, personal relevance, and need for cognition predicted attitude change, but found that none of these factors had an effect. However, the intervention group exhibited more attitude change and increased knowledge than did the control group, presumably as a result of the interaction of factors that, separately, did not account for change.

Other studies have addressed attitude changes toward gay and lesbian persons. Tucker and Potocky-Tripodi (2006) reviewed 17 published studies reporting interventions meant to change heterosexuals' attitudes toward gay and lesbian persons and concluded that the interventions failed to change these attitudes. Oles, Black, and Cramer (1999) suggested that a potentially more effective strategy than attempting to change negative gay/lesbian attitudes would be to anticipate behavior change regarding interacting with gay/lesbian persons. Oles et al. were, indeed, effective at improving the behaviors that participants anticipated exhibiting toward gay/lesbian persons in the future. Overall, this area of research suggests that a direct attempt to change deeply held and highly personal attitudes, even if they might be dysfunctional, may not be as effective as attempting to change something closely related, such as one's anticipated future behavior.

## Persuasion in Psychotherapy

Some of the recent research more directly addresses persuasion and influence in psychotherapy. For example, Hoyt (1996) performed a meta-analysis that supported aspects of Strong's (1968) two-phase model of interpersonal influence in counseling. This review examined published studies on perceived therapist credibility, which was found to be moderately related to credibility cues and a strong predictor of therapist influence, though, as Hoyt cautioned, "the direction of causation in this relation cannot be inferred from most of these studies" (p. 440). Therefore, it may be that clients who are persuaded by therapists think more favorably of them as a result, rather than that therapist credibility *causes* attitude change, as Strong (1968) posited. Hoyt also concluded that Strong's mediational model was insufficient to account for the complex relationships among credibility, cues, and influence.

Houser, Feldman, Williams, and Fierstien (1998) addressed interpersonal influence in counseling by examining psychotherapists' reported use of social influence/persuasion tactics. These authors asked 499 clinicians to rate the frequency with which they used 15 social influence strategies, to indicate their theoretical orientations, and to report their number of years in practice. Behavioral and cognitive-behavioral therapists reported using more influence/persuasion strategies than did psychodynamic, phenomenological, systemic, or eclectic therapists. Also, psychodynamic therapists reported using persuasion strategies less frequently than did therapists from all other theoretical approaches. However, there was no relationship between the use of persuasion/influence strategies and number of years in clinical practice. Some of the influence strategies used most often were metaphors, noting negative consequences of actions, noting positive rewards, reasoning, encouraging clients to compare real self to ideal self, and modeling. Strategies that were used least frequently included appealing to the client to change in order to please significant others and appealing to the client's loyalty to the therapist. The authors suggested that therapists can become more aware of which influence strategies they use and, as a result, may enhance their treatment methods by increasing their use of those that are more effective. The authors also suggested using source-based tactics (e.g., influencing the client through the perception of the therapist as an expert) early in treatment, and message-based persuasion (e.g., influencing the client through message arguments that elicit agreement from the client) later in treatment.

McCarthy and Frieze (1999) examined the other side of the therapeutic relationship by assessing clients' perceptions of their therapists' social influence, burnout, and quality of care by collecting data on the experiences of 131 undergraduate students who were, or had been, therapy clients. The study specifically looked at the relationships among clients' perceptions of their therapists' use of social influence strategies, clients' perceptions of therapist burnout, and clients' perceptions of the quality of their therapy. The influence strategies examined were personal coercive influence, personal reward influence, expert influence, and compromise influence strategies. Results showed that clients who reported therapist use of personal coercive influence and expert influence believed that their therapy was less successful, reported less satisfaction with the therapeutic relationship, viewed their therapist as less effective, and were more likely to leave therapy early, than those who did not report therapist use of coercive and expert influence. Clients viewed therapists as more effective when they used personal reward and compromise strategies. Therapist burnout was associated with less favorable client perceptions of therapeutic outcomes. Evidence suggests the effect of burnout on client favorability perceptions was mediated by clients' perceptions of the therapists' use of expertise, personal reward, and compromise strategies. As burnout increased, use of these techniques decreased. Based on these findings, therapists should use personal coercive influence and expert influence sparingly. Therapists experiencing burnout should be especially vigilant about underusing personal reward and compromise with clients.

## WHERE ARE SOCIAL INFLUENCE AND PSYCHOTHERAPY NOW?

Research at the interface of social influence and psychotherapy in the last 15 years has primarily focused on psychoeducation and prevention, rather than on psychotherapy. Moreover, several articles specifically on psychotherapy published during the period did not report original research, but instead reviewed previously published literature. Typically these articles devoted substantial portions of the text to explaining what had already been done in the field and providing suggestions for the future, suggestions that, for the most part, were not followed in subsequently published work. Tellingly, Heppner and Frazier (1992) gave more suggestions for the future than the total number of empirical studies we uncovered about this topic since their review. As far as we can ascertain, few, if any, of the Heppner–Frazier suggestions have been carried out, at least not in accessible scholarly publications.

In the section that follows we focus on culture because we think it represents an enduring shift of emphasis in clinical and counseling psychology. We suspect that the limited recent emphasis on social influence processes in traditional psychotherapy is directly related to the increased emphasis on multicultural sensitivity and competence in clinical and counseling psychology over the same period. Social influence perspectives and multicultural perspectives are not inherently competing frameworks, as our later discussion underscores. Moreover, social persuasion theory and research could be very useful from a multicultural perspective, as a tool to study and ameliorate misuses of power, both intentional and unintentional. Nonetheless, we do have the sense that as clinical and counseling psychologists *generally* understand social persuasion theory, it may be seen as challenging rather than complementing multicultural sensitivity and competence.

### Social Influence and Multiculturalism

Since the 1980s the research and practice focus of counseling psychology has shifted toward issues related to multiculturalism and diversity. Pederson (1991) has called multiculturalism the "fourth force in counseling," suggesting that all helping is culturally bound. Sue, Bingham, Porché-Burke, and Vasquez (1999) have dubbed the current era in psychology the "multicultural revolution." This shift anticipates the rapid growth of racial and ethnic minority populations in the United States. It also reflects the fact that people of color underuse mental health resources, terminate psychotherapy prematurely (Wu & Windle, 1980), and "receive unequal and poor mental health services" (Sue, 1977, p. 116). Thus, practicing counseling psychologists are now required to demonstrate multicultural competence and seek to fulfill their profession's core values by working with clients from populations that experience societal oppression, financial and political underrepresentation, and, thus, marginalization. Multicultural competence includes awareness of one's own biases, values, and assumptions; knowledge of culturally different clients' worldviews; the ability to develop culturally appropriate interventions; and understanding of organizational forces and how they can hinder or advance multicultural competencies (Sue et al., 1998).

Clinical psychology, too, has seen an increased emphasis in multicultural competence. For example, two recent volumes (Dana, 2000; Kazarian & Evans, 1998) underscore the need for more general cultural competence among practitioners of clinical psychology. These and other indicators suggest that clinical psychology, too, has a growing commitment to multicultural awareness and competence.

Despite the increased emphasis in the psychotherapy literature on multiculturalism, research at the interface of social influence theory and multiculturalism has been sparse, perhaps because the basic tenets of multicultural psychotherapy put it at odds with the traditional application of social influence theory to counseling and psychotherapy. Specifically, multiculturalism heightens psychologists' sensitivity to the power differential and to power dynamics between psychotherapist and client. As a result, clinicians who work with minority populations are more likely to recognize their privileged status relative to clients, especially relative to racial and ethnic minority clients. Given this heightened awareness of differential privilege, both researchers and practicing psychologists may be much less comfortable than they were in the past with the notion of exerting direct and intentional influence over a person lacking societal privilege. It could be argued that what a psychologist is comfortable with is less important than what the research shows is most likely to help. Likewise, one person's "influence" is another person's "coercion." Still, we think that a sense of discomfort made salient by an increased emphasis on multicultural sensitivity may have led to reduced interest in social influence approaches.

One of the major goals of multiculturalism in psychotherapy is to empower marginalized clients. Therefore, multiculturally aware psychologists could readily interpret the traditional application of social influence theory to psychotherapy as oppression in the form of a person of privilege inappropriately influencing clients to accept dominant-culture-based attitudes—a form of psychotherapeutic colonialism, according to Tom Strong (2000). From this perspective, the clinician gains power by not only holding but purveying "correct" attitudes, whereas the client loses power by initially holding "incorrect" attitudes and ultimately embracing the privileged clinician's "correct" attitudes.

Social influence scholars and practitioners are unlikely to embrace or intend such colonial motives. However, the assumption that the therapist has the "correct" set of attitudes, beliefs, and behaviors toward which the client should be persuaded may strike people as colonial, especially in relation to marginalized and disenfranchised people. Indeed, psychologists often do have new and helpful ways of understanding and valuing situations and experiences, and psychologists do embrace individual differences and diversity in clients. So what is needed is articulation of a new perspective, one in which the top-down aspect of social influence by therapists toward clients is deemphasized and a more interactive, reciprocal, collegial influence process is given renewed emphasis (see Beck, 1976, for an example of such a perspective in cognitive-behavioral psychotherapy and Smith, 2005, for an example with financially impoverished clients). Such a new perspective may help therapists and clinical researchers understand forces that seem to call for a different approach to social influence, an approach that reflects the field's important multicultural advances. Embracing this new perspective may facilitate and even reinvigorate a fruitful area of theory and research, reframing social influence in a way that empowers clients and thus makes social influence approaches more helpful in actual therapy.

Heesacker, Conner, and Prichard (1995) and Strong (2000) have attempted to incorporate multiculturalism into this interface by suggesting that research and theory conceptualize the client's level of cognitive processing as the critical mechanism for his or her own attitude change, and by allowing for client individual differences and for racial, ethnic, and other forms of diversity. Multiculturalists advocate acceptance of differences among people with regard to gender, ethnicity, age, religion, physical or mental (dis)abilities, sexual orientation, acculturation, and socioeconomic status, among others.

One important tool for practitioners in addressing clients' individual differences and racial and ethnic diversity is the ELM, because it conceptualizes clients' levels of cognitive processing as the central mechanism for their attitude change. Through this conceptualization, the model accounts for both client individual differences and important aspects of ethnic diversity. There are three ways in which these client differences can influence attitude change from an ELM perspective. First, the therapist's own ethnicity can elicit positive or negative associations in clients, which in turn create positive or negative peripheral-route attitudes. Second, ethnicity (either the client's or the therapist's) can influence the client's overall *type* of cognitive processing (mostly antagonistic to whatever the therapist says or mostly supportive of what the therapist says), which can powerfully affect central-route attitudes. Third, individual differences (again, either the client's or the therapist's) can influence the client's *extent* of cognitive processing. Successful application of the ELM to psychotherapy requires therapists to tailor interventions to specific situations, use longer interventions, and conduct live, face-to-face interventions that allow therapists to make on-the-spot assessments of client reactions and adjustment to those reactions (see Heesacker, Conner, & Prichard, 1995, for a more detailed treatment of these issues).

Tom Strong's (2000) ideas mirror multiculturalism's acceptance of multiple legitimate viewpoints. His discussion of the use of influence in collaborative psychotherapy includes the suggestion that, because therapist influence over the client is unavoidable, therapists should share their influence intentions with their clients. In other words, clients and therapists should collaboratively choose a goal, methods for treatment, homework, and conversational focus. Collaborative therapists customize their efforts in response to client preferences and attend to clients' often-present sensitivity to misunderstandings, according to Strong. When there are misunderstandings, resistance, or implied disagreements, Strong argued, the therapist is not customizing the treatment appropriately, and the therapist needs to renegotiate a way back to shared intentionality and collaboration or accept an end of collaboration. When therapists go outside of shared intentionality, clients remind therapists by resisting. In effect, Strong acknowledged the possibility that therapists' values will not always be congruent with clients'. He asserted that collaborative therapists, then, are not experts; their goal is to acquire a masterful knowing of clients' worlds from clients' points of view. He suggested "customizing our work to the specifics of clients' preferences and their reported circumstances—and accepting that clients' responses are what informs good customizing efforts—helps to move us out of undue influence" (p. 145). Strong also asserted that because psychology originates from a predominantly male and Eurocentric value system, it can be considered "colonisation," and "psychology can be impositional when proffering its views of, and means for achieving, 'the good and proper life' " (p. 145). Strong posited that a therapist engaged in collaborative therapy is more sensitive to those outside of the mainstream. He concluded by saying: "My choice in becoming a collaborative therapist had much to do with finding a way to share my influence comfortably. Not having to be an expert was a huge relief, and so has been experiencing that I can help clients make differences they choose for their lives by aligning my influence with theirs" (p. 147).

Devotees of multiculturalism have suggested that incorporation of individual differences could result in social influence research that more highly values marginalized clients and the attitudes that these clients bring to psychotherapy. Clinicians who simply attempt to change client's attitudes that are discrepant from their own may be less likely *to* succeed than clinicians who first embrace their clients' diversity—and may disserve their clients if they *do* succeed. A shift in perspective from first altering attitudes to first embracing diversity could facilitate more precise, more effective, and more affirming attitude changes with culturally and ethnically diverse clients.

## FUTURE DIRECTIONS FOR SOCIAL INFLUENCE AND PSYCHOTHERAPY

The future vitality of the interface of social influence processes and counseling/psychotherapy processes is uncertain. To remain viable as clinically relevent, theory-based empirical studies, not just thought pieces and reviews, informed by multicultural perspective, must proliferate. We believe that the proliferation of empirical studies and the implementation of social influence approaches in psychotherapy depend on social influence science and application reflecting the recently emergent importance of multicultural perspectives in psychotherapeutic psychology. In so doing, the field must shift from the assumption that the attitude change process relies on the therapist holding and purveying correct attitudes. We have identified three ways to shift this literature toward a more multiculturally sensitive approach. The first is a more thorough empirical examination of the influence *clients have over clinicians'* attitudes. The second is the empirical investigation of the processes by which clients' and psychotherapists' attitudes converge and diverge over time. The third and perhaps most important is an examination of the influence clients have over *their own* attitudes, making explicit the fact that clients may be more responsible for affecting their own attitude changes than are their therapists. One goal of therapy is the empowerment of clients, who often come into therapy because they feel socially or personally disempowered. Believing in and facilitating clients' self-determined attitude change may constitute an essential step in the empowerment process.

## CLINICAL IMPLICATIONS

In this section we highlight information of interest to practitioners in clinical and counseling psychology regarding social influence processes. First, we identify book chapters and an article that practitioners may find helpful in practice. Second, we describe a case that contrasts the traditional application of the ELM to counseling and psychotherapy with a more multiculturally sensitive approach.

### Helpful Case Materials and Step-by-Step Approaches

Heesacker and Mejia-Millan (1996, pp. 67–75) detailed an 11-step approach to applying Petty and Cacioppo's ELM model to psychotherapy with a brief clinical example (see Heesacker &

Shanbhag, 2002, pp. 318–321, for a simpler, four-step approach to the same process with no clinical example). Practitioners in continuing education have responded favorably to training in this approach (for details, see Heesacker & Harris, 1993). Second, we direct practitioners' attention to an article in which a decision tree for working with clients integrates the ELM with instructional and self-consistency approaches to counseling/psychotherapy (Heesacker & Harris, 1993, pp. 698–705). The decision tree is accompanied by step-by-step application instructions, to facilitate effective application to various client situations.

## Reconceptualizing the ELM's Approach to Psychotherapy

In this section we describe an approach with a case example that contrasts with the traditional application of the ELM in psychotherapy (e.g., Heesacker & Harris, 1993; Heesacker & Mejia-Millan, 1996; Heesacker & Shanbhag, 2002). This new approach emphasizes a two-way, dynamic interplay between the client's central- and peripheral-route processing. Both approaches are consistent with the ELM, but the second approach, we believe, may be more responsive to the multicultural, person-focused, and constructivistic threads that have become increasingly important in counseling and psychotherapy.

### *Traditional Application of the ELM to a Case Example*

Mindy is a client whose husband secretly had sexual intercourse with other women on multiple occasions during their 10-year marriage, resulting in a divorce 3 years ago when Mindy discovered her husband's infidelity. Mindy now has difficulty building new romantic relationships with men because she does not trust them, though none has cheated on her since her divorce. Whenever she starts to develop strong romantic feelings for men, she becomes scared and sabotages the relationships by avoiding them and not returning their phone calls. Now, she is seeking psychotherapy because she wants to understand this pattern in hopes of eventually developing other close, meaningful romantic relationships.

One of the traditional applications of the ELM to psychotherapy might suggest that Mindy is dysfunctionally responding to simple cues. Because men have cheated on her in the past, she fears men might cheat on her again in the future. The traditional ELM approach might focus on central-route attitude change designed to alter her maladaptive and incorrect assumptions about men in an enduring way. Therefore, her therapist might focus on (1) Mindy's motivation to think about the issue, (2) her ability to cognitively process the therapist's message to her, (3) her likelihood of generating thoughts that support more adaptive and accurate assumptions about men, and (4) her consolidation of those adaptive and accurate assumptions into long-term memory. Although this type of intervention has intrinsic value, it may not take into account the whole therapeutic picture.

### *A More Culturally Sensitive Approach: The Route-Shift Approach to Psychotherapy*

The traditional ELM application to psychotherapy asserts that clients like Mindy should abandon their surface-level and peripheral attitude processing, moving instead to a deeper and more central-route processing, one that results in lasting attitude and behavior change. The route-shift approach we introduced earlier, however, values both clients' peripheral-route and their central-route processing, positing that at its core psychotherapy involves a dynamic and two-way interplay between clients' central and peripheral processing.

The route-shift approach also holds that lasting attitude change may not occur without the clinicians' validation and acceptance of the clients' peripheral-route processing. The automatic peripheral processing in which Mindy is engaging, for example, is viewed as maladaptive because her fear of infidelity and lack of trust are keeping her from forming lasting and meaningful romantic relationships. Therefore, it makes sense to challenge Mindy's processing, bringing it to a deeper cognitive level. However, peripheral processing is also adaptive in Mindy's life because her fear is preventing her from being hurt in future relationships. Mindy, in fact, may need this fear to allow herself time to grieve; she may not yet be ready to have another serious relationship.

As in Mindy's case, it is important for clients to engage in peripheral-route processing in their everyday lives, but it is also important during psychotherapy. Attempting to restructure Mindy's attitude about potential romantic partners using only the central route may be premature. Doing so initially fails to acknowledge the validity and utility of her fear, because the therapist's focus is on her thinking when Mindy's focus is on her feelings. Peripheral processing has a place in therapy with Mindy. Valuing Mindy's cue-based attitude may allow her to accept and process her fear more deeply and perhaps in a more emotionally genuine way. "Most people," Elliott Aronson (2002) has written, "are more deeply influenced by one clear, vivid, personal example than by an abundance of statistical data" (p. 74). Sometimes even more powerful is one very intense personal experience that creates a strong association between an emotional state and a stimulus. Accordingly, presenting Mindy with persuasive arguments regarding the likelihood of other men cheating on her in a relationship may do little to assuage the intense emotional reaction conditioned from her previous marital experience. Said differently, Mindy may not have the motivation, ability, or memory encoding capacity to engage in central-route attitude change while she is having such intense personal emotions. Likewise, her ability to engage in balanced or bias-free processing is likely to be impaired under those circumstances.

The effective roles of central- and peripheral-route processing can be thought of as generally conforming to the Yerkes–Dodson law (Yerkes & Dodson, 1908). Moderate levels of arousal are likely to allow the operation of both central-route and peripheral-route processing, whereas very high or very low levels of arousal are likely to result in reliance primarily on only peripheral-route processing. Very low levels of arousal are likely to result in inadequate *motivation* to process therapist remarks centrally, whereas very high levels of arousal are likely to result in inadequate *ability* to process those remarks centrally. Optimal therapeutic work occurs, according to this perspective, when both central- and peripheral-route processes are working in dynamic balance. A shift in the balance may occur, but neither process dominates. If a client engages only in central-route processing, there is a risk of *central* saturation, relying only on cognition for therapeutic change, perhaps obsessively or ruminatively so or perhaps at the expense of being aware of one's affective state. On the other hand, if a client engages only in peripheral-route processing—as could readily occur under conditions of either very high or very low arousal—there is a risk of *peripheral* saturation, an overreliance on heuristics and affect-based cues for therapeutic change.

People are often best served by a balance of central and peripheral processing and by the ability to employ each type of processing in harmony with the demands of the situation. If clients centrally processed all the content in a therapy session, the drain on cognitive resources might be so great that they could not be fully present in the moment and experience their feelings. Central-route processing is too cognitively demanding to be maintained continuously, so it may make sense to allow and even encourage clients to process therapeutic content peripherally. Clients—and people in general—only have so many resources to use in processing their experiences, so they have to rely on peripheral processing more than central processing. Clinicians may be able to teach clients to step back and assess their reliance on peripheral-route and central-route processing outside of sessions and from time-to-time critically examine whether the cognitive resources allocated in any given situation are appropriate for that situation. "Am I wasting time analyzing something when I don't need to?" "Am I suffering negative consequences for uncritically accepting my first reaction about a person or situation?" These are the kinds of self-evaluation questions that practitioners might teach clients. In other words, practitioners may help their clients by teaching them to use the route-shift approach in their daily lives.

## CONCLUSION

The route-shift approach to psychotherapy builds acceptance into the therapeutic relationship and thus validates the attitudes the client brings to therapy. This approach stands in contrast to traditional applications of attitude change theory, which usually have focused on changing attitudes through central-route influence attempts. Traditional therapy applications of the ELM emphasize psychotherapist knowledge and power, an emphasis that is increasingly out of step with culturally sensitive mental health care. The route-shift approach decreases the emphasis on psychotherapist's knowledge and power, instead contextualizing them within the psychotherapy relationship, where personal and cultural sensitivity are required. This shift of emphasis sacrifices none of the insights and potential of depth-of-processing attitude-change theories, such as the ELM, or of other social influence process models, but instead modernizes their implementation to fit better into current psychotherapeutic contexts.

### ACKNOWLEDGMENTS

Thanks to Taylor Locker for her very helpful comments on earlier drafts of the chapter. Contributions of the first two authors were approximately equal.

### NOTE

1. This section presents a summary of the major theories and research at the social influence and psychotherapy interface published before the early 1990s. For details of the history, we refer readers to two earlier chapters (e.g., Cacioppo et al., 1991; Heppner & Frazier, 1992).

### REFERENCES

Abelson, R. P., Aronson, E., McGuire, W. J., Newcomb, T. M., Rosenberg, M. J., & Tanenbaum, P. H. (Eds.). (1968). *Theories of cognitive consistency: A sourcebook*. Chicago: Rand McNally.

Ajzen, I., & Fishbein, M. (1977). Attitude–behavior relations: A theoretical analysis and review of empirical research. *Psychological Bulletin*, *84*, 888–918.

Ajzen, I., & Fishbein, M. (1980). *Understanding attitudes and predicting social behavior.* Englewood Cliffs, NJ: Prentice-Hall.

Albarracin, D., Durantini, M. R., & Earl, A. (2006). Empirical and theoretical conclusions of an analysis of outcomes of HIV-prevention interventions. *Current Directions in Psychological Science, 15,* 73–78.

Albarracin, D., Kumkale, G. T., & Johnson, B. T. (2004). Influences of social power and normative support on condom use decisions: A research synthesis. *AIDS Care: Psychological and Socio-Medical Aspects of AIDS/HIV, 16,* 700–723.

Albarracin, D., McNatt, P. S., Klein, C. T. F., Ho, R. M., Mitchell, A. L., & Kumkale, G. T. (2003). Persuasive communications to change actions: An analysis of behavioral and cognitive impact in HIV prevention. *Health Psychology, 22,* 166–177.

Aronson, E. (2002). *The social animal.* New York: Worth.

Beck, A. T. (1976). *Cognitive therapy and emotional disorders.* New York: International Universities Press.

Becker, M. H. (1974). The health belief model and personal health behavior. *Health Education Monographs, 2,* 324–473.

Bochner, S., & Insko, C. A. (1966). Communicator discrepancy, source credibility, and opinion change. *Journal of Personality and Social Psychology, 4,* 614–621.

Brinol, P., & Petty, R. E. (2006). Fundamental processes leading to attitude change: Implications for cancer prevention communications. *Journal of Communication, 56,* 81–104.

Brooks-Harris, J. E., Heesacker, M., & Mejia-Millan, C. (1996). Changing men's male gender-role attitudes by applying the elaboration likelihood model of attitude change. *Sex Roles, 35,* 563–580.

Brown, J. H., D'Emidio-Caston, M., & Pollard, J. A. (1997). Students and substances: Social power in drug education. *Educational Evaluation and Policy Analysis, 19,* 65–82.

Burke, K. (2005). Suave power of persuasion. In J. Whitaker & D. Blakesley (Eds.), *Late poems, 1968–1993.* Columbia, SC: University of South Carolina Press.

Cacioppo, J. T., Claiborn, C. D., Petty, R. E., & Heesacker, M. (1991). General framework for the study of attitude change in psychotherapy. In C. R. Snyder & D. R. Forsyth (Eds.), *Handbook of social and clinical psychology* (pp. 523–539). New York: Pergamon Press.

Cappella, J. N. (2006). Integrating message effects and behavior change theories: Organizing comments and unanswered questions. *Journal of Communication, 56,* S265–S279.

Corrigan, J. D., Dell, D. M., Lewis, K. N., & Schmidt, I. D. (1980). Counseling as a social influence process: A review. *Journal of Counseling Psychology, 27,* 395–441.

Crano, W. D., & Prislin, R. (2006). Attitudes and persuasion. *Annual Review of Psychology, 57,* 345–374.

Dana, R. H. (Ed.). (2000). *Handbook of cross-cultural and multicultural personality assessment.* Mahwah, NJ: Erlbaum.

Dillard, J. P., & Nabi, R. L. (2006). The persuasive influence of emotion in cancer prevention and detection messages. *Journal of Communication, 56,* S123–S139.

Donaldson, S. I., Graham, J. W., & Hansen, W. B. (1994). Testing the generalizability of intervening mechanism theories: Understanding the effects of adolescent drug-use prevention interventions. *Journal of Behavioral Medicine, 17,* 195–216.

Donaldson, S. I., Graham, J. W., Piccinin, A. M., & Hansen, W. B. (1995). Resistance-skills training and onset of alcohol-use: Evidence for beneficial and potentially harmful effects in public-schools and in private Catholic-schools. *Health Psychology, 14,* 291–300.

Durantini, M. R., Albarracin, D., Mitchell, A. L., Earl, A. N., & Gillette, J. C. (2006). Conceptualizing the influence of social agents of behavior change: A meta-analysis of the effectiveness of HIV-prevention interventionists for different groups. *Psychological Bulletin, 132,* 212–248.

Festinger, L. (1957). *A theory of cognitive dissonance.* Palo Alto, CA: Stanford University Press.

Floyd D. L., Prentice-Dunn, S., & Rogers, R. W. (2000). A meta-analysis of research on protection motivation theory. *Journal of Applied Social Psychology, 30,* 407–429.

Frank, J. D. (1963). *Persuasion and healing.* New York: Schocken Books.

Girandola, F. (2000). Fear and persuasion: Review and re-analysis of the literature (1953–1998). *Annee Psychologique, 100,* 333–376.

Girandola, F., & Atkinson, D. (2003). Prevention, detection and processing of persuasive information in situations arousing fear. *Canadian Journal of Behavioral Science, 35,* 197–209.

Greenberg, R. P. (1969). Effects of presession counseling on perception of the therapist and receptivity to influence in a psychotherapy analogue. *Journal of Counseling and Clinical Psychology, 33,* 425–429.

Heesacker, M. (1986). Counselor pretreatment and the elaboration likelihood model of attitude change. *Journal of Counseling Psychology, 33,* 107–114.

Heesacker, M., Conner, K., & Prichard, S. (1995). Individual counseling and psychotherapy: Applications from the social psychology of attitude change. *Counseling Psychologist, 23,* 611–632.

Heesacker, M., & Harris, J. E. (1993). Cognitive processes in counseling: A decision tree integrating two theoretical approaches. *Counseling Psychologist, 20,* 687–711.

Heesacker, M., & Mejia-Millan, C. (1996). A research program on attitude change processes and their applications to counseling. In W. Dryden (Ed.), *Research in counselling and psychotherapy: Practical applications* (pp. 49–78). London: Sage.

Heesacker, M., & Shanbhag, M. G. (2002). Social influence in counseling: Application of the elaboration likelihood model to counseling. In G. S. Tryon (Ed.), *Counseling based on process research: Applying what we know* (pp. 298–324). Boston: Allyn & Bacon.

Heppner, P. P., & Claiborn, C. D. (1989). Social influence research in counseling: A review and critique. *Journal of Counseling Psychology, 36,* 365–384.

Heppner, P. P., & Dixon, D. N. (1978). Effects of client perceived need and counselor role on clients' behaviors. *Journal of Counseling Psychology, 25,* 514–519.

Heppner, P. P., & Dixon, D. M. (1981). A review of the interpersonal influence processes in counseling. *Personnel and Guidance Journal, 59,* 542–550.

Heppner, P. P., & Frazier, P. A. (1992). Social psychological processes in psychotherapy: Extrapolating basic research to counseling psychology. In S. D. Brown & R. W. Lent (Eds.), *Handbook of counseling psychology* (2nd ed., pp. 141–175). New York: Wiley.

Higgins, E. T., Klein R., & Strauman, T. (1985). Self-concept discrepancy theory: A psychological model for distinguishing among different aspects of depression and anxiety. *Social Cognition, 3,* 51–76.

Hochbaum, G. (1956). Why people seek diagnostic x-rays. *Public Health Reports, 71,* 377–380.

Houser, R., Feldman, M., Williams, K., & Fierstien, J. (1998). Persuasion and social influence tactics used by mental health counselors. *Journal of Mental Health Counseling, 20,* 238–249.

Hovland, C. I., Janis, I. L., & Kelley, H. H. (1953). *Communication and persuasion.* New Haven, CT: Yale University Press.

Hoyt, M. F., & Janis, I. L. (1975). Increasing adherence to a stressful decision via a motivational balance-sheet procedure: A field experiment. *Journal of Personality and Social Psychology, 31,* 833–939.

Hoyt, W. T. (1996). Antecedents and effects of perceived therapist credibility: A meta-analysis. *Journal of Counseling Psychology, 43,* 430–447.

Hwang, M. S., Yeagley, K. L., & Petosa, R. (2004). A meta-analysis of adolescent smoking prevention programs between 1978 and 1997 in the United States. *Health Education and Behavior, 31,* 702–719.

Janis, I. L., & Feshbach, S. (1953). Effects of fear-arousing communications. *Journal of Abnormal and Social Psychology, 48,* 78–92.

Kazarian, S. S., & Evans, D. R. (1998). *Cultural clinical psychology: Theory, research, and practice.* New York: Oxford University Press.

Krosnick, J., Chang, L., Sherman, S. J., Chassin, L., & Presson, C. (2006). The effects of beliefs about the health consequences of cigarette smoking on smoking onset and quitting. *Journal of Communication, 56,* S18–S37.

Langer, E., Blank, A., & Chanowiu, B. (1978). The mindlessness of ostensibly thoughtful action. *Journal of Personality and Social Psychology, 36,* 635–642.

Levy, L. H. (1963). *Psychological interpretation.* New York: Holt, Rinehart & Winston.

Lira, M. T., Kunstmann, S., Caballero, E., Guarda, E., Villarroel, L., & Molina, J. C. (2006). Cardiovascular prevention and attitude of people towards behavior changes: State of the art. *Revista Medica de Chile, 134,* 223–230.

Lord, C. G., Ross, L., & Lepper, M. R. (1979). Biased assimilation and attitude polarization: The effects of prior theories on subsequently considered evidence. *Journal of Personality and Social Psychology, 37,* 2098–2109.

McCarthy, W. C., & Frieze, I. H. (1999). Negative aspects of therapy: Client perceptions of therapists' social influence, burnout, and quality of care. *Journal of Social Issues, 55*(1), 33–50.

McGuire, W. J. (1985). Attitudes and attitude change. In G. Lindzey & E. Aronson (Eds.), *Handbook of social psychology* (3rd ed., Vol. 2, pp. 233–346). New York: Random House.

McNeil, B. W., & Stoltenberg, C. D. (1988). A test of the elaboration likelihood model for therapy. *Cognitive Therapy and Research, 12,* 69–80.

Oles, T., Black, B., & Cramer, E. (1999). From attitude change to effective practice: Exploring the relationship. *Journal of Social Work Education, 35*(1), 87–100.

Pederson, P. (1991). Multiculturalism as a generic approach to counseling. *Journal of Counseling and Development, 70*(a), 6–12.

Petty, R. E., & Cacioppo, J. T. (1981). *Attitudes and persuasion: Classic and contemporary approaches.* Dubuque, IA: Brown.

Petty, R. E., & Cacioppo, J. T. (1986). *Communication and persuasion: Central and peripheral routes to attitude change.* New York: Springer/Verlag.

Prochaska, J. O., DiClemente, C. C., & Norcross, J. C. (1992). In search of how people change: Applications to addictive behaviors. *American Psychologist, 47,* 1102–1114.

Shepherd, R. (1999). Social determinants of food choice. *Proceedings of the Nutrition Society, 58,* 807–812.

Slater, M. D. (1999). Integrating application of media effects, persuasion, and behavior change theories to communication campaigns: A stage-of-change framework. *Health Communication, 11,* 335–354.

Smith, L. (2005). Psychotherapy, classism, and the poor: Conspicuous by their absence. *American Psychologist, 60,* 687–696.

Sprafkin, R. P. (1970). Communicator expertise and change in word meaning in psychological treatment. *Journal of Counseling Psychology, 17,* 191–196.

Strong, S. R. (1968). Counseling: An interpersonal influence process. *Journal of Counseling Psychology, 15,* 215–224.

Strong, S. R., & Schmidt, L. D. (1970). Expertness and influence in counseling. *Journal of Counseling Psychology, 17,* 81–87.

Strong, T. (2000). Collaborative influence. *Australian and New Zealand Journal of Family Therapy, 21,* 144–148.

Sue, D. W., Bingham, R. P., Porché-Burke, L., & Vasquez, M. (1999). The diversification of psychology: A multicultural revolution. *American Psychologist, 54,* 1061–1069.

Sue, D. W., Carter, R. T., Casas, J. M., Fouad, N. A., Ivey, A. E., Jensen, M., et al. (1998). *Multicultural counseling competencies.* Thousand Oaks, CA: Sage.

Sue, S. (1977). Community mental health services to minority groups: Some optimism, some pessimism. *American Psychologist, 32,* 616–624.

Tucker, E. W., & Potocky-Tripodi, M. (2006). Changing heterosexuals' attitudes toward homosexuals: A systematic review of the empirical literature. *Research on Social Work Practice, 16,* 176–190.

Visser, A. P., & Vanbilsen, P. (1994). Effectiveness of sex-education provided to adolescents. *Patient Education and Counseling, 23,* 147–160.

Withers, G. F., Twigg, K., Wertheim, E. H., & Paxton, S. J. (2002). A controlled evaluation of an eating disorders primary prevention videotape using the elaboration likelihood model of persuasion. *Journal of Psychosomatic Research*, *53*, 1021–1027.

Witte, K., & Allen, M. (2000). A meta-analysis of fear appeals: Implications for effective public health campaigns. *Health Education and Behavior*, *27*, 591–615.

Wu, I. H., & Windle, C. (1980). Ethnic specificity in the relative minority use and staffing of community mental health services. *Community Mental Health Journal*, *16*, 156–168.

Yerkes, R. M., & Dodson, J. D. (1908). The relationship of strength of stimulus to rapidity of habit-formation. *Journal of Comparative Neurology of Psychology*, *18*, 459–482.

# 25 Implicit Processes in Social and Clinical Psychology

Joel Weinberger
Caleb Siefert
Gregory Haggerty

At first blush, it might appear that clinical psychology and social psychology have little in common. The fields differ substantially in their focus, in the methods employed to investigate their interests, and in the manner in which they strive to intervene and produce change. Further, the day-to-day professional life of the average social and clinical psychologist could not be more different. For example, the former tends to focus on groups of people, makes use of highly controlled research designs (i.e., experimental designs), and studies nonclinical populations. The latter tends to focus on individuals (i.e., patients) and typically conducts research on clinical populations. Despite these differences, the similarities between the two fields are striking. Both are heavily involved in identifying factors that influence motivation, perception, behavior, interpersonal relationships, and change. Both have a strong interest in the role of nonconscious processes (typically referred to as *implicit processes* in social psychology and as *unconscious processes* in clinical psychology) in understanding human behaviors and change. In light of their differences, in fact, precisely because of their differences, each field has much to offer the other.

In this chapter we have attempted to limit our focus to a few areas of social psychology likely to be of interest to clinical psychologists. To this end, we review the areas of implicit learning, automaticity, and attribution theory. We have also included a brief review of some research demonstrating how social psychological methods can be used to study mental processes uncovered by clinical investigation (e.g., Andersen, Reznik, & Glassman, 2005). We have two hopes for this chapter: First, that it will encourage clinical psychologists to read outside of their primary area of expertise and learn a bit about social psychology. Second, we hope that social psychologists will think and write more about the clinical implications of their work.

## IMPLICIT LEARNING

Explicit learning can influence behavior, perception, and expectations. We are, however, also capable of learning without intention or awareness. In fact, in some cases, what we learn without awareness can directly oppose what we are aware of having learned and what we feel we believe. Such discrepancies can lead to inconsistencies in behavior. Although variations in behavior across time and context are normal, they can sometimes be problematic. This is particularly likely to be the case when our intentions and behaviors are repeatedly in conflict. It is common for patients to present for psychotherapy complaining of just such a discrepancy (i.e., explicitly stating a desire for one thing, while behaving in a manner that would appear to directly oppose this desire). This is often experienced as uncomfortable and perplexing. Further, patients often attribute a variety of explanations (some more problematic than others) as the origin of these discrepancies. After many failed attempts to address the issue on their own, it is common for patients to begin to feel that they are stuck, destined for such behavior, or to locate the origin of the issue within themselves (i.e., as a trait) rather than viewing it as arising from previous learning. Indeed, since patients are often unaware that any previous learning took place, it would be quite difficult for them to locate, let alone verbalize, the origin of their difficulties.

What often goes unappreciated by patients is that learning without awareness is not pathological but one way in which the human brain garners information. Further, although a patient may be unable to uncover or verbalize the experience that produced the learning that is resulting in the problem, there are methods designed to help patients become more aware of what has been learned (e.g., thought monitoring, behavioral monitoring, free association). Clinical psychologists are cognizant of the fact that patients are often unaware of what they have learned (particularly in childhood) and how this is influencing them (e.g., Wachtel, 1993; see also Shorey, Chapter 9, this volume, for discussion of attachment theory and research). Researchers in the field of *implicit learning* have done much to substantiate the notion that individuals are capable of learning complex patterns without realizing that they have done so. These researchers have also empirically demonstrated that learning without awareness (i.e., implicit learning) is not necessarily pathological, occurs in nonclinical populations, is not limited to childhood, and can influence a variety of human experiences.

### Illustrative Data

As it is usually studied, *implicit learning* involves picking up relations between stimuli without intention, without knowing that one is doing so, and without being able to verbalize what one has learned (Berry & Dienes, 1993; Seger, 1994). Implicit learning capabilities are fully formed very early in life. In fact, there is evidence that implicit learning arises before the development of formal language skills. This could explain why very young infants are found to "babble" in the language of their culture. (For a review of this research, see Jusczyk, 1997). Understanding the underlying structure and grammar of language is another example. Children learn the rules of language yet cannot articulate them. This is also true for most adults. People just "know" when something is stated properly and when it is not, even if they cannot explain why.

Reber showed that the tendency to automatically pick up "rules" or "patterns" from experience is not limited to children or to the learning of language. (See Reber, 1989, for a review of his early work.) Reber exposed his participants to strings of letters. Unbeknownst to the participants, these strings were organized according to arbitrary rules governing the associations between the letters. Typically, no instruction or explanation was given. After several trials in which participants were simply exposed to letter strings, they were presented with new strings and asked to judge which were consistent with the set previously viewed. They were able to do this at significantly greater than chance levels, despite being unable to articulate the rules. In fact, they did not even realize that any rules applied. Similar results have been obtained for tasks other than grammar and using senses other than sight. For example, Rubin, Wallace, and Houston (1993) had individuals who were not familiar with writing music listen to a series of ballads. They were then asked to compose ballads of their own. Participants' ballads were found to follow twice as many rules for ballads as they could actually articulate. Again, this research suggests that people automatically pick up very complex patterns and incorporate them into behavior without realizing it.

Lewicki (1986) expanded the purview of implicit learning to socially related phenomena. He and his colleagues showed that people learn, through concrete experiences, that certain qualities or characteristics go together or covary. This learning involves inferring relationships between abstract qualities by generalizing from specific concrete instances. In other words, people unconsciously engage in induction. These unconscious inferences and inductions can be quite complex and sophisticated. For example, Lewicki (Experiment 4.2) read participants concrete descriptions of people in which certain types of behavior went together or covaried. The nature of the covariations was designed to lead to certain trait inferences. In one set of examples, a studious person who rarely socialized did poorly on a test, whereas a person who attended many parties rather than study did well on the same exam. The inference implied by the descriptions was that introversion is associated with low intelligence whereas extraversion is associated with high intelligence. Afterward, participants were asked to rate 10 people they knew on various traits. As predicted, participants rated introverts as less intelligent than extraverts, demonstrating that they had "learned" the association. However, no participant associated his or her evaluations with the preceding experimental manipulation. Thus, they were not aware of having "learned" anything, let alone aware that their perception had been influenced by this learning.

Lewicki also showed that the unconscious inductions of implicit learning did not have to be logical or even sensible. In another study, he combined auditorally presented threatening words with photos of someone carrying a book. Participants learned to associate book carrying with threats, although they could not correctly state what they found to be threatening. This finding suggests that, although the ability to form connections implicitly is powerful and sophisticated, *the ability to critically evaluate those connections is weak*. The inductions made from implicit learning are purely empirical in the strict sense of the word and unrelated to what is consciously and logically known to make sense. And this is normal. It is not a consequence of conflict or even of disruptive affective arousal. It is simply one way in which humans process information. Whatever covaries in the environment is what the person will implicitly learn, whether sensibly related or not. Further, people will be unable to report on having made such a connection. They will not know what they have learned or even that they have learned anything at all. They will not be aware that their implicitly learned associations may contradict beliefs and knowledge they consciously hold.

Once established, implicitly learned information can bias the processing of subsequent information so that what has been learned persists, even if the environment does not strongly support it subsequently. Hill, Lewicki, Czyzewska, and Boss (1989) showed that once an initial contingency between two events has been unconsciously detected, people tend to behave as if that relationship still exists long after the contingency has been removed. In other words, people will continue to act as though something is so when it patently is not. Once something has been learned implicitly, it is difficult to unlearn even when there is evidence that would suggest that what has been learned is faulty. It would appear that this resistance to change is amotivational. That is, it is not triggered by conflict, defense, or desire. It is just how the system operates.

Lewicki argued that implicit learning is ubiquitous and not restricted to the lab. If he is correct, as a person develops, he or she builds up a whole repertoire of implicitly learned behaviors and representations that resist change and are applied to the world, sometimes maladaptively. Of particular interest to clinicians would be implicitly learned patterns for relating to others. Children have numerous experiences with their caregivers that likely result in implicit learning about the self, others, and the self in relation to others. At times, these implicitly learned expectations are applied to current relationships, even when circumstances do not support it. Psychoanalysts have termed this *transference*, and this too has been studied empirically.

Andersen and her colleagues expected that adults' concrete experiences in close relationships would produce implicitly learned expectancies for how personality qualities should covary. (See Miranda & Andersen, Chapter 26, this volume, for a review of their work and theorizing.) They argued that adults would be prone to "errors" that make sense, in much the same way that the errors in the implicit learning studies of Lewicki or the grammatical errors of children make sense. Based on the notion that people implicitly develop mental models of important others, these researchers hypothesized that those models, when active, would influence how new people are perceived. They predicted that individuals would see new people as more similar to significant others from the past than they actually are. In an early investigation (Andersen & Cole, 1990, Study 3), participants completed the tasks described above and then took part in a "second study" in which they were asked to read a series of statements about a person they had not met. Embedded in these statements were descriptions of some traits that the participant had identified as highly descriptive of a significant other, as well as some traits identified as irrelevant. After reading the statements, participants completed a distraction task. They where then shown descriptive statements and asked to determine whether they had seen them when reading about the person they had not met. When the original statements incorporated traits of a significant other, participants were more likely to endorse having seen statements containing traits of the significant other that were *not actually presented during the task* (i.e., false positives). This did not happen when the embedded traits were not related to a significant other (i.e., irrelevant). These findings conform to implicit learning principles in that they suggest that, without intention or realization, people made "errors" on the memory task that reflect a bias to view certain traits as covarying.

Andersen's group also demonstrated that these covariation patterns could be activated via subliminal exposure. For example, Glassman and Andersen (1999) had participants generate descriptions of significant others, as described above. A week later, they were subliminally exposed to one of the following: (1) features from their descriptions of the significant other; (2) features from another participant's significant other; or (3) features identified as irrelevant. Subliminal exposure occurred while participants engaged in a computer game in which they were told that a partner in another room was attempting to send them messages. Participants then rated statements for how descriptive they were of the nonexistent game partner. Results indicated that participants who were subliminally exposed to features from their descriptions of significant others were more likely to rate features of their significant others, which had not been presented, as more descriptive of the fictional game partner. Participants exposed to features of someone else's significant other or exposed to irrelevant features did not demonstrate this effect.

Andersen and colleagues have suggested that these results support clinicians' observations of "transference" phenomena in clinical work. Additionally, their results support Westen and Gabbard's (2002) hypothesis that the actions of therapists may serve to activate transference and can do so without the patient's awareness. That is, the therapist may do something that is similar to one of the patient's significant others. This then activates the significant-other representation, thereby increasing the patient's tendency to develop expectations of, and responses to, the therapist in a manner consistent with the patient's model of the significant other.

## Clinical Implications

What holds true for people generally ought to hold true for patients treated by psychotherapists. Patients have arrived at all sorts of unconscious conclusions about the world. Some will be accurate; some may be wildly off. Some may blatantly contradict strongly held conscious beliefs. If events repeatedly covaried in a nonsensible or maladaptive fashion, that is what the person will have learned. And, the patient will often be unable to report such unconscious conclusions. This is not because of conflict or defense; it is because this is how implicit learning operates. This could explain some of the discrepant connections by which people seem to live their lives but deny, seem oblivious to, or find themselves unable to change. They are not necessarily resisting knowing; they really do not know.

When therapists help people make these connections through the use of behavior monitoring, thought monitoring, confrontation (i.e., inquiring about discrepancies between actual behaviors and stated goals/beliefs), transference interpretations, or Socratic dialogue, they are not always breaking through resistances or defenses to make patients realize something that they already knew. Instead, they are helping people make *wholly new connections* that allow them to understand their experiences. They are making patients aware of implicitly learned assumptions and beliefs. In modern social psychological parlance, they are making the implicit explicit.

A continued finding across psychotherapies is the importance of the therapeutic relationship in producing optimal outcomes (Weinberger, 1995; Weinberger & Rasco, 2007). A variety of theories has attempted to explain the power of this relationship. One possibility is that the relationship may produce changes in the patient via implicit learning. That is, many aspects of the therapist's stance and approach to therapy (e.g., empathic, nonjudgmental, warm, goal oriented) may produce implicit learning of new covariations on the part of the patient. Although patients may never become fully aware of, and may never be able to verbalize precisely, what was learned and how, this type of learning in therapy should not be discounted. What is explicitly learned through therapy may be enhanced by what is implicitly learned.

Finally, research from social psychology also indicates that implicit learning is not, in and of itself, a pathological process. The majority of studies demonstrating implicit learning have utilized nonclinical populations, suggesting that learning implicitly is a normative process. Providing patients with education about implicit learning might therefore be helpful. For example, normalizing patients' inability to fully explain discrepancies between their beliefs and behaviors, while validating their desire for change, can help patients to reconceptualize their difficulties and relocate their efforts. If patients view their problems in dispositional terms only (e.g., "I feel sad because I am a depressed person"), then it is difficult for them to appreciate how change can take place and to have a sense of how best to direct efforts. If the problem is conceptualized in terms of past learning (e.g., "I feel sad because I may have learned things in the past that I am unaware of having learned that are influencing my current views and behaviors"), then the patient's effort can be redirected toward uncovering the implicitly learned associations and contingencies and then working to problem-solve around changing them.

## AUTOMATICITY

As stated previously, it is common for patients to present for psychotherapy with problematic patterns of behavior or thought that have become highly distressing to them. As suggested above, learning that has occurred implicitly can result in exactly such patterns. However, even when individuals are well aware of problematic patterns of thought or behavior, and even when they have a clear sense of what they need to do, they often find themselves unable to change old patterns. Or, they find that they are able to engender change for some time, only to have the problem resurface at a later date. For many patients, this relapse results in feelings of hopelessness, ineptness, or a sense that they are destined for failure. Patients are often unaware that repetitive behavior patterns are frequently activated automatically and are difficult to change. Additionally, patients frequently underestimate the degree to which problems are likely to resurface in the face of stress or even when their attention is simply directed elsewhere. Finally, many patients are unaware that patterns of behavior can be *activated* by a variety of factors and then run on automatic pilot unless something intervenes. Researchers interested in automaticity have studied precisely these issues.

### Illustrative Data

Notions of automaticity practically dominate social psychological writings on nonconscious processes (see e.g., Wegner & Bargh, 1998). In simple language, automatic processing involves the activation of well-learned behavioral, cognitive, and/or emotional patterns. These patterns are activated by the perception of cues that prime them. It is very important to note that the perception of these cues often occurs outside of the individual's awareness (Bargh & Chartrand, 1999). Once such patterns have been activated, they proceed mechanically, almost reflexively. There is usually little or no need to attend to or monitor them.

Virtually anything can become automatic. All that is required is sufficient practice and, in some cases, a trigger or stimulus cue to activate the pattern. Many of our everyday activities are automatic (e.g., making coffee, tying shoelaces) but automaticity does not relate only to simple or reflex-like behaviors. Because it can also account for very complex multistep patterns of thought and behavior, automaticity makes for a powerful explanatory concept in social behavior (Wegner & Bargh, 1998).

Once begun, automatic patterns tend to "run off" with little or no need for active attention, monitoring, or control. Automaticity makes functioning more efficient and easy, until one tries to change. It is difficult to stop or alter an automatic pattern; efforts to do so are experienced as highly unpleasant, even frightening (like trying to resist a compulsion). Automatic patterns are inflexible and rigid, like obsessive thoughts, compulsions, or rituals. A nonclinical example should make the nature of automaticity clear. Think of trying to drive on the left side of the road in England, if you are from the United States and are used to driving on the right side. Even though failing to make this change is life-threatening, it is almost impossible and the effort is unpleasant.

Automaticity is not restricted to once-voluntary behaviors. If a person repeats what he or she has implicitly learned often enough, it too will become automatic and therefore extremely resistant to change. There is evidence from brain imaging data that, as individuals become more skilled in performing a task, such as reading words backwards, activation in the cortex decreases and activation in the basal ganglia increases (Poldrack, Desmond, Glover, & Gabrieli, 1998). The basal ganglia has been implicated in procedural learning, which is typically considered a form of implicit learning or memory (Butters, Heindel, & Salmon, 1990). Thus, implicit learning and automaticity are likely to be highly related. Complex behaviors or patterns that are learned implicitly may rapidly become automatic. Such behaviors can include interpersonal enactments, ways of relating, and nonverbal behaviors such as manners of speech and carriage. Most of the time, such behaviors are not problematic. For example, people of different cultures learn to stand at different distances from one another when speaking. These distances vary from culture to culture, as becomes apparent when people from different cultures with different appropriate distances for social intercourse try to carry on a conversation. People are often unaware that they have learned any rules regarding acceptable social intercourse distance until they experience this kind of situation. Nonetheless, the behavior of individuals from different cultures clearly indicates that a "rule" has been learned and is being applied to behavior in an *automatic* fashion.

Automatic behaviors can become problematic and may need to be changed. Because they are automatic, even if the person knows what needs to be changed, changing them is likely to be difficult. Further, automaticity is not restricted to physical activities. Habits of thought can also become automatic (Bargh & Ferguson, 2000) and also sometimes problematic. Maladaptive behaviors and thoughts that clinicians see in treatment are often so well-practiced that they have become automatic (e.g., enactments, styles of relating, obsessions, delusions, negative thoughts).

Automatic processes can be overridden by what are termed *control processes*. Control processes tend to be voluntary, flexible, and most often under conscious control. Their function is to help the person adapt to novel situations, and they are well suited to correct automatic processes that have gone awry or that are no longer adaptive. Control processes have costs, however. They require that mental resources (e.g., attention) be available. This generally means that the person must be aware that control processes are needed and that he or she must be able to figure out which control process would best do the job. He or she then must be willing, motivated, and able to consistently apply the appropriate control process (cf. Fazio & Towles-Schwen, 1999).

Awareness and motivation are needed if a control process is to override an automatic process. This is not always enough, however. Control processes must be attended to and monitored if they are to be effective. If attention or monitoring flags, control processing is disrupted and automatic processing can return, often with a vengeance. According to Wegner (1994), in order to control and prevent unwanted thoughts or behavior, two processes must operate. One, a conscious controlled process, involves behaving in the desired manner and correcting for unwanted behaviors and thoughts. The other is an unconscious process that monitors the environment and mental states for the unwanted thoughts and behaviors. The latter is an "ironic" process because a part of the mind is focused on exactly what is to be avoided. This latter unconscious process does not require much in the way of mental resources, whereas the former, conscious, process does require concentration and resources. If the conscious controlled process goes offline for any reason, the action of the unconscious monitoring process leads to exactly the behavior or thought the person is trying to avoid. Thus distractions, stress, or anything that taxes mental resources (termed *cognitive load* in the social psychological literature) can disrupt controlled processing. When this happens, the automatic patterns comes to the fore.

Examples may help make this phenomenon clearer. Wegner, Ansfeld, and Pilloff (1998) asked participants not to move a handheld pendulum in a particular direction. Participants were able to comply unless they were burdened cognitively. Under a cognitive load condition, the pendulum tended to swing in the undesired direction. Counterintuitively, this effect was greater when participants were allowed to monitor their action visually than when they could not. In common sense terms, ironic effects are like asking someone not to think of a white bear. Once someone has asked you not to think about it, the white bear keeps popping up in your mind. In order to avoid something like a white bear, you have to be on the lookout for it. Wegner, Schneider, Carter, and White (1987) examined this phenomenon empirically and found that people could not help but think of white bears except for short periods during which they actively distracted themselves from the thought.

Research shows that, although application of controlled processing can override automatic behaviors, strong motivation and constant monitoring are needed to maintain such processing. This requires a lot of mental resources and is easily disrupted in the face of stress. Once such disruption occurs, the individual is vulnerable to the old automatic pattern returning. Given this understanding of human functioning, changing behaviors and thoughts is understandably very difficult. Since stress and distractions are inevitable, one cannot count on controlled processing as a permanent and infallible solution to maladaptive automatic processes. It is more a stopgap. Clinical psychologists are unlikely to be surprised by the fact that controlled processing is usually not sufficient to end longstanding (automatic) maladaptive thoughts and behaviors. If patients could simply stop doing the things they wanted to stop doing and thinking the thoughts they wanted to stop thinking, many of them would not seek psychotherapy. One solution is to replace a maladaptive automatic response with an adaptive one. And the way to do that is to practice a controlled response often enough for it to become automatic (cf. Devine & Monteith, 1999).

Research indicates that replacing one automatic process with another is arduous and time-consuming. Shiffrin and Schneider (1977) and Schneider and Shiffrin (1977), two pioneers in the field of automaticity, employed relatively simple perceptual search tasks to study automatic responding. After participants had built up automatic responses in these tasks, it took many hundreds of trials to eliminate them. These automatic behaviors were relatively short-term, only learned in the course of their experiments. Further, the learning and elimination of these automatic responses took place in a controlled lab setting, not in the real world with all of its distractions and stresses (cognitive load). We believe that it is safe to assume that automatic behaviors that have operated for years in the real world would be even harder and take longer to eliminate or change. Prejudice is an obvious and everyday example. Despite societal and personal efforts to combat prejudice, it remains powerful in our society. Although the literature shows that explicitly prejudicial attitudes have diminished considerably in recent years (Schuman, Steeh, Bobo, & Kryson, 1997), possibly due to these efforts, implicit attitudes are difficult to alter (Wilson, Lindsey, & Schooler, 2000). Some prominent social psychologists are quite pessimistic about the possibility of such change (e.g., Bargh, 1999). Others (e.g., Devine & Monteith, 1999) offer a more optimistic point of view that matches our own, below (i.e., make counterattitudinal responding automatic). But whatever position is espoused, changing implicit attitudes is not an easy task.

## Clinical Implications

Many maladaptive patterns of behavior and thought that bring patients to psychotherapy may fall into the category of automatic behaviors. Even when the person recognizes that the pattern is problematic or maladaptive and knows what needs to be done, change is difficult. Control processes are not easy to implement and can be easily disrupted by stress. They would have to be successfully practiced for extended periods of time to be regularly effective. This could help explain some of the difficulty patients have in trying to engage in behaviors that are obviously beneficial to them. They know what they have to do—but doing it is difficult, frustrating, unpleasant, and takes time. The more established the automatic behaviors, the more time it should take to eliminate or alter them, and the longer the unpleasantness and frustration last. Discomfort, frustration, and resistance are necessary byproducts of trying to change automatic processes, not a result of motivated dynamic resistance or unconscious needs to be punished by functioning poorly. Likewise, relapse becomes easier to understand. Under stress, people revert to previous, automatic means of responding (cf. Wilson et al., 2000). Control processes are more easily disrupted by load than are automatic processes. This means that we can expect regression under stress and relapse with time and stress.

Finally, since changing automatic behavior is time-consuming and unpleasant, differences in patients' motivational states over time leave them vulnerable to failures and relapses. Anyone who has purchased a 6-month gym membership, only to use it consistently for 1 month, inconsistently for another, and not at all for the remaining 4, is aware that although the cognition "it is important to exercise" remains stable over time, the motivation to *act* on this understanding fluctuates. And much like the process of going to the gym, normal fluctuations in patients' motivational states increase the likelihood that they will return to their former automatic behavior at some point. All of this suggests that treatment, with the goal of more lasting change, may need to be more long-term than most therapy researchers are currently willing to admit and/or that booster sessions and "retreatments" at times of stress ought to be built into our protocols. Also, therapists should work hard to keep patients motivated, while remaining realistic that setbacks are a part of the process. In fact, teaching patients how to cope with setbacks is likely as important to successful long-term outcomes as increasing patients' insight into the nature of their difficulties and learning new behavioral skills. Additionally, increasing patients' awareness regarding their fluctuations in motivation, the effects of these fluctuations on them, and the things that contribute to these motivational changes, as well as their cognitive and affective responses to their failures, may need to be targeted *early* in treatment.

Change is likely to be even more difficult to effect when automaticity develops out of implicit learning. In such cases, the patient does not even know what needs changing. For example, in Ainsworth's Strange Situation (Ainsworth, Blehar, Waters, & Wall, 1978), 18-month-old infants demonstrate automatically activated behavioral patterns in reaction to mild stressors. Infants are obviously unable to articulate how these patterns have developed, but it is widely accepted that infants' relational experiences with their caretakers are critical to long-term social and emotional adjustment. Ainsworth et al. (1978) have demonstrated that variations in these behavioral patterns are related to actual variations in the quality of the caregiver–child relationship, strongly suggesting that they are likely to be learned, at least in part, implicitly. A large body of research (e.g., Fraley & Shaver, 2000; Waters, Merrick, Treboux, Crowell, & Albersheim, 2000) has suggested that these implicitly learned and remembered patterns continue to influence behavior in adolescence and adulthood and are fairly resistant to change. This is one example of how implicit learning and automaticity can converge to exert a longstanding influence on the behavior of an individual.

Before automatic patterns based on implicit processes can be changed, a preliminary step may be necessary. Before any interventions can be offered, before controlled processing can be brought into play, patients may first need to make the appropriate connections. They may need to know what they are doing and how it is affecting their lives. Here is a place for making the unconscious conscious (or in social psychological parlance, the explicit implicit) and for insight. That is, the person needs to know what needs changing. Once these connections are made, the person will be in a better position to know which control processes can work to override implicitly learned behaviors and, with a lot of work, develop them into adaptive automatic behaviors. Implicit automatic maladaptive behaviors, by this analysis, would be even harder to change than consciously available maladaptive behaviors. It may be harder to change a habitual way of relating (e.g., avoidant) or thinking (self-denigration) than to learn to drive on the left side of the road when you are used to driving on the right.

Another clinical implication of this research is that generating insight (i.e., making the implicit explicit) may be only the first step in helping the individual to change maladaptive behaviors. Once a patient is capable of recognizing a previously unconscious maladaptive pattern, he or she can begin to work toward behaving in a different fashion. At this point, the work may actually involve making the patient's explicit adaptive behaviors implicit, that is to say, automatic, through repetition and practice.

## ATTRIBUTION THEORY

Previous sections of this chapter have examined nonconscious cognitive processes that are likely to be heavily influenced by previous experiences. However, social psychology can also be helpful to clinical psychologists in highlighting characteristic patterns of thought and behavior that are typical of most adults and are not necessarily "learned" in the strict sense of the word. The identification of such processes in nonclinical populations can be helpful in identifying how certain clinical syndromes may result in variations from the norm, can help therapists make sense of how patients view patient–therapist interactions, and can also alert therapists to typical styles of thinking or ways of processing information that might influence the way the therapist sees the patient. Though there are many fields in social psychology that address these issues, we have chosen to briefly discuss attribution theory, as research in this realm focuses heavily on how individuals (be they therapists or patients) tend to understand and interpret the behavior and intentions of themselves as well as others.

## Illustrative Data

Attribution theory assumes that people are strongly motivated to explain the behavior of themselves and others (Jones & Davis, 1965; Weiner, 1986). In fact, the literature suggests that people may care more about why people do things than what it is they do (Gilbert & Malone, 1995). People tend to interpret other people's behavior as the result of their disposition and/or the situation they were in when they behaved as they did. Logically, a person *should not* make use of dispositions to explain behavior when that behavior occurs in the presence of a strong situational force. Similarly, a person *should* make a dispositional attribution when a person behaves in a way that is not in accord with situational norms (e.g., makes a racist comment in a public media outlet). Jones and Davis (1965) were the first to formally name this the *law of noncommon effects*. Kelley (1967) broadened and codified it as the *discounting principle*.

The research indicates that people are not consistent in their use of the discounting principle. They often see others' behavior as dispositionally motivated even when situational factors could explain it. This is so pervasive that it has been labeled the "fundamental attribution error" (Ross, 1977). Nowadays, the more modest term *correspondence bias* tends to be employed (Gilbert & Malone, 1995). Whatever it is called, this tendency is pervasive and powerful. Jones and Harris (1967) and others (Ross, Amabile, & Steinmetz, 1977) reported that even when participants were made aware of situational factors (the person was instructed to make a pro-choice or pro-Castro speech), they still inferred dispositional characteristics (i.e., they thought the person giving the speech was pro-choice or pro-Castro). A recent study (Bargh, Williams, & Huang, 2007) found that dispositional attributions can be made in response to the flimsiest of evidence. When a participant was asked to hold a cold cup of coffee for a confederate who had his hands full, the confederate was judged negatively (i.e., aloof and cold), whereas confederates that asked participants to hold a warm cup of coffee were seen in more positive terms (i.e., pleasant and warm). Clearly, this effect is nonconscious as no one would (or did, in this experiment) declare that they were basing their conclusions on coffee temperature.

Skinner (1971) felt that one of the main reasons people misattribute behavior to personality is that situational constraints are not easily perceived by viewers. For example, it is difficult to concretize a situational constraint such as "audience pressure" because it is not something you can hear, see, or touch. Yet anyone who has spoken publicly can attest to being cognizant of it. The inability to sense the totality of the situation the person is in makes it difficult to judge accurately (cf. Gilbert & Malone, 1995).

The other side of the attributional coin is that people tend to explain their own behavior in terms of situational constraints. The tendency to explain one's own behavior in terms of situations while attributing the behavior of others to personality dispositions has been termed the *actor–observer bias* (Jones & Nisbett, 1971). A great deal of research supports the actor–observer bias. For example, college students are likely to explain others' performance on an intelligence test in terms of the test takers' ability but to explain their own performance on the same test as due to the difficulty of the test items (Jones, Rock, Shaver, Goethals, & Ward, 1968; McArthur, 1972; Nisbett, Caputo, Legant, & Marecek, 1973). They also believe a peer's future behavior is likely to mirror his or her current behavior. In contrast, these same college students stated that they would behave differently in the future. Students also described their friend's choice of girlfriend and college major in terms of their friend's personality. Yet, they described their own choice of girlfriend in terms of her personality and their major in terms of its qualities. In sum, college students (and presumably people in general) understand the behavior of others in terms of enduring personality traits, whereas they see their own behaviors as reactions to the situations they face.

### Clinical Implications

Clinicians often ascribe their patients' behavior to their personality or disposition. The patient is depressed or anxious or has a personality disorder. This has been codified as diagnoses (American Psychiatric Association, 2000), although, to be fair, there is a category termed *adjustment disorder* that allows for situational diagnosis. The patient, on the other hand, is likely to explain his or her behavior as situational. The clinician may (and often does) see this as defense and/or resistance. The patient may see the therapist as not appreciating the situation with which he or she has had to deal. This can then result in a sense of being misunderstood, which can seem like further resistance to the therapist. Attribution theory suggests that the different points of view of therapist and patient may not represent lack of empathy on the part of the therapist or resistance on the part of the patient, but may instead be a product of how humans understand the behavior of self and others (i.e., actor–observer bias). Some of the relationship ruptures that are endemic to clinical work (Safran & Muran, 1995, 1996) might be avoided if clinicians had a greater appreciation of this bias. This is not to say that resistance, defense, and lack of empathy do not occur. Rather, by being aware of the actor–observer bias as a fundamental human propensity, the therapist might be more effective in identifying genuine resistance and defense, thereby being more effective and also avoiding alienating the patient with a perceived lack of empathy.

## SUMMARY AND CONCLUSIONS

The above sections discussed the implications of implicit learning, automaticity, and attribution theory for clinical psychology. Our reading of the literature led us to certain conclusions: Attributional and implicit processes are ubiquitous, begin early in life, continue throughout life, are self-perpetuating, and are long-lasting. They are not necessarily the result of, nor do they inevitably result in, pathology. They become pathological and need to be addressed clinically when the thoughts, feelings, and behaviors they trigger are maladaptive. The actor–observer bias can lead to difficulties between therapist and patient, as the former sees the patient as dispositionally motivated whereas the latter sees him- or herself as reacting to situational exigencies. The therapist may therefore see the patient as defensive and resistant; the patient may see the therapist as unempathic. Sensitivity to this human tendency might improve the process and outcome of psychotherapy.

Implicit learning may underlie some of the maladaptive life choices people make. Implicit learning becomes connected to whatever is most salient in the environment. Treatment that educates patients with regard to the nature of implicit processes and then uses this information to help patients understand how they can understand and work to solve their difficulties has a greater chance to result in a positive outcome. This way of understanding people is implicit in both psychodynamic (Westen, Weinberger, & Bradley, 2007) and cognitive (Beck, Rush, Shaw, & Emery, 1979) approaches to psychotherapy. Well-practiced behaviors and thoughts become automatic. So does oft-repeated implicit learning. Changing automatic behaviors is labor-intensive and unpleasant. Changing automatic behaviors learned implicitly involves first bringing them to light (i.e., making them explicit) so that they can be overridden through conscious attention and effort (controlled processing). The resulting, more adaptive behavior then needs to be repeatedly practiced until it becomes automatic, otherwise regression and relapse are likely. This process suggests that therapy may need to be more long-term than is currently in vogue and/or that several courses of treatment may be necessary, especially if stressful life events intervene. Finally, we strongly believe that that the apparently contradictory views of clinicians and social psychologists (i.e., that dispositions and coping styles are paramount vs. situations are paramount, respectively) are in fact complementary and that each discipline can learn much from the other to the betterment of both. We hope that this chapter has made some small contribution in this direction.

## REFERENCES


Ainsworth, M. D. S., Blehar, M. C., Waters, E., & Wall, S. (1978). *Patterns of attachment: A psychological study of the strange situation.* Hillsdale, NJ: Erlbaum.

American Psychiatric Association. (2000). *Diagnostic and statistical manual of mental disorders* (4th ed., text rev.). Washington, DC: Author.

Andersen, S. M., & Cole, S. W. (1990). "Do I know you?" The role of significant others in social perception. *Journal of Personality and Social Psychology, 59,* 384–399.

Andersen, S. M., Reznik, I., & Glassman, N. S. (2005). The unconscious relational self. In R. Hassin, J. S. Uleman, & J. A. Bargh (Eds.), *The new unconscious* (pp. 421–481). New York: Oxford University Press.

Bargh, J. A. (1999). The cognitive monster: The case against the controllability of automatic stereotype effects. In S. Chaiken & Y. Trope (Eds.), *Dual processing theories in social psychology* (pp. 361–382). New York: Guilford Press.

Bargh, J. A., & Chartrand, T. L. (1999). The unbearable automaticity of being. *American Psychologist, 54,* 462–479.

Bargh, J. A., & Ferguson, M. J. (2000). Beyond behaviorism: On the automaticity of higher mental processes. *Psychological Bulletin, 126,* 925–945.

Bargh, J. A., Williams, L. E., & Huang, J. H. (2007, September). *Mating and metaphors.* Symposium presentation at the annual meeting of the Society of Experimental Social Psychology, Chicago.

Beck, A. T., Rush, J. A., Shaw, B. F., & Emery, G. (1979). *Cognitive therapy of depression.* New York: Guilford Press.

Berry, D. C., & Dienes, Z. (1993). *Implicit learning: Theoretical and empirical issues.* Hillsdale, NJ: Erlbaum.

Butters, N., Heindel, W. C., & Salmon, D. (1990). Dissociation of implicit memory in dementia: Neurological implications. *Bulletin of the Psychodynamic Society, 28,* 359–366.

Devine, P. G., & Monteith, M. J. (1999). Automaticity and control in stereotyping. In S. Chaiken &

Y. Trope (Eds.), *Dual process theories in social psychology* (pp. 339–360). New York: Guilford Press.

Fazio, R. H., & Towles-Schwen, T. (1999). The MODE model of attitude–behavior processes. In S. Chaiken & Y. Trope (Eds.), *Dual process theories in social psychology* (pp. 97–116). New York: Guilford Press.

Fraley, R. C., & Shaver, P. R. (2000). Adult romantic attachment: Theoretical developments, emerging controversies, and unanswered questions. *Review of General Psychology, 4,* 135–154.

Glassman, N., & Andersen, S. (1999). Activating transference without consciousness: Using significant-other representations to go beyond what is subliminally given. *Journal of Personality and Social Psychology, 77,* 1146–1162.

Gilbert, D. T., & Malone, P. S. (1995). The correspondence bias. *Psychological Bulletin, 117,* 21–38.

Hill, T., Lewicki, P., Czyzewska, M., & Boss, A. (1989). Self-perpetuating development of encoding biases in person perception. *Journal of Personality and Social Psychology, 57,* 373–387.

Jones, E. E., & Davis, K. E. (1965). From acts of dispositions: The attribution process in person perception. In L. Berkowitz (Ed.), *Advances in experimental social psychology* (Vol. 2, pp. 219–266). San Diego, CA: Academic Press.

Jones, E. E., & Harris, V. A. (1967). The attribution of attitudes. *Journal of Experimental Social Psychology, 3,* 1–24.

Jones, E. E., & Nisbett, R. E. (1971). The actor and the observer: Divergent perceptions of the causes of behavior. In E. E. Jones et al. (Eds.), *Attributions: Perceiving the causes of behavior* (pp. 79–94). Morristown, NJ: General Learning Press.

Jones, E. E., Rock, L., Shaver, K. G., Goethals, G. R., & Ward, L. M. (1968). Patterns of performance and ability attribution: An unexpected primacy effect. *Journal of Personality and Social Psychology, 10,* 317–349.

Jusczyk, P. W. (1997). *The discovery of spoken language.* Cambridge, MA: MIT Press.

Kelley, H. H. (1967). Attribution theory in social psychology. In D. Levine (Ed.), *Nebraska symposium on motivation* (Vol. 15, pp. 192–238). Lincoln: University of Nebraska Press.

Lewicki, P. (1986). *Nonconscious social information processing.* New York: Academic Press.

McArthur, L. (1972). The how and what of why: Some determinants and consequences of causal attribution. *Journal of Personality and Social Psychology, 22,* 171–193.

Nisbett, R. E., Caputo, C., Legant, P., & Marecek, J. (1973). Behavior as seen by the actor and as seen by the observer. *Journal of Personality and Social Psychology, 27,* 154–164.

Poldrack, R. A., Desmond, J. E., Glover, G. H., & Gabrieli, J. D. (1998). The neural basis of visual skill learning: An fMRI study of mirror reading. *Cerebral Cortex, 8,* 1–10.

Reber, A. S. (1989). Implicit learning and tacit knowledge. *Journal of Experimental Psychology, 118,* 219–235.

Ross, L. (1977). The intuitive psychologist and his shortcomings: Distortions in the attribution process. In L. Berkowitz (Ed.), *Advances in experimental social psychology* (Vol. 10, pp. 173–220). New York: Academic Press.

Ross, L., Amabile, T. M., & Steinmetz, J. L. (1977). Social roles, social control, and biases in social-perception processes. *Journal of Personality and Social Psychology, 35,* 485–494.

Rubin, D., Wallace, W., & Houston B. (1993). The beginnings of expertise for ballads. *Cognitive Science, 17,* 435–462.

Safran, J. D., & Muran, J. C. (1995). Resolving therapeutic alliance ruptures: Diversity and integration. *In Session: Psychotherapy in Practice, 1* 81–92.

Safran, J. D., & Muran, J. C. (1996). The resolution of ruptures in the therapeutic alliance. *Journal of Consulting and Clinical Psychology, 64,* 447–458.

Schneider, W., & Shiffrin, R. M. (1977). Controlled and automatic human information processing: Detection, search, and attention. *Psychological Review, 84,* 1–66.

Schuman, H., Steeh, C., Bobo, L., & Kryson, M. (1997). *Racial attitudes in America: Trends and interpretations* (rev. ed.). Cambridge, MA: Harvard University Press.

Seger, C. A. (1994). Implicit learning. *Psychological Bulletin, 115,* 163–196.

Shiffrin, R. M., & Schneider, W. (1977). Controlled and automatic human information processing: II. Perceptual learning, automatic attending, and a general theory. *Psychological Review*, *84*, 127–190.

Skinner, B. F. (1971). *Beyond freedom and dignity.* New York: Knopf.

Wachtel, P. (1993). *Therapeutic communication.* New York: Guilford Press.

Waters, E., Merrick, S., Treboux, D., Crowell, J., & Albersheim, L. (2000). Attachment security in infancy and early adulthood: A twenty-year longitudinal study. *Child Development*, *71*, 684–689.

Wegner, D. M. (1994). Ironic processes in mental control. *Psychological Review*, *101*, 34–52.

Wegner, D. M., Ansfeld, M., & Pilloff, D. (1998). The putt and the pendulum: Ironic effects of mental control of action. *Psychological Science*, *9*, 196–199.

Wegner, D. M., & Bargh, J. A. (1998). Control and automaticity in social life. In D. T. Gilbert & S. E. Fiske (Eds.), *The handbook of social psychology* (4th ed., Vol. 2, pp. 446–496). New York: McGraw-Hill.

Wegner, D. M., Schneider, D. J., Carter, S. R., & White, T. L. (1987). Paradoxical effects of thought suppression. *Journal of Personality and Social Psychology*, *53*, 5–13.

Weinberger, J. (1995). Common factors aren't so common: The common factors dilemma. *Clinical Psychology: Science and Practice*, *2*, 45–69.

Weinberger, J., & Rasco, C. (2007). Empirically supported common factors. In S. Hoffmann & J. Weinberger (Eds.), *Art and science in psychotherapy* (pp. 103–130). New York: Routledge.

Weiner, B. (1986). *An attributional theory of motivation and emotion.* New York: Springler-Verlag.

Westen, D., & Gabbard, G. O. (2002). Developments in cognitive neuroscience: II. Implications for theories of transference. *Journal of the American Psychoanalytic Association*, *50*, 99–134.

Westen, D., Weinberger, J., & Bradley, R. (2007). Motivation, decision making, and consciousness: From psychodynamics to subliminal priming and emotional constraint satisfaction. In P. D. Zelazo, M. Moscovitch, & E. Thompson (Eds.), *The Cambridge handbook of consciousness* (pp. 673–702). New York: Cambridge University Press.

Wilson, T. D., Lindsey, S., & Schooler, T. Y. (2000). A model of dual attitudes. *Psychological Review*, *107*, 101–126.

# 26 The Social Psychology of Transference

Regina Miranda
Susan M. Andersen

Theories of personality and psychopathology have long focused on the influence of past relationships with significant persons on an individual's emotional and relationship functioning in the present. From the early 20th century onward, various models of personality have assumed that interpersonal processes are at the heart of personality. (See also Benjamin, Chapter 19, this volume.) This idea was initiated by Freud (1912/1958, although he disavowed it), developed by subsequent psychodynamic theorists (e.g., Fairbairn, 1952; Kernberg, 1976; Sullivan, 1953), adopted by cognitive therapists (e.g., Safran, 1990; Safran & Segal, 1990), and extended still further by work on attachment theory (Bowlby, 1969, 1973, 1980). More recently, research grounded in social cognition (e.g., Andersen & Chen, 2002; Baldwin, 1992) has examined the proposition that people hold mental representations of important individuals from their past in memory, which then influence their present experiences and interpretations of self and others, how they view new others in the present, and how they view themselves. Indeed, research in both social cognition and clinical psychology has focused intensively on characteristics of the individual (e.g., personality traits, self-schemas). Extending this research to the individual in the context of his or her relationships, in our work we have focused on the social cognitive process of *transference* and *the relational self*—as they transpire in everyday social relations.

We conceptualize and examine transference in terms of social cognitions, proposing that an individual's identity is inextricably bound to how he or she comes to view the self in relationships with significant others both from the past and in the present. We argue that this process is evident in everyday interpersonal relations as well even when the significant other is not there. That is, an individual's view of new relationships and of new encounters, and also of the self in the context of each, is shaped by prior experiences with significant others.

This shaping occurs as a function of knowledge stored in memory about those who have mattered greatly to an individual in his or her life. The social cognitive process of transference plays out in everyday life among perfectly normal people as they encounter new people or new relationships. Relationships from the past (or present) come to shape views of the self and of others in the present moment.

In this chapter we describe a social cognitive model of transference and its implications for the self as well as for emotional and motivational experience, and we present evidence from a program of laboratory-based research that supports the approach. Research from other laboratories making related assumptions have obtained compatible findings, suggesting that this is indeed a phenomenon relevant to people's lives, and potentially relevant to the degree of their own suffering and resilience. Both adaptive and maladaptive processes are evoked in transference, including those that are affectively and motivationally laden and those that are self-regulatory. We discuss these in turn and conclude with the potential clinical implications of the findings.

## THE SOCIAL COGNITIVE MODEL OF TRANSFERENCE AND THE INTERPERSONAL NATURE OF SELF

In our work, we assume that individuals have a fundamental need for human connection (Andersen, Reznik, & Chen, 1997; Chen & Andersen, 1999; see also, Baumeister & Leary, 1995), an assumption long held by classical models of personality (e.g., Adler, 1927/1957; Bakan, 1966; Batson, 1990; Bowlby, 1969; Deci, 1995; Fairbairn, 1952; Greenberg & Mitchell, 1983; Guisinger & Blatt, 1994; Horney, 1945; Rogers, 1951; Safran, 1990; Sullivan, 1953). This assumption is of special relevance because this need is likely to shape the nature of the mental representations individuals come to hold about themselves and others. We propose that the knowledge that people ultimately hold in memory about themselves is acquired and changed in the context of past and present relationships with significant others that matter to individuals and who are influential in their lives (e.g., family members, romantic partners, friends). In short, people hold mental representations of the self, as is commonly assumed, and we argue that these representations are tied to mental representations of significant others as well as representations of individuals' unique relationship with each significant other. Thus, cues that trigger the significant-other representation also activate the particular view of the self one holds while with the significant other. In this way, significant-other relationships, when activated, come to shape the working view of the self in the moment. Knowledge about the self stored in memory is "entangled" with knowledge about significant others (Andersen & Chen, 2002; Andersen et al., 1997), with people holding a number of differing relational selves in memory. Activating a particular significant other activates the relevant aspect of the self.

This model is similar to other social cognitive models such as those concerned with relational schemas (e.g., Baldwin, 1992; Baldwin & Sinclair, 1996). Our model simply emphasizes the unique and idiosyncratic nature of the relational representations stored in memory, whereas related models emphasize generic knowledge in relational schemas. The literature nonetheless contains many methodological and conceptual parallels that converge on the same kind of evidence about the effects of activating a significant-other representation and the relational dynamics with that significant other.

The broader field of social cognition emphasizes the basic mental processes by which various representations stored in memory ultimately shape perception and interpretation. Research offers strong evidence that human thought takes place automatically, that is, without investment of energy or even attention. When mental processes are relatively automatic in how they operate, or relatively implicit, this tells us something about how ideas in the mind are interconnected and that meaning is made on the spot as people try to make sense of their current experience. (For an integrative review of representations and processes typically studied, see Andersen, Moskowitz, Blair, & Nosek, 2007; see also, Bargh, 1997; Higgins, 1996a; Higgins & King, 1981.)

In our work, as elsewhere in the social cognition field, we assume that situational cues (e.g., a situation with a new person) will trigger or *activate* preexisting mental representations, making them ready for use in interpreting the new person or situation. This activation will occur quite automatically, without thought, effort, attention, control, or awareness (Bargh, 1997; see also, Andersen, Moskowitz, et al., 2007). The mental processes involved are best characterized as (1) the *activation* process, by which stored knowledge is readied for use; (2) the *application* process, by which the activated representation is actually used in interpretation and response; and (3) the *applicability* process, by which the nature of a stimulus person and of other elements in the situation make the particular knowledge *applicable* in some manner to this new stimulus (Higgins, 1996a). If a representation is not applicable at all, it obviously is less likely to be used.

Existing evidence supports such processes. In our work, we also assume that significant-other representations are activated and used automatically. This assumption is supported by our research, particularly direct evidence that the process of transference is provoked without conscious awareness (Glassman & Andersen, 1999a; see Andersen, Reznik, & Glassman, 2005). This and other evidence shows clearly that these basic automatic processes that occur with other mental representations in memory (e.g., stereotypes, trait-labeled social categories, evaluations) are also at work in relation to significant-other representations (Chen, Fitzsimons, & Andersen, 2007; see Andersen, Moskowitz, et al., 2007).

## LINEAGE IN PSYCHOANALYTIC THOUGHT

As originally proposed by Freud, transference was considered the individual's transfer of childhood fantasies and unconscious conflicts about parental figures onto the psychoanalyst or to another new person. Freud termed the "mental representations" of parental figures that formed the basis of transference *imagoes*. However, Freud did not view transference as mental representational, but rather saw it as rooted in psychosexual conflict and as a defense, and while he believed it occurred in everyday life, he particularly focused on its occurrence in psychoanalytic treatment (Freud, 1912/1958).

Our view of the relational self and transference is more consistent with that of Harry Stack Sullivan (1953). Sullivan posited the existence of two basic interpersonal needs: for felt security (i.e., feeling safe from harm) and for satisfaction (i.e., personal growth and connection to others). As a result of these needs, individuals developed mental representations of important others, which Sullivan termed *personifications*, and of relationship patterns with these significant others, or *dynamisms*. Sullivan used the term *parataxic distortion* to refer to the process by which attributes of a new person activated mental representations of individuals with similar characteristics, which, in turn, led people to interpret the new person's behavior based on those characteristics (Sullivan, 1953).

We also conceptualize significant others as bound up with motivational and emotional relevance for the person. We assume that transference takes place in everyday life among nonclinical populations and can be defined in social cognitive terms—in terms of mental representations (i.e., stored knowledge in memory). Our research offers considerable support for this view, and we believe that the research has implications for clinical work. We describe the evidence and its meaning for the self and for human suffering and resilience in the pages that follow, and we draw out their clinical implications.

## HOW WE STUDY TRANSFERENCE: OUR LABORATORY-BASED SOCIAL COGNITION PARADIGM

In our social cognitive model, we operationalize transference as the degree to which individuals "go beyond the information given" (Bruner, 1957) about a new person (i.e., ascribe characteristics to the person) based on a significant other's characteristics, when the representation of this significant other has been activated (Andersen & Chen, 2002). Activation of a significant-other representation provokes particular inferences about the new person, as well as expectancies, motivations, affective experiences, and behaviors associated with the relationship with the significant other. Moreover, given the link between self and other in memory, this process also provokes shifts in the working view of the self that one experiences—that is, it provokes a similar view of self as that experienced when with the significant other.

We demonstrate transference in laboratory experiments that rely on what we term an *idiographic–nomothetic* procedure—one that uses information unique to the individual as well as a standard experimental paradigm that allows generalizable processes to be assessed. We can thus trigger distinct significant-other representations, defined as a personally known important other in an individual's life, and measure the occurrence of transference in terms of basic mental processes. The methodology involves two laboratory sessions that are separated by a period of at least 2 weeks and assumed by participants to be unrelated. As part of their ongoing requirements as undergraduate students taking introductory psychology, all research participants take part in numerous other studies during the same period, which also likely leads to memory interference between all the various studies.

In the first session participants are asked to describe two of their significant others—usually one who is very loved or liked and one who is disliked—by listing an equal number of positive and negative phrases that characterize each significant other. Participants later take part in the seemingly unrelated experimental session in which they are told that they will soon be interacting with a new person—a "potential buddy" in a university mentoring program we are testing—and that they will do so in a "getting acquainted" conversation. This individual, they are informed, was just interviewed in an adjacent room by an interviewer who provided a description of this person which participants are then given to read. This description, in fact, includes a minimal number of phrases—in one condition of the experiment—drawn from the participants' previous description of their own significant other. The phrases are allegedly about the new person next door, and participants in all conditions are asked to imagine themselves interacting with this person.

In the transference (experimental) condition, as noted, the phrases participants in the experiment read are those that they had listed in the first session as characterizing their positive or negative significant other. In the control condition, participants are yoked to a participant in the experimental condition so that they read descriptions about the new person drawn from this other participant's significant other. That is, individuals in these conditions are yoked as pairs and presented with the same set of phrases. However, in one case the individual described minimally resembles the participant's own significant other, whereas in the other case the new person minimally resembles someone else's significant other.

After learning about the new person and imagining interacting with him or her, participants complete a number of ratings that assess their evaluations of the potential buddy, expectancies about being accepted or rejected by the person, motivation to approach versus avoid the new person, and present views of the self (depending on the purposes of the study). We typically measure whether or not transference occurs and how much individuals "go beyond the information given" (Bruner, 1957) about the potential buddy by using a recognition memory task in which participants are asked to rate how confident they are that certain phrase descriptors were presented as descriptions of the new person. Transference is evident when participants report that they were presented with representation-consistent features that were not, in fact, presented in describing the new person. Transference is also evident when they evaluate a new person especially positively or negatively, liking or taking an aversion to him or her, with minimal information, or quickly expecting to be embraced and accepted or rejected.

## Transference and the Relational Self: Bias in Inferences and Memory

Our first experimental evidence of transference occurred in the study of schema-triggered memory (Andersen & Baum, 1994; Andersen & Cole, 1990). We expected that information stored about a significant other could be triggered by information from the environment that activates a particular relational schema. We have found this to be the case, using both explicit and implicit memory measures. Individuals express more confidence in having been presented with information about a new person if the person resembles their own, rather than another participant's, significant other—regardless of whether the representation triggered was of a positive or a negative significant other (Andersen, Reznik, & Manzella, 1996; Berenson & Andersen, 2006; Berk & Andersen, 2000; Hinkley & Andersen, 1996). This is the case both when they expect to interact with a new person (Andersen & Baum, 1994) and when they are merely reading about a fictional character with whom they do not expect to interact (Andersen & Cole, 1990; Andersen, Glassman, Chen, & Cole, 1995; Chen, Andersen, & Hinkley, 1999; Glassman & Andersen, 1999b). Such memory effects seem to be automatic in that they are also found when the significant-other features are presented outside of participants' conscious awareness—as with a subliminal computer presentation (Glassman & Andersen, 1999a). Furthermore, these effects have been demonstrated using indirect measures of memory activation. In a recent study (Miranda, Andersen, & Edwards, 2009), we found that triggering a significant-other representation led dysphoric individuals to make faster lexical decisions about adjectives that they had previously rated to be descriptive of their negative significant other, compared to a condition in which the significant other was not triggered.

### Eliciting Positive and Negative Evaluation and Affect

Evidence suggests that people evaluate all stimuli that they encounter as either positive or negative, and they appear to do this automatically—that is, quickly and without much effort (Bargh, Chaiken, Raymond, & Hymes, 1996; Duckworth, Bargh, Garcia, & Chaiken, 2002). When encountering a new person, individuals may immediately have some idea how they will feel about the person, even without having much information about him or her. At the same time, knowledge held in memory about a particular stimulus can come to be associated with an affective state, such that triggering a mental representation also evokes the affect associated with the representation. This *schema-triggered affect* (Fiske & Pavelchak, 1986) arises when a mental representation of a certain valence is activated.

We have found both of these to be the case in transference, depending on whether a new person one expects to encounter resembles a positive or negative significant other from one's life. When a participant expects to encounter someone whose characteristics resemble those of a positively toned significant other (i.e., someone who is liked or loved and who has made an impact in the person's life), they evaluate this new person more positively than do participants who expect to encounter someone who resembles a negatively toned significant other (i.e., someone who is disliked and not loved but has had an impact in the person's life) (Andersen et al., 1996; Andersen & Baum 1994; Berk & Andersen, 2000) and more positively than those who expect to interact with a person who resembles someone else's positive significant other (Baum & Andersen, 1999; Reznik & Andersen, 2007). These findings suggest that automatic evaluations of new people are affected by prior knowledge that becomes triggered in memory by external cues.

Furthermore, we have evidence that schema-triggered affect is elicited in transference. In one study, participants' facial expressions, which were recorded while they were reading descriptions of their "potential buddy," were later rated by independent judges. Participants who read descriptions of a person who resembled a positive significant other showed more positive facial affect than did participants who read descriptions of someone who resembled a negative significant other—despite the fact that an equal number of positive and negative descriptors were included in the characteristics that they read. That is, their facial expressions took on the overall affect associated with the representation, and this appeared to occur relatively automatically (Andersen et al., 1996).

Such automatic evaluations may influence the moods people experience and the goals they pursue. For example, a recent study found that continual activation of positive and negative evaluations resulted in the induction of a mood of the same valence and impacted whether individuals processed information heuristically and effortlessly, versus analytically and cautiously (Chartrand, van Baaren, & Bargh, 2006). Continual activation of negative significant-other representations by contextual cues may contribute to chronically experienced negative affective states and thus to difficulties in emotion regulation, particularly among individuals whose repertoire of significant others is negatively toned. At the same time, stimuli that are evaluated positively are more likely to give rise to the motivation to approach a stimulus rather than avoid it (Chen & Bargh, 1999).

## Eliciting Expectancies

Because evaluations of new people are made based on affective information stored in memory about significant others, experiences with significant others should also translate into expectancies for acceptance and rejection by new others. Research in social cognition suggests that expectations about being accepted or rejected by others may be stored in memory as part of relational schemas—that is, as part of mental representations of regular relationship patterns (Baldwin & Sinclair, 1996). People might expect acceptance from significant others whom they like or love and rejection from significant others whom they dislike and do not love, and these expectancies may be triggered in a new interpersonal encounter with someone who resembles one of these types of significant others. This is what we have found in our work. Participants who read descriptions of a new person who resembled their own positively toned significant other and imagined interacting with the person rated themselves as expecting that this new individual would be more accepting of them and less rejecting than individuals who expected an interaction with someone who resembled a negatively toned significant other. This differential activation of expectancies did not occur in the yoked control condition (Andersen et al., 1996; Berk & Andersen, 2000).

## Triggering Motivational States

In the past decade, there has been increasing interest in the way in which motivational states (just like cognitions and affective states) might also be activated outside of conscious awareness and impact behaviors. For example, Bargh's theory of *auto-motives* suggests that goals can be triggered automatically by contextual cues previously associated with those goals (Bargh, 1990). Research has found that these nonconsciously activated goals can influence behavior in such domains as memorization and impression formation (e.g., Chartrand & Bargh, 1996). This research has been extended to interpersonal relationships (Fitzsimons & Bargh, 2003). Given our assumption that one human motivation is that of connection to others, activating a representation of someone to whom an individual is motivated to be close—such as a significant other who is liked or loved—should result in the corresponding activation of the motivation to approach or to be close to someone whose characteristics resemble a positive significant other. This is what our work has found. When individuals expect to interact with someone who resembles a positively toned significant other, they report a higher level of motivation to approach the new individual than when they anticipate an interaction with someone who resembles a negatively toned significant other. This effect does not occur when individuals expect to interact with someone who resembles another participant's positive or negative significant other (Andersen et al., 1996; Berk & Andersen, 2000). Such approach or avoidance motivations, once activated, may then come to guide subsequent behavior.

## Evoking Behavioral Confirmation

Transference has consequences for interpersonal behavior with another person. For example, in Berk and Andersen (2000) participants who learned about a new person who either resembled their own or another participant's positive or negative significant other participated in a brief telephone conversation with another naïve participant. Later, independent judges—blind to the condition—rated the content of this verbal exchange. These judges tended to rate the conversation elicited from the new person more positively when a positive significant-other representation was triggered, compared to when the representation was of a negative significant other. This was not the case in the nontransference (control) condition. That is, participants in the transference condition appeared to elicit conversational behavior from a new individual that was consistent in tone with that of the overall significant-other representation (Berk & Andersen, 2000). This study provided evidence that behavioral confirmation (Snyder, 1992; Snyder, Tanke, & Berscheid, 1977) occurs in transference.

## Eliciting Working Views of the Self

Given the close link between representations of the self and those of significant others, triggering views of unique significant others should activate corresponding views of the self in those relationships—both in the characteristics that comprise one's view of the self and in feelings about the self. We have found, in fact, that triggering significant-other representations in transference results in changes in the working self-concept—that is, in characteristics of the self that are present in working memory at a particular time (Ogilvie & Ashmore, 1991). For example, in one study (Hinkley & Andersen, 1996) participants were asked to list general characteristics of themselves and descriptions of the self when with a positive and a negative significant other. In a second session they were randomly assigned to either a transference or control condition in which they expected to interact with someone who resembled either their own or someone else's positive or negative significant other. They were instructed to imagine themselves interacting with this person, to list phrase descriptors of how they viewed themselves at the present moment, and to classify these self-descriptors as either positive or negative. Participants showed shifts in the working self-concept in the direction of the self-when-with-the-significant-other. That is, individuals in the transference condition showed more overlap between the features they listed as true of themselves in the present moment during the second study session and those that they listed as true of themselves when with their significant other in the initial study session than did participants in the control condition, even after adjusting for participants' general self-concept. Additionally, the valence of the self-concept also shifted, depending on whether the representation triggered was of a positive or a negative significant other, in that individuals in the positive transference condition reported a more positive working self-concept than did individuals in the negative transference condition. This effect was not found in the control condition.

Similar changes in the evaluative tone of the working self-concept were found in a study in which either a desired or a dreaded version of the self was triggered (Reznik & Andersen, 2004). When a significant-other representation involved a dreaded self, the self-view in the present moment was evaluated more negatively than when the representation triggered was of a desired self and also more negatively than that of yoked control participants.

## Eliciting Self-Regulatory Processes in Transference

A characteristic of healthy adjustment is the ability to regulate the self. Self-regulation can involve efforts to control or manage aspects of the self—including self-views and emotional experiences, in order to achieve particular outcomes (Carver, 2004; Gollwitzer, 1996; Higgins, 1998; Doerr & Baumeister, Chapter 5, this volume), such as maintaining positive views of the self and others. We have evidence that not only self-protective but also other-protective regulatory responses occur in transference.

### *Self-Regulation That Is Self-Protective*

As noted previously, both positive and negative transferences result in shifts in the working self-concept in the direction of the self-when-with-the-significant-other, such that aspects of the self that overlap with the self in the context of the relationship are consistent with the tone of the significant-other representation. However, this same study found that in a negative transference (i.e., when a negative significant-other representation was triggered), individuals rated nonoverlapping aspects of the working self-concept (i.e., characteristics they listed as being true of themselves in the present moment but that were not consistent with the self-when-with-the-significant-other) more positively than in other conditions. That is, they demonstrated compensatory self-inflation or self-enhancement (see Greenberg & Pyszczynski, 1985) in the face of a negative transference—thus regulating their overall working view of the self.

### *Other-Protective Self-Regulation*

Individuals also appear to regulate their views of significant others in transference. When presented with positive and negative features of a new person resembling a positively toned significant other, participants display the most positive facial affect when reading negative features that describe the new person. This does not occur, however, when the representation triggered is of a negative significant other, nor does it occur in the nontransference (control) condition (Andersen et al., 1996). Such affective shifts may be a method of protecting the overall view of someone who is liked or loved.

### *Potentially Maladaptive Other-Protective Processes and History of Abuse*

In some instances, other-protective self-regulation may be maladaptive. Indeed, there may be instances in which disruptions in relationships with significant others may result in maladaptive self-regulation patterns, as might be the case when a person experiences psychological, physical, or sexual abuse. This idea was examined in a study of female college students with and without a history of physical and psychological abuse by a parent who was regarded positively (Berenson & Andersen, 2006). Participants were assigned to learn about a new person who resembled this parent or to a yoked control condition in which the person resembled another participant's abusive or nonabusive parent. In addition, individuals were told that the person about whom they were learning was becoming increasingly tense and irritable while waiting in the next room. Participants in the transference condition involving an abusive but positively regarded parent displayed more positive facial affect when reading descriptions about the new person and after learning that the person was becoming tense and irritable than did the corresponding control condition. (In fact, more positive facial affect was displayed in the transference condition than in the control condition, regardless of abuse history.) At the same time, individuals with an abuse history who were in the transference condition also reported greater mistrust, rejection expectancies, and emotional indifference toward the new person than did nonabused individuals in the transference condition. These differences were not evident in the control condition. Thus, despite subjective experience consistent with the experience of threat in transference, individuals with a history of abuse seemed to use self-regulation strategies that serve to protect a relationship with a positively regarded parent, even though the parent had been abusive. Such other-protective self-regulation may be maladaptive in cases in which it leads individuals to be protective of later abusive relationships, thus increasing vulnerability to revictimization (see Classen, Field, Koopman, Nevill-Manning, & Spiegel, 2001).

Indeed, it is adaptive for people to "want" to control their affect as well—to self-regulate. That is, as these data suggest, transference should be relevant to how individuals learn to regulate emotions in their lives. Some evidence also suggests that emotion regulation patterns may be learned in primary relationships with caretakers such that these patterns are evoked indirectly later under the right conditions in transference (Carter & Andersen, 2009). For example, such socialization may punish the expression of particular emotions such as sadness with the result that when sadness cues are encountered in the context of transference, down-regulation of such emotions occurs. One source of people's regulatory competencies, then, for good or for ill, are the relationships with important others they have had and the resources or constraints learned in those relationships.

We turn now to problematic emotions that may be experienced in transference. We know that negative significant others evoke discomfort when their representations are activated. However, there may also be conditions in which positive significant others evoke plenty of discomfort on their own, and this discomfort may deflect or replace any positive affect that might otherwise have been elicited by a positive significant-other representation. What are these conditions?

## How Can a Positive Transference Be Disturbing?

So far we have primarily discussed ways in which transference involving a positive significant other may result in positive affect. However, in some situations, positive transference might disrupt a positive mood.

### *Unsatisfied Goals and Hostility*

One instance in which positive transference can disrupt a positive mood is when it involves a representation of a significant other with whom the individual has a chronically unsatisfied goal for love and acceptance (Berk & Andersen, 2008). Individuals who expect to encounter someone resembling a positively regarded significant other with whom they have such a chronically unsatisfied goal report higher degrees of hostility than do those who expect to encounter someone resembling another person's comparable significant other. Additionally, this increased hostility appears to be associated with overt behaviors designed to gain acceptance from the new person, suggesting that approval-seeking behavior may be triggered by the negative affect.

### *Role Violation and Dysphoria*

Another instance in which a positive transference can lead to mood disruptions is when the transference involves a new person who violates the interpersonal role associated with the significant other (Baum & Andersen, 1999). We assume that representations of significant-other relationships include the interpersonal role the other occupies, and hence, the other's interpersonal role is indirectly activated when the significant-other representation is activated, along with role-based expectations. For instance, an individual who meets a new person who reminds her of a highly regarded authority figure (e.g., her mentor) should expect the new person to act with authority. As a result, if this new person were to violate the role expectation by having no formal expertise or otherwise being clueless, it would be a role violation and should lead to discomfort. Consistent with this, individuals expecting to encounter a new person who resembles a positive authority figure (a significant other) report a decline in positive affect if the new person is in a contradictory role (a novice vs. an authority). Hence, the significant other's role was indirectly activated when the significant-other representation was triggered, and this role violation evoked discomfort.

### *Self-Discrepancies and Depression or Hostility*

Transference also should evoke a significant other's standards, which may, in some instances, include the sense that one is meeting these standards—resulting in positive affective consequences—or, in other cases, falling short of these standards (Reznik & Andersen, 2007)—leading to negative affective consequences. According to self-discrepancy theory (Higgins, 1987), individuals hold in memory particular standards from their own point of view or from another person's point of view. "Ideals" are standards, for example, that a significant other hopes or wishes one to meet, whereas "oughts" are standards that involve a sense of duty and obligation. Discrepancies between these standards and a person's actual self are associated with particular emotional vulnerabilities. Specifically, self-discrepancies involving one's ideal standards for the self are associated with changes in depression-related affect, whereas discrepancies involving "ought" standards are associated with changes in agitation-related affect (see Higgins, 1996b)—although these relationships are not always observed (e.g., Tangney, Niedenthal, Covert, & Barlow, 1998), which has prompted examination of the conditions under which these effects do and do not occur (see Boldero, Moretti, Bell, & Francis, 2005).

Given the relationship linking views of the self with views of significant others in memory, it stands to reason that particular views of the self can be activated when a significant-other representation is cued by features in a new person, because the activation spreads to the self experienced with the significant other. This self-with-significant-other should include self-discrepancies, and activation of the self-discrepancy should result in corresponding changes in affect. The evidence shows that an ideal–actual self-discrepancy or an ought–actual self-discrepancy will be activated indirectly when a significant-other representation is triggered, provoking different mood states as a function of individual differences in such discrepancy (i.e., whether an individual has an ideal–actual vs. an ought–actual discrepancy) and whether this self-discrepancy is triggered in transference (Reznik & Andersen, 2007). College students with an ideal discrepancy (i.e., individuals who scored high on a measure of ideal discrepancy and low on a measure of ought discrepancy) or an ought discrepancy (i.e., individuals who scored high on a measure of ought discrepancy and low on a measure of ideal discrepancy) were randomly assigned to a transference condition involving a positive significant-other representation, from whose perspective they perceived this discrepancy, or to a yoked control condition. Among ideal-discrepant individuals, a positive transference resulted in more self-reported dysphoric mood than did the control condition. Among ought-discrepant participants, however, positive transference resulted in higher self-reported resentful and hostile mood (i.e., an agitation-related affect) and less relaxation relative to the control condition. The latter was not observed among ideal-discrepant individuals.

### *The Attachment System and Anxiety and Hostility*

Attachment models have focused on how internal working models of the self and others develop through relationships with early caregivers (Ainsworth, Blehar, Walters, & Wall, 1978; Bowlby, 1969). There is evidence that early attachment styles can come to influence later relationships (e.g., Simpson & Rholes, 1998). Whereas earlier research on attachment theory focused on attachment styles as stable characteristics—as examined in work with infants (Ainsworth et al., 1978; Barnett & Vondra, 1999) and adults (Bartholomew & Horowitz, 1991; Hazan & Shaver, 1987)—recent research also suggests that people have different attachment styles with different people and that attachment can be activated by cues in the environment (Baldwin, Keelan, Fehr, Enns, & Koh-Rangarajoo, 1996; Mikulincer, Gillath, & Shaver, 2002; Pierce & Lydon, 2001). That is, such research has examined the attachment system as contextual. We assume that mental representations of self and others include attachment styles, and that attachment styles can be triggered in the social cognitive process of transference.

Recent research has examined the notion that the attachment system may be evoked when a significant-other representation is activated and that the particular response will depend on the particular attachment style with that significant other (Andersen, Bartz, Berenson, & Keczkemethy, 2006). Triggering a parental representation designating a parent with whom the participant has a particular attachment style indirectly activated an emotional state indicative of the attachment style. Specifically, when expecting to encounter someone resembling a parent with whom the individual had a secure versus an insecure attachment, participants experienced more positive mood than did participants in a corresponding yoked control condition. The difference occurred only for those securely attached in the relationship and not for those who had an avoidant, anxious-ambivalent, or fearful attachment in the relationship. Moreover, activation of a parental representation in transference involving a preoccupied attachment relationship resulted in increased anxious mood in transference compared to a control condition. No such difference in anxiety of this kind occurred among securely attached, avoidantly attached, or fearfully attached persons. Finally, when transference involved a dismissive (or dismissive-avoidant) attachment relationship, it resulted in the down-regulation of hostility relative to a control condition, presumably because eschewing emotional vulnerability in attachment relationships is crucial for these individuals. No such pattern was observed among people with other attachment styles. This finding is consistent with the characteristic suppressed emotional reactivity that is thought to define avoidant attachment.

In short, differences in one's attachment styles with different significant others will predict the affective states one experiences when the mental representations of these significant others are triggered.

### *Rejection Expectancies in Depressed Individuals*

Transference processes should also be important to the emotional experience of individuals suffering from depression. Interpersonal models of depression suggest that depression is associated with disruptions in interpersonal relationships (Coyne, 1976; Joiner, Coyne, & Blalock, 1999) and that individuals who are depressed have maladaptive ways of seeking support and reassurance from others that might even maintain or exacerbate their symptoms (Davila, 2001; Joiner, Metalsky, Gencoz, & Gencoz, 2001). We hypothesized that due to past problems in relationships, including rejection, depressed individuals would be especially vulnerable to experiencing rejection in the context of transference, particularly if the significant other whose representation is triggered is one from whom they have experienced rejection.

In this research, we asked moderately depressed and nondepressed college students to describe positive and negative significant others from whom they had experienced rejection (Miranda et al., 2009; see also Andersen & Miranda, 2005). We defined rejection as not having received the desired level of acceptance from the person. We also asked these individuals to describe how they viewed themselves when with each significant other. They were then randomly assigned to a positive transference condition, a negative transference condition, or a yoked control condition.

The moderately depressed individuals experienced greater mood disruptions and greater shifts in their working self-concept in the context of the positive transference than did participants in the control condition, whereas nondepressed individuals did not show such mood disruption. The effect only occurred when a positive significant other who was rejecting was triggered and did not extend to the condition in which a person's own negative significant other who was also rejecting was activated. That is, these depressed individuals experienced increases in their degree of depressed mood in this condition (relative to baseline), and other participants did not. In addition, in this condition participants freely described themselves in the experiment using features that independent judges rated as indicating more of a sense of rejection, adjusting for their self-concept ratings at pretest. These findings did not occur among nondepressed individuals. Thus, depressed individuals appear to be particularly sensitive to cues suggesting interpersonal rejection when they involve a significant other who is liked or loved versus when they involve someone else's significant other.

## SUMMARY OF RESEARCH

Our program of research suggests that a new person triggering a significant-other representation results in biases in inferences and memory, elicitation of positive and negative evaluations of the new person, an emotional tone associated with the representation, and expectancies for acceptance versus rejection by the new person who resembles a positive versus a negative significant other. An individual is also more motivated to approach (vs. avoid) a new person depending on the representation that is triggered, and individuals will tend to elicit representation-consistent behavior from a new person who resembles an important other. Furthermore, individuals' working views of the self shift in the direction of the self-when-with-the-significant-other. Finally, self-regulatory responses—both adaptive and maladaptive—can be triggered in transference, and positive transference can disrupt mood when the significant-other representations triggered involve unsatisfied goals, role violations, self-discrepancies, insecure attachments, and rejection expectancies (in depression).

## CLINICAL IMPLICATIONS

Transference is a phenomenon that occurs in everyday life and not merely in the context of a psychoanalytic session. The program of research we have presented constitutes the first experimental evidence that transference occurs using a method that allows clear causal conclusions about the importance of cognitions and emotions regarding past significant others in people's reactions to new persons and new relationships. Our research with nonclinical populations should apply also to people who meet formal diagnostic criteria for mental disorders, particularly in light of the growing research on the continuity between normal problems in living and mental disorders (see Maddux, Chapter 22, this volume). Although our studies have been restricted perhaps—by not focusing exclusively on people in psychotherapy or on those diagnosed with a particular disorder—the evidence has clear clinical implications (see Andersen & Berk, 1998; Miranda & Andersen, 2007). Although there are likely to be cultural differences, gender differences, and individual differences in *how* transference is experienced and expressed, there is unlikely to be much variability in *whether* it occurs. Furthermore, transference is a process that is likely to be a part of the therapeutic process, regardless of a clinician's theoretical orientation. The implications we offer below for psychopathology and psychotherapy are compatible with a variety of theoretical orientations, including cognitive-behavioral, interpersonal, and psychodynamic orientations.

As noted previously, in some situations transference may become pathological. It can lead individuals to respond to a new interpersonal situation in a manner that is not optimal for that current encounter and hence may disrupt a positive mood, exacerbate a negative emotional state, or lead to other kinds of problematic changes, such as in a person's working view of the self or in self-regulatory (e.g., in affect regulation) responses that may be problematic for the present encounter. Applying the significant-other representation to a new person and relationship can result in negative interpersonal outcomes. Moreover, because these negative outcomes can happen habitually and without awareness, they may be hard to correct. For this reason, it may be valuable for a clinician to help a client identify the relevant cues that provoke the maladaptive response pattern.

A transference that is dysfunctional or inflexible might be the focus of discussion in psychotherapy. Also, in some conditions the individual may have difficulty separating real from imagined aspects of a new person and, likewise, more common and central aspects of the self from those made temporarily accessible (and seemingly highly relevant) in the new encounter. For instance, when encountering a new individual who resembles a significant other with whom one has typically experienced a negative view of the self, the individual is apt to experience changes in the self-concept that are consistent with the representation, and the individual may even elicit behaviors from a new person consistent with that self-view. In the case of depression, for example, this may take the form of eliciting from others negative feedback that may not otherwise have occurred or expecting rejection from new people as a result of the activation of a working self-concept involving a sense of rejection. Complementary research suggests that depressed people have difficulty accepting positive feedback from others, as cognitive-interpersonal models suggest (Joiner, Alfano, & Metalsky, 1993). There is further evidence suggesting that depressed individuals respond to negative feedback from relationship partners by seeking even more negative feedback (Casbon, Burns, Bradbury, & Joiner, 2005), which can perhaps exacerbate symptoms. We show relevant variability as a function of the transference process. As another example, in the case of individuals with an early history of abuse, activating the representation of the abusive other in a new encounter or relationship might involve the same kind of protection of the abusive other as is present in most significant relationships, leading to a failure to take seriously cues in the relationship that may indicate a potential for revictimization. In addition, individuals with preoccupied attachment styles may respond anxiously in new interpersonal encounters when a significant-other representation is triggered—even if the representation is of a positive significant other—leading them to be on guard in their relationships and to have difficulty experiencing a sense of closeness, security, and safety. Those with a dismissive attachment with the significant other may become inexpressive with a new person in transference.

Transference also has implications both for the therapeutic relationship and for techniques likely to be therapeutic for the individual beyond the relationship with the therapist (see Miranda & Andersen, 2007). An individual's comfort in disclosing personal information to a therapist may depend, in part, on the person's early response to the therapeutic interaction and on the mental representations that are triggered in the course of therapy. Just as the triggering of a positive significant-other representation may result in greater trust of the therapist and the expectation that the therapist will be accepting of the client, activating a negative significant-other representation may lead an individual to avoid sharing personal information with the therapist, perhaps due to the expectation that the clinician will respond with rejection or disapproval. Such immediate, often implicit, responses to the therapist may be evident in the client's nonverbal behaviors, such as automatically elicited facial expressions of positive or negative affect, posture, eye contact, and in shifts in the nature of the material revealed in the session. For this reason, clinicians should be attentive to such responses and view them not as an indication of pathology but as an indication of the meaning systems from the client's own life that may have been triggered by the therapist. Initial openness or guardedness in treatment and changes in these responses over the course of treatment may reveal (1) therapeutically relevant material that has been triggered from memory (concerning a specific significant-other representation and relationship) and (2) the kinds of interpersonal cues coming from the therapist that may have activated those representations.

Clients' descriptions of their everyday relationships and encounters and their response to the therapist may be useful in identifying and modifying maladaptive patterns of interaction. Interpersonal psychotherapy (IPT) used in the treatment of depression, for example, conceptualizes depression as occurring in the context of relationships, and thus the techniques are directed toward modifying interpersonal patterns that are assumed to underlie the individual's symptoms (Weissman, Markowitz, & Klerman, 2000). Focusing primarily on present (rather than past) relationships, the early phase of this treatment asks clients to identify important people in their lives, along with positive and negative characteristics of each significant other (in a manner not unlike the methodology we use in our laboratory-based experiments). This information is then used to construct an interpersonal formulation of the person's symptoms. For instance, among the interpersonal problem areas addressed within the IPT framework, a person's depression might be conceptualized in the context of a *role dispute* or relationship conflict, and treatment would assist the individual in examining the relationship and considering ways to change the relationship in order to resolve the dispute (Weissman et al., 2000). A role dispute that might arise as a result of transference could be addressed by making the client aware of characteristics of the relationship partner that may resemble a significant-other representation and the circumstances under which significant-other resemblance may lead to maladaptive interpretations. This kind of procedure may prove a valuable tool for clinicians making use of any number of different theoretical orientations. Similarly, certain cognitive-behavioral treatments for trauma include the identification and modification of maladaptive relationship schemas (see Cloitre, Cohen, & Koenen, 2006), as do some other cognitive approaches (Safran & Segal, 1990; Young, Klosko, & Weishaar, 2003). (See also Benjamin, Chapter 19, this volume.)

In addressing transference in such treatments, a clinician might identify instances in which the individual responds to a new person with the same pattern of expectancies, motivations, emotions, and behaviors that he or she typically experiences with a particular significant other. This information can enable both the clinician and the individual in therapy to become more aware of the precise cues in a new person's tone of voice, facial expression, actions, or statements that may set in motion this transference response. Becoming increasingly aware of the cues that provoke a maladaptive response can help the person to become more aware, at the time of encountering such cues, that the old, familiar pattern is about to occur. Even if during the early stages of therapy, the response still plays out in full, it can enable the individual to become more cognizant the next time such cues are encountered that a more adaptive response is possible. The old familiar refrains might always have a special resonance for the individual, but he or she can learn how to better regulate just exactly how and when prior experience is applied to contemporary interpersonal relations. The fact that the self and personality and behavior vary by situational cues (e.g., Mischel & Shoda, 1995; Kross, Mischel, & Shoda, Chapter 20, this volume)—in the case of transference, interpersonal cues (Andersen & Chen, 2002; Andersen & Saribay, 2005; Andersen, Saribay, & Kooij, 2008)—suggests that therapeutic attention to such cues and to what one might do instead upon encountering such cues could be helpful.

It may also be useful to identify a relationship that is particularly problematic for the individual or a representation that is applied too ubiquitously, creating problems in a number of relationships. Treatment may also include identifying thoughts about the self and others that arise automatically in relation to new people when a problematic significant-other representation is activated and applied in a new interpersonal context. Assisting the client in becoming aware of these thoughts and addressing them as they arise, perhaps in the manner of a number of recent mindfulness-based therapies (Segal, Williams, & Teasdale, 2002; Teasdale et al., 2000) or in a formal restructuring of these thoughts, may also be helpful by enabling awareness of the phenomenon in principle and cue recognition in particular. For instance, an individual who experiences the expectation that he or she will be rejected by a new person whom he or she has recently met, if made aware of the connection of such an expectation to a particular significant-other representation, may be instructed to be aware that this thought arises in response to this representation and, as a result, choose the appropriate reaction to such a thought (see Segal et al., 2002). Such awareness could lead to cognitive, emotional, and behavioral changes.

## CONCLUSION

Transference is a normal, social cognitive process that occurs commonly in everyday life. It is largely implicit in that it occurs without people having much awareness of it. The process by which transference occurs involves the activation of a significant-other representation, often cues in a new person or in other aspects of the situation. These representations designate those individuals—from one's past or present—with whom the individual has a degree of interdependence and whom he or she feels is important to him or her in some way—whether the individual is someone liked or loved versus disliked and not loved. When a new person triggers these representations, it results in the activation of a set of associated inferences and shifts in memory, feelings, expectancies, motivations, goals, self-regulatory attempts, and behaviors that are applied to that new person. In the process, one comes to experience the version of the self typically experienced and expressed with the significant other, even though the significant other is not there. Although future research is necessary to determine whether the effects generalize beyond the laboratory, the body of work described in this chapter represents the first experimental demonstration that the longstanding clinical concept of transference does, in fact, occur as a basic process in everyday interpersonal encounters. Because the kinds of emotional and motivational shifts that arise in transference are linked sometimes to human suffering, this research offers a number of potential clinical uses.

## ACKNOWLEDGMENT

This research was funded in part by a grant from the National Institute of Mental Health (No. R01-MH48789).

## REFERENCES

Adler, A. (1957). *Understanding human nature.* New York: Fawcett. (Original work published 1927)

Ainsworth, M. D. S., Blehar, M. C., Walters, E., & Wall, S. (1978). *Patterns of attachment: A psychological study of the strange situation.* Hillsdale, NJ: Erlbaum.

Andersen, S. M., Bartz, J., Berenson, K., & Keczkemethy, C. (2006). *Triggering the attachment system in transference: Evoking specific emotions through implicit activation of a parental representation.* Unpublished manuscript, New York University.

Andersen, S. M., & Baum, A. (1994). Transference in interpersonal relations: Inferences and affect based on significant-other representations. *Journal of Personality, 62,* 459–498.

Andersen, S. M., & Berk, M. S. (1998). Transference in everyday experience: Implications of experimental research for relevant clinical phenomena. *Review of General Psychology,* 2, 81–120.

Andersen, S. M., & Chen, S. (2002). The relational self: An interpersonal social-cognitive theory. *Psychological Review, 109,* 619–645.

Andersen, S. M., & Cole, S. W. (1990). "Do I know you?": The role of significant others in general social perception. *Journal of Personality and Social Psychology, 59,* 383–399.

Andersen, S. M., Glassman, N. S., Chen, S., & Cole, S. W. (1995). Transference in social perception: The role of chronic accessibility in significant-other representations. *Journal of Personality and Social Psychology, 69,* 41–57.

Andersen, S. M., & Miranda, R. (2006). Through the lens of the relational self: Triggering emotional suffering in the social-cognitive process of transference. In R. Kreuger & J. Tackett (Eds.), *Personality and psychopathology* (pp. 292–334). New York: Guilford Press.

Andersen, S. M., Moskowitz, D. B., Blair, I. V., & Nosek, B. A. (2007). Automatic thought. In E. T. Higgins & A. W. Kruglanski (Eds.), *Social psychology: Handbook of basic principles* (2nd ed., pp. 138–175). New York: Guilford Press.

Andersen, S. M., Reznik, I., & Chen, S. (1997). The self in relation to others: Motivational and cognitive underpinnings. In J. G. Snodgrass & R. L. Thompson (Eds.), *The self across psychology: Self-recognition, self-awareness, and the self-concept.* New York: New York Academy of Science.

Andersen, S. M., Reznik, I., & Glassman, N. S. (2005). The unconscious relational self. In R. Hassin, J. S. Uleman, & J. A. Bargh (Eds.), *The new unconscious*. New York: Oxford University Press.

Andersen, S. M., Reznik, I., & Manzella, L. M. (1996). Eliciting facial affect, motivation, and expectancies in transference: Significant-other representations in social relations. *Journal of Personality and Social Psychology*, *71*, 1108–1129.

Andersen, S. M., & Saribay, S. A. (2005). The relational self and transference: Evoking motives, self-regulation, and emotions through activation of mental representations of significant others. In M. W. Baldwin (Ed.), *Interpersonal cognition* (pp. 1–32). New York: Guilford Press.

Andersen, S. M., Saribay, S. A., & Kooij, C. S. (2008). Contextual variability in personality: The case of the relational self and the process of transference. In F. Rhodewalt (Ed.), *Personality and social behavior* (pp. 79–116). New York: Psychology Press.

Bakan, D. (1966). *The duality of human existence*. Chicago: Rand McNally.

Baldwin, M. W. (1992). Relational schemas and the processing of information. *Psychological Bulletin*, *112*, 461–484.

Baldwin, M. W., Keelan, J. P. R., Fehr, B., Enns, V., & Koh-Rangarajoo, E. (1996). Social-cognitive conceptualization of attachment working models: Availability and accessibility effects. *Journal of Personality and Social Psychology*, *71*, 94–109.

Baldwin, M. W., & Sinclair, L. (1996). Self-esteem and "if ... then" contingencies of interpersonal acceptance. *Journal of Personality and Social Psychology*, *71*, 1130–1141.

Bargh, J. A. (1990). Auto-motives: Preconscious determinants of social interaction. In E. T. Higgins & R. M. Sorrentino (Eds.), *Handbook of motivation and cognition: Foundations of social behavior* (Vol. 2, pp. 93–130). New York: Guilford Press.

Bargh, J. A. (1997). The automaticity of everyday life. In R. S. Wyer, Jr. (Ed.), *Advances in social cognition* (Vol. 10, pp. 1–61). Mahwah, NJ: Erlbaum.

Bargh, J. A., Chaiken, S., Raymond, P., & Hymes, C. (1996). The automatic evaluation effect: Unconditionally automatic attitude activation with a pronunciation task. *Journal of Experimental Social Psychology*, *32*, 185–210.

Barnett, D., & Vondra, J. I. (1999). Atypical patterns of early attachment: Theory, research, and current directions. In J. I. Vondra & D. Barnett (Eds.), Atypical attachment among children (pp. 1–24). *Monographs of the Society for Research in Child Development*, *64*(3, Serial No. 209).

Bartholomew, K., & Horowitz, L. M. (1991). Attachment styles among young adults: A test of a four-category model. *Journal of Personality and Social Psychology*, *61*, 226–244.

Batson, C. D. (1990). How social an animal? The human capacity for caring. *American Psychologist*, *45*, 336–346.

Baum, A., & Andersen, S. M. (1999). Interpersonal roles in transference: Transient mood states under the condition of significant-other activation. *Social Cognition*, *17*, 161–185.

Baumeister, R. F., & Leary, M. R. (1995). The need to belong: Desire for interpersonal attachments as a fundamental human motivation. *Psychological Bulletin*, *117*, 497–529.

Berenson, K., & Andersen, S. M. (2006). Childhood physical and emotional abuse by a parent: Transference effects in adult interpersonal relations. *Personality and Social Psychology Bulletin*, *32*, 1509–1522.

Berk, M. S., & Andersen, S. M. (2000). The impact of past relationships on interpersonal behavior: Behavioral confirmation in the social-cognitive process of transference. *Journal of Personality and Social Psychology*, *79*, 546–562.

Berk, M., & Andersen, S. (2008). The sting of lack of affection: Chronic goal dissatisfaction in transference. *Self and Identity*, *7*, 393–412.

Boldero, J., Moretti, M. M., Bell, R. C., & Francis, J. J. (2005). Self-discrepancies and negative affect: A primer on when to look for specificity, and how to find it. *Australian Journal of Psychology*, *57*, 139–147.

Bowlby, J. (1969). *Attachment and loss: Vol. 1. Attachment*. New York: Basic Books.

Bowlby, J. (1973). *Attachment and loss: Vol. 2. Separation: Anxiety and anger.* New York: Basic Books.

Bowlby, J. (1980). *Attachment and loss: Vol. 3. Loss: Sadness and depression.* New York: Basic Books.

Bruner, J. S. (1957). Going beyond the information given. In H. E. Gruber, K. R. Hammond, & R. Jessor (Eds.), *Contemporary approaches to cognition* (pp. 41–69). Cambridge, MA: Harvard University Press.

Carter, C., & Andersen, S. M. (2009). *Parental socialization and emotion regulation: Activating a parental representation evokes parallel affect-regulatory processes.* Manuscript in preparation.

Carver, C. S. (2004). Self-regulation of action and affect. In R. F. Baumeister & K. D. Vohs (Eds.), *Handbook of self-regulation: Research, theory, and applications* (pp. 13–39). New York: Guilford Press.

Casbon, T. S., Burns, A. B., Bradbury, T. N., & Joiner, T. E. (2005). Receipt of negative feedback is related to increased negative feedback seeking among individuals with depressive symptoms. *Behaviour Research and Therapy, 43,* 485–504.

Chartrand, T. L., & Bargh, J. A. (1996). Automatic activation of impression formation and memorization goals: Nonconscious goal priming reproduces effects of explicit task instructions. *Journal of Personality and Social Psychology, 71,* 464–478.

Chartrand, T. L., van Baaren, R. B., & Bargh, J. A. (2006). Linking automatic evaluation to mood and information processing style: Consequences for experienced affect, impression formation, and stereotyping. *Journal of Experimental Psychology: General, 135,* 70–77.

Chen, M., & Bargh, J. A. (1999). Consequences of automatic evaluation: Immediate predispositions to approach or avoid the stimulus. *Personality and Social Psychology Bulletin, 25,* 215–224.

Chen, S., & Andersen, S. M. (1999). Relationships from the past in the present: Significant-other representations and transference in interpersonal life. In M. P. Zanna (Ed.), *Advances in experimental social psychology* (Vol. 31, pp. 123–190). San Diego, CA: Academic Press.

Chen, S., Andersen, S. M., & Hinkley, K. (1999). Triggering transference: Examining the role of applicability and use of significant-other representations in social perception. *Social Cognition, 17,* 332–365.

Chen, S., Fitzsimons, G. M., & Andersen, S. M. (2007). Automaticity in close relationships. In J. A. Bargh (Ed.), *Social psychology and the unconscious: The automaticity of higher mental processes* (pp. 133–172). New York: Psychology Press.

Classen, C., Field, N. P., Koopman, C., Nevill-Manning, K., & Spiegel, D. (2001). Interpersonal problems and their relationship to sexual revictimization among women sexually abused in childhood. *Journal of Interpersonal Violence, 16,* 495–509.

Cloitre, M., Cohen, L. R., & Koenen, K. C. (2006). *Treating survivors of childhood abuse: Psychotherapy for the interrupted life.* New York: Guilford Press.

Coyne, J. C. (1976). Toward an interactional description of depression. *Psychiatry, 39,* 28–40.

Davila, J. (2001). Refining the association between excessive reassurance seeking and depressive symptoms: The role of related interpersonal constructs. *Journal of Social and Clinical Psychology, 20,* 538–559.

Deci, E. L. (1995). *Why we do what we do.* New York: Putnam.

Duckworth, K. L., Bargh, J. A., Garcia, M., & Chaiken, S. (2002). The automatic evaluation of novel stimuli. *Psychological Science, 13,* 513–519.

Fairbairn, W. R. D. (1952). *Psychoanalytic studies of personality.* London: Tavistock.

Fiske, S. T., & Pavelchak, M. (1986). Category-based versus piecemeal-based affective responses: Developments in schema-triggered affect. In R. M. Sorrentino & E. T. Higgins (Eds.), *Handbook of motivation and cognition* (pp. 167–203). New York: Guilford Press.

Fitzsimons, G. M., & Bargh, J. A. (2003). Thinking of you: Nonconscious pursuit of interpersonal goals associated with relationship partners. *Journal of Personality and Social Psychology, 84,* 148–164.

Freud, S. (1958). The dynamics of transference. In J. Strachey (Ed. & Trans.), *The standard edition of the complete psychological works of Sigmund Freud* (Vol. 12, pp. 97–108). London: Hogarth. (Original work published 1912)

Glassman, N. S., & Andersen, S. M. (1999a). Activating transference without consciousness: Using significant-other representations to go beyond what is subliminally given. *Journal of Personality and Social Psychology*, *77*, 1146–1162.

Glassman, N. S., & Andersen, S. M. (1999b). Transference in social cognition: Persistence and exacerbation of significant-other based inferences over time. *Cognitive Therapy and Research*, *23*, 75–91.

Gollwitzer, P. M. (1996). The volitional benefits of planning. In P. M. Gollwitzer & J. A. Bargh (Eds.), *The psychology of action: Linking cognition and motivation to behavior* (pp. 287–312). New York: Guilford Press.

Greenberg, J. R., & Mitchell, S. A. (1983). *Object relations in psychoanalytic theory.* Cambridge, MA: Harvard University Press.

Greenberg, J., & Pyszczynski, T. (1985). Compensatory self-inflation: A response to the threat to self-regard of public failure. *Journal of Personality and Social Psychology*, *49*, 273–280.

Guisinger, S., & Blatt, S. J. (1994). Individuality and relatedness: Evolution of a fundamental dialectic. *American Psychologist*, *49*, 104–111.

Hazan, C., & Shaver, P. R. (1987). Romantic love conceptualized as an attachment process. *Journal of Personality and Social Psychology*, *52*, 511–524.

Higgins, E. T. (1987). Self discrepancy: A theory relating self and affect. *Psychological Review*, *94*, 319–340.

Higgins, E. T. (1996a). Knowledge: Accessibility, applicability, and salience. In E. T. Higgins & A. W. Kruglanski (Eds.), *Social psychology: Handbook of basic principles* (pp. 133–168). New York: Guilford Press.

Higgins, E. T. (1996b). Ideals, oughts, and regulatory focus: Affect and motivation from distinct pains and pleasures. In P. M. Gollwitzer & J. A. Bargh (Eds.), *The psychology of action* (pp. 91–114). New York: Guilford Press.

Higgins, E. T. (1998). Promotion and prevention: Regulatory focus as a motivational principle. In M. P. Zanna (Ed.), *Advances in experimental social psychology* (Vol. 30, pp. 1–46). New York: Academic Press.

Higgins, E. T., & King, G. (1981). Accessibility of social constructs: Information processing consequences of individual and contextual variability. In N. Cantor & J. F. Kihlstrom (Eds.), *Personality, cognition and social interaction* (pp. 69–121). Hillsdale, NJ: Erlbaum.

Hinkley, K., & Andersen, S. M. (1996). The working self-concept in transference: Significant-other activation and self change. *Journal of Personality and Social Psychology*, *71*, 1279–1295.

Horney, K. (1945). *Our inner conflicts.* New York: Norton.

Joiner, T. E., Jr. (1994). Contagious depression: Existence, specificity to depressed symptoms, and the role of reassurance seeking. *Journal of Personality and Social Psychology*, *67*, 287–296.

Joiner, T. E., Jr., Alfano, M. S., & Metalsky, G. I. (1993). Caught in the crossfire: Depression, self-consistency, self-enhancement, and the response of others. *Journal of Social and Clinical Psychology*, *12*, 113–134.

Joiner, T. E., Jr., Coyne, J. C., & Blalock, J. (1999). On the interpersonal nature of depression: Overview and synthesis. In T. E. Joiner & J. C. Coyne (Eds.), *The interactional nature of depression: Advances in interpersonal approaches* (pp. 3–19). Washington, DC: American Psychological Association.

Joiner, T. E., Jr., Metalsky, G. I., Gencoz, F., & Gencoz, T. (2001). The relative specificity of excessive reassurance-seeking to depressive symptoms and diagnoses among clinical samples of adults and youth. *Journal of Psychopathology and Behavioral Assessment*, *23*, 35–41.

Kernberg, O. (1976). *Object relations theory and clinical psychoanalysis.* New York: Aronson.

Mikulincer, M., Gillath, O., & Shaver, P. R. (2002). Activation of the attachment system in adulthood: Threat-related primes increase the accessibility of mental representations of attachment figures. *Journal of Personality and Social Psychology*, *83*, 881–895.

Miranda, R., & Andersen, S. M. (2007). The therapeutic relationship: Implications from social-cognition and transference. In P. Gilbert & R. L. Leahy (Eds.), *The therapeutic relationship in the cognitive-behavioral psychotherapies* (pp. 63–89). New York: Routledge.

Miranda, R., Andersen, S. M., & Edwards, T. (2009). *Exacerbated dysphoria among depressed individuals based on implicit activation of significant–other representations.* Manuscript submitted for publication.

Mischel, W., & Shoda, Y. (1995). A cognitive-affective system of personality structure. *Psychological Review, 102,* 246–268.

Ogilvie, D. M., & Ashmore, R. D. (1991). Self-with-other representation as a unit of analysis in self-concept research. In R. C. Curtis (Ed.), *The relational self: Theoretical convergencies in psychoanalysis and social psychology* (pp. 282–314). New York: Guilford Press.

Pierce, T., & Lydon, J. E. (2001). Global and specific relational models in the experience of social interactions. *Journal of Personality and Social Psychology, 80,* 613–631.

Reznik, I., & Andersen, S. M. (2004). *Becoming the dreaded self: Diminished self-worth with positive significant others in transference.* Unpublished manuscript, New York University, New York.

Reznik, I., & Andersen, S. M. (2007). Agitation and despair in relation to parents: Activating emotional suffering in transference. *European Journal of Personality, 21*(3), 281–301.

Rogers, C. (1951). *Client-centered therapy.* Boston: Houghton-Mifflin.

Safran, J. D. (1990). Toward a refinement of cognitive therapy in light of interpersonal theory: I. Theory. *Clinical Psychology Review, 10,* 87–105.

Safran, J. D., & Segal, Z. V. (1990). *Interpersonal process in cognitive therapy.* New York: Basic Books.

Segal, Z. V., Williams, J. M. G., & Teasdale, J. D. (2002). *Mindfulness-based cognitive therapy for depression: A new approach to preventing relapse.* New York: Guilford Press.

Simpson, J. A., & Rholes, W. S. (1998). *Attachment theory and close relationships.* New York: Guilford Press.

Snyder, M. (1992). Motivational foundations of behavioral confirmation. In M. P. Zanna (Ed.), *Advances in experimental social psychology* (Vol. 25, pp. 67–114). New York: Academy Press.

Snyder, M., Tanke, E. D., & Berscheid, E. (1977). Social perception and interpersonal behavior: On the self-fulfilling nature of social stereotypes. *Journal of Personality and Social Psychology, 35,* 656–666.

Sullivan, H. S. (1953). *The interpersonal theory of psychiatry.* New York: Norton.

Tangney, J. P., Niedenthal, P. M., Covert, M. V., & Barlow, D. H. (1998). Are shame and guilt related to distinct self-discrepancies? A test of Higgins's (1987) hypotheses. *Journal of Personality and Social Psychology, 75,* 256–268.

Teasdale, J. D., Segal, Z. V., Williams, J. M. G., Ridgeway, V. A., Soulsby, J. M., & Lau, M. A. (2000). Prevention of relapse/recurrence in major depression by mindfulness-based cognitive therapy. *Journal of Consulting and Clinical Psychology, 68,* 615–623.

Weissman, M. M., Markowitz, J. C., & Klerman, G. L. (2000). *Comprehensive guide to interpersonal psychotherapy.* New York: Basic Books.

Young, J. E., Klosko, J. W., & Weishaar, M. E. (2003). *Schema therapy: A practitioner's guide.* New York: Guilford Press.

# 27 Group Processes and Group Psychotherapy

## *Social Psychological Foundations of Change in Therapeutic Groups*

Donelson R. Forsyth

Social psychology and clinical psychology share an interest in change. Rather than assuming that people are static and that psychological systems are immutable, social psychologists track the shifts in social attitudes, actions, values, and beliefs that result from individuals' everyday interactions in their social worlds. Similarly, clinical psychologists examine changes in adjustment, well-being, and dysfunction that are evidenced as people develop psychologically and physically, confront new life circumstances, or react effectively or less adaptively to daily life events.

Social and clinical psychologists also recognize that such changes often result from group-level processes. Cooley, an early social psychologist, noted in 1909 that groups play a primary role in forming the "social nature and ideals of the individual" (p. 29). Subsequent studies of beliefs, values, actions, and attitudes returned again and again to the group as the agent of change, eventually leading Lewin to conclude that "it is usually easier to change individuals formed into a group than to change any one of them separately" (1951, p. 228). Clinical psychologists, too, recognized, if somewhat grudgingly, the influence of groups on members. Freud (1922, p. 1), for example, wrote that individuals cannot be understood if separated from the groups to which they belong: "Individual Psychology is concerned with the individual man and explores the paths by which he seeks to find satisfaction for his instincts; but only rarely and under certain exceptional conditions is Individual Psychology in a position to disregard the relations of this individual to others." Maslow (1937) opined that "every human adult living is a member of a particular cultural group and has the social norms characteristic of this group" (p. 487). Similarly Laing (1969, pp. 81–82) concluded that "we cannot give an undistorted account of 'a person' without giving an account of his relation with others. Even an account of one person cannot afford to forget that each person is always acting upon others and acted upon by others. The others are there also."

Social psychology and clinical psychology also seek ways to promote change in others. Both fields recognize that change often occurs spontaneously as a result of some life experience, but that in other cases change can be achieved through explicit, intentionally designed interventions. Social psychologists, for example, have long been interested in how people's attitudes are changed by other people. Some of the earliest work in the field concerned explicit attempts to change the beliefs of others, including interventions aimed at making bigoted people less prejudiced, increasing citizens' civic engagement in military efforts, or convincing consumers to purchase one brand over another. In like fashion, clinical psychologists' interest in change reflects a practical concern; far from passive spectators of change, clinical psychologists seek to develop and refine the methods that will promote adaptive, healthy, and desirable change in their clients.

This chapter examines the obvious implication of these three intersecting similarities: the use of groups to achieve therapeutic change. It begins with a brief survey of group-level interventions before asking, What social psychological processes are at work in these groups that provide them with their transformative power? The chapter then concludes by considering the effectiveness of group interventions and ways to further enhance the curative efficacy of groups.

## THE USES OF GROUPS TO PROMOTE CHANGE

Most general texts on psychotherapeutic treatments sequester group approaches near the end of the book, sandwiched between sections with titles such as "Alternative Approaches," "Sociocultural Perspectives," "Family Therapy," or "Couples Counseling." Group therapists are sometimes portrayed as innovators, rebels, or even radicals who are willing to take risks in their work. Yet, group therapists are in most respects similar to other mental health practitioners. Rarely do they endorse some unique, unusual, and unproven set of assumptions in their work, but instead they base their approach to change on such traditional psychotherapeutic perspectives as psychodynamic, cognitive-behavioral, and interpersonal/existential orientations (DeLucia-Waack & Kalodner, 2005).

### Psychodynamic Group Therapy

Psychoanalysis is, by tradition, conducted in the smallest of all groups: the dyad comprising client and therapist. This method can, however, guide therapeutic practices carried out with larger assemblages. Freud (1922) himself, in his *Group Psychology and the Analysis of Ego*, recognized that groups provide a buffer against psychological threat, and as a result, membership in a cohesive group may promote adjustment: "Where a powerful impetus has been given to group formation neuroses may diminish and at all events temporarily disappear" (p. 124). In *Civilization and Its Discontents* he suggests that although one who is suffering psychologically may be tempted to seek isolation, "there is, indeed, another and better path: that of becoming a member of the human community, and, with the help of a technique guided by science, going over to the attack against nature and subjecting her to the human will. Then one is working with all for the good of all" (1961, pp. 24–25).

Psychoanalytic group therapy is usually a leader-centered method, for the psychoanalyst actively and obviously organizes, directs, coordinates, supports, and motivates the members' efforts. Rather than encouraging group discussion, traditional group psychoanalysts focus the group's attention on specific members, with this attention shifting from person to person throughout the course of the session. This procedure allows members to act in the role of the client for a time, but also to take on the role of observer of others' attempts to gain insight into the causes of their life difficulties. Groups also stimulate the transference processes that occur, in any case, in therapy. As Freud's (1922) replacement hypothesis suggests, the group can become a surrogate family for members, and the emotions linking members are like the ties that bind siblings together, with the group therapist taking on the role of the primal authority figure. As transference unfolds, the group provides the therapist with the means of exploring the childhood roots of current adult anxieties.

Just as free association provides the therapist with the means of gaining insight into the hidden motivations and conflicts of the ego, so the exchanges among group members provide data for the therapist's exploration of the workings and contents of the conscious and unconscious mind (Langs, 1973). The conversation among the members may, at a superficial level, appear to focus on banalities and pleasantries, but the subliteral text of the conversation carries with it information about unstated and often unrecognized motives and fears. The verbal exchanges among members offer many opportunities to ask "What did you mean by that?" and "Why did you say that?" According to psychoanalytic theory, the answers to these questions reveal the way each person's unconscious motivations and preconceptions influence their perceptions, emotions, and actions (Haskell, 1999). Therapists working one on one with a client tend to rely on dreams and free associations to chart the unconscious mind, whereas group psychodynamic theorists consider the ordinary dialogue of interacting group members to be an alternate route to the unconscious (Weiss, 2006).

## Cognitive-Behavioral Therapy Groups

Therapists who question the value of Freudian theories and methods often base their interventions on principles of learning and cognition. Such approaches assume that problematic thoughts and behaviors are acquired through experience, so interventions are based on principles derived from learning theories and the expansion of these theories into cognitive realms. Behavioral and cognitive-behavioral therapies eschew a search into clients' pasts for the ultimate cause of their problems, and instead focus pragmatically on encouraging healthy, desirable cognitions and behaviors (e.g., expressing positive emotions) and discouraging undesirable, harmful cognitions and behaviors (e.g., drinking alcohol).

The earliest group psychotherapies used methods that were simplified versions of cognitive-behavioral interventions. Joseph Hersey Pratt's groundbreaking work with group approaches, for example, stressed teaching and learning rather than interpretation and analysis. He initially used the group format for its efficiency—"I originally brought the patients together as a group simply with the idea that it would save my time" (Pratt, 1922, p. 403)—but he was impressed by the group-level processes that increased patient compliance. Pratt gradually enlarged his focus from physical illness to psychological disorders and took to calling his sessions "Thought Control Classes" (Pratt, 1922). He used psychoeducational methods, including short lectures and demonstrations, to help clients recognize self-defeating, unhealthy ways of dealing with their illnesses and called on more successful group members to model the ways they were achieving their successes.

Modern behavioral and cognitive-behavioral group therapists focus, as Pratt did, on explicit, observable behaviors, such as social or relationship skills, and the cognitions that sustain these behaviors. Behavioral approaches include systematic desensitization training, behavior modification, and skills training. Cognitive-behavioral approaches, such as rational–emotive therapy, cognitive-behavioral modification, and cognitive therapy, focus on changing cognitive processes (Emmelkamp, 2004; Hollon & Beck, 2004). These therapies were initially developed as one-on-one therapies, but they have been used with great success in groups. McDermut, Miller, and Brown's (2001) meta-analysis of group approaches to the treatment of depression, for example, found that nearly all of the experimental studies that examined group methods included at least one treatment condition that made use of cognitive-behavioral therapy.

### Interpersonal (Existential) Therapy Groups

Psychodynamic and cognitive-behavioral methods consider and make use of group processes, but some group therapists focus more squarely on the group and relations among group members as the means for achieving change. This third cluster of group therapies is a very heterogeneous one, containing approaches that differ in many ways from one another but are usually based on principles derived from clinical and personality theories that stress the interpersonal and existential roots of adjustment and disorder (Elliott, Greenberg, & Lietaer, 2004). Humanistic, third-force theories such as Rogers's (1940) person-centered theory, Moreno's (1934) psychodrama, Gestalt methods (Perls, Hefferline, & Goodman, 1951), human potential movement methods such as growth and encounter groups (Lakin, 1972), and Yalom's (1995) interpersonal, or interactive, group psychotherapy assume that individuals are, at core, searching for ways to improve their current functioning and maximize their potentialities. Such approaches are often phenomenological and experiential and underscore the importance of a strong, positive, empathic therapeutic environment for facilitating personal and collective growth.

The humanistic therapist Carl Rogers (1970), for example, traced most dysfunction to a loss of self-worth due to the conditional nature of acceptance by others. Rogers treated people by providing them with unconditional positive regard in an accepting therapeutic group encounter. Rogers thought that groups help members experience their emotions more fully and learn to deal with other people in authentic, open ways (Page, Weiss, & Lietaer, 2002). Similarly Gestaltist Fritz Perls frequently conducted his therapeutic sessions in groups rather than with single individuals. In some cases, Gestalt group therapy is one-to-one Gestalt therapy conducted in a group setting, with members observing one another's "work" but not interacting with each other. More frequently, however, interaction takes place among group members, with the therapist actively orchestrating the events. Many group therapists make use of unstructured interpersonal activities to stimulate members' emotional understanding, but Gestalt therapists generally resist offering interpretations to their patients (Goulding & Goulding, 1979; Greve, 1993).

Psychodrama, developed by Jacob Moreno, also makes use of exercises to stimulate emotional experiences in group members. Moreno (1932) conducted therapeutic groups perhaps as early as 1910, and he used the term *group therapy* in print in 1932. Moreno believed that the interpersonal relations that developed in groups provide the therapist with unique insights into members' personalities and proclivities and that by taking on roles the members become more flexible in their behavioral orientations. He made his sessions more experientially powerful by developing psychodrama techniques. When role playing, for example, members take on the identity of someone else and act as he or she would in a simulated social situation. Moreno believed that psychodrama's emphasis on physical action was more involving than passive discussion and that the drama itself helped members overcome their reluctance to discuss critical issues (Kipper & Ritchie, 2003; Rawlinson, 2000).

Yalom's (1995) interpersonal group psychotherapy is perhaps the most influential of the interpersonal approaches to groups. Yalom views the group as a social microcosm where individuals gain a profound awareness of how they are coming across to others interpersonally and the disruptive impact of their mistaken assumptions about other people on their relationships (parataxic distortions). Because they respond to one another in ways that are characteristic of their interpersonal tendencies outside of the group, Yalom encourages members to focus on the here and now of their group experience, rather than on problems they may be facing at home or at work. When, for example, one member of a group displays self-contempt and is challenged by another member, or when one member responds actively only to questions asked by the leader rather than other group members, the group can review these tendencies and explore their adaptiveness. As the group grapples with personal conflicts, problems of organization, goal setting, and communication failures, the members reveal their preferred interaction styles to others and to themselves. They also learn to disclose their feelings honestly, gain conflict reduction skills, and find enjoyment from working in collaborative relationships.

Yalom (1995) believes that a number of curative factors underlie change in a variety of group settings: the installation of hope, universality, imparting of information, altruism, the corrective recapitulation of the primary family group, development of socializing techniques, imitative behavior, interpersonal learning, group cohesiveness, catharsis, and existential factors. Some of the factors on Yalom's list are mechanisms that facilitate change, whereas others describe the general group conditions that should be present within effective therapeutic groups. Yalom's list, as the section that follows suggests, is consistent with social psychological analyses of the influential processes that occur in groups.

## THE SOCIAL PSYCHOLOGICAL BASES OF CHANGE IN THERAPEUTIC GROUPS

What is the best restorative method to help people regain and maintain their mental well-being? A group-level approach offers an answer that is, in some ways, at variance with psychology's traditional emphasis on psychogenic solutions. Asked why an individual is depressed, addicted, or engaged in aberrant actions and how that individual can be helped, psychologists tend to focus their attention on intrapsychic, individualistic processes, such as personality traits, past events, and biological processes. In contrast, a group-level, sociogenic approach complements and enriches the psychogenic perspective. Such an analysis assumes that each person is nested in a hierarchy of increasingly complex and inclusive social aggregates, such as groups, organizations, and communities. The unique qualities of each individual cannot be ignored, but neither can the processes operating within the groups that enfold the individual members. Here we look again at the personal and interpersonal processes examined earlier in this book—self and identity, self-esteem, self-regulation, self-efficacy, self-awareness, social cognition, and interpersonal relations—and the role therapeutic groups play in shaping these socially and clinically significant processes.

## Personal Process in Groups

A group-level analysis of change does not ignore individual-level processes but instead seeks to integrate these processes into a multilevel analysis. This perspective recognizes the reciprocal nature of the individual-to-group connection: Individuals' thoughts, actions, and emotions are shaped by group-level processes, but each member also influences every other member as well as the group as a whole. Social psychologists realize that if one is to understand processes that unfold *between* people in groups, then one must also understand the processes that occur *within* the individuals who are members of the groups.

### *Self and Identity*

Sages throughout history have championed the adaptive value of self-knowledge, and contemporary clinical wisdom similarly urges those who are seeking to strengthen their resilience to stressful life events or enhance their psychological well-being to know themselves thoroughly. But even though people often believe that they can best learn who they are through self-reflection (Sedikides & Skowronski, 1995), a group-level analysis suggests that the self is as much a social creation as an intrapsychic one. To answer questions such as, "What is my personal worth?", "Do people like me?", and "Am I an introvert or an extravert?", one must rely on information provided through interaction with other people.

Psychotherapeutic groups, as groups, thus provide members with information that allows them to construct an answer to the question "Who am I?" In some cases, the group may provide explicit information about one's personal qualities, but it also provides indirect feedback by responding in certain ways. When a person is treated in a certain way by others—if, for example, other people respond as if one is intelligent, friendly, confused, or clumsy—then in time these qualities will be incorporated into the self. When members see themselves acting in a particular way consistently—say, by dominating the group interaction, constantly criticizing others, displaying strong emotions, or expressing concern for others' well-being—then they will, in time, come to realize that they are dominant, critical, emotional, or caring, respectively. Because in most cases members of therapeutic groups are known to one another as individuals rather than as the occupants of a particular social role (e.g., parent, child, boss, or employee), members can no longer attribute their actions to the requirements placed on them by the roles in which they find themselves. Ed may typically blame his gruffness on the demands made by his role as boss and Edwina may think her moodiness is caused by her family, but if Ed is gruff and Edwina is moody in group, then they must consider the possibilities that these qualities are part of who they are.

Members also provide one another with explicit verbal and nonverbal feedback about how they are coming across in the group. John may, in time, realize that he lacks social skills when he finally notices that no one in the group will look him in the eye or sit near him, but he might also get this message when members criticize him for speaking too harshly and for failing to show concern for others' feelings. Individuals are, in fact, somewhat leery of joining therapeutic groups because they recognize that the group may see them for what they are—and that this accurate appraisal may not match their own sense of self (Ringer, 2002). They may find, however, that as they act in ways that are inconsistent with their original self-conception, their self becomes increasingly complex and, in consequence, stabler (Vickery, Gontkovsky, Wallace, & Caroselli, 2006). A simple view of the self may be just as valid as a complex one, but the advantage of a complex view is this: When people who are high in self-complexity experience a negative event in their life, they can cope by focusing on the more positive aspects of their life. Also, because individuals who are high in self-complexity differentiate between their various self-views, a catastrophe in one arena is less likely to spill over and contaminate their other self-views (Dixon & Baumeister, 1991).

Research does not clearly confirm the mental health benefits of accurate, detailed self-knowledge (Sedikides & Strube, 1997), but members of therapy groups nonetheless believe that groups provide them with self-diagnostic data that are, in themselves, therapeutic. When Kivlighan and his colleagues asked participants in therapeutic groups to identify events that took place in their groups that helped them the most, members most frequently mentioned the feeling that their problems were shared with others (universality), the opportunities to learn interpersonal skills, the group's acceptance of them, and the insight into themselves that they gained from the group experience (Kivlighan & Mullison, 1988; Kivlighan, Multon, & Brossart, 1996). When researchers ask members to rank or rate the importance of various curative factors in the group, usually using the list developed by Yalom (1995), they generally find that group members emphasize self-understanding, interpersonal learning, and catharsis, and that clients rate self-understanding as increasingly important as their therapy progresses. In general, individuals who stress the value of self-understanding tend to benefit the most from participation in a therapeutic group (Butler & Fuhriman, 1983a, 1983b; MacNair-Semands & Lese, 2000; Rugel & Meyer, 1984).

### *Self-Esteem*

*Knowing* the self may promote better adjustment, but *valuing* the self may be equally essential to psychological well-being (Swann, Chang-Schneider, & Larsen McClarty, 2007). A number of psychological problems, including depression, anxiety, alcohol abuse, masochism, and eating disorders such as bulimia, are rooted in a devalued self. (See Dijkstra, Gibbons, & Buunk, Chapter 11, this volume; Leary & Tate, Chapter 2, this volume.) Individuals suffering from depression, for example, report confusion about identity and purpose in life, a sense of emptiness when they turn their attention toward the self, and strong, unrelenting feelings of worthlessness and inadequacy. They often talk of feeling little self-confidence and how this uncertainty leaves them dependent on, and easily influenced by, other people.

Group therapy offers members a means to regain a sense of self-worth. Self-esteem is linked, at a basic psychological level, to inclusion in stable, clearly defined groups. As Baumeister and Leary's belongingness hypothesis argues, "Human beings have a pervasive drive to form and maintain at least a minimum quantity of lasting, positive, and impactful interpersonal relationships" (1995, p. 497). Just as exclusion from a group can trigger a loss in self-esteem, so can inclusion in a group contribute to more positive feelings of self-worth. Leary and Baumeister's (2000) sociometer model goes so far as to suggest that inclusion in a group raises self-esteem, since self-esteem is not an index of self-appraisal but a monitor of inclusion in social groups (Leary, Tambor, Terdal, & Downs, 1995).

Groups also raise members' sense of worth by ritualizing the exchange of praise and positive feedback among the members. Group members often exchange corrective, and in some cases negative, feedback, but such exchanges are usually counterbalanced by substantial doses of congratulatory, positive evaluations. The group format also provides members with (1) information about other people's failings and faults, setting the stage for the realization that their problems are not unique but instead universal; (2) the chance to help others, thereby establishing their value to the group and its members; and (3) a range of individuals who can be used as targets of social comparison.

Therapeutic groups also enhance self-esteem by providing members with a positive group-level, or social, identity. Although a psychogenic viewpoint typically stresses the importance of the personal, individualistic aspects of the self, the self includes a social side. This collective identity is based on connections to other people and groups, including roles, memberships, and interpersonal relations. Social psychological researchers have repeatedly found that even though individuals may have qualities that are stigmatized by society (e.g., psychological problems; see Corrigan, Larson, & Kuwabara, Chapter 4, this volume), when these individuals identify strongly with their group, their self-esteem increases rather than decreases (Twenge & Crocker, 2002). Marmarosh and Corazzini (1997) examined the impact of membership in a therapy group on social identity by asking the members of some groups to carry a symbol of their group with them (a group card) at all times. The card was to serve as a reminder that they were valued members of their therapy group and that they should know that their group was with them all the time. Those group members given a group identity card reported greater collective self-esteem and displayed more positive treatment gains than members in a no-card control condition.

### *Self-Regulation*

The capacity to control oneself is considered an essential element of mental health, but self-regulation, for some people, is a difficult, complex, and daunting task (see Doerr & Baumeister, Chapter 5, this volume). Depressed individuals may want to regain a sense of purpose and energy. Obsessive–compulsive individuals may wish to limit their repetitive tendencies. People who abuse alcohol may want to control how much they drink. Socially phobic individuals may hope that they can socialize easily with others. Yet, when these individuals try to control their thoughts, emotions, and actions, they are disappointed in the results and in themselves.

It might seem paradoxical to suggest that individuals can enhance their self-regulation by relying on a group, for *self-regulation* implies control of the self by the self rather than by others (Muraven & Baumeister, 2000, p. 247). Indeed, most theories of self-regulation draw a distinction between goals individuals set for themselves and those that are pressed upon them by outside agents. Therapeutic groups, however, blur the distinction between self and other. For example, Kelman (1963), in his analysis of psychotherapy groups, concluded that group members initially merely comply with the demands of the group and its leader. They may act as the group requires, but when the group's restraint is relaxed, they often revert to their original ways. In time, however, they often begin to identify with the group, and their self-image changes as they take on the behaviors, characteristics, and roles of influential group members. They regulate their actions to reduce the discrepancy between their personal state and the state required by the group. As members become more firmly embedded in the group, they eventually internalize the group's values, so that their personal beliefs, opinions, and goals become one with the group's standards. Over time, group control is transformed into self-control (Kelman, 2006). Similarly, self-determination theory (SDT; Ryan & Deci, 2000) proposes that goals cannot always be clearly divided into those set by the self for personal reasons and goals that originate outside the self. SDT identifies four types of goals that vary in the degree to which regulation is external to the person or integrated internally: external regulation, introjection (complying, often unknowingly, with the external demand but not fully accepting it as one's own), identification, and integration (integrating requirements that were once externally imposed within the self-system).

### *Self-Efficacy*

Groups are not only the source of the individual's goals, but they also play a major role in generating a sense of efficacy about the behaviors one needs to perform to be successful in reaching those goals. As Maddux and Lewis (1995, p. 37) note, self-efficacy and competence are not sufficient conditions for psychological well-being, but "adjustment is difficult, if not impossible, without such beliefs." Individuals who are high in self-efficacy are likely to view their setbacks as challenges rather than as threats. Instead of focusing on their problems and shortcomings, they focus their efforts on identifying ways to achieve their goals and solve their problems. Those who are low in self-efficacy, in contrast, lose their confidence when facing a challenge and become self-focused rather than task-focused.

Groups contribute to members' sense of self-efficacy by helping them learn the specific skills they are seeking. In therapy groups members can observe the actions of others and learn from those who model healthy ways of dealing with interpersonal situations. Members can also practice and receive feedback about their success in performing specific behaviors, so that in time they should feel that they are capable of performing the actions that they (and their therapist) feel they need to develop. Yalom (1995) refers to this increase in self-efficacy as the "installation of hope," and research confirms that group-derived self-efficacy contributes to well-being, as assessed by measures of life satisfaction, depression, and group-derived hope for the self (Cameron, 1999; Marmarosh, Holtz, & Schottenbauer, 2005). Cheavens, Feldman, Gum, Michael, and Snyder (2006), for example, discovered that members of a short-term therapeutic group that focused directly on members' sense of hope reported more optimism about reaching their goals, as well as reduced anxiety and depression, than did members of a waiting-list control group.

Groups are also a source of *collective efficacy* for members. Unlike esprit de corps or liking for other group members, collective efficacy is the belief that group members can work together effectively to reach the group's goals. Members of a psychotherapy group with collective efficacy are optimistic about their group's specific skills and competencies, and these beliefs should help members maintain a higher level of motivation as they seek to attain their goals (Forsyth, 2010).

### *Self-Awareness*

Most analyses of the self-regulation process suggest that individuals monitor the match between their current state and their desired state and, based on that assessment, then initiate changes in their current state or revise their conception of the desired state to minimize the discrepancy (e.g., Carver & Scheier, 1981). Because increased self-awareness tends to be associated with increased self-regulation and goal attainment, the effectiveness of groups can be traced, in part, to their impact on members' discrepancy-monitoring process. Groups create an audience for individual members and thereby generate increases in self-focus; when people join with others, their self-awareness tends to increase. Group activities also trigger increases in self-awareness; if members engage in role playing, structured awareness activities, or physical activities, they are likely to feel more self-aware. The tendency for groups to trigger increased self-awareness also accounts for some of the negative side effects of therapeutic groups. Since self-focus can exacerbate negative psychological states such as depression, the relationship between positive change and self-focused attention may be curvilinear: To be effective, group members must become self-aware, but this awareness should not be so strong that it engenders social anxiety (Leary & Kowalski, 1995; Leary & Tate, Chapter 2, this volume).

## Interpersonal Processes in Groups

Interpersonal theorists suggest that psychological disturbances such as depression, anxiety, and personality disorders can be traced back to relational sources—particularly interactions with peers, coworkers, friends, relatives, and acquaintances (e.g., Sullivan, 1953). Because people's problems stem from their "failure to attend to and correct the self-defeating, interpersonally unsuccessful aspects" of their interpersonal acts (Kiesler, 1991, pp. 443), therapies that focus specifically on groups and social relationships are particularly potent since they highlight the origin of the dysfunction. As noted above, psychotherapeutic groups are thought to profoundly affect the selves of the group members: their self-knowledge, self-esteem, self-efficacy, and self-awareness. But these groups are also interpersonal microcosms, and a skilled therapist can harness the social processes in these groups to help individuals achieve the therapeutic goals they have set for themselves. This assumption is summarized in the mantra of group psychotherapists who take an interpersonal approach to treatment: by the group they have been broken, and by the group they will be healed (Marsh, 1931).

### *Social Learning in Therapeutic Groups*

When clients meet one on one with their therapist, they can discuss problems, identify solutions, and receive support and encouragement. But even in the best of circumstances, this exchange is limited, because only one other person acts as listener, mentor, helper, critic, and advisor. In a group, in contrast, individuals can learn not only from the therapist but also from the other group members. When, for example, a group member who has been struggling to express a feeling or painful thought to the group discloses, at last, this message, other members may learn how they too can put their feelings into words. When the leader of the group gradually helps a member understand his or her angry reaction to another member, those watching this process unfold learn how they can help others resolve interpersonal conflicts. When members treat one another in positive, respectful ways and are rewarded by the group leader for doing so, their actions serve as a model for others (Dies, 1994).

Falloon, Lindley, McDonald, and Marks (1977) confirmed the value of modeling in their study of individuals with marked social skills deficits. Those assigned to a simple group discussion treatment showed some improvement over time, but not as much as clients who observed their group leaders demonstrate skillful social interaction before role-playing these actions themselves. Groups that used explicit modeling methods showed greater improvement than others, and these changes were stable for all but the clients diagnosed with schizophrenia. These findings, and others, prompted Lambert and Ogles (2004) to identify *modeling* and the *social learning* it facilitates as key factors common to effective therapies.

### *Guidance and Leadership*

Unlike support or self-help groups, psychotherapy groups have a designated leader: the therapist who is charged with guiding the others in their pursuit of improved mental health. Group psychotherapists, as the recognized leaders in their groups, can make use of the power of that role to increase their impact on the individual members, and on their groups as a whole. Given individuals' tendency to recognize the authority of leaders, clients who are unmoved by a therapist who meets with them one on one may, in contrast, comply with therapeutic directives when they are offered by someone who is not just a therapist but also a group leader. Therapists, as group leaders, may also enhance their impact by harnessing group pressure to serve therapeutic purposes.

Even though most would agree that the therapist-leader strives to stimulate a change in the client's behavior, there is little consensus concerning the methods the leader should use to achieve this goal. As in individual therapy (Strupp, 1986), no one technique has emerged as clearly superior to other techniques. Many group therapists, for example, advocate the leader-centered approaches typical of psychoanalytic, Gestalt, and behavioral groups. In such groups, the leader controls the course of the interaction, assigns various tasks to the group members, occupies the center of a centralized communication network, and offers interpretations of the causes of clients' problems. In some instances, group members may communicate with only the group leader and not each other. In contrast, other therapists advocate a nondirective style of leadership in which all group members communicate with one another. These group-oriented approaches encourage the analysis of the group's processes, with the therapist-leader sometimes facilitating process but at other times providing no direction whatsoever. In general, so long as leaders are perceived to be caring, to help members interpret the cause of their problems, to keep the group on course, and to meet the members' relationship needs, the group will prosper (Lieberman & Golant, 2002; Lieberman, Yalom, & Miles, 1973).

### *Cohesive Groups and Social Support*

Psychotherapeutic groups offer members something that groups, in general, offer their members: social support. When people find themselves facing difficult life experiences, they often suffer psychological and physical illness. But members of supportive groups are protected against these negative consequences in some ways (Herbert & Cohen, 1993; Uchino, Cacioppo, & Kiecolt-Glaser, 1996; Wills & Cleary, 1996; Lakey, Chapter 10, this volume). Most people turn to familiar groups such as friendship cliques and family for their social support, but members of therapeutic groups frequently turn to one another and offer help by providing advice, guidance, direction, and emotional support (e.g., LaBarge, Von Dras, & Wingbermuehle, 1998).

Studies of the capacity of therapeutic groups to provide support to members suggest that the more cohesive the group, the more likely its members will feel as though the group serves as a buffer against stress and anxiety (Burlingame, Fuhriman, & Johnson, 2001). Hence, therapists who help the group move through periods of uncertainty and conflict to a stage of cohesion and performance may find that their members gain more from membership (Kivlighan & Mullison, 1988; MacNair-Semands, 2002). A cohesive therapy group functions like a team: The members are engaged in the group and its change-promoting processes. They rarely miss meetings, they take part in the planning of the group's topics and activities, and they may even explicitly mention the group's esprit de corps and sense of camaraderie (Kivlighan & Tarrant, 2001; Ogrodniczuk & Piper, 2003).

### *Self-Disclosure*

Studies of reactions to stressful events suggest that self-disclosure about these events promotes adjustment for a variety of psychological reasons. Disclosing troubling, worrisome thoughts also reduces the discloser's level of tension and stress. Individuals who keep their problems secret but continually ruminate about them display signs of physiological and psychological distress, whereas individuals who have the opportunity to disclose these troubling thoughts are healthier and happier (Pennebaker, 1997; Sloan, Chapter 12, this volume). Speculating, since self-disclosure to a single person (or to an unknown audience) is healthy, then disclosure to a group should be particularly beneficial. When groups first convene, members usually focus on superficial topics and avoid saying anything too personal or provocative; but as cohesion increases, members begin to feel that they can share very personal information with other members. As a result, self-disclosure and cohesion are reciprocally related. Each new self-disclosure deepens the group's intimacy, and this increased closeness then makes further self-disclosures possible (Agazarian, 2001). By sharing information about themselves, members are expressing their trust in the group and signaling their commitment to the therapeutic process. Members can also vent strong emotions in groups, although the value of such emotional venting continues to be debated by researchers, since "blowing off steam" heightens members' psychological distress and degree of upset (Ormont, 1984).

## THE EFFECTIVENESS OF GROUP TREATMENTS

Therapeutic groups capitalize on a range of interpersonal processes common to groups, in general, to promote the functioning and adjustment of members. Yet when earlier adopters of this format suggested treating people's psychological problems by having them gather together in a group, this idea was considered radical and risky. History, however, proved the skeptics wrong. Group psychotherapy is currently used to treat all types of psychiatric problems, including addictions, thought disorders, depression, eating disorders, posttraumatic stress disorder, and personality disorders (Barlow, Burlingame, & Fuhriman, 2000; Forsyth & Corazzini, 2000).

But how effective is group psychotherapy? Meta-analytic reviews, including those that code studies for methodological rigor, generally suggest that group approaches are as effective as individual methods. Earlier reviews (e.g., Fuhriman & Burlingame, 1994; Smith & Glass, 1977) found that individual and group treatments were roughly equivalent in terms of effectiveness, and more recent reviews have confirmed those conclusions (e.g., Burlingame, Fuhriman, & Mosier, 2003; Burlingame & Krogel, 2005; Kösters, Burlingame, Nachtigall, & Strauss, 2006). Burlingame and his colleagues (McRoberts, Burlingame, & Hoag, 1998), in a particularly careful analysis, tracked a number of treatment and procedural variables that past researchers identified as key determinants of therapeutic success, but the only factors that covaried significantly with outcome were client diagnosis, number of treatment sessions, and the year in which the study was conducted. Group therapies were more effective with clients who were not diagnosed clinically, and the more sessions, the better. Studies conducted prior to 1980 were more likely to favor group over individual approaches.

Burlingame, MacKenzie, and Strauss (2004, p. 652), in summarizing the outcome literature on group therapy, conclude that "group psychotherapy is potent enough to be the sole or primary treatment for patients suffering from a psychiatric disorder," but they temper their positive conclusion by noting that group approaches work better for some disorders than for others. In particular, in both outpatient (Burlingame et al., 2003) and inpatient (Kösters et al., 2006) settings, individuals experiencing mood disorders (anxiety, depression) respond better to group psychotherapies than individuals experiencing other types of disorders (e.g., thought and dissociative disorders).

Burlingame and his colleagues (2004) reiterate a conclusion reached by Bednar and Kaul (1979): too little is known about the psychological and social processes that sustain the changes that are produced by group therapy. Do group-level processes such as social influence (informational, normative, and interpersonal), group cohesion, group norms, and social networking operate to shape the structure and function of therapeutic groups? If so, how do these group-level processes combine to influence outcome? Which group-level processes are most responsible for attitudinal and behavioral change, and which are less critical? Researchers have only begun to answer questions pertaining to the factors that mediate the treatment–outcome relationship.

Second, much of the evidence that is available is tainted by methodologically limited procedures. Groups are difficult to study, and so studies of their effectiveness often suffer from fatal flaws in design and execution. Treatment fidelity is difficult to verify, as each treatment session is influenced not only by the therapist but also by the clients themselves. In many cases, too, no attempt is made to measure group-level processes, such as cohesiveness or emerging networks of influence within the group, as researchers' rely only on each individual members' perceptions of these qualities. Researchers, too, often study so few groups that they have problems separating out the effects of the treatment from the unique effects of a particular group or group member on members. It is common, for example, for a researcher to assign one therapy group to the treatment condition and a second therapy group to a control condition. Since this design confounds treatment and group, the relative effectiveness of the treatment cannot be ascertained.

These two significant limitations aside, the available evidence prompts a guardedly optimistic conclusion about the therapeutic use of groups. Groups often exert an unrelenting influence on their members. Nearly all human societies are organized around small groups, and these groups shape their members' psychological adjustment and dysfunction. Given their ubiquity, people generally respond positively when presented with the opportunity to work in a group to achieve mental health goals. Far more research is needed to analyze the nature of the therapeutic group and its impact on members, but given the powerful self-processes and interpersonal processes that such groups instigate and the positive findings already reported by researchers, groups should be considered a treatment of choice rather than a radical alternative.

## REFERENCES


Agazarian, Y. M. (2001). *A systems-centered approach to inpatient group psychotherapy*. Philadelphia: Jessica Kingsley.

Barlow, S. H., Burlingame, G. M., & Fuhriman, A. (2000). Therapeutic applications of groups: From Pratt's "thought control classes" to modern group psychotherapy. *Group Dynamics, 4*, 115–134.

Baumeister, R. F., & Leary, M. R. (1995). The need to belong: Desire for interpersonal attachments as a fundamental human motivation. *Psychological Bulletin, 117*, 497–529.

Bednar, R. L., & Kaul, T. J. (1979). Experiential group research: What never happened! *Journal of Applied Behavioral Science, 15*, 311–319.

Burlingame, G. M., Fuhriman, A., & Johnson, J. E. (2001). Cohesion in group psychotherapy. *Psychotherapy: Theory, Research, Practice, Training, 38*, 373–379.

Burlingame, G. M., Fuhriman, A., & Mosier, J. (2003). The differential effectiveness of group psychotherapy: A meta-analytic perspective. *Group Dynamics, 7*, 3–12.

Burlingame, G. M., & Krogel, J. (2005). Relative efficacy of individual versus group psychotherapy. *International Journal of Group Psychotherapy, 55*, 607–611.

Burlingame, G. M., MacKenzie, K. R., & Strauss, B. (2004). Small group treatment: Evidence for effectiveness and mechanisms of change. In M. J. Lambert (Ed.), *Bergin and Garfield's handbook of psychotherapy and behavior change* (5th ed., pp. 647–696). New York: Wiley.

Butler, T., & Fuhriman, A. (1983a). Curative factors in group therapy: A review of the recent literature. *Small Group Research, 14*, 131–142.

Butler, T., & Fuhriman, A. (1983b). Level of functioning and length of time in treatment variables influencing patients' therapeutic experience in group psychotherapy. *International Journal of Group Psychotherapy, 33*, 489–505.

Cameron, J. E. (1999). Social identity and the pursuit of possible selves: Implications for the psychological well-being of university students. *Group Dynamics, 3*, 179–189.

Carver, C. S., & Scheier, M. F. (1981). *Attention and self-regulation: A control-theory approach to human behavior*. New York: Springer-Verlag.

Cheavens, J. S., Feldman, D. B., Gum, A., Michael, S. T., & Snyder, C. R. (2006). Hope therapy in a community sample: A pilot investigation. *Social Indicators Research, 77*, 61–78.

Cooley, C. H. (1909). *Social organization: A study of the larger mind*. New York: Scribner's.

DeLucia-Waack, J. L., & Kalodner, C. R. (2005). Contemporary issues in group practice. In S. A. Wheelan (Ed.), *The handbook of group research and practice* (pp. 65–84). Thousand Oaks, CA: Sage.

Dies, R. R. (1994). The therapist's role in group treatments. In H. S. Bernard & K. R. MacKenzie (Eds.), *Basics of group psychotherapy* (pp. 60–99). New York: Guilford Press.

Dixon, T. M., & Baumeister, R. F. (1991). Escaping the self: The moderating effect of self complexity. *Personality and Social Psychology Bulletin, 17*, 363–368.

Elliott, R., Greenberg, L. S., & Lietaer, G. (2004). Research on experiential psychotherapies. In M. J. Lambert (Ed.), *Bergin and Garfield's handbook of psychotherapy and behavior change* (5th ed., pp. 493–540). New York: Wiley.

Emmelkamp, P. M. G. (2004). Behavior therapy with adults. In M. J. Lambert (Ed.), *Bergin and Garfield's handbook of psychotherapy and behavior change* (5th ed., pp. 393–446). New York: Wiley.

Falloon, I. R. H., Lindley, P., McDonald, R., & Marks, I. M. (1977). Social skills training of outpatient groups: A controlled study of rehearsal and homework. *British Journal of Psychiatry, 131*, 599–609.

Forsyth, D. R. (2010). *Group dynamics* (4th ed.). Belmont, CA: Wadsworth/Thompson.

Forsyth, D. R., & Corazzini, J. G. (2000). Groups as change agents. In C. R. Snyder & R. E. Ingram (Eds.), *Handbook of psychological change: Psychotherapy processes and practices for the 21st century* (pp. 309–336). New York: Wiley.

Freud, S. (1922). *Group psychology and the analysis of the ego* [*Massenpsychologie und ich-analyse.*]. London/Vienna: International Psychoanalytical Press.

Freud, S. (1961). *Civilization and its discontents* (J. Strachey, Trans. & Ed.). New York: Norton.

Fuhriman, A., & Burlingame, G. M. (Eds.). (1994). *Handbook of group psychotherapy: An empirical and clinical synthesis*. New York: Wiley.

Goulding, R. L., & Goulding, M. M. (1979). *Changing lives through redecision therapy*. New York: Brunner/Mazel.

Greve, D. W. (1993). Gestalt group psychotherapy. In H. I. Kaplan & B. J. Sadock (Eds.), *Comprehensive group psychotherapy* (3rd ed., pp. 228–235). Baltimore: Williams & Wilkins.

Haskell, R. E. (1999). *Between the lines: Unconscious meaning in everyday conversation*. New York: Plenum Press.

Herbert, T. B., & Cohen S. (1993). Stress and immunity in humans: A meta-analytic review. *Psychosomatic Medicine*, *55*, 364–379.

Hollon, S. D., & Beck, A. T. (2004). Cognitive and cognitive behavioral therapies. In M. J. Lambert (Ed.), *Bergin and Garfield's handbook of psychotherapy and behavior change* (5th ed., pp. 447–492). New York: Wiley.

Kelman, H. C. (1963). The role of the group in the induction of therapeutic change. *International Journal of Group Psychotherapy*, *13*, 399–432.

Kelman, H. C. (2006). Interests, relationships, identities: Three central issues for individuals and groups in negotiating their social environment. *Annual Review of Psychology*, *57*, 1–26.

Kiesler, D. J. (1991). Interpersonal methods of assessment and diagnosis. In C. R. Snyder & D. R. Forsyth (Eds.), *Handbook of social and clinical psychology: The health perspective* (pp. 438–468). New York: Pergamon Press.

Kipper, D. A., & Ritchie, T. D. (2003). The effectiveness of psychodramatic techniques: A meta-analysis. *Group Dynamics*, *7*, 13–25.

Kivlighan, D. M., Jr., & Mullison, D. (1988). Participants' perception of therapeutic factors in group counseling: The role of interpersonal style and stage of group development. *Small Group Research*, *19*, 452–468.

Kivlighan, D. M., Jr., Multon, K. D., & Brossart, D. F. (1996). Helpful impacts in group counseling: Development of a multidimensional rating system. *Journal of Counseling Psychology*, *43*, 347–355.

Kivlighan, D. M., Jr., & Tarrant, J. M. (2001). Does group climate mediate the group leadership–group member outcome relationship? A test of Yalom's hypotheses about leadership priorities. *Group Dynamics*, *5*, 220–234.

Kösters, M., Burlingame, G. M., Nachtigall, C., & Strauss, B. (2006). A meta-analytic review of the effectiveness of inpatient group psychotherapy. *Group Dynamics*, *10*, 146–163.

LaBarge, E., Von Dras, D., & Wingbermuehle, C. (1998). An analysis of themes and feelings from a support group for people with Alzheimer's disease. *Psychotherapy: Theory, Research, Practice, Training*, *35*, 537–544.

Laing, R. D. (1969). *Self and others*. London: Penguin Books.

Lakin, M. (1972). *Experiential groups: The uses of interpersonal encounter, psychotherapy groups, and sensitivity training*. Morristown, NJ: General Learning Press.

Lambert, M. J., & Ogles, B. M. (2004). The efficacy and effectiveness of psychotherapy. In M. J. Lambert (Ed.), *Bergin and Garfield's handbook of psychotherapy and behavior change* (5th ed., pp. 139–193). New York: Wiley.

Langs, R. J. (1973). *The technique of psychoanalytic psychotherapy*. New York: Aronson.

Leary, M. R., & Baumeister, R. F. (2000). The nature and function of self-esteem: Sociometer theory. *Advances in Experimental Social Psychology*, *32*, 1–62.

Leary, M. R., & Kowalski, R. M. (1995). *Social anxiety*. New York: Guilford Press.

Leary, M. R., Tambor, E. S., Terdal, S. K., & Downs, D. L. (1995). Self-esteem as an interpersonal monitor: The sociometer hypothesis. *Journal of Personality and Social Psychology*, *68*, 518–530.

Lewin, K. (1951). *Field theory in social science: Selected theoretical papers*. New York: Harper.

Lieberman, M. A., & Golant, M. (2002). Leader behaviors as perceived by cancer patients in professionally directed support groups and outcomes. *Group Dynamics*, *6*, 267–276.

Lieberman, M. A., Yalom, I. D., & Miles, M. B. (1973). *Encounter groups: First facts*. New York: Basic Books.

MacNair-Semands, R. R. (2002). Predicting attendance and expectations for group therapy. *Group Dynamics*, *6*, 219–228.

MacNair-Semands, R. R., & Lese, K. P. (2000). Interpersonal problems and the perception of therapeutic factors in group therapy. *Small Group Research*, *31*, 158–174.

Maddux, J. E., & Lewis, J. (1995). Self-efficacy and adjustment: Basic principles and issues. In J. E. Maddux (Ed.), *Self-efficacy, adaptation, and adjustment: Theory, research, and application* (pp. 37–68). New York: Plenum Press.

Marmarosh, C. L., & Corazzini, J. G. (1997). Putting the group in your pocket: Using collective identity to enhance personal and collective self-esteem. *Group Dynamics*, *1*, 65–74.

Marmarosh, C. L., Holtz, A., & Schottenbauer, M. (2005). Group cohesiveness, group-derived collective self-esteem, group-derived hope, and the well-being of group therapy members. *Group Dynamics*, *9*, 32–44.

Marsh, L. C. (1931). Group treatment for the psychoses by the psychological equivalent of revival. *Mental Hygiene*, *15*, 328–349.

Maslow, A. H. (1937). The comparative approach to social behavior. *Social Forces*, *15*, 487–490.

McDermut, W., Miller, I. W., & Brown, R. A. (2001). The efficacy of group psychotherapy for depression: A meta-analysis and review of the empirical research. *Clinical Psychology: Science and Practice*, *8*, 98–116.

McRoberts, C., Burlingame, G. M., & Hoag, M. J. (1998). Comparative efficacy of individual and group psychotherapy: A meta-analytic perspective. *Group Dynamics*, *2*, 101–117.

Moreno, J. L. (1932). *Group method and group psychotherapy* (Sociometry Monograph No. 5). New York: Beacon House.

Moreno, J. L. (1934). *Who shall survive? A new approach to the problem of human interrelations*. Washington, DC: Nervous and Mental Disease Publishing.

Muraven, M., & Baumeister, R. F. (2000). Self-regulation and depletion of limited resources: Does self-control resemble a muscle? *Psychological Bulletin*, *126*, 247–259.

Ogrodniczuk, J. S., & Piper, W. E. (2003). The effect of group climate on outcome in two forms of short-term group therapy. *Group Dynamics*, *7*, 64–76.

Ormont, L. R. (1984). The leader's role in dealing with aggression in groups. *International Journal of Group Psychotherapy*, *34*, 553–572.

Page, R. C., Weiss, J. F., & Lietaer, G. (2002). Humanistic group psychotherapy. In D. J. Cain & J. Seeman (Eds.), *Humanistic psychotherapies: Handbook of research and practice* (pp. 339–368). Washington, DC: American Psychological Association.

Pennebaker, J. W. (1997). *Opening up: The healing power of expressing emotions* (rev. ed.). New York: Guilford Press.

Perls, F., Hefferline, R., & Goodman, P. (1951). *Gestalt therapy: Excitement and growth in the human personality*. New York: Julian Press.

Pratt, J. H. (1922). The principles of class treatment and their application to various chronic diseases. *Hospital Social Services*, *6*, 401–417.

Rawlinson, J. W. (2000). Does psychodrama work? A review of the literature. *British Journal of Psychodrama and Sociodrama*, *15*, 66–101.

Ringer, T. M. (2002). *Group action: The dynamics of groups in therapeutic, educational, and corporate settings*. Philadelphia: Jessica Kingsley.

Rogers, C. R. (1940). The processes of therapy. *Journal of Consulting Psychology*, *4*, 161–164.

Rogers, C. R. (1970). *Carl Rogers on encounter groups*. New York: Harper & Row.

Rugel, R. P., & Meyer, D. J. (1984). The Tavistock group: Empirical findings and implications for group therapy. *Small Group Research, 15*, 361–374.

Ryan, R. M., & Deci, E. L. (2000). Intrinsic and extrinsic motivations: Classic definitions and new directions. *Contemporary Educational Psychology, 25*, 54–67.

Sedikides, C., & Skowronski, J. J. (1995). On the sources of self-knowledge: The perceived primacy of self-reflection. *Journal of Social and Clinical Psychology, 14*, 244–270.

Sedikides, C., & Strube, M. J. (1997). Self evaluation: To thine own self be good, to thine own self be sure, to thine own self be true, and to thine own self be better. *Advances in Experimental Social Psychology, 29*, 209–269.

Smith, M. L., & Glass, G. V. (1977). Meta-analysis of psychotherapy outcome studies. *American Psychologist, 32*, 752–760.

Strupp, H. H. (1986). The nonspecific hypothesis of therapeutic effectiveness: A current assessment. *American Journal of Orthopsychiatry, 56*, 513–520.

Sullivan, H. S. (1953). *The interpersonal theory of psychiatry*. New York: Norton.

Swann, W. B. J., Jr., Chang-Schneider, C., & Larsen McClarty, K. (2007). Do people's self-views matter? Self-concept and self-esteem in everyday life. *American Psychologist, 62*, 84–94.

Twenge, J. M., & Crocker, J. (2002). Race and self-esteem: Meta-analyses comparing whites, blacks, Hispanics, Asians, and American Indians and comment on Gray-Little and Hafdahl (2000). *Psychological Bulletin, 128*, 371–408.

Uchino, B. N., Cacioppo, J. T., & Kiecolt-Glaser, J. K. (1996). The relationship between social support and physiological processes: A review with emphasis on underlying mechanisms and implications for health. *Psychological Bulletin, 119*, 488–531.

Vickery, C. D., Gontkovsky, S. T., Wallace, J. J., & Caroselli, J. S. (2006). Group psychotherapy focusing on self-concept change following acquired brain injury: A pilot investigation. *Rehabilitation Psychology, 51*, 30–35.

Weiss, D. S. (2006). Psychodynamic group treatment. In L. A. Schein, H. I. Spitz, G. M. Burlingame, & P. R. Muskin (Eds.), *Psychological effects of catastrophic disasters: Group approaches to treatment* (pp. 787–839). New York: Haworth Press.

Wills, T. A., & Cleary, S. D. (1996). How are social support effects mediated? A test with parental support and adolescent substance use. *Journal of Personality and Social Psychology, 71*, 937–952.

Yalom, I. D. (1995). *The theory and practice of group psychotherapy* (4th ed.). New York: Basic Books.

# PART V

# CURRENT STATUS AND FUTURE DIRECTIONS

# 28 Social Psychological Foundations of Clinical Psychology

## *Initial Trends, Current Status, and Future Directions*

June Price Tangney

Many of the most significant advances in clinical psychology over the past several decades have roots in social psychological theory and associated basic research. First, social psychological constructs have been employed in assessments of, and interventions for, a number of important problems frequently presented in clinical settings. For example, modern cognitive conceptualizations of depression and anxiety, informed by social psychologists' attribution theory (e.g., Abramson, Seligman, & Teasdale, 1978; Peterson & Seligman, 1984; Weiner, 1986), have led to a range of theoretically informed, clinically useful assessment methods—such as the Attributional Style Questionnaire (Peterson et al., 1982), assessing depressogenic styles of thinking, and the Looming Questionnaire (Riskind, Williams, Gessner, Chrosniak, & Cortina, 2000), assessing anxiety-specific patterns of cognition and biased perception. In turn, these assessment methods have worked hand in hand with the development of powerful cognitive-behavioral treatment approaches aimed at modifying clearly operationalized dysfunctional patterns of thinking, with the ultimate goal of reducing human suffering. The recognition of social cognitive distortions uniquely prevalent among depressed and anxious individuals has paved the road to some of our most efficacious treatments, as demonstrated by numerous rigorous clinical trials (Butler, Chapman, Forman, & Beck, 2006). Attribution theory has also been employed in the assessment and treatment of marital dysfunction (e.g., Fincham & Bradbury, 1987, 1990). This work has identified attributional patterns characteristic of both distressed and nondistressed couples and has led to the development of effective interventions aimed at changing those of distressed couples.

A second major contribution of social psychology is an unwavering emphasis on the importance of the situation—in interaction with (not instead of) personality characteristics (Reis, 2008). Whereas for many years, traditional clinical approaches to assessment (and, by extension, treatment) focused on stable traits that presumably influenced behavior and dysfunction across time and space, social psychological theories such as Bandura's (1986) social cognitive theory and Mischel and Shoda's (1995) Cognitive–Affective Processing Systems (CAPS) have underscored the joint interaction between individual traits and social situations in influencing and understanding human affect and behavior. The impact of this "trait by situation" approach to treatment has been profound. No longer are clinicians rigidly focused on overgeneralized individual proclivities to misinterpret, overreact to, or otherwise maladaptively respond to life in general. Rather, clinical conceptualizations and associated assessments and interventions more effectively focus on particular problems in perceiving and reacting to particular kinds of (typically social) situations. In addition to resolving the great "trait–situation" debate of the 1970s, modern social psychology has helped clinicians to consider sophisticated processes of social influence and learning. And rather than dismissing the absence of broad cross-situational consistency as an irritating error in assessment or client self-report, modern clinicians can effectively draw on Mischel and Shoda's sophisticated and compelling notions of *if . . . then . . .* relations and the concept of "consistent inconsistencies"—inconsistencies made consistent by considering the structure and/or psychological meaning of situations to which clients respond (see Kross, Mischel, & Shoda, Chapter 20, this volume). Well-articulated theory—and assessments adapted accordingly—that consider situational factors help clinicians to sort effectively through the complexity of client presentations, to better understand and identify more precise interventions tailored to the individual and his or her interaction with the social world, as idiographically defined.

A third major contribution of social psychology concerns the notion of continuity between normal and abnormal behavior (see Maddux, Chapters 1 and 22, this volume). Ironically, Freud and the neo-Freudians following him also emphasized this continuity—for example, in the notion of normative psychosocial conflicts across a universal set of developmental stages, and in viewing psychological defenses as a normal and necessary feature of human psychological functioning that occurs substantially outside of conscious awareness (i.e., in the unconscious). Pathology, from this perspective, arose from arrested development at early stages of childhood; from consequently rigid, constricted defensive structures typically relying too heavily on "primitive," less efficient forms of defense; and a resulting weak ego ill-prepared to negotiate and resolve conflicts among the demands of reality, moral imperatives, and basic human instinctual impulses.

The notion of continuity between normal human processes and "abnormal" psychological symptoms declined precipitously in the post-Freudian era. A new conception of "normal psychology" as qualitatively distinct from "abnormal psychology" took hold, due to a number of converging factors (see Maddux, Chapter 1, this volume). These include, but are not limited to, the rise of psychiatric nosology (e.g., the DSM, across additions) designed to assign people to categorical disorders. As a consequence, approaches to clinical assessment shifted toward identifying disorders and distinguishing between the disordered and the nondisordered (the abnormal and the normal). With these changes came the understandable, but unfortunate, tendency of clinical psychologists and psychiatrists to apply labels to *people*, (*schizophrenics*, *borderlines*) rather than describe symptoms *experienced by* people (e.g., people *with* current symptoms of schizophrenia, people exhibiting borderline personality characteristics). Perhaps clinical psychology might have unfolded differently had the 1921 experiment to integrate clinical and social psychology under the umbrella of the *Journal of Abnormal and Social Psychology* succeeded. But by the 1960s, colleges and universities offered undergraduate courses in clinical psychology and in social psychology that had remarkably little overlap—in terms of theory, in coverage of empirical research, and in discussions of real-life application. Graduate programs in clinical psychology and social psychology were equally divorced, with clinical doctoral programs often housed in separate quarters, apart from more "scientific" psychology programs.

Several significant changes in social psychology from 1985 to the present have brought social psychology much closer to the concerns and needs of clinical psychology. An emerging synergy between social and clinical psychology, articulated by Leary and Maddux (1987) in the *American Psychologist*, is now in full bloom. The current volume summarizes many exciting new advances that have enriched inquiry in both fields. Here, I mention just a few themes highlighted within and across chapters.

## WHAT'S NEW AT THE INTERFACE BETWEEN SOCIAL AND CLINICAL PSYCHOLOGY?

### The Self

For many years, social psychology's efforts to understand "the self" focused almost exclusively on self-esteem—a rather thin strand of a multifaceted construct that could not possibly do justice to a construct of "self" central to many clinical theories and therapeutic approaches. Beginning in the 1980s, social psychology delved into the depths of the self, including, to name a few, Linville's (1985) work on self-complexity; Higgins's (1987) work on self-discrepancies, Markus and Nurius's (1986) possible selves; Greenberg, Pyszczynski, and Solomon's (1986) terror management theory; and Baumeister's (1987) analysis of the problems posed by the self's very existence. The *Handbook on Self and Identity* (Leary & Tangney, 2003) is a treasure trove of social psychological research aimed at unraveling, theoretically and empirically, the many clinically useful aspects of modern self psychology, much of it directly relevant to applied clinical conceptions of the self (e.g., narcissism, defensive structure, ego resilience). It is no coincidence that fully one-third of this volume focuses specifically on matters related to the self (Chapters 2, 3, and 4 on self and identity; Chapters 5, 6, 7, and 8 on self-regulation). Most other chapters integrate a consideration of the self in authors' discussion of other clinically relevant social psychological phenomena.

### Emotion

As an undergraduate in the late 1970s, I was dismayed to learn from my introductory psychology textbook that psychology was "the science of behavior." Just *behavior*?! Much of psychology at that time eschewed nonobservable psychological events that might (or might not) occur in the netherworld of the "black box." The cognitive revolution soon legitimized some portions of the black box—namely, cognitive processes. Largely absent, however, was the meat of emotion. All the while, practicing clinicians were dealing routinely with their clients' emotions using either psychodynamic theories or cognitive theories that were developed apart from mainstream scientific psychology (e.g., Ellis's rational–emotive therapy, Beck's cognitive therapy). Emotions were regarded by many as "mere epiphenomena" of cognition, and largely unamenable to empirical study, except to the extent that they could be reliably coded (behaviorally) as expressed via facial expression (e.g., the pioneering work of Ekman & Friesen, 1978; Izard, 1972). How psychological science has changed! Human emotion, in all its richness—as encountered daily by clinicians in applied practice—has become a respectable topic of inquiry. No longer are we restricted solely to consideration of "basic" emotions with presumably hardwired behavioral (and codable) facial expressions. Clinically relevant emotions sans clear facial markers, such as shame, guilt, embarrassment, pride, hubris, jealousy, and envy, have been scientifically examined by social psychologists with results directly informing clinical intervention (see Tangney & Salovey, Chapter 14, this volume; also Miller, 1986; Tracy & Robins, 2004). In short, recent social psychological research has expanded its analysis of the broad palate of human emotions with an emphasis on the implications for both individual and interpersonal adjustment. Perhaps of special interest to practicing clinicians are the "emotions of the imperiled ego"—jealousy, envy, shame, and guilt.

## The Unconscious

In 1997 Roy Baumeister chaired a provocative social psychological symposium at the American Psychological Associated entitled "*Was Freud right? Psychoanalytic theories in modern social-personality research.*" The surprising answer: For the most part, "Yes." In particular, modern social psychological research has lent strong support for the existence of an "unconscious." Although today's social psychologists may employ more modern terms (e.g., *implicit processes*, *automaticity*, *subliminal effects*), the data strongly support the notion that significant cognitive events occur routinely beyond our awareness. People subliminally primed with words associated with old age walk more slowly when exiting an experimental room (Bargh, Chen, & Burrows, 1996). People consciously professing nonprejudicial beliefs toward minorities display unconsciously measured prejudices (Banaji & Greenwald, 1994). There is compelling modern scientific evidence for the "return of the repressed," as seen in Wegner's (1989) work on "ironic processes." In short, social psychologists have empirically documented the existence of an unconscious well known by psychodynamically oriented clinicians. And they have offered new insights into methods that may help laypersons and clinicians alike to capture and harness the power of the unconscious (see Miranda & Andersen, Chapter 26, this volume).

## Positive Psychology

Although social psychology has been traditionally focused on normative interpersonal and intrapersonal processes, for decades, theory and research have been somewhat skewed toward the negative. Just as clinical psychologists focused on mental disorder, many social psychologists were naturally drawn to topics relevant to understanding and ameliorating society's ills—aggression, prejudice, dyadic and intergroup conflict, biases, and so forth. In recent years, social psychology has given birth to "positive psychology," a burgeoning scientific effort that has brought new insights into the critical functions of positive affect, moral virtues, psychological well-being, and cooperative social relations (Lopez & Snyder, 2009). Social psychology's recent emphasis on positive psychology challenges the "illness ideology" that has colored much of clinical psychology over the past century (Maddux, 2008), and it promises to work hand in hand with new emphases in clinical psychology on psychological resilience and the strengths that come from experiencing and overcoming traumatic experiences and various forms of mental illness.

### Mediation and Moderation

Social psychologists have been among the leaders in developing powerful new models (conceptual and statistical) that help scientists to develop and test complex explanatory mechanisms. With social psychologists Baron and Kenny's (1986) landmark article on mediation and moderation, followed by important developments and refinements by social psychologist MacKinnon (2008) and others, we are no longer satisfied with knowledge that *X* is related to *Y* (and we no longer use the terms *mediation* and *moderation* interchangeably!). Having demonstrated that *X* is related to *Y*, these models press us to specify and test "Via what mechanisms?" (mediation) such relations exist, and they press us to examine "For whom and under what conditions?" (moderation) *X* is in fact related to *Y*. These conceptual and statistical tools are ideally suited to addressing critical issues in clinical psychology. They provide a framework for specifying and testing "mechanisms of action" (MOAs) in the context of psychotherapy, which greatly enhances clinical scientists' ability to evaluate new treatment approaches and to then fine-tune such approaches to maximize impact. Once a new treatment approach has been demonstrated to be effective, a meditational framework greatly simplifies this task, relative to the more traditional "decomposition of treatment" approach that can take decades of painstaking research. It is perhaps no surprise that in recent years, the National Institutes of Health (NIH) have emphasized the importance of explicitly measuring and analyzing hypothesized MOAs (also referred to as "mechanisms of change") in proposals focused on treatment development and evaluation.

## WHY IS SYNERGY BETWEEN SOCIAL AND CLINICAL PSYCHOLOGY ESPECIALLY IMPORTANT NOW?

### Managed Care and the Changing Roles of Clinical Psychologists

In the wake of managed care, the role of PhD-level psychologists has changed dramatically. Whereas once doctoral-level clinical psychologists could reasonably look forward to a successful private practice, seeing readily treatable, verbal, insight-oriented clients with the means (personal finances or via insurance) to embark on long-term therapy (perhaps augmented by an occasional intellectual or personality assessment), doctoral-level clinical psychologists of today are less apt to be engaged solely in direct service in private settings. Their roles are likely to be more diverse—demanding of a much broader range of skills. First, clinical psychologists of today and tomorrow need to be prepared to answer higher levels of accountability regarding treatment efficiency and efficacy. They need to be well versed in empirically supported assessment and treatment methods, and to be able to justify techniques and procedures with reference to the scientific literature. Second, rather than serving as rank-and-file clinicians, doctoral-level clinical psychologists are frequently called upon to manage clinical settings, to supervise master's-level clinicians, and to engage in structured clinical training. Third, doctoral-level clinical psychologists need to be prepared to develop and evaluate new treatment initiatives. This is not the job description of clinical psychologist that was in place in 1949, when the field's visionaries met in Boulder Colorado to adopt the "scientist-practitioner" model that has shaped so many clinical training programs since.

## The Emergence of a New Model of Clinical Training: "Clinical Science"

As the needs of society have changed, as the roles of clinical psychologists have broadened and developed, a new model of clinical training has emerged, termed "clinical science." Emanating in part from "cross-over" clinical research psychologists who had a foot in both social and clinical psychology, the clinical science model is designed to train professionals uniquely positioned to develop, evaluate, and disseminate new theoretically derived empirically supported treatments (McFall, 1991).

## What Can Social Psychology Offer?

As demonstrated throughout this volume, social psychology has much to offer clinical psychology as it refocuses in a new direction. Social psychology's potential contributions to clinical science (current and future) can be summarized in three categories: (1) sophisticated theory, (2) conceptual and statistical models for enhancing treatment efficacy, and (3) scientific approaches to measure and document treatment efficacy at multiple levels.

The chapters in this volume summarize a rich range of clinically relevant social psychological theories that can help inform the development of new treatments. Drawing on these theories, in combination with social psychology's emphasis on meditational models and methods for testing such models (e.g., Baron & Kenny, 1986; MacKinnon, 2008), clinical scientists are now well equipped to identify MOAs (e.g., changes in attributions, self-related processes, interpersonal patterns of behavior) that account for treatment effectiveness. By modeling and honing in on theoretically specified mechanisms of action, treatment strategies can be refined to further enhance effectiveness. Moreover, models of moderation (close cousin of mediation) provide a framework for optimally matching client issues with treatment approach. Tests of moderation answer the question "For whom, and under what conditions, does this treatment work best?" (as well as "For whom, and under what conditions, might this treatment be counterproductive?). Models of mediation and moderation are just one component of a larger treatment evaluation approach that requires clearly articulated constructs, closely matched operationalizations, and psychometrically sound assessments of psychological, interpersonal, and situational factors—all hallmarks of social psychological science as practiced for decades. These are powerful tools ideally suited to the tasks facing the new clinical scientists of the 21st century.

At last, decades since the dissection of clinical and social psychology (see Maddux, Chapter 1, this volume), clinical and social psychology are again reuniting to scientifically address the challenges of mental illness, mental distress, and optimal human functioning and experience in this new complex world.

## REFERENCES

Abramson, L. Y., Seligman, M. E. P., & Teasdale, J. (1978). Learned helplessness in humans: Critique and reformulation. *Journal of Abnormal Psychology, 87*, 49–74.

Banaji, M. R., & Greenwald, A. G. (1994). Implicit stereotyping and unconscious prejudice. In M. P. Zanna & J. M. Olson (Eds.), *The psychology of prejudice: The Ontario symposium* (Vol. 7, pp. 55–76). Hillsdale, NJ: Erlbaum.

Bandura, A. (1986). *Social foundations of thought and action.* New York: Prentice-Hall.

Bargh, J. A., Chen, M., &Burrows, L. (1996). Automaticity of social behavior: Direct effects of trait construct and stereotype activation on action. *Journal of Personality and Social Psychology, 71*, 230–244.

Baron, R. M., & Kenny, D. A. (1986). The moderator–mediator variable distinction in social psychological research: Conceptual, strategic, and statistical considerations. *Journal of Personality and Social Psychology, 51*, 1173–1182.

Baumeister, R. F. (1987). How the self became a problem: A psychological review of historical research. *Journal of Personality and Social Psychology, 52*, 163–176.

Butler, A. C., Chapman, J. E., Forman, E. M., & Beck, A. T. (2006). The empirical status of cognitive-behavior therapy: A review of meta-analyses. *Clinical Psychology Review, 26*, 17–31.

Ekman, P., & Friesen, W. V. (1978). *Facial Action Coding System: A technique for the measurement of facial movement.* Palo Alto, CA: Consulting Psychologists Press.

Fincham, F. D., & Bradbury, T. N. (1987). Cognitive processes and conflict in close relationships: An attribution–efficacy model. *Journal of Personality and Social Psychology, 53*, 1106–1118.

Fincham, F. D., & Bradbury, T. N. (Eds.). (1990). *The psychology of marriage: Basic issues and applications.* New York: Guilford Press.

Greenberg, J., Pyszczynski, T., & Solomon, S. (1986). The causes and consequences of self-esteem: A terror management theory. In R. F. Baumeister (Ed.), *Public self and private self* (pp. 189–212). New York: Springer-Verlag.

Higgins, E. T. (1987). Self-discrepancy: A theory relating self and affect. *Psychological Review, 9*, 319–340.

Izard, C. E. (1972). *Patterns of emotion.* New York: Academic Press.

Leary, M. R., & Maddux, J. E. (1987). Progress toward a viable interface between social and clinical-counseling psychology. *American Psychologist, 42*(10), 904–911.

Leary, M., & Tangney, J. P. (Eds.). (2003). *Handbook of self and identity.* New York: Guilford Press.

Linville, P. W. (1985). Self-complexity and affective extremity: Don't put all your eggs in one cognitive basket. *Social Cognition, 3*, 94–120.

Lopez, S. J., & Snyder, C. R. (Eds.). (2009). *Oxford handbook of positive psychology* (2nd ed.). New York: Oxford University Press.

MacKinnon, D. P. (2008). *Introduction to statistical mediation analysis.* Mahwah, NJ: Erlbaum.

Maddux, J. E. (2008). Positive psychology and the illness ideology: Toward a positive clinical psychology. *Applied Psychology: An International Review, 57*, 54–70.

Markus, H., & Nurius, P. S. (1986). Possible selves. *American Psychologist, 41*, 954–969.

McFall, R. M. (1991). Manifesto for a science of clinical psychology. *The Clinical Psychologist, 44*, 75–88.

Miller, R. S. (1996). *Embarrassment: Poise and peril in everyday life.* New York: Guilford Press.

Mischel, W., & Shoda, Y. (1995). A cognitive–affective system theory of personality: Reconceptualizing situations, dispositions, dynamics and invariance in personality structure. *Psychological Review, 102*(2), 246–268.

Peterson, C., & Seligman, M. E. P. (1984). Casual explanations as a risk factor for depression: Theory and evidence. *Psychological Review, 91*, 347–374.

Peterson, C., Semmel, A., von Baeyer, C., Abramson, L. Y., Metalsky, G. I., & Seligman, M. E. P. (1982). The Attributional Style Questionnaire. *Cognitive Therapy and Research, 6*, 287–299.

Reis, H. T. (2008). Reinvigorating the concept of situation in social psychology. *Personality and Social Psychology Review*, *12*, 311–329.

Riskind, J. H., Williams, N. L., Gessner, T., Chrosniak, L. D., & Cortina, J. (2000). The looming maladaptive style: Anxiety, danger, and schematic processing. *Journal of Personality and Social Psychology*, *79*, 837–852.

Tracy, J. L., & Robins, R. W. (2004). Show your pride: Evidence for a discrete emotion expression. *Psychological Science*, *15*(3), 194–197.

Wegner, D. M. (1989). *White bears and other unwanted thoughts*. New York: Viking/Penguin.

Weiner, B. (1986). *An attributional theory of motivation and emotion*. New York: Springer-Verlag.

# Author Index

# Subject Index